BMA

Psychiatry

Psychiatry

FIFTH EDITION

EDITED BY

Rebecca McKnight

General Adult Psychiatrist, Warneford Hospital, Oxford, UK

Jonathan Price

Formerly Director of Medical Studies, Department of Psychiatry,
Oxford University, UK

John Geddes

Professor of Epidemiological Psychiatry, Oxford University, UK

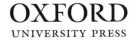

OXFORD
UNIVERSITY PRESS

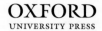

OXFORD
UNIVERSITY PRESS

Great Clarendon Street, Oxford, OX2 6DP,
United Kingdom

Oxford University Press is a department of the University of Oxford.
It furthers the University's objective of excellence in research, scholarship,
and education by publishing worldwide. Oxford is a registered trade mark of
Oxford University Press in the UK and in certain other countries

First Edition Published in 1994
Second Edition Published in 1999
Third Edition Published in 2005
Fourth Edition Published in 2012
Fifth Edition Published in 2019

Impression: 1

Published in the United States of America by Oxford University Press
198 Madison Avenue, New York, NY 10016, United States of America

British Library Cataloguing in Publication Data
Data available

Library of Congress Control Number: 2018964333

ISBN 978–0–19–875400–8

Printed in Great Britain by
Bell & Bain Ltd., Glasgow

Preface: fifth edition

The fifth edition has been thoroughly updated to reflect developments in research and clinical practice since the last edition. We have continued to try to tie theoretical study to clinical practice, and provide practical guidance for patient management. For example, one emerging area is the finding that some cases of first-episode psychosis are caused by an antibody-mediated encephalitis: this theoretically challenges the way we think about the aetiological basis of psychosis and has already changed the investigation and potential treatment options for patients with psychosis (Chapter 22). We have also considered students' feedback on the fourth edition in our revision: providing information in 'easily digestible' formats, completely rewriting the chapters on 'Sexual disorders' and trying to be less UK-centric in our approach. We hope that this edition remains true to the principles of Professors Gelder, Mayou, and Gath, our retired co-authors, but the updates render it more useful to a modern student cohort.

We are grateful to everyone who has helped us in writing this new edition and to our colleagues at OUP for their ongoing commitment to our project. Particular thanks go to Dr Agnes Ayton, Professor Kate Saunders, Dr Gail Critchlow, and Dr Susan Shaw for their comments on specific chapters and/or expert guidance during the writing process.

Rebecca McKnight, Jonathan Price, and John Geddes

Contents

Abbreviations

5-HT	5-hydroxytryptamine (serotonin)
AA	Alcoholics Anonymous
ADHD	attention deficit hyperactivity disorder
AMHP	Approved Mental Health Professional
AMTS	Abbreviated Mental Test Score
ARFID	avoidant–restrictive food intake disorder
ASD	autistic spectrum disorders
ASPD	antisocial personality disorder
BED	binge eating disorder
BMI	body mass index
BNF	*British National Formulary*
CAMHS	child and adolescent mental health services
CBT	cognitive behavioural therapy
CD	conduct disorder
CMHT	community mental health team
CPAP	continuous positive airway pressure
CPN	community psychiatric nurse
CSF	cerebrospinal fluid
CT	computed tomography
DALY	disability-adjusted life year
DoLS	Deprivation of Liberty Safeguarding
DSH	deliberate self-harm
DSM	*Diagnostic and Statistical Manual of Mental Disorders*
ECG	electrocardiogram
ECT	electroconvulsive therapy
EEG	electroencephalogram
EUPD	emotionally unstable personality disorder
FGA	first-generation antipsychotic (drug)
GABA	gamma-aminobutyric acid
GAD	generalized anxiety disorder
GID	gender identity disorder
GMC	General Medical Council
GnRH	gonadotropin-releasing hormone
GP	general practitioner
HPA	hypothalamic–pituitary–adrenal
IAPT	Improving Access to Psychological Therapies
IBS	irritable bowel syndrome
ICD	International Classification of Diseases
ICSD	International Classification of Sleep Disorders
IPT	interpersonal therapy
IV	intravenous/intravenously
LD	learning disability
LPA	lasting power of attorney
LSD	lysergic acid diethylamide
MAOI	monoamine oxidase inhibitor
MHA	Mental Health Act
MHRT	Mental Health Review Tribunal
MMSE	Mini Mental State Examination
MRI	magnetic resonance imaging
MSE	mental state examination
NHS	National Health Service
NICE	National Institute for Health and Care Excellence
NMDA	*N*-methyl-d-aspartate
NNT	number needed to treat
NREM	non-rapid eye movement
NSAID	non-steroidal anti-inflammatory drug
OCD	obsessive–compulsive disorder
ODD	oppositional defiance disorder
PHQ	Patient Health Questionnaire
PTSD	post-traumatic stress disorder
RCT	randomized controlled trial
REM	rapid eye movement

SCN	suprachiasmatic nuclei	**SPC**	Summary of Product Characteristics
SGA	second-generation antipsychotic (drug)	**SSRI**	selective serotonin reuptake inhibitor
SNRI	serotonin and noradrenaline reuptake inhibitor	**U&Es**	urea and electrolytes
		WHO	World Health Organization

Part 1   Introduction

1 Introduction to psychiatry

Psychiatry is the branch of medicine which specializes in the treatment of those brain disorders which primarily cause disturbance of thought, behaviour, and emotion. These are often referred to as *mental*, or *psychiatric*, disorders. The boundary with the specialty of neurology, which also deals with disorders of the central nervous system, is therefore indistinct. Neurology mainly focuses on brain disease with clear physical pathology and/or obvious peripheral effects on, for example, motor function.

Mental disorders such as depressive disorder and psychoses have been recognized since antiquity. Modern epidemiological studies have demonstrated that they are both highly prevalent and widely distributed across all societies. Overall, mental disorders account for a very high proportion of the disability experienced by the human race (see Chapter 2). Unfortunately, in most societies mental disorders still do not receive the recognition or a level of health service commensurate with their public health importance. There are several reasons for this. Probably most importantly, the brain is a vastly complex organ and the neural systems underlying mental disorders remain poorly characterized. This inevitably means that our understanding of the pathophysiology is relatively poor compared to disorders such as diabetes or heart disease. The absence of a clear body of reliable scientific evidence means that competing unscientific views—and stigma—can flourish. Recently, however, our neurobiological techniques have improved in sophistication and sensitivity to the extent that

mental disorders have become *tractable* problems. Phenomena such as mood symptoms, anxiety, and even psychosis seem to exist on a continuum in the population, and the absence of reliable neurobiological measures creates difficulties in determining where the thresholds lie in the gradual change from normality to illness. In clinical practice, the use of diagnostic criteria can increase the reliability of diagnoses and reduce the variations between clinicians. However, small changes in diagnostic criteria can have large effects on the resulting estimates of the prevalence of disorders. Unfortunately, the criteria themselves are based on very imperfect knowledge about the natural history or boundaries of the disorders.

This combination of limited understanding of pathophysiology, widespread prevalence, and efflorescence of competing unscientific or folk explanations (which a post-modern culture accords equal status) could lead to pessimism about the potential of psychiatry to help people suffering from the reality of mental disorders. It is remarkable therefore that such effective treatments *do* exist which, properly implemented, can produce worthwhile clinical benefits. We may not yet have arrived at the stage of rational therapies based on fundamental scientific understanding. Nonetheless, through a combination of speculative creativity and guided serendipity coupled with rigorous evaluation in clinical trials, we have a range of valuable interventions. Moreover, although again not based on pathophysiological markers reflecting the underlying neurobiology, psychiatry has developed reliable diagnostic systems that create a common language to facilitate communication between clinicians and patients, clinicians and clinicians, and researchers.

There are compelling reasons for *all* doctors to have at least a basic awareness of mental disorders and their assessment and effective management. This text aims to provide that basic knowledge. We hope that students will be inspired to follow a career in psychiatry—which can be a rocky road but one that amply repays the efforts spent both by satisfying intellectual curiosity and by providing the unique reward of relieving the suffering of fellow humans.

2 The scale of the problem

One in four individuals suffer from a psychiatric disorder at some point in their life, with 15–20 per cent fitting criteria for a mental disorder at any given time. The latter corresponds to around 450 million people worldwide, placing mental disorders as one of the leading causes of global morbidity. Mental health problems represent five of the ten leading causes of disability worldwide. The World Health Organization (WHO) reported in mid 2016 that 'the global cost of mental illness is £651 billion per year', stating that the equivalent of 50 million working years was being lost annually due to mental disorders. The financial global impact is clearly vast, but on a smaller scale, the social and psychological impacts of having a mental disorder on yourself or your family are greater still.

It is often difficult for the general public and clinicians outside psychiatry to think of mental health disorders as 'diseases' because it is harder to pinpoint a specific pathological cause for them. When confronted with this view, it is helpful to consider that most of medicine was actually founded on this basis. For example, although medicine has been a profession for the past 2500 years, it was only in the late 1980s that *Helicobacter pylori* was linked to gastric/duodenal ulcers and gastric carcinoma, or more recently still that the *BRCA* genes were found to be a cause of breast cancer. Still much of clinical medicine treats a patient's symptoms rather than objective abnormalities.

The WHO has given the following definition of mental health:

> **Mental health is defined as a state of well-being in which every individual realizes his or her own potential, can cope with the normal stresses of life, can work productively and fruitfully, and is able to make a contribution to her or his community.**

This is a helpful definition, because it clearly defines a mental disorder as a condition that disrupts this state in any way, and sets clear goals of treatment for the clinician. It identifies the fact that a disruption of an individual's mental health impacts negatively not only upon their enjoyment and ability to cope with life, but also upon that of the wider community.

The rest of this chapter will consider the epidemiology of mental disorders, the impact that these have on both individuals and society, and the public perception of psychiatry and the effect that this has on those with mental disorders.

Worldwide prevalence of mental disorders

Psychiatric disorders are among the most prevalent causes of ill health in humans. They are found in

Table 2.1 World prevalence of mental health disorders

Condition	World prevalence (millions)
Unipolar depressive disorders	311.1
Anxiety disorders	267.0
Alcohol use disorders	63.5
Schizophrenia	23.4
Bipolar affective disorder	44.0
Alzheimer's and other dementias	24.2
Learning disability	92.0
HIV/AIDS	37.3
Malaria	295.7
Chronic obstructive pulmonary disease	174.5
Osteoarthritis	237.4
Ischaemic heart disease (all causes)	1.1 billion
Diabetes mellitus	435.0

Reproduced from *The Lancet*, 388, GBD 2015 Disease and Injury Incidence and Prevalence Collaborators, Global, regional, and national incidence, prevalence, and years lived with disability for 310 diseases and injuries, 1990–2015: a systematic analysis for the Global Burden of Disease Study 2015, pp. 1545–602. © 2016 The Authors. Published by Elsevier Ltd. Reproduced under the terms of the Creative Commons Attribution 4.0 International (CC BY 4.0) License. https://creativecommons.org/licenses/by/4.0/.

Table 2.2 Epidemiology of mental disorders in the USA, adults from 18 years, 2014

Condition	Prevalence (% population)	Median age of onset (years)
Any mental illness meeting DSM-IV criteria, excluding substance misuse	18.1	–
Anxiety disorders	16.1	21
All mood disorders	9.5	30
Unipolar depression	6.7	32
Post-traumatic stress disorder	3.5	23
Eating disorders	1–7 (females)	17
Bipolar disorder	2.6	25
Schizophrenia	1.1	20
Obsessive–compulsive disorder	1.0	19
ADHD	4.1	7
Autism	0.34	3
Alzheimer's disease	10% of over 65s	72

ADHD, attention deficit hyperactivity disorder; DSM-IV, *Diagnostic and Statistical Manual of Mental Disorders*, fourth edition.
Source data from the US National Institute for Mental Health, www.nimh.nih.gov

all parts of the world, in both economically developed and developing countries. Table 2.1 outlines the worldwide prevalence of the major psychiatric disorders, with some common physical disorders for comparison. Depression is one of the most prevalent diseases currently seen in humans, only superseded by conditions associated with poverty and poor access to healthcare (e.g. infection, iron-deficiency anaemia, and low vision). Approximately 6 per cent of the population have a severe, enduring psychiatric disorder which impacts their functioning in the long term. Schizophrenia, bipolar disorder,

and unipolar depression make up the majority of these cases.

As an example of the relative prevalence of common mental health disorders seen in developed countries, Table 2.2 shows epidemiological data from the USA collected in 2014. Always remember that patients frequently fit the diagnostic criteria for more than one diagnosis—for example, social phobia and major depressive disorder—and that this is especially true for the mood, anxiety, and behavioural conditions. Rates of most conditions appear to have been rising slowly since the mid twentieth century: it is unclear at the moment if this is a true representation or merely a diagnostic artefact. Time will tell.

Global service provision for mental health disorders

As psychiatry is a medical specialty that affects such a large proportion of the population, it would seem logical for there to be health services at least equivalent to those for other medical conditions available. However, this is not the case. WHO data from 2014 suggest that the global provision of psychiatric services is woefully inadequate. The WHO Mental Health Global Action Programme (mhGAP) has been designed to try and tackle this problem. The following are key statistics:

- Only 68 per cent of countries (including 77 per cent of the world population) have a specific mental health policy outlining provision of services.

- In 18% of countries, the primary source of funding for mental health is private households. Looking only at 'high-income' countries, approximately one-third of funding is from non-governmental, not-for-profit organizations.

- Twenty-six per cent of the world's population are not covered by a dedicated mental health law or legislation covering involuntary treatment and human rights.

- The global median of mental health workers (nurses and doctors) is 9 per 100,000 population (range 1–53.2).

- The mean number of psychiatric beds per 10,000 people worldwide is 6.5, compared with 292 for physical and mental health conditions combined.

- There are just 0.9 psychiatrists per 100,000 population worldwide, of whom 90 per cent work in high-income countries.

Table 2.3 lists some drugs that are commonly used in psychiatry, and the percentage of countries with easy access to them. Most of the older typical antipsychotics are now widely available, but other 'basics' such as lithium and sodium valproate are still limited to two-thirds of the world. There are currently no data

Table 2.3 Availability of common psychiatric drugs worldwide

Drug	Countries with availability (%)
Carbamazepine	91.4
Valproate	67.4
Amitriptyline	86.4
Diazepam	96.8
Haloperidol	91.8
Lithium	65.4
Levodopa	61.9
Chlorpromazine	91.4

Reprinted from *WHO Mental Health Atlas*. Copyright (2005) World Health Organization.

published for selective serotonin reuptake inhibitors (SSRIs) or atypical antipsychotics. Access to medications is a good marker for the level of development of health services. If a doctor does not have access to antidepressants, it is very unlikely that they will have other more complex treatments available, for example, cognitive behavioural therapy (CBT).

In the UK, which has a National Health Service (NHS) funded from taxation, 13 per cent of the health budget is allotted to mental health services. This is the highest proportion in Europe, but still there is a distinct shortage of facilities, especially for psychological therapies and specialty services such as those for adolescents or eating disorders.

The impact of mental health disorders upon individuals and society

With so many people suffering from mental health disorders, it is unsurprising that these disorders have a major impact on society. Disability is defined as 'a loss of health', and is usually used to describe impairments in activities of daily living caused by physical

Table 2.4 Non-communicable causes of disability in descending order by global prevalence

Conditions	DALYs (thousands)
Mental health disorders	149,977.9
Endocrine disorders (incl. diabetes)	66,092.0
Unintentional injuries	30,679.5
Chronic respiratory disorders	30,465.9
Cardiovascular disorders	25,620.1
Gastrointestinal disorders	12,142.8
Intentional injuries to self or others	1077.5
Neoplasms	8569.3
Dementia	6851.2

DALYs, disability adjusted life years.
Reproduced from *The Lancet*, 388, GBD 2015 Disease and Injury Incidence and Prevalence Collaborators, Global, regional, and national incidence, prevalence, and years lived with disability for 310 diseases and injuries, 1990–2015: a systematic analysis for the Global Burden of Disease Study 2015, pp. 1545–602. © 2016 The Authors. Published by Elsevier Ltd. Reproduced under the terms of the Creative Commons Attribution 4.0 International (CC BY 4.0) License. https://creativecommons.org/licenses/by/4.0/.

or mental disorders. The disability-adjusted life year (DALY) is a measure of the overall burden of a disease, combining morbidity and mortality into one number. Table 2.4 shows the latest WHO data from the Global Burden of Disease study, which has produced a list of disease areas and the burden of disability they represent worldwide. Part of the high burden of disability is related to the chronic nature of many mental disorders. Depression is currently the second leading cause of disability globally.

While the majority of physical diseases tend to be more common in older people, psychiatric conditions predominantly affect the young and middle aged. Table 2.2 shows the median age of onset of various conditions in the USA; most are between 18 and 30 years. This means that mental health disorders tend to affect people when they are in the later stages of education, starting a career, and setting up home. In the UK, 48 per cent of claimants of incapacity benefit in 2015 stated a mental health or behavioural disorder as the principal reason for their disability leading to an inability to work. The impact of psychiatric disorders on the economic success and social coherence of a country is therefore great.

Mortality associated with mental health disorders is very variable, depending upon the condition. The most important area is that of deliberate self-harm and completed suicide. Globally, it is estimated that 800,000 people complete suicide each year, 90 per cent of whom have a diagnosable mental health disorder. Two-thirds of those who commit suicide are aged between 15 and 44 years. Suicide is the leading cause of death in men aged 15–34 years in the UK, and for women it is the second most prevalent cause. Three times as many men die by suicide as women, although more women make attempts. WHO data from 2016 report suicides accounted for 1.4 per cent of global deaths in 2012–2014, making it the 15th leading cause of death. These statistics are rarely appreciated by the general public.

The public perception of mental health

It is an unfortunate truth that individuals with mental health disorders are subject to significant negative stigma within society. This is a worldwide phenomenon, with many people experiencing victimization, difficulty accessing employment, or losing the support of their family members and friends. This also occurs in medicine. Even in developed countries, young doctors who express an interest in being psychiatrists are often deemed to be either 'mad' themselves, or unable to get another job. The WHO programme Mind the Gap and the UK charity Time to Change are just two initiatives to try and reduce stigma. Some recent findings from a report entitled *Attitudes to Mental Illness* (2011), a large cross-sectional study of UK adults, included the following:

- Twenty-one per cent of respondents felt that an individual with a history of mental disorder should not be allowed to work in the public sector.

- Sixteen per cent thought that the main cause of mental illness was a lack of self-discipline and personal will power.

- Only twenty-five per cent of people felt that a woman who had previously had inpatient treatment for 'a mental disorder' could be trusted to use as a babysitter.

- Only 72 per cent of respondents thought that people with mental health problems should have the same right to a job as those without them.

- Twenty-eight per cent of respondents felt that 'all people with mental health problems are prone to violence'.

- Two-thirds of people said they were scared of those with psychiatric illnesses, and would not want to live next door to one of them.

- Eighty per cent of respondents underestimated the prevalence of mental health disorders in the UK by at least a factor of ten.

One positive finding is that the majority of adults agree that community and outpatient-based interventions are preferable to prolonged hospitalizations. Data for less economically developed countries are more difficult to find, but common situations for people suffering from mental disorders include:

- the belief from others that all people with mental disorder are aggressive and dangerous;

- the idea that patients with psychosis are bewitched by evil spirits, are possessed by the devil, or did bad things in a previous life;

- in areas of arranged marriage, difficulties getting married;

- trouble accessing education;

- a lack of psychiatric facilities in rural areas.

Education surrounding mental health is badly needed the world over, both to help the vast number of people with mental health disorders to cope with them more productively, and to allow the rest of society to include them in a cohesive manner.

Further reading

Office for National Statistics (UK). Mental health: mental health of children, adolescents and adults. https://www.ons.gov.uk/peoplepopulationandcommunity/healthandsocialcare/mentalhealth.

National Institute for Mental Health (USA). Statistics. https://www.nimh.nih.gov/health/statistics/index.shtml.

The World Health Organization website provides copious reading material on all aspects of mental health epidemiology, including a searchable database of psychiatric service provision for all countries: http://www.who.int/topics/mental_health/en/.

http://www.euro.who.int/en/health-topics/noncommunicable-diseases/mental-health.

http://www.who.int/topics/global_burden_of_disease/en/.

Time to Change: http://www.time-to-change.org.uk/.

3 Mental disorder and you

Facts, beliefs, and prejudices

People's attitudes to mental disorder vary widely. Often this is because of the extent of their personal experience of mental illness. Some people have experienced a mental illness themselves while others may well have experience of mental illness in a friend or relative. If you have been lucky enough to avoid these personal experiences, it is almost inevitable that you will be exposed to one or the other during your lifetime, and, perhaps, several times. Of course, because you are reading this book, it is likely that you are, or want to be, a healthcare professional. In whatever area of healthcare you work, you will encounter hundreds or thousands of people with mental illness in your professional lifetime. The beliefs that you hold about mental illness and people with mental illness will influence how you respond. It is therefore important that you assess your existing beliefs and, if necessary, consider changing some of them.

Assessing and altering our beliefs is difficult. We all tend to assume that what we believe—about ourselves, others, or the world around us—is true. However, only some beliefs are facts. Despite this, our beliefs tend to be 'static' and resistant to change. One reason for this is the kind of cognitive biases that operate, unconsciously but persistently, to maintain our system of beliefs. Cognitive therapists use a model which they call 'the prejudice model' to describe these biases: most evidence which *conflicts with* our core beliefs is either not noticed, or is altered in order to fit our core beliefs; whereas most evidence which *fits with* our core beliefs is noticed and used to bolster those beliefs. In this way, the beliefs that we hold tend to be stable through time.

Common prejudices

This section describes a short exercise for you to complete, with three stages:

1 In Box 3.1, we list several common prejudices about mental illness. Rate each of those statements from 0 to 100 per cent, where the percentage is the extent to which you hold that belief. For example, if you believe that mental illness is a sign of weakness in most cases, you might answer 80 percent. It is important to be honest, rather than give what you believe to be the 'correct' answer.

2 Continue to read this chapter, where we challenge some of these prejudices, largely by comparing mental illness with physical illness. Think carefully about the comparisons and arguments, and how they fit with or contradict your own beliefs.

3 Finally, re-rate the six statements in Box 3.1. Are there any differences from your initial ratings?

Box 3.1 Common prejudices about mental illness

1 Mental illness is a sign of weakness
2 Mental illness is something that affects other people
3 People with mental illness should just pull themselves together
4 There are no effective treatments for people with mental illness
5 People with mental illness should be kept in hospital
6 People with mental illness are a risk to others

This three-part strategy is identical to one used by cognitive therapists when attempting to tackle 'negative automatic thoughts' which contribute to common problems such as anxiety or depression. The bottom line is that much of what we *believe* to be true is not actually *factual,* but is subject to biases and subjective interpretation.

Mental illness is a sign of weakness

Is physical illness a sign of weakness? We do not commonly associate a fractured neck of the femur, a myocardial infarction, or diabetes mellitus with 'weakness', and yet people with mental illness may well be judged to be weak in some way. As you will see, the causes of mental illness are complex, involving physical, psychological, and social factors. In many cases, mental illness appears to have a strong genetic basis, and this is particularly likely in some illnesses, such as bipolar disorder. Furthermore, many people whose lives have demonstrated personal strength or extraordinary ability have also suffered from mental illness. These include Winston Churchill (who, besides his successes as a wartime politician, won the Nobel Prize for Literature), Florence Nightingale (pioneer of modern nursing), Vincent Van Gogh (artist), Isaac Newton (scientist), Freddie Flintoff (sportsman), Oprah Winfrey (talk show host), and JK Rowling (author). It is difficult, in these circumstances, to argue that mental illness is a sign of weakness. Indeed, one common mental illness—bipolar disorder—appears to be strongly represented among successful people, and it has been argued that mood disorder persists in populations because mood variability may present a selective advantage in evolution.

Mental illness is something that affects other people

Many of us are rather blasé about our health, both physical and mental. This may change when we receive an 'early warning' that something is wrong (such as high blood pressure or impaired glucose tolerance). Many of us have had short or mild periods of emotional distress, often in the context of personal difficulty such as the end of a relationship or the death of a close relative. Such an episode indicates that we are vulnerable. However, few of us, in those circumstances, seek help or advice, yet mental illness is often seen in healthcare professionals, including doctors and psychiatrists. Mood disorder, anxiety disorder, eating disorder, and alcohol and substance misuse are common. Unfortunately, healthcare professionals can be very slow in acknowledging that there is a problem and in obtaining effective assessment and care.

People with mental illness should just pull themselves together

If only this were possible! We know from personal experience that, when we have received some kind of setback, or when our energy or confidence is at a low ebb, achieving our goals is more difficult. By its nature, depression is associated with physical fatigue, mental fatigue, pervasive low mood, and powerful negative biases about self, world, and future. Imagine how difficult it is to engage with treatment, and to continue with those aspects of life that are either essential or help to keep us going, during such an illness. The more depressed the person's mood, the more difficult it is for that person to 'just pull themselves together', and the more dependent they are on others, including healthcare professionals, for support, tolerance, and the instillation of hope (a core psychotherapeutic task).

There are no effective treatments for people with mental illness

There is no doubt that mental illness can be difficult to treat and that, sometimes, the resulting distress and disability are long-standing. However, this is similar to the

Box 3.2 Numbers needed to treat (NNTs)

The NNT is a potentially helpful way of presenting the comparative effectiveness of a treatment. It represents the number of patients who need to be treated with a treatment to achieve one additional good outcome. So, if we know, from randomized evidence, that a patient has a 60 per cent chance of a bad outcome without the treatment, and that this decreases to 40 per cent with the treatment, their absolute risk reduction (ARR) is 20 per cent, and we would need to treat five patients (100/20 per cent) to gain one whole additional good outcome. So, the NNT is 5.

If an NNT is quoted, it should relate to five specific pieces of context: (a) the patient group, (b) the experimental treatment, (c) the comparison treatment, (d) the timepoint of the comparison, and (e) the outcome. So, for example, in a randomized controlled trial in (a) adults with panic disorder, comparing (b) individual CBT with (c) individual supportive therapy, (d) at 8 weeks, the (e) proportion of patients still with panic attacks was 29 per cent in the CBT group and 75 per cent in the supportive group. The ARR is 46 per cent, and so the NNT = 100/46 per cent = 2.2.

treatment and prognosis of physical disorders. Some physical illnesses, such as appendicitis, can be cured by a clear, discrete intervention. However, others, such as rheumatoid arthritis or multiple sclerosis, can often not be cured, and the focus of most treatments is on reducing disability rather than eliminating disease. Psychiatric treatments, such as SSRIs, have proven effectiveness for anxiety and depression, with a number needed to treat (NNT) of 5–8 versus placebo in panic disorder and 5 versus placebo for treatment response in moderately severe depression. Box 3.2 gives more details about NNTs.

People with mental illness should be kept in hospital

Perhaps it is helpful to ask, first, whether people with *physical* illness should be kept in hospital. Clearly, in some cases, they should. However, in most cases, we will want to manage physical disorder in primary care, in outpatients, or through day care, with the patient spending most of their life at home. The treatment of mental illness is similar. Most psychiatric patients will at no time need to be admitted to hospital, and even those patients who need inpatient care will, for the vast majority of their lives, be managed as outpatients.

People with mental illness are a risk to others

The proportion of people with mental illness who present a risk to others is small. Even when a particular

mental illness is associated with violence, the majority of people with that disorder are not violent. Indeed, people with mental illness are more likely to be the victims of violence than the perpetrators. The vast majority of people who are violent do not suffer from mental illness. Unfortunately, the public perception of this issue is maintained by some of the prejudices or cognitive biases that we mentioned earlier and, perhaps, by selective reporting in the media.

People with mental illness don't make good doctors

It is perfectly possible for people with diabetes, hypertension, or asthma to be good doctors, so why not people with anxiety disorder or depressive disorder? Just as the experience of physical illness may help to develop some important insights and skills, which can enhance good medical practice, so the experience of mental illness may help to develop individuals so that they can deliver particularly insightful and compassionate care. The General Medical Council accepts that doctors in training and qualified doctors may be or become ill, and offers guidance in *Good Medical Practice*.

Your mental health

It is quite possible that you have had mental illness in the past, or that you are currently suffering from one. If so, you may well have sought help and advice from healthcare professionals. However, you may well have avoided seeking help. Perhaps you feared that your medical career would be in peril; that you couldn't be helped; that the problem was not very serious, and you would be wasting someone's time; that you were too busy and could not afford the time; or that your fellow students, or others, might find out about your difficulties, and think badly of you. Whatever the reason or reasons, now is a good time to seek advice. Often, the experience of psychiatry as a trainee healthcare professional brings one's own emotions and emotional problems to the fore. Furthermore, you are early in your professional career, and seeking to understand and deal with any difficulties makes good sense at this stage. You will be able to learn the knowledge and skills to help to keep you well during the challenging early years of your career, and for the rest of your life. Finally, you may be able to consider important life and career decisions (such as location, choice of specialty, and choice of full- or part-time training) in the light of your greater understanding of your health.

Your first step should be to arrange to talk to your general practitioner (GP) about your problems. To make the consultation easier for you, it can be helpful to write down your concerns on paper, and take these with you. As you will see later in this textbook, our day-to-day worries are *maintained* (kept going, sustained) by *avoidance*. Facing up to your concerns is therefore the first step towards managing them effectively. Cognitive therapists know, through extensive experience with their patients (and themselves!), that fears about an event are often much greater than the reality of that event. By *avoiding avoiding*, by seeking help for your difficulties, you may well experience great relief that you have taken the first steps forward. So, if you're concerned about your emotional health, don't delay—get in touch with your GP today.

Further reading

Hodgson R, Cookson J, Taylor M. Numbers needed to treat analysis: an explanation using antipsychotic trials in schizophrenia. *Advances in Psychiatric Treatment* 2011;17:63–71.

Wikipedia, The Free Encyclopedia. Number needed to treat. https://en.wikipedia.org/wiki/Number_needed_to_treat.

Part 2 Assessment

Assessment

4 Conducting the assessment: setting it up and taking a history

Assessment prepares the way for management. The form and detail of an assessment depends therefore on the management that is likely to be needed, and this depends in turn on the nature of the problem. Although the basic structure will be the same, the length and focus of the assessment will differ in each case. For example:

- After assessing a severely depressed patient, the GP may need to arrange for admission or arrange further focused support at the patient's home. The assessment will therefore focus on the level of risk in the short term, and the resources available to support the patient in their home.

- After arriving to assess a disturbed patient in the emergency department, the doctor's first action will be to attempt to calm the patient and ensure their own safety and the safety of others. Only then will they start to gather information about possible physical and psychological causes of disturbed behaviour, perhaps focusing on sources of information that do not rely on the patient's cooperation—hospital records, GP records, or family informant, for example.

- After assessing an adolescent with the eating disorder bulimia nervosa who has been brought to the clinic by a parent, the psychiatrist needs to determine the patient's insight into their problems, their motivation to change, and their ability to engage with a self-help cognitive behavioural programme.

Diagnosis begins as soon as the presenting problem is known—it does not wait until all the relevant data have been collected. From the start of the interview, the assessor begins to think what disorders could account for the presenting problem and what data will be required to decide. Assessment is not a fixed procedure, carried out in the same way with every patient. It is a *dynamic* process in which healthcare professionals make, test, and modify hypotheses as they gather information.

Although the details of the assessment vary in this way, the *general aims* are always the same. These are to:

- begin to form a *therapeutic relationship* with the patient;
- understand the *problem*, the *symptoms*, and their *functional impact*, from the patient's perspective, including their *concerns*;
- understand these issues from the *perspective of the relatives/carers*, if appropriate;
- consider the *course of the illness*—compare the present condition of the patient with their former state or states;
- enquire about *treatments*—current and past, physical and psychological;
- consider the patient's social and family circumstances, including sources of support.

Whenever possible, history from the patient is supplemented by history from another *informant* or *corroborant*. History taking is followed by an examination of the mental and physical state and, in some cases, by psychological or physical investigations. At this stage, the assessment may be complete or incomplete, depending on the complexity of the problem, the time available, and the information immediately accessible. The full assessment will inform the diagnosis and differential diagnosis (see Chapter 6), aetiology (see Chapter 7), prognosis (see Chapter 8), risks to the patient and others (see Chapter 9), and a plan of management (see chapters relating to specific disorders). When the assessment has been made, the results are discussed with the patient and often with a relative, and communicated to other relevant healthcare professionals (see Chapter 10).

The clinical skills required to elicit symptoms and signs and to make a diagnosis are similar to those used in other branches of medicine—careful *history taking*, systematic *clinical examination*, and sound *clinical reasoning*. The only substantial difference is that the clinical examination includes the mental as well as the physical state of the patient.

However, eliciting the signs and symptoms of mental disorder, and considering diagnoses, are only part of the assessment of patients. The assessment should never lose sight of the patient as a unique individual. For example:

- What impact is there on the patient's feelings about life (e.g. making them feel like a failure, and letting down their partner/children)?
- What impact is there on their social roles (e.g. affecting their caring for their small children)?
- What impact is there on their livelihood (e.g. making it difficult to drive to work)?
- What attitudes do they have to psychiatric treatments, and why (e.g. rejection of anti-depressants because of intolerable side effects in a close relative)?

The more that interviewers gain insight into such personal experiences, the more they can help their patients. Because such understanding is equally important when caring for patients with physical illnesses, the experience gained during training in psychiatry is of value in every kind of clinical work. This understanding cannot be acquired solely from books—it is learnt though listening to patients as they describe their lives. Some students are reluctant to do this, fearing that psychiatric patients may behave in odd, unpredictable, or alarming ways. In fact this is uncommon. **Students should therefore take every opportunity to talk to patients**: no textbook can ever replace this experience.

Indeed, students should also take every opportunity to talk to their friends and relatives about their emotional lives, and to consider their own emotional reactions and coping with adversity. This is because one of the most challenging tasks for any healthcare professional is deciding the boundary between 'normal' and 'abnormal'. To succeed in this task, it is vital to have an understanding of 'normal' emotional reactions to difficult circumstances.

This chapter and Chapters 5–10 are concerned primarily with the general assessment of adult patients. The assessment of children is described in

Chapter 17, and of people with a learning disability in Chapter 19. Assessment of suicide risk is on p. 72, of alcohol problems on p. 423, and of sexual dysfunction on p. 457.

Starting to assess patients

Very early in your psychiatry attachment, you should feel confident enough to begin to interview patients, and to present your (initially very limited) findings in a structured and coherent way. Some of the language and the ideas will be new to you. You will not understand everything straight away, so don't be disgruntled. Most importantly, meet and talk to patients informally about their situation. Many of you will want to avoid seeing patients until you can do a 'good' assessment, but this is a mistake. *We recommend that you regard your initial meetings with psychiatric patients as being, simply, conversations with fellow human beings about their predicament—their experience of their illness, what led up to it, the impact that it has had on their lives, and their experience of treatment, including admission.* Only subsequently should you aim, with the help of this chapter, and Chapters 5–10, to be able to conduct and present a more formal and comprehensive assessment.

We therefore suggest three stages when practising interviewing patients:

- First, meet several patients and become comfortable talking to them informally, enquiring about their lives outside hospital, their lives inside hospital, their problems, and their hopes and fears for the future.
- Then, steadily introduce more structure, and start to ask specific questions, until you are confident with conducting a full psychiatric assessment.
- Finally, practise being flexible, so that you are equally confident conducting a very short screening assessment, a brief assessment, or a thorough assessment, depending on the circumstances.

Staying safe

Only a very small minority of patients with psychiatric illness are potentially dangerous, although this proportion depends on the setting (risk is greater in inpatients than outpatients) and subspecialty (greater in forensic psychiatry than old age psychiatry). Nevertheless, it is imperative that a brief risk assessment is *always* done before seeing *any* patient, in *any* setting, no matter how busy you are. Only then will you get into the habit of thinking about, assessing, and managing the risk posed to you by patients and, of course, by their family and their acquaintances.

In some circumstances, it is obvious that risks need to be assessed and managed. For example:

- assessment of a disturbed patient, not known to health services, in an A&E department;
- assessment of a man with a long history of violent offences who has presented to his GP surgery without an appointment as the surgery is closing for the evening and reception staff are leaving;
- assessment of a woman with schizophrenia, and a history of violence when unwell, who is thought to have relapsed, and needs to be seen at home;
- assessment late at night at her home of an elderly lady who is medically unwell, who lives in an area where street robbery and assault are very frequent;
- assessment of a woman with severe abdominal pain, whose cohabitee has a history of violence when stressed at her home.

In many other cases, though, it is not clear that there are significant risks. If you do not prepare properly, you are at much greater risk if there is an incident. Simple risk management strategies should therefore be part of your daily routine, in whichever branch of medicine you practise.

The simple approach outlined in Table 4.1 will ensure that you are considering the relevant issues.

Table 4.1 A plan to stay safe

Who?	Who is the patient?
	• Ask someone who knows them, such as a member of the nursing staff on the ward, and/or read medical notes/letters
	• Are they currently aggressive, irritable, or disinhibited? Do they have a history of harming others? Are they considered to be low risk to others?
Where?	Where will you interview?
	• Which room? A room down a long corridor with no other offices nearby, or in an interview room adjacent to the nursing station, with a viewing window so that other staff can observe proceedings while patient confidentiality is maintained?
	• Where in the room? In a corner where your exit is obstructed by the patient, or adjacent to the door? Think about setting up the room to your requirements in advance, by moving furniture. If the patient sits in 'your' chair, politely ask them to move
	• With weapons or missiles? As part of your preparation of the room, consider removing objects that could be used as weapons, such as paperweights or letter openers
With whom?	With whom will you interview?
	• You may be fine on your own
	• Alternatively, you may need to take another student, or a member of staff, so that if something does go wrong, one of you can go to fetch help
With alarm?	Will you take an alarm?
	• Many psychiatric wards now have 'pinpoint' alarm systems, where staff wear alarms on their belts which can be activated when necessary, and help other staff to locate (pinpoint) a staff member in trouble. An alarm is no use, however, if (1) it is forgotten, (2) it cannot be reached easily by the carrier, or (3) the carrier does not know how to activate it
	• Some rooms, such as in Accident and Emergency departments, have alarm buttons fixed to walls. Again, this is of no use if staff members do not know where they are, or are not close enough to operate it
	• In the community, remember to carry a mobile phone, and consider carrying a personal attack alarm
With knowledge?	Do other staff know where you are?
	• This is particularly important in the community, where you should make sure that your team base knows (1) where you are going, (2) who you are going to see, (3) when you are due back, and (4) how you are contactable, e.g. mobile phone number
	• On the ward, it can be as simple as saying to the patient's keyworker that you will be interviewing patient X in room Y until time Z
With insight?	• Our communication, both verbal and non-verbal, within the assessment can 'wind up' or 'wind down' patients. Avoid actions that might provoke anger, such as approaching too close, prolonging eye contact, or avoiding eye contact altogether. Be aware of changes in the patient's emotional state and, in particular, their state of arousal
	• Finally, IF IN DOUBT (about your safety), GET OUT!

Interviewing

Approach

The interview serves not only to collect information, but also to establish a therapeutic relationship. Hence, the clinician's approach to the patient is critical. This is described next, but it can only guide readers, who should take every opportunity to watch experienced interviewers at work and to practise under supervision. Psychiatric interviews are carried out in many different settings including patients' homes, the wards of a general hospital, primary care clinics, and police station custody suites. The advice that follows cannot be followed completely in every setting and situation but it is, nevertheless, important to follow it whenever possible.

Starting the interview

It is important to work hard to form a successful working relationship with the patient. This will not always be possible, but, if such a relationship is formed, the assessment will be easier and more will be revealed, such a relationship can be therapeutic in itself, and compliance (concordance) with treatment is enhanced.

The interview should be carried out in a place where it cannot be overheard and is, as far as possible, free from interruptions. If these requirements are difficult to meet, as in a medical ward, the interview should, if possible, be moved—for example, to a side room. Patients should be seated comfortably, with the chairs arranged so that the interviewer sits at an angle to, and no higher than, the patient.

Interviewers should welcome the patient, introduce themselves by name, and explain their role (e.g. medical student). They should greet anyone who is accompanying the patient, and explain how long they can expect to wait, and whether they too will be interviewed. It is usually better to see the patient on their own first, and to interview any accompanying person later. Exceptions are made if that person has to leave early, and when the patient is unable to give an account of the problems. Interviewers should explain briefly:

- how long the interview will last;
- how it will proceed;
- the need to take notes;
- the confidentiality of these notes but the need to share certain information with others directly involved in treatment.

Interviews are more likely to be effective if the interviewer:

- appears relaxed and unhurried—even when time is short;
- maintains appropriate eye contact and does not appear engrossed in the notes;
- is alert to non-verbal as well as to verbal cues and shows an understanding of the patient's feelings;
- attends to emotional problems and makes empathic responses to indications of distress, for example, 'I'm sure that was very upsetting for you';
- intervenes appropriately when patients are over-talkative, or have departed from or avoided the subject;
- has a systematic but flexible plan.

The interviewer *begins with a general question* to encourage patients to express their problems in their own words: for example, 'Tell me about your recent problems', 'Tell me what you have noticed wrong', or 'Tell me why you're here'. During the reply, interviewers should notice whether their patients are calm, or distressed despite their efforts to put them at ease. If the latter, interviewers should try to find the nature of the difficulty and attempt to overcome it.

Continuing the interview

Having elicited the complaints, the next step is to enquire into them systematically. In doing this, the interviewer should as far as possible *avoid closed and leading questions*. A *closed* question allows only a brief answer, usually 'Yes' or 'No'; whereas a *leading* question suggests the answer. 'Do you wake early?' is both closed and leading. 'At what time do you wake?' is both open and non-leading. If there is no alternative to a leading question, it should be followed by a request for an example. The only way to ask about an important symptom of schizophrenia (the first-rank symptom of 'made actions') is to use the leading, closed question 'Have you ever felt that your actions were being controlled by another person?' If the answer is yes, the interviewer should ask for one or more examples of the experience, and should conclude that the symptom is present only if the examples are convincing. Leading questions can be avoided by prompting the patient indirectly by:

- repeating what the patient has said, but in a questioning tone, for example, 'Feeling low ...?'; or

- restating the problem in other words, for example (after a patient has spoken of sadness), 'You say you have been feeling low';

- asking for clarification, for example, 'Could you say more about that?'

It is important to *establish when each symptom and problem began* as well as if and when it became worse or better. If a patient finds it difficult to remember these dates, it may be possible to relate the events to others that are more easily remembered, such as a birthday or a public holiday.

As the interview progresses, the interviewer has a number of tasks:

- *To help patients to talk freely* by interrupting only when necessary, by nodding, and by saying, for example, 'Go on', 'Tell me more about that', or 'Is there more to say?'

- *To keep patients to relevant topics* in part with non-verbal cues such as leaning forward or nodding to encourage the patient to continue with the topic.

- *To make systematic enquiries* but without asking so many questions that other—unanticipated—aspects of the problem are not volunteered.

- *To check their understanding* by summarizing key points back to the patient, and saying 'Is that right?—Does that sum it up?'

- *To select questions according to the emerging possibilities* regarding diagnoses, causes, and plans of action. The choice of questions is modified progressively as additional information is gathered.

As explained previously, *interviewing is an active and selective process, not the asking of the same set of questions to every patient.* The shorter the time available for the interview, the more important it is to proceed in this focused and targeted way. Occasionally, the patient is so disturbed that it is impossible to follow an orderly sequence of questioning. In such cases, it is even more important to keep the diagnostic possibilities in mind so that the most relevant questions are selected and the most relevant observations are carried out.

Ending the interview

Before ending the interview, the interviewer should summarize the main points and ask whether the patient has anything to add to the account that he or she has given. The interviewer should then explain what will happen next.

Taking notes

Whenever possible, notes should be taken during the interview because attempts to memorize the history and make notes later are time-consuming and liable to error. Exceptions may, however, have to be made when patients are very restless or agitated. At the start of the interview, note taking may be deferred for a few minutes so that patients can feel that they have the undivided attention of the interviewer. However, experienced interviewers can often achieve both tasks.

Challenges

Interviewing patients from another culture

If the patient and the interviewer do not speak a common language, it is obvious that an interpreter will be needed. However, language is not the only problem in such cases; cultural differences are also important, and interpreters may share the patient's language but not their culture. Issues such as the following may be understood best by talking with someone from the patient's cultural group:

- *Cultural beliefs* may explain why certain events are experienced as more stressful or shameful than they would be in the host culture.
- *Roles* within the family may differ from those in the host culture.
- *Distress may be shown in different symptoms*. In some cultures, distress is often expressed in physical rather than mental symptoms, for example, sadness may manifest as 'heartache'.
- *Distress may be shown in different behaviours*. In some cultures, unrestrained displays of emotion that would suggest illness in the host culture are socially acceptable ways of expressing distress.
- *Cultural beliefs* may include ideas that would suggest delusional thinking in the host culture, such as being under the influence of spells cast by neighbours.
- *Expectations about treatment* may be based on experiences of very different traditions of medical care.

Ideally the interpreter should be a member of a health profession who knows both the language and the culture of the patient. This ideal arrangement is not easy to achieve and often the only available interpreter is a family member. Although a family member will know both the language and the culture, patients may not talk freely about personal matters through such a person, especially when their genders differ, or when there are problems within the family.

Patients who appear anxious or angry

The first step is to discover the reason for the anxiety or anger. The cause might be, for example, that the patient has come to the interview reluctantly, and at the insistence of another person (e.g. when there is an alcohol problem). Some patients are worried that their employers could learn about the interview. Once the problem is understood, appropriate reassurance usually reduces distress enough for the interview to proceed.

Patients who appear confused

Sometimes the patient's initial responses are muddled and confused. This problem can be caused by *anxiety, low intelligence*, or *cognitive impairment*—the latter due to delirium or dementia. If cognitive impairment seems possible, brief tests of concentration and memory should be carried out before continuing (see Chapter 5). If the results are abnormal, it is usually better to interview an informant before continuing with the patient.

Taking a history

Basic structure of the psychiatric history

The amount of detail and the focus of the psychiatric history varies from case to case but the basic aims are the same—it is not necessary to learn a separate interview for each condition. These common aims are reflected in the basic structure of the interview shown in Box 4.1. When time is short, parts of the background

Box 4.1 The elements of the psychiatric history

- History of the presenting problems
- Background history
- Family history
- Personal history
- Social history
- Past medical history
- Past psychiatric history
- Medicines
- Personality
- Corroborative history

history should be covered only in outline. It is important to be flexible and able to adopt any of the following three approaches: (1) to spend 2 minutes screening patients for mental disorder; (2) to spend 5–10 minutes undertaking a shortened, focused history in an emergency; or (3) to spend 20 minutes or longer obtaining a full history. Note that the most important investigation in psychiatry is always obtaining a *corroborative history* from someone who knows the patient well.

Screening questions

In primary care and general hospital medicine, psychiatric disorder is common. When a patient complains of symptoms of physical illness, for example, it is often appropriate to check for evidence of a psychiatric disorder since this may be present as the cause or a consequence of the symptoms. For this purpose, a brief screening interview is required to detect any symptoms and problems that have not been complained of spontaneously. The following seven domains are helpful:

- **General well-being:** fatigue, irritability, poor concentration, poor sleep, not coping.
- **Anxiety:** repeated worrying thoughts; avoidance; physical symptoms (e.g. headache), shortness of breath, sweating, palpitations.
- **Depression:** persistent low mood, low energy, loss of interest, loss of confidence, and hopelessness.
- **Elation:** abnormally elevated mood, irritability, increased energy, disinhibition, talkativeness.
- **Memory:** difficulty in recalling recent events, difficulty in performing everyday tasks (note that this is an area in which a corroborative history is especially important).
- **Alcohol and illicit drugs:** extent of use of alcohol and drugs, physical/psychological/social problems arising from use of alcohol and drugs.
- **Eating:** distress arising from perceived shape and weight; presence and extent of weight-control behaviours; concerns of others.

Shortened history taking in an emergency

When urgent action is required, the interview has to be *brief* (focused on the basic points set out earlier) and *effective* (leading to a provisional diagnosis and a plan of immediate action). The information needed includes, at the least:

- the *presenting problem* in terms of symptoms or behaviours, together with their onset, course, and present severity;
- *other relevant symptoms*, with their onset, course, and severity, including an assessment of risks, to self (e.g. self-harm/suicide/neglect) and others (e.g. assault or homicide, childcare, driving, operating machinery);
- *stressful circumstances* around the time of onset and at the present time;
- *previous and current physical or mental disorders* and how the patient coped with them;
- *current medicines*;
- the use of *alcohol and illicit drugs*;
- *family and personal history*, covered with a few salient questions;
- *social circumstances*, and the possibilities of support;
- *personality*—this is valuable although it may be difficult to obtain this information in the circumstances of an emergency.

Throughout, the interviewer should think which questions need to be answered at the time and which can be deferred. If the patient has had previous treatment, efforts should be made to contact a professional who knows the patient. However short the time, the patient should feel that he has the interviewer's undivided attention and an opportunity to say what is important.

The full psychiatric history

The structure of the full psychiatric history is shown in Box 4.2. Readers may find it helpful to copy this page and refer to it when they interview their first

Box 4.2 The psychiatric history

Name, age, and address of the patient; name of any informants, and their relationship to the patient.

History of presenting problems

- Patient's description of the presenting problems—nature, severity, onset, factors making the problem worse or better
- Other problems and symptoms
- Treatment received to date

Background history

Family history

- Parents: age (now or at death), occupation, personality, and relationship with the patient
- Similar information about siblings
- Social position; atmosphere of the home
- Mental disorder in other members of the family, abuse of alcohol/drugs, suicide

Personal history

- Mother's pregnancy and birth
- Early development, separation, childhood illnesses
- Educational history
- Occupational history
- Intimate relationships

Social history

- Living arrangements
- Financial problems
- Alcohol and illicit drug use
- Forensic history

Past medical history

Past psychiatric history

Medicines

Personality

Corroborative history

patients. The amount of detail required in a particular case varies with the diagnostic possibilities of the case and the time available. Experienced interviewers focus on the most relevant items but students should practise the full history until they are confident in its use, before they learn the more selective approach.

History of the presenting problems

Patient's description of the presenting problems

The interviewer should allow patients adequate time to talk spontaneously before asking questions, otherwise they may not reveal all their problems. For example, a patient who begins by describing depression may also have a marital problem that she is hesitant to reveal. If the interviewer asks questions about depression as soon as this is mentioned, the marital problem may not be revealed. To avoid overlooking problems, when patients have finished speaking spontaneously the interviewer should summarize the problems that have been mentioned, and ask if there are any others. The interviewer's subsequent questions are designed to understand the following issues:

- **Nature** of the problem. For example, a patient who complains of worrying excessively could be describing anxiety, obsessional symptoms, or intrusive thoughts occurring in a depressive disorder.

- **Severity** of the problem, which will be related to (1) the amount of **distress** caused by the problem, and (2) the amount of **functional impairment**/interference with day-to-day activities.

- **Onset**—how long ago it started, and whether this was spontaneous ('out of the blue') or related to stressful events.

- **Course** of the problem—whether it is static, worsening, improving, or fluctuating in severity; whether it has worsened gradually or in a stepwise fashion; whether it is present continuously or intermittently.

- **Factors making the problem worse or better**. For example, low mood might be worse on workdays, due to problems at work such as poor relationships with colleagues, and the presence of a supportive relationship at home. Alternatively, low mood might be better on workdays, due to the structure and sense of purpose that work can bring, and the presence of a difficult marital relationship at home.

Other problems and symptoms

The interviewer should now enquire about the symptoms and problems that he or she judges relevant and that have not yet been volunteered by the patient. These further enquiries are guided by the interviewer's knowledge of the disorders in which the presenting symptoms and problems can occur (this information will be found in subsequent chapters). For example, if the presenting problem is poor sleep, the interviewer would ask about the symptoms of depressive and anxiety disorders, and about pain, all of which can cause insomnia. If the presenting problem is depression, a variety of physical, psychological, and social symptoms should be assessed (Box 4.3).

The *date of onset* and *sequence* of the various symptoms should also be noted; for example, whether obsessional symptoms began before or after depressive symptoms is relevant to diagnosis and treatment. The sequence of problems is similarly important; for example, whether abuse of alcohol began before or after marital difficulties.

Treatment received to date

Finally, a note should be made of any *treatment already received*, its effectiveness or ineffectiveness, side

Box 4.3 Associated symptoms of depression

Physical: low energy, poor (or increased) sleep, poor (or increased) appetite, loss (or gain) of weight, constipation, amenorrhoea, reduced libido
Psychological: diurnal mood variation (typically mood lower in the morning), hopelessness, suicidal thoughts, helplessness, low self-esteem, reduced confidence, guilt, agitation, poor concentration
Social: social withdrawal, work absence, impaired work performance

effects, and adherence. For example, a patient may report that they took fluoxetine for low mood, for about 1 month, but this made them feel anxious and worsened their sleep, so they stopped taking it despite their GP advising them to continue, and that their GP also recommended that they read a named self-help book, but they have not yet obtained this.

Some specific symptoms

- **Pathological depression** is a pervasive lowering of mood accompanied by feelings of sadness and a loss of the ability to experience pleasure (*anhedonia*).

- **Pathological elation** is a pervasive elation of mood accompanied by excessive cheerfulness, which in extreme cases may be experienced as *ecstasy*.

- **Pathological anxiety** is a feeling of apprehension that is out of proportion to the actual situation. This is usually associated with autonomic changes, manifest by pale skin and increased sweating of the hands, feet, and axillae (see Chapter 24).

- **Depersonalization and derealization** are less easy to understand than anxiety and depression because they are less often experienced by healthy people. They are experienced occasionally by healthy people, sometimes when they are very tired. They occur as symptoms of many kinds of psychiatric disorder, especially anxiety disorders, depressive disorders, and schizophrenia, and occur also in temporal lobe epilepsy.

- **Depersonalization** is the experience of feeling unreal and detached. People who experience depersonalization often have difficulty in describing it and use similes such as 'It feels *as if* I were cut off by a wall of glass'. An 'as if' description of this kind must not be confused with a delusion (see p. 39), when the person lacks insight into their actual situation.

- **Derealization** is a similar experience but occurs in relation to the environment rather than the self: for example, the feeling that other people seem '*as if* made of cardboard' or that things no longer evoke any emotional response.

Background history

Family history

This part of the background history concerns the patient's father, mother, siblings, and other relatives. Enquiries about the patient's spouse or partner, and children are made later. The family history is important for several reasons:

- Psychiatric disorder in other family members may point to *genetic causes*.
- Past events in the family, such as the divorce of parents, are the background to the patient's *psychological development*.
- Past events in the family may help to *explain the patient's concerns*. For example, the discovery that a brother died of a brain tumour may help to explain a patient's seemingly excessive concerns about headaches.
- Current events in the family may be *stressful*.
- A history of *completed suicide in a first-degree relative* increases the patient's risk of suicide.

The amount of detail required varies from case to case. It is unlikely to be profitable to spend time in detailed enquiries about the childhood of an elderly patient seeking help for poor memory, but it could be highly relevant to obtain this information about a young adult whose behaviour is unusual.

A useful introduction to this part of the enquiry is: 'I would like to ask about the family into which you were born. Let us start with your father—is he still alive?' If the father is alive, his age, state of health, and job are recorded. If the father has died, the cause of death, and his age and that of the patient at the time of the death should be determined. The father's personality and relationship with the patient can be elicited by asking 'What was your father like when you were a child?', 'What is he like now?', 'How did you get on when you were a child?', and 'How do you get on now?' Similar enquiries are made about the mother, siblings, and other important figures in the patient's early life, such as a stepfather or a grandmother living with the patient.

Personal history

The aims in taking the personal history are to describe and understand the following:

- The *life story*, including any influences that help to explain the patient's personality, concerns, and preferences. For example, sexual abuse in childhood may help explain a woman's low self-esteem and sexual difficulties in adult life, and being the unwanted child of an unaffectionate mother may partly explain a man's fear of rejection.
- Any *stressful circumstances*, including how the patient reacted to them.

The amount of detail required to achieve these aims varies from patient to patient.

Pregnancy and birth

The mother's health during pregnancy and the nature of the patient's delivery can be important in the context of learning disability. Information from the patient may be unreliable and should be checked whenever possible with the mother or with hospital records made at the time of the event. In most other cases, it is necessary to enquire only about any major problems.

Early development, separation, and childhood illnesses

The comments in the previous paragraph about the relevance and reliability of information about pregnancy and delivery apply equally to developmental milestones, which are seldom important except when the patient is a child or an adult with a learning disability. A note should be made of any *prolonged separation* from either parent for whatever reason. Since the effects of separation vary considerably, it is important to find out whether the patient was distressed at the time and for how long. If possible, this information should be checked with the parents. Serious and prolonged *childhood illnesses* may have affected the patient's emotional development. Diseases of the central nervous system in this period may be relevant to learning disability.

Educational history

The history of school and, if applicable, college and university education gives a general indication of intelligence and achievements, and contributes to an understanding of personality. As well as academic, artistic, and sporting achievement, enquiries are made about friendships, sociability, aggressive behaviour, bullying, leadership, and relationships with fellow students and with teachers.

Occupational history

The occupational history throws light on abilities and achievements, and on personality. Frequent changes of job, failure to gain promotion, or arguments with senior staff, may reflect negative aspects of personality (although there are, of course, many other reasons for these events). Persistence with jobs or degrees that are poorly rewarded financially, and associated with frustrations and difficulties, may reflect more positive aspects of personality.

Intimate relationships

This part of the history includes the success and failure of intimate relationships, as well as sexual preferences and behaviour. Detailed enquiries are not needed in every case, but when they are relevant, the interviewer should be able to make them sympathetically, objectively, and without embarrassment. Common-sense judgement and a knowledge of clinical syndromes will indicate how much to ask. If the patient is sexually active, questions about the patient's attitude to pregnancy and contraception are relevant. Detailed questions about sexual preferences and behaviour may be relevant when one of the problems is a sexual one; in other cases, it is usually enough to ask more generally whether there are any sexual problems. These are often relevant in patients with mental illness—for example, depression is associated with low sexual interest, and antidepressants can have sexual side effects including delayed orgasm. Women should be asked about *menstrual problems* appropriate to their age, including psychological and other symptoms of the premenstrual syndrome and the menopause.

The interviewer should ask about long-term relationships, including marriage and civil partnerships, whether same-sex or otherwise. Ask whether the partnership is happy; how long it has lasted; about the partner's work and personality; and about the sex, age, parentage, health, and development of any children. Similar enquiries are made about any previous partnership(s). If the partnership is unhappy, further questions should be asked about the nature and causes of this unhappiness, how the couple came together, and any periods of separation or plans for future separation or divorce. These enquiries may also throw light on the patient's personality, which may be relevant to the management plan

Social history

This section is important. Without the following topics being addressed, an overview of the patient's problems is not possible, and important aspects of the management plan will not be addressed:

- **Living arrangements.** Potentially relevant enquiries include the size and quality of the patient's home; whether it is owned or rented; who else lives with the patient; and how these people relate to one another, and to the patient.
- **Financial problems.** Does the patient have financial difficulties and, if so, what kind, and what steps are they taking to deal with them.
- **Alcohol and illicit drug use.** These are often associated with mental disorder, and a careful alcohol and drugs history should be taken in every case. A screening question will often suffice for illicit drug use.
- **Forensic history.** This concerns behaviour that breaks the law. Common sense should be used to judge its relevance, but it is important in all cases of alcohol or drug misuse. For example, a young man who binge drinks on Friday and Saturday nights may have convictions for assault and criminal damage while intoxicated with alcohol, and one or more

convictions for drink driving, and yet be denying that he has an alcohol problem. If the patient has a criminal record, note the charges and the penalties, and find out whether other such acts have gone undetected.

Past medical history

Medical illnesses, past and current, should be asked about in every case. Medical problems are often a cause or a consequence of mental disorder. For example: (1) in many cases, people with mental illness and physical illness receive poor-quality care for their physical illness; (2) endocrine disorders such as hypothyroidism are associated with mental illness; and (3) psychiatric medications such as antipsychotics have metabolic side effects.

Past psychiatric history

When there is a past psychiatric history, careful notes should be taken of the nature of the illness, the number and severity of episodes, any association with risks to self (e.g. self-harm) or to others, and success or otherwise of treatments, including inpatient admission.

Medicines

A careful medicine history should be recorded. Which medicine is the patient taking, at what dose, and at what frequency? Is the patient non-adherent and, if so, to what extent? Does the patient know why they are prescribed? Does the patient use tablets prescribed for someone else, such as using a relative's antidepressants as an occasional pick-me-up, or benzodiazepines to calm nerves? Does the patient buy other pills or remedies from the chemist, including herbal remedies such as St John's wort or valerian? St John's wort is a popular herbal remedy for depression, but it interacts with the metabolism of many medicines, including anti-AIDS drugs, the combined oral contraceptive, and immunosuppressants, and so potential risks include progression from HIV to AIDS, unwanted pregnancy, and organ rejection. A careful medicine history is essential.

Personality

Personality assessment is discussed more fully in Chapter 31 and only salient points will be mentioned here. Enquiries should begin by asking patients to describe their personality. Subsequent questions are concerned with education, work, social relationships, leisure activities, prevailing mood, character, attitudes and standards, and habits. Whenever possible, an informant should be interviewed since few people can give a wholly objective account of their own personality. Sometimes, the interviewer's impressions of the patient formed during the interview are useful, but these impressions can be misleading, especially when the patient is very distressed or suffering from a psychiatric disorder. GPs are able to build up a picture of their patients' personalities over years of occasional medical contacts. This information is valuable and should be passed on if the patient is referred to a psychiatrist.

Corroborative history
What informants can contribute

In every case, informants can provide useful information about the patient's personality. Their information is essential when the patient is unable or unwilling to reveal important information, for example when the patient:

- is unaware of the nature and extent of their abnormality (e.g. a demented patient);
- knows the extent of the problem but is unwilling to reveal it (e.g. a patient with an alcohol problem);
- cannot say reliably when the disorder started.

The need for consent

With few exceptions, the patient's consent should be obtained before interviewing informants. The interviewer should explain that the interview is to obtain information that will help to decide how best to help the patient, and that information given to the interviewer by the patient will not be revealed to the informant unless the patient has agreed. The *exceptions to the need for consent* are when patients cannot provide an adequate history because they are: (1) confused, stuporose, extremely retarded, or mute (and therefore lack capacity); (2) extremely agitated or violent; or (3) depending on specific local mental health law, being assessed with a view to detention against their will (the Mental Health Act of England and Wales requires consultation with the 'nearest relative' in every case, even if the patient rejects this). A further exception is usually made for children.

Arranging the interview

It is generally better to interview relatives or other informants after the interview with the patient. It is usually better to see them away from the patient so that they can speak freely: for example, a wife may be reluctant to talk in her husband's presence about his heavy drinking. The purpose of the interview should be explained because relatives sometimes expect that they are about to be blamed for the patient's problems, or asked to give help that they are not prepared to provide.

Confidentiality

Unless informants have agreed to disclosure, the interviewer should not tell the patient what they have said. This rule applies even when the relative has spoken of something that the interviewer needs to discuss with the patient, such as heavy drinking that has been denied. If the relative has refused permission for the information to be disclosed, the interviewer can only try to help the patient reveal the information himself. In view of this and because patients may ask to see their case notes, it is better to record the interview with the informant on a separate sheet. The law regarding access to notes is complex, and differs between countries, in some of which specific safeguards are in place to protect information given by relatives.

The informants' concerns

As well as asking for information about the patient, the interviewer should find out how the informants view the problem, how it affects them, and what help they are seeking.

Helping the informants

When the interview with informants reveals that they too have emotional problems, either as a result of the patient's illness or for other reasons, the interviewer should either offer help or assist them to obtain help from another professional.

Further reading

Harrison P, Cowen P, Burns T, Fazel M. Assessment. In: *Shorter Oxford Textbook of Psychiatry*, 7th ed. Oxford: Oxford University Press; 2017:35–70.

Harrison P, Cowen P, Burns T, Fazel M. Signs and symptoms of psychiatric disorders. In: *Shorter Oxford Textbook of Psychiatry*, 7th ed. Oxford: Oxford University Press; 2017:1–20.

5 Conducting the assessment: examining the patient

Psychological ('mental state') examination

Terminology

In general hospital and community settings, the term 'physical examination' is almost always applied to the procedures used by medical and other staff to examine the body, including the nervous system, of patients. In mental health settings, the terms 'psychological examination' or 'mental examination' might seem most appropriate for the procedures used to examine the mind. However, the lengthier term 'mental state examination' is usually used, often with capitals, for reasons of tradition. This term is often shortened to MSE.

You will find that effective communication of the results of the MSE requires familiarity with many new terms and with their precise meanings. It is important that you grapple with these issues early on in your training. Like specific diagnostic terms, the terms for

specific abnormalities of mental state become an effective shorthand, aiding communication between healthcare professionals.

Goals

The goal of the MSE is to elicit the patient's **current psychopathology**, that is, their abnormal subjective experiences, and an objective view of their mental state, including abnormal behaviour. It therefore includes both **symptoms** (what *the patient reports* about *current* psychological symptoms, such as mood, thoughts, beliefs, abnormal perceptions, cognitive function, etc.) and **signs** (what *you observe* about the patient's behaviour *during the interview*).

Inevitably, the MSE (i.e. now) merges at the edges with the history of the presenting problems (recently). Behavioural abnormalities which the patient reports as still present, but which cannot be observed at interview (e.g. disturbed sleep, overeating, cutting) are part of the history of the presenting illness. A symptom which has resolved, such as an abnormal belief held last week but not today, should usually form part of the history, but will not be reported in the MSE. In contrast, an abnormal belief held last week which is still held today will be reported in both the history of the presenting problems and the MSE.

How to conduct a mental state examination

The components of the MSE are listed in Box 5.1. In taking the history, the interviewer will have learnt about the patient's symptoms up to the time of the consultation. Often the clinical features on the day of the examination are no different from those described in the recent past, in which case the mental state will overlap with the recent history.

Several aspects of the MSE do not require specific questions, and can be assessed by conversation with the patient and careful observation. These include appearance and behaviour, speech, the 'objective' assessment of mood, and the assessment of the 'form' and 'stream' of thoughts. However, other aspects do require specific questioning, including mood—subjective, thoughts—content, perceptions, cognition, and insight.

Performing the MSE is a practical skill that can be learnt only by observing experienced interviewers and by practising alone and under supervision. This chapter can assist the reader with this training but cannot replace it. Do not be intimidated by the apparent complexity of the MSE. It is simply a structured conversation with a patient, with the aim of understanding their mental world in order to determine whether mental illness exists and, if it does, to characterize that illness. Students should learn how to conduct a *complete* MSE with every patient. With increasing experience, they will become able to focus on items judged from the history to be of particular relevance and importance.

Box 5.1 Mental state examination

Appearance and behaviour
- General appearance
- Facial expression
- Posture
- Movements
- Social behaviour

Speech
- Quantity
- Rate
- Spontaneity
- Volume

Mood
- Subjective
- Objective:
  - Predominant mood
  - Constancy
  - Congruity

Thoughts
- Stream
- Form
- Content:
  - Preoccupations
  - Morbid thoughts including suicidality
  - Delusions and overvalued ideas
  - Obsessional symptoms

Perceptions
- Illusions
- Hallucinations
- Distortions

Cognition
- Orientation
- Attention and concentration
- Memory
- Language functioning
- Visuospatial functioning

Insight

Form and content of psychiatric signs

Many psychiatric signs have two aspects: form and content. The distinction can be explained with the help of clinical examples:

- A patient says that, when alone and out of hearing distance of other people, he hears voices telling him that he is changing sex. The *form* of his experience is an auditory hallucination (a sensory perception in the absence of an external stimulus, see p. 45), and the *content* is the idea that he is changing sex.

- A patient hears voices saying that he is about to be killed by persecutors. The *form* of this symptom is again an auditory hallucination, but the *content* is different.

- A patient experiences repeated intrusive thoughts that he is changing sex but realize that these thoughts are untrue. The *content* of this symptom is the same as that of the first patient, but the *form* is different—it is an obsessional thought (see p. 43).

In making a diagnosis, the form of the sign is important: delusions and obsessional features have a different diagnostic significance. In helping patients, the content is important as a guide to how they may respond (e.g. whether or not they might consider attacking a supposed persecutor) and in understanding their experience of the illness.

Difficulties in the mental state examination

Apart from the obvious problem of examining patients who speak little or no English—which requires the help of a skilled interpreter, preferably familiar with both cultures—difficulties can arise with patients who are unresponsive, overactive, or confused.

- **Unresponsive patients.** When patients are mute or stuporous (conscious but not speaking or responding in any other way), it is possible only to make observations of behaviour. Nevertheless, these observations can be informative. Since stuporous patients can sometimes become suddenly violent, it is prudent to be accompanied when examining such a patient.

Before deciding that the patient is mute, it is important that the interviewer (1) establishes that he or she is speaking a language that the patient understands, (2) has allowed adequate time for reply (delay can be lengthy in severe depressive illness), (3) has tried a variety of topics, and (4) has found out whether the patient will communicate in writing.

As well as making the observations of behaviour described previously, the interviewer should note whether the patient's eyes are open or closed. If they are open, he or she should note whether they follow objects, move apparently without purpose, or are fixed. If the eyes are closed, the interviewer should note whether they are opened on request and, if not, whether attempts at opening them are resisted.

Physical examination, including neurological assessment, is essential in all such cases, which should be seen, whenever possible, by a specialist who will look for certain additional, uncommon signs found in catatonic schizophrenia (e.g. **waxy flexibility** of muscles, **negativism**). In all such cases it is essential to interview an informant to discover the onset and course of the condition.

- **Overactive patients.** When the patient is overactive (e.g. because of mania), questions have to be limited to a few that seem particularly important, and conclusions have to be based mainly on observations of behaviour and on spontaneous utterances. Sometimes the overactivity has been made worse by attempts at physical restraint. A quiet, confident approach by the interviewer may calm the patient enough to allow adequate examination.

- **Confused patients.** When patients give the history in a muddled way, and especially when they appear perplexed or frightened, cognitive function should be tested early in the interview. If there is evidence of impairment, a corroborative history is essential.

If consciousness is impaired, try to orientate the patient and reassure them, and then start the interview again in a simplified form.

Appearance and behaviour

Much can be learnt from general appearance, facial expression, posture, voluntary or involuntary movements, and social behaviour. Relevant features should be summarized in a few phrases that give a clear picture to someone who has not met the patient. For example, 'a tall, gaunt, stooping, and dishevelled man, who looks much older than his 40 years, and who displays some parkinsonian features'.

General appearance includes physique, hair, make-up, and clothing. Manic patients may dress incongruously in brightly coloured or oddly assorted clothes. Signs of *self-neglect* include a dirty, unkempt appearance and stained, crumpled clothing. Self-neglect suggests alcoholism, drug addiction, dementia, or schizophrenia. An appearance of *weight loss* is as important in psychiatry as it is in general medicine, suggesting *physical* disorder (e.g. cancer, hyperthyroidism), *psychological* disorder (e.g. anorexia nervosa, depressive disorder), or *social* problems such as financial difficulty or homelessness.

Facial expression Mood states are accompanied by characteristic facial expressions and postures (Box 5.2). For example, turning down of the corners of the mouth and vertical furrows in the brow suggest *depression*; whereas horizontal furrows on the brow, wide palpebral fissures, and dilated pupils suggest *anxiety*. An unchanging 'wooden' expression may result from a *parkinsonian syndrome*, either primary or caused by antipsychotic drugs.

Posture may also give indications of prevailing mood. A depressed patient characteristically sits with shoulders hunched, and with the head and eyes 'downcast'. An anxious patient typically sits upright, with the head erect and the hands gripping the chair.

Movement Manic patients are overactive, restless, and move rapidly from place to place and task to task.

Box 5.2 Association between mood and appearance

- **Depression.** The corners of the mouth are turned down and the centre of the brow has vertical furrows. The head is inclined forward with the gaze directed downwards, and shoulders are bent. The patient's gestures are reduced.
- **Elation.** A lively, cheerful expression. Posture and expressive movements are normal or exaggerated.
- **Anxiety.** The brow is furrowed horizontally, the posture is tense, and the person is restless and sometimes tremulous. Often there are accompanying signs of autonomic overactivity, such as pale skin and increased sweating of the hands, feet, and axillae.
- **Anger.** The eyebrows are drawn down, with widening of the palpebral fissure, and a squaring of the corners of the mouth that may reveal the teeth. The shoulders are square and the body tense as if ready for action.

Depressed patients are inactive and move slowly. Rarely, a depressed patient becomes completely immobile and mute, a condition known as *stupor*. Anxious or agitated patients are restless, and sometimes tremulous. Any involuntary movements should be noted, including tics, choreiform movements, dystonia, or tardive dyskinesia.

Social behaviour Manic patients are disinhibited, and may break social conventions, for example, by being unduly familiar. Some demented and some schizophrenic patients are disinhibited, while others are withdrawn and preoccupied. In describing these behaviours, a clear and accurate description of what is done or not done is more scientific than subjective terms such as 'disinhibited' or 'bizarre'.

Signs of impending violence include restlessness, sweating, clenched fists or pointed fingers, intrusion into the interviewer's 'personal space', and a raised voice.

Motor symptoms and signs such as mannerisms, stereotypies, and catatonic symptoms are briefly described in the chapter on schizophrenia (see p. 289) and more extensively in the *Shorter Oxford Textbook of Psychiatry*. Here we define three movement disorders:

- **Tics** are irregular repeated movements involving a group of muscles (e.g. a sideways movement of the head).
- **Choreiform movements** are brief involuntary movements that are coordinated but purposeless, such as grimacing or movements of the arms.
- **Dystonia** is a muscle spasm, which is often painful and may lead to contortions.

Speech

The physical characteristics of a patient's speech come under this heading; the 'form' and 'content' of the thoughts they express through the medium of speech are recorded later under 'Thoughts'. Here, we describe changes to speech that are often seen in patients with depression or mania:

- **Quantity.** Depressed patients speak less than usual; manic patients speak more. Occasionally a patient does not speak at all (**mutism**).
- **Rate.** Depressed patients speak more slowly than usual. Manic patients speak faster. Copious rapid speech which is hard to interrupt is called **pressure of speech**.
- **Spontaneity.** Patients with depression or intoxicated patients may have a **long answer latency**; they are asked a question, but it can be many seconds, or longer, before an answer is forthcoming. Patients with mania will answer promptly, and often very quickly, if they are able to attend for long enough to the interview.
- **Volume.** Depressed patients may speak quietly; manic patients may often be heard far down the corridor.

Abnormalities of the *continuity* of speech, including any sudden interruptions, rapid shifts of topic, and lack of logical thread, should be recorded under 'thoughts—form'.

Mood

Changes in mood are the most common symptoms of psychiatric disorder. They are the principal symptoms of depressive and anxiety disorders, but they may occur in every kind of psychiatric disorder, during physical illness, and in healthy people encountering stressful events. Terminology can be confusing. The term *affect* is used by some professionals instead of *mood*, and the term *affective disorder* is an alternative name for *mood disorder*. We recommend using the terms **mood** and **mood disorder**, as mood is a word which is in common use in the general population, and is therefore widely understood.

The patient's 'subjective' mood and the professional's 'objective' assessment of mood should be documented. Mismatch between the two can be useful in the assessment of diagnosis and risk.

Subjective mood

Ask the patient 'What is your mood just now?', or 'Can you tell me how you're feeling … in your spirits?' or '… in yourself?' Record the patient's responses without altering them, so record (for example) 'Great, never felt better', or 'OK, not too bad', or 'Awful, terrible, desperate'. Often, patients will need some encouragement to report their feelings. Be sensitive to this need.

Further questions can then be asked about the patient's recent mood, and about symptoms associated with particular mood states. These are aspects of history, and should be recorded there rather than within the MSE. However, it may help rapport within the interview to link questions about emotions here and now, within the interview, with questions about emotional experiences in recent days and weeks. If a **depressed** mood is reported, the associated symptoms may include a feeling of being ready to cry, lack of interest and enjoyment, and pessimistic thoughts, including thoughts of suicide. When **anxiety** is reported, associated symptoms include palpitations, dry mouth, tremor, sweating, and worrying thoughts. When **elevated mood** is reported, associated symptoms include excessive self-confidence, grandiose plans, and an inflated assessment of the person's own ability. These manic symptoms have, of course, to be elicited indirectly, for example, by asking the patient about his plans and his assessment of his abilities.

Objective mood

The nature, constancy, and congruity of a patient's observed mood should be described:

1 **Nature of mood or moods.** What mood or moods appear to predominate within the interview? These might include *depression, elation, anger, anxiety, suspicion*, or *perplexity*. It is possible to record more than one; a patient might appear depressed and perplexed, for example. Of course, the patient may exhibit no particular emotions, and not appear, in particular, either depressed or elated. In this circumstance, many psychiatrists use the term '**euthymic**', but, as this term is unusual outside psychiatry, we prefer the term '*unremarkable mood*'. As described earlier, mood states are accompanied by characteristic facial expressions and postures, which can help to identify the mood of a patient who is denying emotion (e.g. denying that he is angry).

2 **Constancy of mood.** In healthy people, mood varies from day to day and hour to hour—it is normal for mood to fluctuate in reaction to internal circumstances (e.g. what the person is thinking about) and external circumstances (e.g. reminders of a failed relationship, or of recent exam success). However, this normal emotional reactivity is limited in extent and limited in time. This normal spectrum of change may be increased (**emotional liability**) such as in dementia, mania, or after a stroke, and, when it is extreme, may be called **emotional incontinence**. Alternatively, it may be decreased (**reduced reactivity, blunting**, or **flattening**), such as in depression, when smiles or laughter do not follow a shift to a positive or amusing topic. **Irritability** is a term which spans two components of the objective assessment of mood—predominant moods (in irritability, this might include tension and anger) and variation in mood (in irritability, this would be labile, with anger triggered easily).

3 **Congruity of mood.** Normally, our *mood*, our *thoughts*, and our *perceptions* are closely associated, and 'fit' together logically. For example, if we are watching news scenes from a natural disaster, we are *seeing* scenes of destruction and suffering, we are *thinking* about how difficult this must be for the people involved, and we are likely to be *feeling* subdued, contemplative, and maybe depressed. Equally, an elated person will be thinking happy thoughts and perceiving all the good, positive things in the world around them. In these cases, there is '**congruity of mood**', which is normal. Very occasionally, such as in schizophrenia, this linkage is lost, and there is '**incongruity of mood**', so that, for example, a person appears cheerful while describing sad events. This is different to the apparent cheerfulness that hides embarrassment (which is commonly experienced, and normal), and also different to the lack of outward show of emotion in people who feel it inwardly—a condition that occurs in some depressed patients.

Thoughts

Accessing thoughts

If we want to know what someone is thinking, we can work it out in several ways. The first and most obvious is to listen to what they are saying, either spontaneously or in response to our or someone else's questions. The next is to read what they are writing, whether that is on paper, on a computer, or in a text message. Finally, we can observe their appearance and behaviour, and use clues from that to guide our

A patient's thoughts

John is a 21-year-old university physics student, who has been locking himself in his room, refusing to come out, except from time to time when he went around the house systematically switching off electrical items such as mobile phones, televisions, and computers. He refused to tell his housemates or his parents why he was doing this. His parents were called to his shared house by his housemates, and called his GP, Dr Jones, who has now attended for an assessment. On careful and supportive questioning by the GP, John explained his concern that he would be harmed by secret services from another country, which he would not name. He was wanted by them because of his new invention, which had arisen out of his final year project, and which would revolutionize warfare in the years to come. Switching off all electrical devices was his way of preventing secret services locating him through electronic means. Dr Jones expressed some surprise that John's degree project had generated such an important finding, but John remained adamant that this was the case. Dr Jones asked if he might speak to John's research supervisor, to corroborate his account, and, after insisting on some safeguards, John reluctantly agreed.

understanding of what might be in their mind (see Case study box 5.1).

Abnormalities of thought

Disorders of thinking can be of several kinds:

1 Abnormality of the **stream** of thought (its amount and speed).

2 Abnormality of the **form** of thought (the ways in which thoughts are linked together).

3 Abnormality of the **content** of thought (preoccupations, morbid thoughts, delusions, overvalued ideas, obsessional and compulsive symptoms).

Abnormalities of the stream of thought

In disorders of the stream of thought, both the amount and the speed of thoughts are changed. There are three main abnormalities: *pressure, poverty* and *blocking* of thought.

1 **Pressure of thought.** Thoughts are unusually rapid, abundant, and varied. The disorder is characteristic of mania but also occurs in schizophrenia.

2 **Poverty of thought.** Thoughts are unusually slow, few, and unvaried. The disorder is characteristic

of severe depressive disorder but also occurs in schizophrenia.

3 **Blocking of thought** refers to an experience in which the mind is suddenly empty of thoughts. The symptom of thought blocking should not be confused with the normal experiences of sudden distraction, the intrusion of a different line of thinking, or the experience of losing a particular word or train of thought while other thoughts continue. Thought blocking is the experience of an abrupt and complete emptying of the mind. It occurs especially in schizophrenic patients, who may interpret the experience in a delusional way (see 'Delusional themes')—believing, for example, that their thoughts have been removed by another person (delusion of thought withdrawal).

Abnormalities of the form of thought

There are three main abnormalities of the ways in which thoughts are linked together: *flight of ideas, loosening of associations*, and *perseveration*.

1 **Flight of ideas.** In this abnormal state, characteristic of mania, thoughts and any accompanying spoken words move quickly from one topic to another, so that one train of thought is not completed before the next begins. Because topics change so rapidly, the links between one

topic and the next may be difficult to follow. Nevertheless, recognizable and understandable links are present, though not always in the form of logical connections. Instead the link may be through (1) *rhyme*, for example when an idea about chairs is followed by an idea about pears (rhyming links are sometimes called *clang associations*); (2) *puns*, that is two words that have the same sound (e.g. male/mail); and (3) *distraction*, for example, a new topic suggested by something in the interview room.

2 **Loosening of associations** is a lack of logical connection between a sequence of thoughts, not explicable by the links described under flight of ideas. This lack of logical association is sometimes called *knight's move thinking* (referring to the sudden change of direction of the knight in chess). Usually, the interviewer is alerted to the presence of loosening of associations because the patient's replies are hard to follow. This difficulty in understanding differs from that experienced when interviewing people who are very anxious or are of low intelligence. Anxious people become more coherent when put at ease, and people of low intelligence do so when questions are simplified. When there is loosening of associations, the links between ideas cannot be made more understandable in either of these ways. Instead, the interviewer has the experience that the more he tries to clarify the patient's thinking, the less he understands it. Loosening of associations occurs most often in schizophrenia. It is often difficult to distinguish loosening of associations from flight of ideas, and when this happens it is often helpful to tape-record a sample of speech and listen to it carefully.

3 **Perseveration** is the persistent and inappropriate repetition of the same sequence of thought, as shown either in speech or actions. It can be demonstrated by asking a series of simple questions: the patient repeats his answer to the first question as his response to all subsequent questions even though these require different answers. Perseveration occurs most often in dementia but may occur in other disorders.

Preoccupations

Preoccupations are thoughts that recur frequently but can be put out of mind by an effort of will. They are a part of normal experience—students, for example, who are concerned about an imminent exam are likely to be preoccupied with thoughts and concerns about their preparation, likely exam questions, and the consequences of a poor performance. They are clinically significant only if they contribute to distress or disability. They are commonly seen in psychiatric disorders, including (1) *depressive disorders*, where preoccupations about suicide should be explored carefully (see p. 261); (2) *anxiety disorders*, where preoccupations may prolong the disorder (see p. 329); and (3) *sexual disorders* where preoccupations may influence behaviour (see p. 457). Some preoccupations are noticed during history taking; others may be revealed by asking 'What sort of things do you worry about?', or 'What sort of thoughts occupy your mind?'

Morbid thoughts

These are thoughts particularly associated with specific illnesses, through either their nature, for example, *suicidality*, or their severity, for example *self-criticism*—it is normal, and can be helpful, to be self-critical, but in a depressive illness such self-criticism can be severe and pervasive, and help to maintain the disorder. Other morbid thoughts in depression include:

- *hopelessness* (negativity about the future);
- *helplessness* (negativity about the prospects for being helped by healthcare professionals, medicines, or psychological treatment);
- *low self-esteem* (negativity about the self);
- *guilt* (negativity about actions in the past, such as in relationships).

The depressed patient is likely to consider their negative thoughts to be entirely reasonable, because they are interpreting evidence relating to themselves, the people around them, and the world around them, through 'grey-coloured spectacles', which emphasize the negative and minimize the positive. In contrast, the thoughts of a person with elated mood are distorted positively, through 'rose-coloured spectacles', which give them an overly positive view of themselves, the world, and the future.

Enquiring about **thoughts and plans of suicide** is an essential component of the MSE, and should always be asked about and recorded. Suicidal thoughts are a personal and sensitive matter, and it is important to practise asking about them in a supportive but rigorous way. Some interviewers are reluctant to ask about suicide, in case the questions should suggest the idea, but there is no evidence to support this. Approach the topic in stages:

1 Ask about feelings of depression, and then hopelessness ('Have you felt that you have lost hope for the future?'), before

2 Moving onto 'passive' suicidal ideas ('Have you thought life is not worth living?', 'Have you wished you might not wake up one morning?'), and finally

3 Asking about 'active' suicidal ideas ('Have you thought of taking steps to end your life?', 'Have you thought how you might do this?', 'What thoughts did you have?', and 'How close have you got to doing something about it?').

Delusions

A delusion is *a belief that is held firmly but on inadequate grounds; is not affected by rational argument or evidence to the contrary; and is not a conventional belief that the person might be expected to hold given his cultural background and level of education.* This rather lengthy definition is required to distinguish delusions, which are indicators of mental disorder, from other kinds of strongly held belief found among healthy people, such as religious or political views. A delusion is nearly always a false belief but not always so (see later in this section). There are several problems surrounding the definition

Box 5.3 Some problems surrounding the definition of delusions

Delusions are arrived at through abnormal thought processes. This is the fundamental point that characterizes delusions but it cannot be observed directly. The various clauses in the definition of a delusion are intended to provide indirect criteria to establish the point but there are some problems with each of them.

Delusions are held firmly despite evidence to the contrary. This is the key to the definition and it is often revealed through the person's words and actions. For example, a person with the delusion that persecutors are in the next room will not alter his belief when shown that the room is empty; instead, he may say that the persecutors left before he arrived. However, not all beliefs that are impervious to contrary evidence are delusions: some non-delusional beliefs are of this kind. For example, a convinced spiritualist hangs on to his belief in spiritualism when presented with contrary evidence that would convince a non-believer. These strongly held non-delusional beliefs are called *overvalued ideas*. When deluded patients recover, either with treatment or spontaneously, they pass through a stage of increasing doubt in the truth of their delusions. This stage of partial conviction in a belief

that was previously a full delusion is called a *partial delusion*.

Delusions are false beliefs. Some definitions of delusion include this point. It is not included in our definition because, very occasionally a delusional belief is either true from the onset, or subsequently becomes true. For example, a man may develop the delusional belief that his wife is unfaithful despite a complete lack of evidence of infidelity or of any other rational reason for holding the belief. The belief has been arrived at in an abnormal way and is delusional even if, unbeknown to him, the wife is unfaithful. The point is of mainly theoretical importance but it is sometimes brought up in discussions of delusion since it highlights the fact that the essential criterion for delusion is that it was arrived at in an abnormal way.

Delusions are usually odd and improbable beliefs. However not all odd and improbable beliefs are delusional. Some people express seemingly improbable beliefs (e.g. that they are being poisoned by close relatives), which are subsequently proved to be true. Apparently odd beliefs should be investigated most carefully before they are accepted as delusional.

of delusions and these are considered briefly in Box 5.3.

Conviction in the truth of a delusion does not necessarily influence all the person's feelings and actions, especially when the delusion has been present for a long time, as in chronic schizophrenia. For example, such a patient may have the delusion that he is a member of the Royal Family and yet live contentedly in a hostel for discharged psychiatric patients.

We distinguish between primary and secondary delusions. A **primary delusion** is one that *occurs suddenly without any other abnormal mental event leading to it*. For example, a patient may suddenly develop the unshakable conviction that he is changing sex, without ever having thought of this before and without any reason to do so at the time. Primary delusions are rare, and when they occur they strongly suggest schizophrenia. However, this is not very useful in practice because few patients can give a reliable account of how they first had a delusional idea. A **secondary delusion** *arises from some previous abnormal idea or experience*, which may be (1) a *hallucination*: for example, a person hears a voice and believes he is being followed; (2) a *mood*: for example, a person with deep depression feels worthless and believes that other people think the same about him; or (3) *another delusion*. Secondary delusions occur in a variety of severe psychiatric disorders. When one delusion gives rise to another in a sequence, the resulting network of interrelated ideas is known as a **delusional system**, in which many abnormal beliefs fit together into a coherent whole. This is common in paranoid schizophrenia.

Other mental phenomena related to delusions

There are three mental phenomena which are closely related to delusions, but are not delusional in nature, despite their names incorporating the term 'delusional'. These are:

- **Delusional mood.** This is an inexplicable feeling of apprehension that is followed before long by a delusion that explains it. For example, a person is feeling inexplicably frightened, and then suddenly gains the belief that someone is following him with the intent to harm him.

- **Delusional perception.** This is the misinterpretation of the significance of something perceived normally. For example, a patient may suddenly be convinced that the particular arrangement of objects on his desk indicates that his life is threatened.

- **Delusional memory.** This is the retrospective delusional misinterpretation of memories of actual events. For example, the conviction that on a previous occasion when the patient felt ill his food had been poisoned by persecutors, though previously and at the time of the illness he did not believe this.

Shared delusions

Usually, other people recognize delusional beliefs as false and they argue with the deluded persons in an attempt to correct them. Occasionally, a person who lives with or is otherwise in a close relationship with a deluded patient comes to share the delusional beliefs. This person is then said to have shared delusions or *folie à deux*. The affected person's conviction may be unshakable while they remain with the patient, but usually weakens quickly on separation.

Box 5.4 Delusional themes

- Persecutory (paranoid)
- Reference
- Grandiose and expansive
- Guilt and worthlessness
- Nihilistic
- Hypochondriacal or dysmorphophobic
- Jealousy
- Sexual or amorous
- Religious
- Control
- The possession of thoughts

Delusional themes

Delusions are usually grouped according to their main themes (Box 5.4). There is some correspondence between delusional theme and type of disorder.

1 **Persecutory delusions** are often (but incorrectly) called **paranoid delusions**. Used strictly, 'paranoid' refers not only to persecutory but also to grandiose, jealous, amorous, and hypochondriacal delusions. However, this strict usage is seldom adopted. Persecutory delusions are ideas that people or organizations are trying to inflict harm on the patient, damage his reputation, or make him insane. It is important to remember that it is normal in some cultures to ascribe misfortunes to the malign activities of other people, for example, through witchcraft. Such ideas are not delusions. Persecutory delusions are common in *schizophrenia*, and occur also in *organic states* and *severe depressive disorders*. When the delusions are part of a depressive disorder, the patient characteristically accepts that the supposed actions of his persecutors are justified by his own wickedness; in schizophrenia, however, he characteristically resents them.

2 **Delusions of reference** are concerned with the idea that objects, events, or the actions of other people have a special significance for the patient. For example, a remark heard on television is believed to be directed specifically to the patient; or a gesture by a stranger is believed to convey something about the patient. Delusions of this kind are associated with *schizophrenia*.

3 **Grandiose and expansive delusions** are beliefs of exaggerated self-importance. Patients may think themselves wealthy, endowed with unusual abilities, or in other ways special. Such ideas occur mainly in *mania* and sometimes in *schizophrenia*.

4 **Delusions of guilt and worthlessness** are beliefs that the person has done something shameful or sinful. Usually the belief concerns an innocent error that caused no guilt at the time, for example, a small error in an income tax return, which the patient now fears will be discovered and lead to

prosecution. This kind of delusion occurs most often in *severe depressive disorders*.

5 **Nihilistic delusions** include beliefs that the patient's career is finished, that he is about to die or has no money, or that the world is doomed. Nihilistic delusions occur most often in *severe depressive disorders*.

6 **Hypochondriacal delusions** are false beliefs about the presence of disease. The patient believes, in the face of convincing medical evidence to the contrary, that he has a disease. Such delusions are more common among the elderly, reflecting the increasing concerns about ill health in later life. Related **dysmorphophobic delusions** are concerned with the appearance of parts of the body, for example, the belief that the person's (normally shaped) nose is seriously misshapen. Hypochondriacal delusions occur in *depressive disorders* and *schizophrenia*.

7 **Delusions of jealousy** are more common among men. 'Morbid (pathological) jealousy' may lead to dangerously aggressive behaviour towards the person who is believed to be unfaithful.

8 **Sexual or amorous delusions** are more frequent among women. Usually, the woman believes that she is loved by a man who has never spoken to her and who is inaccessible—for example, an eminent public figure.

9 **Religious delusions** may be concerned with guilt (e.g. divine punishment for minor sins) or with special powers. Before deciding that such beliefs are delusional, it is important to determine whether they held by other members of the patient's religious or cultural group.

10 **Delusions of control** are beliefs that personal actions ('made acts'), impulses, or thoughts are controlled by an outside agency. This experience has to be distinguished from (a) voluntary obedience to commands given by hallucinatory voices, and (b) culturally normal beliefs that human actions are under divine control. Delusions of control strongly suggest *schizophrenia*.

11 **Delusions concerning the possession of thoughts.** Healthy people have no doubt that their thoughts are their own and that other people can know them only if they are spoken aloud or revealed through actions. Delusions of thought possession are found most often in schizophrenia, and include:

- **delusion of thought insertion**—some of the person's thoughts have been implanted by an outside agency;
- **delusion of thought withdrawal**—some of their thoughts have been taken away;
- **delusion of thought broadcasting**—some of their thoughts are known to other people through telepathy, radio, or some other unusual way.

Asking about delusions

Often the first indication of the presence of delusions is during history taking, either from the patient or from an informant. When there is no such indication, judgement should be used about whether to enquire about delusions, because the questions may antagonize patients who have come for help for another problem. Questions should be asked whenever there is evidence of a *severe depressive disorder*, when *schizophrenia* enters the differential diagnosis, or in cases of doubt. It is often difficult to elicit delusions during the MSE because the patient does not regard them as abnormal. A good way of starting the enquiry is to ask for an explanation of any unusual statements, unpleasant experiences, or unusual events that the patient has mentioned. For example, a patient may say that his headaches started when his neighbours caused him trouble; when asked why the neighbours should do this, he may say they are conspiring to harm him. Patients often hide delusions, and the interviewer needs to be alert to evasions, vague replies, or other hints that information is being withheld.

Having discovered an unusual belief, the interviewer has to decide three things:

1 *Is the belief true?* Some beliefs are clearly false; for example, that persecutors are damaging the patient's brain by beaming radio waves on him. Other beliefs need to be checked—for example, that neighbours are collaborating in harassing the patient.

2 *How strongly are the beliefs held?* Considerable tact is required when finding out. The patient should feel that he is having a fair hearing, and that the interviewer's response is enquiring, rather than argumentative or dismissive. The interviewer should question the reasons for the beliefs gently but persistently.

3 *Are the beliefs culturally determined?* Are the beliefs accepted by others sharing the patient's cultural background or religious beliefs? In some cultures, beliefs in evil forces or witchcraft are widespread. Doubt can usually be resolved by finding another person from the same religion or culture, and asking whether the patient's ideas are held by them or others.

Delusions of *thought broadcasting, thought insertion, thought withdrawal*, or *control* can usually be elicited only by asking direct questions. Since their presence strongly suggests schizophrenia, it is essential to check any positive answer by asking for examples. Appropriate questions include: 'Do you ever think that other people can tell what you are thinking, even though you have not told them?', 'Do you ever think that thoughts have been put into your mind?', 'Why is that?', and 'How does that happen?'

Overvalued ideas

An overvalued idea is:

- an isolated, preoccupying, and strongly held belief;
- that dominates a person's life and may affect his or her actions;
- but which (unlike a delusion) has been derived through normal mental processes.

For example, someone whose parents developed cancer within a short time of one another may be convinced that cancer is contagious, despite having been presented many times with evidence to the contrary. It is sometimes difficult to distinguish between overvalued ideas and delusions since the two may be equally strongly held, and the differentiation depends on a judgement of the way in which the idea developed. In practice, this difficulty seldom causes problems since diagnosis does not depend on a single symptom.

Obsessional and compulsive symptoms

Obsessions:

- are recurrent and persistent thoughts, impulses, or images;
- that enter the mind despite efforts to exclude them;
- that the person recognizes are senseless or stupid; and
- that the person recognizes as a product of their own mind.

The obsessions usually concern matters that the person finds distressing or unpleasant, and often feels ashamed to tell others about them. The person has no doubt that the intruding thoughts are their own, in contrast to a person with the delusion of thought insertion, who believes that the ideas have been implanted from outside. A sense of struggling to resist the intrusions

is part of an obsessional symptom. Resistance distinguishes obsessions (in which it is present) from delusions (in which it is absent). However, when obsessions have been present for a long time, resistance may decrease so that this distinction becomes difficult to make. In practice, this decrease seldom leads to diagnostic problems because it takes place late in the course of the disorder, when the diagnosis has already been made.

Obsessional thoughts are repeated, intrusive words or phrases, which take many forms including obscenities, blasphemies, and thoughts about distressing occurrences (e.g. that the patient's hands are contaminated with bacteria that will spread disease). There are several common themes (see Box 5.5). **Obsessional ruminations** are repeated sequences of such thoughts (e.g. about the ending of the world). **Obsessional doubts** are recurrent uncertainties about a previous action (e.g. whether or not the person has switched off an electrical appliance that could cause a fire). **Obsessional impulses** are urges to carry out actions that are usually aggressive, dangerous, or socially embarrassing (e.g. using a knife to stab someone, jumping in front of a moving train, or shouting obscenities in church). Whatever the urge, the person recognizes that it is irrational and does not wish to carry it out ('*ego-dystonic*'). This

---

Box 5.5 Themes of obsessional phenomena

Obsessional thoughts

- **Dirt and contamination,** e.g. the idea that the hands are contaminated with bacteria
- **Aggressive actions,** e.g. the idea that the person may harm another person, or shout angry remarks
- **Orderliness,** e.g. the idea that objects should be arranged in a special way, or clothes put on in a particular order
- **Disease,** e.g. the idea that the person may have cancer
- **Sex,** usually thoughts or images of practices that the person finds disgusting

- **Religion,** e.g. blasphemous thoughts, doubts about the fundamentals of belief, doubts about the adequacy of confession

Compulsions

- **Checking rituals,** which are often concerned with safety (e.g. checking repeatedly that a gas tap has been turned off)
- **Cleaning rituals** such as repeated handwashing or domestic cleaning
- **Counting rituals** such as counting to a particular number or counting in threes
- **Dressing rituals** in which the clothes are always set out or put on in a particular way

is an important point of distinction from delusions, which are regarded as rational by the patient ('*ego-syntonic*') and which may lead to action, such as aggression against a supposed persecutor. **Obsessional images** are recurrent, vivid mental pictures that are unexpected, unselected, usually unwelcome, and usually distressing (e.g. an image of oneself sick and dying in a hospital, or covered in human excrement from an overflowing sewer in the street, or standing mute and helpless while supposed to be giving an important talk to colleagues).

Obsessional symptoms are essential features of obsessive–compulsive disorder. They occur also in other psychiatric disorders, especially anxiety and depressive disorders. They should be distinguished from the following phenomena, which are not regarded by patients as unreasonable, and are not resisted:

- ordinary preoccupations of healthy people;
- intrusive concerns/preoccupations of anxious or depressed patients;
- recurring thoughts and images associated with sexual preference disorders/drug dependence;
- delusions.

Although compulsions are actions not thoughts, it is appropriate to describe them here because most compulsions are associated with and motivated by obsessions. Compulsions are:

- recurrent and persistent actions;
- that the person feels compelled to carry out but resists;
- that the person recognizes are senseless or stupid; and
- that the person recognizes as a product of their own mind.

Compulsions are also known as **compulsive or obsessional rituals**. Sometimes the association between the action and the thought seems understandable, for example, when handwashing is associated with the idea that the hands are contaminated. In other cases, there is no meaningful connection between the actions and the thoughts, for example, when checking the position of objects is associated with aggressive ideas. Most compulsions are followed by an immediate lessening of the distress associated with the corresponding obsessional thoughts. However, the long-term consequence is that the thoughts persist for longer. Compulsions are sometimes accompanied by obsessional thoughts concerned with doubt that the compulsive behaviours have been executed correctly, and this can lead to further repetitions, which may last for hours.

Asking about obsessional phenomena

Ask 'Do any thoughts (images, impulses to act) keep coming repeatedly into your mind, even when you try hard to get rid of them?' Patients who reply yes should be asked for examples. Patients are often ashamed of their obsessional thoughts (e.g. those with aggressive or sexual themes), so questioning needs to be sympathetic and patient. The interviewer should make certain that patients regard the thoughts as their own, rather than as being implanted from outside. Although not strictly disorders of thinking, compulsive rituals are driven by thoughts, and are therefore usually recorded with obsessional phenomena. The following questions are useful: 'Do you ever have to repeat actions over and over, which most people would do only once?' or 'Do you have to go on repeating the same action when you know this is unnecessary?'

Perceptions

There are two important terms, perception and imagery, which need to be explained.

Perception is the process of becoming aware of what is presented to the body through the sense organs (the eyes, the ears, the nose, the tongue, and the skin). You may, for example, go for a walk by a river, and *see* rowing boats, *hear* the chatter of the rowers, *smell* the fresh air, and *feel* the cool breeze on your face. These perceptions are experienced as real, and are real.

Imagery is an experience originating within the mind that usually lacks the sense of reality that is part of perception. After your walk, you may close your eyes and relive it in your 'mind's eye' or imagin-ation; it is *as if* you were walking, but the experience is clearly an internal one rather than being 'real'. Imagery differs from perception in that it can be initi-ated and terminated at will. Almost always, imagery is obliterated when something is perceived in the same modality. A few people experience **eidetic imagery**, which is imagery as vivid and detailed as perception.

Abnormalities of perception are of four kinds: (1) *changes in intensity*, (2) *changes in quality*, (3) *il-lusions*, and (4) *hallucinations*. Each kind of abnor-mality will be described, but particular attention is paid to hallucinations as they are of most significance in diagnosis. Sometimes, perception is *normal* in na-ture, but has a changed *meaning* for the person who experiences it. This phenomenon is called **delusional perception**. Despite this name, it is not a disorder of perception; rather, it is a disorder of thinking and is described with other disorders of thinking.

Changes in the intensity of perception

In mania, perception seems more intense, and, for ex-ample, colours may be particularly bright and vivid, and the sound of a pin dropping can seem loud. In depressive disorder, perception may be less intense, with colours downgraded so that the world seems drab and grey.

Changes in the quality of perception

In some disorders, especially schizophrenia, percep-tions may seem distorted or unpleasant; for example, food tastes unpleasant or flowers smell acrid.

Illusions

An illusion is a *misperception of a real external stimulus*. Illusions are likely if one or more of the following circumstances is present:

1 **Sensory impairment,** such as at dawn or dusk, or if the person is visually or hearing impaired.

2 **Inattention** on the sensory modality, such as when a person whose attention is focused on a book may mistakenly identify a sound as a voice.

3 **Impaired consciousness,** such as delirium.

4 **Emotional arousal,** usually fear.

Healthy people sometimes experience illusions, particularly when more than one of the above-listed circumstances occur together. For example, a young person may be returning home late at night along an unlit rural road (visual impairment), on a windy night (hearing impairment), and become increasingly anx-ious about their personal safety (emotional arousal), such as they perceive a bush on the side of the road as a potentially threatening person.

Illusions may come to notice when the history is taken, or when the patient is being observed, for ex-ample, in a medical ward. Visual illusions can be elicited with a question such as 'Have you seen any-thing unusual?' (or frightening if the patient seems afraid). If the answer is yes, the interviewer should at-tempt to find out whether the experience is based on an actual visual stimulus (e.g. mistaking a shadow for a threatening person).

Hallucinations

A hallucination is a *perception experienced in the ab-sence of an external stimulus to the corresponding sense organ*; for example, hearing a voice when no one is speaking within hearing distance, or seeing bright flashing lights when there is no light source. A hallucination has two qualities which distinguish it from imagery: (1) it is experienced as a true percep-tion, and (2) it seems to come from outside the head. Unless the experience has these two qualities it is not a hallucination. Experiences that possess one of these qualities, but not the other, are sometimes called **pseudohallucinations**.

Although hallucinations are generally regarded as the hallmark of mental disorder, healthy people experience them occasionally, especially when falling asleep (**hypnagogic hallucinations**) or when waking (**hypnopompic hallucinations**). These two kinds of hallucinations are brief and usually of a simple kind, such as a bell ringing or a name being called. Usually the person wakes suddenly and immediately recognizes the nature of the experience. These two kinds of hallucination do not point to mental disorder.

Modalities of hallucination

Auditory and visual hallucinations are the most frequent, but hallucinations can occur in all sensory modalities:

- **Auditory hallucinations** may be experienced as voices, noises, or music. Hallucinatory voices may seem to speak words, phrases, or sentences. Some address the patient as 'you' (*second-person hallucinations*). Others talk about the patient as 'he' or 'she' (*third-person hallucinations*), and these are characteristic of schizophrenia (see p. 289). Sometimes, a voice seems to say what the patient is about to say; and sometimes it seems to repeat what he has just been thinking (*thought echo*).

- **Visual hallucinations** may be *simple*, such as flashes of light, or *complex*, such as the figure of a person. Usually they are experienced as normal in size, but sometimes may seem unusually small or large. Visual hallucinations are associated particularly with organic mental disorders or drug misuse but can occur in other conditions.

- **Hallucinations of smell and taste** are uncommon. The taste or smell may seem to be recognizable, but more often it is unlike any smell or flavour that has been experienced before, and has an unpleasant quality.

- **Tactile hallucinations** are also uncommon. They may be experienced as superficial sensations of being touched, pricked, or strangled. Sometimes, they may be experienced as sensations just below the skin, which may be attributed to insects or other small creatures burrowing through the tissues—in this way, a tactile hallucination may be associated with a delusional interpretation (*dermatozoic delusion, formication, 'cocaine bug'*).

- **Hallucinations of deep sensation** are also uncommon. They may be experienced as feelings of the viscera being pulled or distended, or as sexual stimulation. Again, they may well be associated with delusional interpretation.

Diagnostic associations of hallucinations

Hallucinations occur in organic disorders, severe affective disorders, and schizophrenia. Visual hallucinations occur particularly in organic psychiatric disorders and drug use, but also in severe mood disorders and schizophrenia. Although not specific to organic disorder, they should always prompt a thorough search for other symptoms of an organic disorder. Hallucinations of taste, smell, and deep sensation occur mainly in schizophrenia. Other associations between particular kinds of hallucination and individual disorders are described in the chapters on clinical syndromes.

Asking about hallucinations

Enquiries about hallucinations should be made tactfully, lest patients take offence. With experience, the interviewer will be able to judge when it is safe to omit these enquiries. If enquiry is indicated, questions can be introduced by saying: 'When their nerves are upset, some people have unusual experiences'. Questions can then be asked about hearing voices or sounds when there is nobody within earshot, or about seeing unusual things. If patients say yes to either of these questions, they should be asked whether the voice, sound, or vision appeared to be inside or outside the head. When the history makes it relevant, similar questions should be asked about other kinds of hallucinations. If the patients describe **auditory hallucinations**, further questions should be asked, to determine whether they are of a kind which is characteristic of schizophrenia (see p. 289).

They should be asked whether they hear sounds or voices; if the latter, whether one voice or more, and whether the voices talk to them (second person) or to each other (third person). Hallucinations of voices discussing patients (**third-person hallucinations**) should be distinguished from the delusion that people at a distance are discussing them (**delusion of reference**). If the hallucinatory voices talk to the patient (**second-person hallucinations**), the interviewer should find out whether they give commands, and if so, what kind of commands, and whether the patient feels impelled to obey them. Such '**command hallucinations**' can indicate a high risk of harm to self or others.

Cognition

Assessment of cognitive functioning can appear complex, as it seeks to assess several inter-related aspects of higher cortical functions. Nevertheless, it should be a standard part of the MSE, and it is relatively quick and easy to conduct screening tests. The usual domains which are assessed are *consciousness, orientation, attention* and *concentration, memory, language*, and *visuospatial functioning*.

Consciousness

Consciousness is awareness of self and the environment. Its level varies between the extremes of coma and alertness. Several terms are used for the intervening states of consciousness:

- **Clouding of consciousness** refers to a state of drowsiness with incomplete reaction to stimuli; impaired attention, concentration, and memory; and slow, muddled thinking.
- **Stupor** refers to a state in which the person is mute, immobile, and unresponsive, but appears conscious because the eyes are open and follow objects. Note that this is the use in psychiatry; in neurology the term is used when there is *some* impairment of consciousness.

- **Confusion** refers to muddled thinking. The resulting term '**confusional state**' can be qualified by the term 'acute' or 'chronic', which are alternative terms for **delirium** and **dementia** respectively.

Orientation

Orientation is assessed by asking about awareness of time, place, and person. *Disorientation* is an important symptom that indicates impairment of consciousness or impairment of new learning. Questions begin with the time, day, month, year, and season. In assessing responses to questions about time, the interviewer should remember that many people do not know the exact time of day (although they usually know it to the nearest hour) or the exact date (though they are usually accurate to a few days). Orientation in place is assessed by asking the name of the place in which the interview is being held. If the answer is inaccurate, further questions are asked about the kind of place (e.g. home, a hospital ward, or a home for the elderly), and the name of the town. Personal orientation is assessed by asking about other people present (e.g. relatives in the home, or the staff in a hospital ward). If patients give wrong answers, they should be asked about their own identity—their name, occupation, and role in life.

Attention and concentration

Attention is the ability to focus on the matter in hand, and *concentration* is the ability to sustain that focus. Attention and concentration can be impaired in many kinds of psychiatric disorder but especially in anxiety disorder, depressive disorder, mania, schizophrenia, and organic disorder. Detection of impaired attention or concentration does not help in diagnosis but is important in assessing the patient's disability; for example, poor concentration may prevent a person from working effectively in an office.

While taking the history, the interviewer should look out for evidence of impaired attention and concentration. In the MSE, specific tests are given. It is usual to begin with the '*serial 7s test*'. The patient is asked to subtract 7 from 100 and then to take 7 from the remainder repeatedly until it is less than 7. The interviewer assesses whether the patient can concentrate on this task. Of course, it is quite possible that poor performance could be due to poor arithmetic ability. If so, the patient should be asked to do a simpler subtraction, such as taking 3s from 30; or to avoid a mathematical task and say the months of the year in reverse order, or the simpler task of naming the days of the week in reverse order. Such tests of attention are given before tests of memory because poor attention can lead to poor performance on memory tasks, even when there is no memory deficit.

Memory

Memory problems may come to light during history taking. During the MSE, tests are given to assess *immediate, recent*, and *remote* memory. Note that, although this simple classification is useful in clinical practice, it does not correspond exactly with the types of memory identified through research. No 'memory test' is wholly satisfactory and the results should be assessed cautiously and in relation to other information about the patient's ability to remember. If there is doubt, standardized psychological tests can be given by a clinical psychologist.

Assessment of immediate recall/working memory

This is assessed by asking patients to repeat sequences of digits immediately after they have been spoken slowly enough for them to register the digits (the '*digit span test*'). An easy sequence of three digits is given first to make sure that patients understand the task. Then a new sequence of four digits is presented. If patients can repeat four digits correctly, sequences of five, six, and seven are given. When patients reach a level at which they cannot repeat the digits, a different sequence of the same length is given to confirm the finding. Clearly it is important to use random series of digits, rather than (for example) telephone numbers. Healthy people of average intelligence can repeat seven digits correctly; five or less

suggests impairment. Note that the test involves concentration and, therefore, cannot be used to assess memory when tests of concentration are abnormal.

This can also be assessed through a test of recall of a name and address. Say to the patient 'Please can you repeat back to me the following name and address ... [for example] John Peters, 22 Church Street, Oxford'. Common names and addresses likely to be familiar to a patient should be avoided. If the patient does not correctly repeat the name and address, the same name and address are repeated, and repeated, until the patient repeats all six elements of the name and address correctly. This is a test of *immediate recall*, and a requirement for several repetitions may indicate a deficit in attention and concentration, or in working memory.

Assessment of recent memory

This uses a continuation of the name and address test. When the patient has correctly registered the name and address, do *not* say to them 'Remember that name and address; I will ask you them later'—if you do this, the patient is likely to focus on that task, and performance on other tasks in the interim will be adversely affected. Other topics should then be discussed for 5 minutes, or other cognitive tests undertaken as distracters, and the patient is then asked to repeat the name and address that was given to them earlier. This task generates a score out of 6, of which 5 or 6 would be normal, 3 or 4 might indicate abnormality and would invite further testing, and 0, 1 or 2 would be abnormal. Responses should be recorded verbatim.

Recent memory can also be assessed by asking about news items from the last day or two, or about recent events in the patient's life that are known with certainty to the interviewer (do not ask the commonly used question about what the patient had for breakfast unless you know the answer). Questions about news items should be adapted to the patient's interests, and should have been widely reported in the media. Of course, if the patient has no interest in the news, or no access to newspapers or television, this is an inappropriate task.

Assessment of long-term memory

This can be assessed by asking the patient to recall personal events or well-known public events from some years before. Personal events could be the birth dates of the patient's children or grandchildren (provided these dates are known to the interviewer); public events could be political, sporting, or cultural.

Observations suggesting memory disorder

When a patient is in a general hospital, important information about memory is available from observations made by nurses or other staff. These observations include how rapidly patients learn the daily routine of the ward, and the names of staff and other patients, and whether they forget where they have put things, or cannot find their way about, although apparent deficits in visuospatial memory may indicate a disturbance in visuospatial functioning rather than memory per se. When the patient is at home, relatives may report comparable observations about the patient's ability to learn and remember.

Special tests of memory

Among elderly patients, questions about memory do not distinguish well between those who have cerebral pathology and those who do not. For cases of doubt, there are standardized ratings of memory for recent personal events, past personal events, and general events, which allow a better assessment of severity. Standardized tests of learning and memory can help also in the diagnosis of organic mental disorder, and can be used for quantitative assessments of the progression of memory disorder. These tests are usually administered by a clinical psychologist. In primary care, the *GPCOG* (General Practitioner assessment of COGnition) is an effective cognitive screen and, in secondary care, the *ACE-III* (Addenbrooke's Cognitive Examination III) performs well.

Specific disorders of memory

Memory is affected in several kinds of psychiatric disorder, but is particularly suggestive of organic disorder.

In *depressive disorder,* unhappy or guilt-laden memories are recalled more readily than other kinds of memory. In *organic disorder,* memory of remote events is impaired less than that of more recent memory. Total loss of memory, including memory for personal identity, occurs very rarely in organic conditions and strongly suggests psychogenic causes (see p. 357) or malingering (see p. 359). Some organic causes lead to an *amnesic syndrome* in which short-term memory is severely impaired but longer-term memory is retained (see p. 361). Other abnormalities of memory include the following:

- **Anterograde amnesia.** This occurs after a period of unconsciousness. It is the impairment of memory for events between the ending of complete unconsciousness and the restoration of full consciousness.

- **Retrograde amnesia.** This is the loss of memory for events before the onset of unconsciousness. It occurs after head injury or electroconvulsive therapy (ECT), when patients will be unable to remember events such as waking and showering during the early morning before their treatment.

- **Jamais vu** is a failure to recognize events that have been encountered before, and **déjà vu** is the recognition of events as familiar when they have never been encountered. Both abnormalities may occur in neurological disorders.

- **Confabulation** is the reporting as 'memories' of events that did not take place at the time in question. It occurs in some patients with severe disorders of recent memory (see 'Amnesic syndrome', p. 49).

Language

Language functions can be tested in simple ways. These include the following:

- **Naming**—the patient is asked to name common objects, such as those in the interview room (e.g. pen, chair, and window). It should be straightforward for a patient to name such objects, unless they have a severe deficit. More obscure objects may pick up more subtle deficits—for example, rather than pointing to his shirt, the interviewer might point to his cuff, or cufflink.

- **Verbal instruction**—the patient is asked to carry out a command, which may have several components, such as 'Take this piece of paper, fold it, and place it under your chair'.

- **Written instruction**—the interviewer writes a simple command on a piece of paper (e.g. 'Stand up'), shows it to the patient, and says 'Do what it says'.

- **Writing a sentence**—the interviewer hands the patient a pen and a piece of paper, and says 'Please write a sentence'.

Visuospatial functioning

This can be tested informally or formally. Informally, a patient's carers (whether relatives or healthcare staff such as nurses) can be asked to observe the patient's ability to find their way around, such as from their bed to the toilet and back again. More formally, a patient can be asked to perform the following:

- Copy simple line figures, such as a star, a cube, and the front of a simple house, with windows and doors, as a simple test of visuospatial functioning.

- Recall those simple line figures several minutes later, following distractor tasks (such as some of the language tasks described previously), as a simple test of visuospatial memory.

- The '*clock drawing test*': draw an old-fashioned clock face, with the time showing (for example) 'quarter to three'. This requires quite complex *visuospatial skills*, such as remembering that the '12' goes at the top of the clock, and spacing the numbers appropriately, and *executive functioning skills*, such as the planning and sequencing the different actions—the circle must be drawn first, followed by the numbers, and then the hands.

Insight

This is a term that is used more often in psychiatry than in other areas of medicine. It is akin to 'congruence', or *the extent to which the patient's view of their symptoms, illness, prognosis, and treatment is identical to that of their healthcare professional.* Assessment of insight is extremely important in determining a patient's likely cooperation with treatment. For example, a patient who believes that he is being persecuted and does not accept that his beliefs are a sign of illness, is unlikely to accept treatment readily. Nonetheless, he may be aware that he feels distressed and is sleeping badly, and may agree to accept help with these problems (which he ascribes to the persecution). Assessment of insight can therefore help in two ways. *First*, it suggests how far patients are likely to collaborate with treatment; the greater the degree of 'fit' between the patient's and the professional's views, the better the prognosis is likely to be. *Second*, it provides information on where the patient's and the professional's views differ, and where effort to change the patient's health and illness beliefs should be focused. Psychiatrists and other mental health professionals spend a high proportion of their face-to-face contact with patients working with them to change their attitudes to their symptoms, their illness, and their treatments.

At its briefest, insight can be described as 'good', 'moderate', or 'poor'. However, it is more helpful clinically to provide a short description of the areas in which the patient and the professional hold similar views, and those in which they differ. These might include, for example:

1 *awareness of oneself as presenting phenomena that other people consider abnormal* (e.g. being unusually active and elated);

2 *recognition that these phenomena are abnormal* (versus, for example, being a desirable mental state, of which other people are jealous);

3 *acceptance that these abnormal phenomena are caused by mental illness* (versus, for example, being excited about and energized by a new project or idea, or having a physical illness);

4 *awareness that treatment is required* (versus treatment being unnecessary and undesirable);

5 *acceptance of the professional's specific treatment recommendations* (e.g. admission to hospital and sedative medication).

Physical examination

The extent of the physical examination is decided by considering diagnostic possibilities in the individual case. When there is doubt, a systematic physical examination should be performed, and should include a careful examination of the endocrine and nervous systems. In selected cases, this examination should also include assessment of language, constructional apraxias, and agnosias. The methods of examination are described in textbooks of neurology, and are learnt during neurology training. Readers who have not had this training are advised to refer to the *Shorter Oxford Textbook of Psychiatry*, to consult a textbook of neurology, and to obtain supervised practice of the relevant clinical skills.

Investigations

Investigations are chosen according to the clinical features and the diagnostic possibilities. There is no single set of routine investigations appropriate for every patient.

A corroborative history

In psychiatry, the most important investigation is a corroborative history. If a corroborative history is not obtained, there must be a strong basis for this omission. Often, a corroborative history will give vital additional information or correct errors in the patient's account.

Physical investigations

Often, a focused physical history and examination are all that are needed to exclude the possibility of physical illness. However, sometimes physical investigations are appropriate. These are helpfully divided into *near-patient tests* which can be obtained quickly if the patient is cooperative (e.g. dipstick urinalysis for infection, dipstick urinalysis for illicit drugs, fingertip blood oxygen, weight, and height) and *non-near-patient tests* (e.g. laboratory blood tests, imaging). Relevant physical investigations are discussed in subsequent chapters.

Psychological investigations

- **Questionnaires and rating scales.** These are used in certain cases to either (1) characterize the extent or nature of specific problems, for example, the ACE-III in the assessment of cognitive functioning, or (2) follow the progress of a disorder, such as to monitor response to treatment, for example, the QIDS-SR (Quick Inventory of Depressive Symptomatology-Self Report), as used by the True Colours online mood monitoring system (https://truecolours.nhs.uk/).

- **Neuropsychological tests.** A wide variety of structured, sophisticated tests are available for assessing specific aspects of cognitive function, such as frontal or parietal cortical functioning. These are usually conducted by clinical psychologists with specific training. Although brain imaging methods are generally more useful in diagnosis, neuropsychological tests may be used to follow the progress of the disorder.

- **Tests of intelligence.** In most cases it is not necessary to have a precise assessment of intelligence. If a patient seems to be of low intelligence, or if his psychological symptoms could be a reaction to work beyond his intellectual capacity, intelligence tests may be helpful. In child psychiatry, tests of intelligence are often supplemented by tests of *reading ability*.

Further reading

Harrison P, Cowen P, Burns T, Fazel M. Assessment. In: *Shorter Oxford Textbook of Psychiatry*, 7th ed. Oxford: Oxford University Press; 2017:35–70.

Harrison P, Cowen P, Burns T, Fazel M. Signs and symptoms of psychiatric disorders. In: *Shorter Oxford Textbook of Psychiatry*, 7th ed. Oxford: Oxford University Press; 2017:1–20.

6 Thinking about diagnosis

Why we diagnose

Rationale for diagnosis

Diagnosis performs a useful function because it allows us to classify patients into groups. This enables us to:

- **study** diagnostic groups, so that we can learn more about aetiology, prognosis, risks, and treatment through research;
- **communicate** briefly but effectively with other healthcare professionals about a specific patient—rather than having to list the specific features in every case, we have a convenient shorthand;
- **predict** the likely aetiology, prognosis, risks, and effective treatments in a specific patient, based on evidence from other people with that diagnosis.

Objections to diagnosis

The process of diagnosis in mental health is not universally accepted as being appropriate. This stems from concerns that diagnosis:

- labels people with mental illness with names that may be unhelpful and stigmatizing, such as 'personality disorder' or 'schizophrenia';

- excessively simplifies the details of a particular person's predicament, so that a person's uniqueness is not acknowledged;
- relies upon an understanding of illness (existing classification systems) that does not reflect real illness categories, and therefore has low validity;
- relies upon the interpretation of the individual clinician, and therefore has low reliability—clinicians presented with the same information (the same patient) may draw different diagnostic conclusions.

We would argue that the rationale for diagnosis is strong, that no realistic alternative exists, and that the advantages of this approach far outweigh the disadvantages. When diagnostic assessment is conducted thoroughly and appropriately, it focuses very much on the *detail* of the patient's psychological, physical, and social situation, and emphasizes the *particular* aspects of an individual's case. It is therefore crucial that, when you are presenting a case, you stress those points, so that your case description is rich and individual, rather than being bland and general. The former reflects a real, unique person; the latter reflects a textbook description.

How to diagnose

Addressing complexity

In psychiatry, diagnosis is rarely just one simple term describing the patient's medical situation. As we have seen so far while considering assessment, there is usually more than one issue, and sometimes many, whether within the biological, psychological, or social domains. This complexity needs to be reflected in the shorthand of diagnosis. One way in which psychiatric diagnosis has achieved this in an ordered way is by adopting a *multiaxial* classification, in which several *axes* reflect different aspects of the patient's situation. These axes may include:

- **main psychiatric diagnoses**—usually one or more mental illnesses, such as depressive disorder;
- **other psychiatric diagnoses**—and, in particular, the presence of lifelong diagnoses such as *personality disorder* or *learning disability,* which may modify the presentation and prognosis of other psychiatric diagnoses;
- **physical disorder(s)**—especially those that are relevant to the presentation or prognosis of psychiatric diagnoses, such as cerebrovascular disease or endocrine disorder;
- **social problem(s)**—such as debt, unemployment, poor housing, social isolation, or abusive relationship(s);
- **extent of functional impairment**—the impact of the above-listed psychological, physical, and social problems on day-to-day functioning and responsibilities, whether at home or at work/school/college, and whether to the self or to others such as children. This may be formalized in a rating scale such as the Global Assessment of Functioning, which is a scale from 0 to 100, with written descriptions for each decile. While this approach is helpful in research, in clinical practice it is more common to describe functional impairment as nil, minimal, mild, moderate, or severe.

Diagnostic criteria

Typically, the diagnostic criteria for a particular disorder include five elements:

- **The main features**—those that define the core nature of the disorder and that are often required for the diagnosis to be made.
- **Associated features**—those that are commonly seen in the disorder, but which may be absent; which are often shared with other disorders; and of which only a specific number or proportion may be required for diagnosis.
- **Duration**—usually a minimum duration, but occasionally a maximum, or a minimum and a maximum.
- **Severity**—often expressed as the extent of functional impairment. For a diagnosis to be made, it is usual for there to be functional impairment, although one important exception to this is when the patient has recovered from one or more episodes of illness, but they retain a diagnosis because of the increased risk of recurrence compared to the general population (e.g. '*recurrent depressive disorder, currently in remission*').
- **Exclusions**—other diagnoses which might explain the presentation, and which need to be excluded in order for the diagnosis to be valid.

For example, in a depressive episode:

- *main features* include low mood, reduced enjoyment, and reduced energy;
- *associated features* are multiple, and include *physical* features such as poor appetite, weight loss, amenorrhea, and constipation; *psychological* features such as reduced concentration, guilt, low self-esteem, hopelessness, and suicidal thoughts; and *social* features, such as withdrawal from hobbies and interests, absence from work, and poor performance at work;
- the main features and associated features must have a *duration* of at least 2 weeks;

- there must be at least some *functional impairment*;
- several alternative causes of the depressive syndrome must be *excluded*, including harmful use of alcohol or other substances, physical disorder, prescribed medicines, and schizophrenia.

Variation in diagnostic criteria

Diagnostic systems in psychiatry are currently (2019) quite complex. This is for two reasons:

- There are two widely used systems—the WHO International Classification of Diseases (ICD) and the American Psychiatric Association (APA) *Diagnostic and Statistical Manual of Mental Disorders* (DSM).
- The APA released the latest DSM version, DSM-5, in 2013; the WHO's current version remains the ICD-10, which was released in 1992, and the implementation of ICD-11 is not due until 2022.

Please don't let this worry you:

- The descriptions of syndromes and associated diagnostic criteria are very similar in DSM-5, ICD-10, and draft ICD-11.
- In this textbook, we have used draft ICD-11 criteria.

Occasionally, there is an important difference between the DSM and the ICD. These diagnostic systems have been derived very carefully, through hard work by many experienced mental healthcare professionals. When differences occur, they are often informative, as they may reflect core issues about diagnosis—areas where there are differences of opinion, where it has proved difficult to reliably categorize the complex natural phenomena that are mental illnesses. The durational criterion of schizophrenia is one example. ICD-10 requires more than 1 month of the core symptoms before schizophrenia can be diagnosed; whereas DSM-5 requires 6 months. In a large group of individuals with 'schizophreniform' symptoms, ICD-10 schizophrenia will therefore be more common, as it is diagnosed

sooner. It will also be, on average, a better prognosis: the longer an illness continues, the more likely it is to continue, and so long duration is a predictor of poor prognosis. A rationale to diagnose early (as in ICD-10) is to enable 'possible schizophrenia' to be identified early, and appropriate measures to be put in place to improve prognosis. On the other hand, a pressure to diagnose later (as in DSM-5) is to avoid labelling patients with what is potentially a very stigmatizing illness, and to be more certain that the presenting illness is indeed 'schizophrenia' rather than something from which the patient will recover within weeks or months.

Lifetime diagnoses

Some patients retain a diagnosis even when they are symptom free. For example, people who have had two or more discrete *depressive episodes* will retain the diagnosis of *recurrent depressive disorder* even when they are completely well. This is because the multiple depressive episodes bestow upon that person a lifetime risk of further depressive episodes that is significantly higher than if that person had not had those episodes. The multiple episodes therefore have prognostic significance. Making the diagnosis of recurrent depressive disorder, even in the absence of current symptoms, tells us as mental health professionals that we need to consider management approaches that will help to reduce the risk of recurrence.

How to make a diagnosis

When you first approach a patient, almost any diagnosis is possible. The aim of your assessment is to determine:

1 your *preferred (most likely) diagnosis*;
2 other *differential diagnoses*;
3 *diagnoses which will not be considered further*.

Within a minute or two, you may have been able to rule out several possibilities, and to start to focus your diagnostic radar. The aim is to systematically *rule out* some diagnoses, by which we mean that the chance of them being the 'real' diagnosis shifts progressively towards 0 per cent—although it is unlikely to ever reach 0 per cent. These diagnoses will not be considered further, unless there is a need for subsequent diagnostic review. Simultaneously, the aim is to *rule in* the preferred diagnosis, by which we mean that, by seeking specific, diagnostically relevant information, the chance of one diagnosis being the 'real' diagnosis shifts progressively towards 100 per cent—although it is unlikely to ever reach 100 per cent. Those diagnoses that are neither the preferred diagnosis nor excluded diagnoses form the small number of differential diagnoses. Typically, the differential diagnosis will include no more than two or three other mental illnesses. In addition, it is good practice to include the possibility of physical disorder, no matter how remote you consider this

to be—this helps to keep this important possibility in mind.

Note that this approach prioritizes both explicitly and implicitly. Explicitly, diagnoses are stated as either the preferred diagnosis or (likely or important) differentials. Implicitly, clinical prioritization takes place by not even mentioning diagnoses that are considered to be unlikely and unimportant.

Further reading

American Psychiatric Association. *Diagnostic and Statistical Manual of Mental Disorders*. 5th ed. Washington, DC: American Psychiatric Association; 2013.

World Health Organization. *The ICD-10 Classification of Mental and Behavioural Disorders: Clinical Descriptions and Diagnostic Guidelines*. Geneva: World Health Organization; 1992.

World Health Organization. ICD-11 beta draft. http://apps.who.int/classifications/icd11/.

7 Thinking about aetiology

CHAPTER CONTENTS

Doctors need to be able to combine scientific knowledge with empathic understanding in order to form a coherent account of their patients, their illnesses, and their difficulties. In this chapter, we will describe how this can be achieved in the assessment of the aetiology (cause or causes) of a patient's disorder.

A knowledge of the causes of psychiatric disorders is important for two main reasons:

- It helps the doctor to evaluate possible causes of an individual patient's psychiatric disorder and life difficulties. This is the focus for this chapter.

- It adds to the general understanding of psychiatric disorders, which may contribute to advances in diagnosis, treatment, or prognosis. This is reviewed in subsequent chapters.

Aetiology and the individual patient

When assessing aetiology in a particular patient, we usually structure this by talking of *predisposing*, *precipitating*, and *perpetuating* (often called *maintaining*) factors (see Fig. 7.1 and Box 7.1). These 'three Ps' are often supplemented by a fourth P: *protective* factors. These terms are used most commonly in psychiatry and related disciplines. However, the principles are broadly applicable in medicine. We therefore recommend that you practise their use in long-term physical conditions such as diabetes, asthma, and vascular disease.

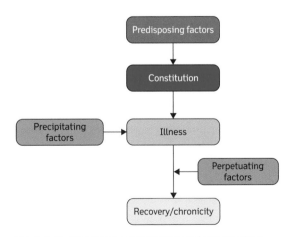

Fig. 7.1 Predisposing, precipitating, and perpetuating factors.

Box 7.1 Predisposing, precipitating, and perpetuating factors in psychiatric disorder

Predisposing factors

- Genetic endowment (informed by family history of illness)
- Environment *in utero*
- Trauma at birth
- Psychosocial factors during childhood/adolescence
- Personality traits

Precipitating factors

- Physical—onset of diseases, new medicines, accidents, acute use of street drugs
- Lifestyle—change in sleep–wake pattern due to shift work
- Psychological/social—life events of any kind

Perpetuating factors (often called maintaining factors)

- Cognitive biases/errors
- Poor compliance with treatment(s)
- Use of alcohol or street drugs as self-medication
- Avoidance of normal activities, at work and at home
- Social isolation
- Relationship problems

Classification of causes

Predisposing factors determine vulnerability to other causes that act close to the time of the illness. Many predisposing factors act early in life. *Physical* factors, for example, include genetic endowment, the environment *in utero*, and trauma at birth. *Psychological* and *social* factors in infancy and childhood are also relevant, such as bullying at school, abuse in its various forms, and family stability. Such factors lead to the development of a person's 'constitution', which leads to wide variability, at a population level, in vulnerability to disorder: some people are highly *vulnerable*, some are highly *resilient*, and most are somewhere in between. Some personality traits increase vulnerability to specific disorders—for example, obsessional traits predispose to depressive illness, perhaps because the

challenges and uncertainty of everyday life inevitably lead to disappointment for those seeking order and perfection at all times.

Precipitating factors are events that occur shortly before the onset of a disorder and appear to have induced it. Again, these may be *physical, psychological*, or *social*. Physical precipitating causes include diseases such as hypothyroidism, myocardial infarction, breast cancer, and stroke, and the effects of drugs taken for treatment or used illegally. Examples of *psychosocial* causes include bereavement, or other loss events such as illness, injury, divorce, redundancy, or retirement; assault; moving home; pregnancy; bankruptcy; or a conviction or prison term. In bipolar disorder, a change in a person's sleep–wake cycle, such as a change in shift pattern from days to nights, or a prolonged period without sleep, may induce mania.

Perpetuating factors (often called maintaining factors) prolong a disorder after it has begun. Perpetuating factors are important when planning treatment because they may be modifiable, and they often therefore form the basis of treatment of an acute episode of illness. They may be a component of the illness:

- In anxiety disorders, *cognitive* factors (thinking errors, e.g. catastrophization) and *behavioural* factors (e.g. avoidance, use of safety behaviours) play important roles, and their understanding has led to the design of CBT, based on challenging unrealistic thoughts and reducing avoidance.

- In depressive disorders, cognitive and behavioural factors are again highly relevant: negative cognitive biases (e.g. *negative mental filter*) and behavioural changes (e.g. *reduction in satisfying/ enjoyable activities*) help to keep the individual in a depressive 'rut', unable to make progress.

- In psychotic disorders, paranoid delusions are self-reinforced by cognitive and behavioural mechanisms. Cognitively, delusions *bias* (in a threatening way) the person's interpretation of other people's (neutral/non-threatening) actions, leading to confirmation and reinforcement of those delusions. Behaviourally, delusions lead to *social avoidance*, so that the person is less likely to observe socially normal behaviour and less likely to receive reassuring comments from others. Delusions may also lead to unusual behaviour, which triggers friends, neighbours, and members of the public to act differently to normal when near the psychotic person. Changes in others' behaviour can reinforce the beliefs held by the psychotic person, by being used as evidence that 'something odd is going on'.

Other perpetuating factors include:

- poor adherence to medication;
- poor relationship with healthcare professionals;
- social isolation;
- unemployment;
- continued alcohol or substance misuse;
- overprotective relatives.

An example from general medicine

For example, in a 56-year-old man with poorly controlled heart failure:

- *predisposing* factors include his male sex, his older age, and his obesity;
- *precipitating* factors include his recent myocardial infarction;
- *perpetuating* factors include:
  - his lack of adherence to cardiac medication due to associated side effects and lack of understanding of their role;
  - the adverse impact of his breathlessness on his activity levels;
  - his low mood and consequent poor motivation to attend cardiac rehabilitation;
  - consequent further reductions in physical fitness and increase in weight.

Identified aetiological factors help to inform our view of prognosis and a management plan. In many cases, the perpetuating factors are particularly relevant, as their successful management enables a return to a higher level of functioning, and enables the clinician and the patient to address longer-term issues. In this cardiac case, prognosis is likely to be poor, with ongoing functional impairment and the likelihood of further cardiac events, unless the patient can be engaged to adhere to the treatment plan. Management, derived from the specific aetiological factors just described, might include:

1 an explanation of what heart failure is, and about the rationale for each cardiac medicine;

2 an explanation of the role of physical activity in training the heart and improving function, accompanied by physical rehabilitation with the aid of a physiotherapist;

3 an appointment with a dietician to help with healthy eating and define a plan for weight loss;

4 a review by the patient's GP with a view to prescribing an SSRI antidepressant for their low mood;

5 a follow-up by a clinician who knows the case and who can continue to endorse lifestyle interventions.

An example from psychiatry

In assessing the causal significance of these events, the clinician can draw on his knowledge of scientific studies of depressive disorders, and on his understanding of human emotional reactions to life events (see Case study box 7.1). These enable the clinician to draw conclusions about likely *predisposing*, *precipitating*, and *perpetuating* factors.

Predisposing factors are those factors which increase an individual's risk above the population average. Genetic epidemiological studies have shown that a predisposition to depressive disorder may be genetically transmitted. It is possible, therefore, that this patient inherited this kind of predisposition from his mother. Is the separation from his mother likely to have been significant? There have been several studies of the long-term effects of separating children from their parents, but they refer to people who

CASE STUDY BOX 7.1

Causes of psychiatric disorder

For 4 weeks, a 38-year-old married man, who has worked for the last 15 years as a supervisor in a car factory, has become increasingly depressed. His symptoms started soon after his wife left him to live with another man. The following points in the history seemed relevant to aetiology. The patient's mother had received psychiatric treatment on two past occasions, once for a severe depressive disorder and once for mania; on neither occasion was there any apparent environmental cause for the illness. When the patient was 14 years old, his mother went to live with another man, leaving the patient, his brother, and his sister with their father. For several years afterwards the patient felt rejected and unhappy but eventually settled down. He married and had two children, aged 13 and 10 at the time of his illness. Two weeks after leaving home, the patient's wife returned saying that she had made a mistake and really loved her husband. Despite her return, the patient's symptoms persisted and worsened. He began to wake early, gave up his usual activities, ruminated about his predicament and found it difficult to be distracted from his difficulties, and spoke at times of suicide.

were separated when younger than the patient was at separation. Nonetheless, extrapolations from this evidence and from human experience suggest that his mother's departure is likely to have been an important event, increasing his emotional vulnerability.

Precipitating factors are those factors that appear to trigger the onset of illness in someone who may or may not have predisposing factors. In this case, it is understandable that a man should feel depressed when his wife leaves him, and this man is likely to be especially affected by this experience because the event repeats the similar distressing separation in his own childhood.

Perpetuating (or maintaining) factors are those factors that keep an illness going, even in the absence of factors that might have precipitated it. In this case, empathy and common sense would suggest that the patient should have felt better when his wife came back, but he did not. This lack of improvement can be explained, however, by evidence that, once a depressive disorder starts, it is established through *physical* means (neurochemical changes are embedded; alcohol is often used as self-medication; helplessness means that compliance with medication is poor), *psychological* means (thinking is pervasively negative, with gloom and despondency affecting motivation and interest; cognitive errors are powerful forces which maintain negative beliefs about the past, the present, and the future), and *social* means (reduced attendance at work, reduced hobbies and interests, and reduced

friendships mean reduced distraction from a person's predicament, and a reduced sense of achievement and purpose). Again, this understanding can inform a simple management plan, in which the patient is informed about:

- the nature of the illness and the role of persistence in its management;
- the depressant effect of alcohol, and the need to reduce consumption;
- the antidepressant effect of medication, and its delayed rather than immediate effect;
- some simple cognitive techniques to make thinking more realistic;
- the relevance of a staged return to work, to hobbies and interests, and to friendships.

Protective factors in this patient would include his employment and employment stability. This suggests that a priority should be discussions with occupational health over a phased return to work, to bolster his self-esteem, and to help to distract him from his depressed and anxious thoughts.

This case study illustrates several important issues concerning aetiology in psychiatry, including:

- the interaction of multiple different causes in a single case;
- the need to identify different causes through time— *predisposing*, *precipitating*, and *perpetuating*;

- the need to identify causes different in nature—*physical, psychological*, and *social*;
- the concept of stress and of psychological reactions to it;
- the roles of scientific evidence and of evaluation based on empathy and common sense;
- the link between an effective understanding of aetiology and an effective management plan.

Explanation and understanding

There are two ways of trying to make sense of the causes of a patient's problems. Both are useful, but it is important to distinguish between them.

- The first approach is quantitative and based on research findings; for example, a person's aggressive behaviour may be explained as the result of an injury to the frontal cortex sustained in a road accident. This statement draws on the results of scientific studies of the behaviour of patients with damage to various areas of the brain. It is conventional to refer to this kind of statement as **explaining** the behaviour.
- The second approach is qualitative and is based on an empathic understanding of human behaviour. We use this approach when we decide, for example, that a person was aggressive because his wife was insulted by a neighbour. The connection between these two events makes sense; it is convincing even though a quantitative study may not have shown a statistical association between aggression and this kind of insult. It is conventional to refer to this kind of statement as **understanding** the cause.

Remote causes, multiple effects, and multiple causes

In psychiatry, certain events in childhood are associated with psychiatric disorder in adult life; the causes are *remote* in time. For example, subjects who develop schizophrenia are more likely than controls to have been exposed to complications of pregnancy and labour. *One cause* can lead to *several effects*: for

example, lack of parental affection in childhood has been reported to predispose to suicide, antisocial behaviour, and depressive disorder. Conversely, a *single effect* can have *several causes*, which act singly or in combination. For example, a learning disability can be caused by any one of several distinct genetic abnormalities, while a depressive disorder can be caused by the combined effects of genetic factors and recent stressful events.

Models

In discussions of aetiology, the word 'model' is often used to mean a way of ordering information. A model seeks to explain certain phenomena and to show the relationships between them. Crucially, a single model is insufficient to fully explain any psychiatric disorder, or to fully explain the predicament of any single person with a psychiatric problem. The following words, by Professor Kenneth Kendler, sum up the challenge, and interested readers are encouraged to read his excellent 2008 essay in the *American Journal of Psychiatry* (see 'Further reading'):

> **Rather than adopting a single explanatory perspective, as is often advocated in traditional theories of science, etiological models for psychiatric disorders need to be pluralistic or multilevel. A range of compelling evidence indicates that these disorders involve causal processes that act both at micro levels and macro levels, that act within and outside of the individual, and that involve processes best understood from biological, psychological, and sociocultural perspectives.**

Several models are in common use in psychiatric practice, and the following examples are not exhaustive:

- The **medical model** is an approach in which psychiatric disorders are investigated in ways that have proved useful in general medicine, such as by identifying regularly occurring patterns of symptoms (syndromes) and relating them to brain pathologies. This model has proved particularly useful in investigating schizophrenia and mood disorders. It has so far proved less useful in the study of anxiety disorders and personality disorders, although rapid advances in functional neuroimaging may change this in the near future.

- The **behavioural model** is an approach in which psychiatric disorders are explained in terms of *adaptive* and *maladaptive* behaviours. For example, if a person is bullied at work by a particular individual, a strategy to discuss this with their manager, and to avoid that person when possible, might be considered *adaptive*; whereas taking time off work might be considered *maladaptive*. Equally, in a depressive illness, *avoidance* of the structure and enjoyment and sense of satisfaction that daily activities can bring is invariably *maladaptive*, unless those activities are placing unreasonable stress on the individual. Reduced activity acts as a depressant via several mechanisms, including *reduced positive social interactions*, and reduced *distraction* from negative thoughts. One important behavioural mechanism is *avoidance*, when the person actively avoids the feared stimulus, to reduce distress or the anticipation of distress. Unfortunately, avoidance is a potent *perpetuating factor* in psychiatric illness: by avoiding, the person cannot learn that the feared stimulus is in fact neutral or helpful, rather than toxic. For example, in the phobic anxiety disorders, behaviour therapy specifically targets a progressive reduction in avoidance with a treatment called 'graded exposure' (to the feared stimulus). Another important behavioural mechanism is *distraction*, whereby a depressed or anxious person may be distracted from their depressed or anxious thoughts in a helpful way, by engaging in a distracting activity, such as work, or being with friends. By identifying maladaptive and adaptive behaviours, and by discouraging the maladaptive and encouraging the adaptive, progress can be made in treating psychiatric disorder and reducing the risk of relapse.

- The **cognitive model** is an approach in which psychiatric disorders are explained in terms of cognitive biases, which influence our thoughts and beliefs, automatically, pervasively, and silently.

These mechanisms influence the way in which we all *select, interpret*, and *act* on information received from the sense organs and from memory. A wide variety of *cognitive distortions* are seen in common psychiatric disorders, and their identification and management forms a core part of *cognitive therapy*. In depression, pervasive negative cognitive biases promote a negative, grey view of the person themselves, as well as their illness, the people around them, and the world. These cognitive biases *predispose* a person to become depressed; may influence the person's interpretation of a life event, so that it is more likely to *precipitate* an illness; and reduce the likelihood of the person engaging in satisfying or enjoyable activities, so that the illness is *perpetuated* (*maintained*). In mania (elevated mood), pervasive positive biases lead to an inflated view of the person's abilities and their life's possibilities, so that they engage in behaviours which may cause embarrassment, relationship breakdown, physical danger, or financial disaster. Anxiety disorders are maintained, in part, by the ways that patients think about the physical symptoms associated with emotional arousal. Normal physical signs of the 'fight or flight' response, such as palpitations and sweating, may be interpreted (*catastrophization*) as signs of a heart attack, rather than as a normal feature of the body's stress/anxiety response. This '*misattribution*' leads to a 'panic attack' (rapid onset of a severe, but time-limited, crescendo of anxiety) due to the fear of sudden death.

Typical coping strategies are often both behavioural *and* cognitive. For example, after bereavement, a person's coping mechanisms might include thinking about religious beliefs about the afterlife (cognitive), joining a social club to combat loneliness (behavioural), and looking at photographs of happy times such as holidays with the deceased person (behavioural).

- The **social model** regards social factors as the important forces in the development and maintenance of psychiatric disorder. It postulates close relationships between the person's mood and behaviour and their social environment. Learning through association (classical conditioning) explains, for example, the development of situational anxiety in phobic patients following an initial attack of anxiety in the situation. The reinforcement of behaviour by its consequences (operant conditioning) explains, for example, the maintenance of disruptive behaviour in some patients (or children) by the extra attention that is provided by staff (or parents) when this behaviour occurs. In depression, 'learned helplessness' may help to explain persistently low levels of social and other behaviours that might otherwise help the person to lift themselves out of a depressive rut.

- Finally, the **biopsychosocial model** is an approach in which psychiatric disorders are explained by carefully integrating physical factors (such as those within the medical model), psychological factors (such as those within the behavioural and cognitive models), and social factors. It is helpful not only in psychiatry, but also in medicine in general, where physical factors derived from a medical model approach often dominate thinking about aetiology and treatment, but where significant improvements in functional outcome can be delivered by attending

to psychological and social factors. Importantly, a similar approach is used when considering and structuring the management plan for a particular patient. Indeed, the physical, psychological, and social aetiological perpetuating factors in any patient often map closely onto a sensible physical, psychological, and social initial management plan. For example, a young man with depression, who is drinking too much alcohol (physical), thinking pervasively negatively about his situation and future (psychological), and avoiding work and workmates (social), should be encouraged to stop drinking (physical), identify and challenge his negative automatic thoughts (psychological), and consider a phased return to work and to his social life (social).

Further reading

Gelder MG, Andreasen NC, López-Ibor JJ, Geddes JR, eds. New Oxford Textbook of Psychiatry. 2nd ed. Oxford: Oxford University Press; 2012. [This textbook includes an extensive section on the scientific basis of psychiatric aetiology, divided up into subsections, each of which is easily digestible for those interested in a particular topic.]

Kendler KS. Explanatory models for psychiatric illness. American Journal of Psychiatry 2008;165:695–702.

8 Thinking about prognosis

The role of prognostic assessment

The prognostic assessment of a patient aims to predict the future, using the range of evidence available. This evidence relates to:

- **the individual patient** (e.g. their own history of illness, and their compliance with medication);

- **groups of patients like the individual patient**, that is, diagnostic and subdiagnostic groups (e.g. in depressive disorder, the risk of recurrence; and in anorexia nervosa, the risk of suicide or of death by starvation);

- **psychiatric patients in general** (e.g. the importance of good relationships with healthcare professionals, supportive family and friends, and insight into illness).

Prognostic assessment results in an understanding of the following:

- **What outcomes are likely to happen?** Relevant outcomes can be related to *the illness* (relapse and recurrence, for example—see 'Terminology'

for definitions), to *treatments* (such as side effects or complications), to *risks* (to self, to others—see Chapter 7), or to *important social outcomes* (such as return to work, marital break-up, or permission to drive a car, bus, or lorry).

- **How likely are they to happen, and when/over what time period?** An estimate of both *likelihood* and *timeline* is helpful. So, for example, in a patient with recurrent depressive episodes, who is now well, we may view that their lifetime risk of suicide is significantly higher than the population risk, that they are not currently at increased risk, and that suicide attempts are likely to occur in the context of depressive recurrence.

- **What can change the nature or likelihood of the outcomes?** For example, in the case just mentioned, we may view that the lifetime risk of recurrence can be reduced by training the patient and family to spot the early warning signs of illness, by reducing daily consumption of alcohol, and by finding regular, stable employment. In addition, we can reduce suicidal risk by ensuring that the patient is prescribed medicines that are relatively safe in overdose (e.g. SSRI antidepressants rather than tricyclics), and by making family members aware of the risk of their own medication being used in an overdose.

The prognostic assessment therefore relates closely to the assessment of diagnosis, of risks, of the patient's social situation, and of a suitable management plan. Indeed, the prognosis in a specific case helps to guide us in determining (1) whether any management is necessary, (2) the nature and intensity of that management, and (3) the extent of healthcare resources that it would be appropriate to use. It also helps to guide the patient to make decisions, based upon their own values and priorities. In a situation where the emotional impact is usually self-limiting, such as bereavement, the prognosis is good without medical management focused on the cause, and so reassurance, explanation, and simple advice are all that are required. In an illness with greater consequences, such as moderate depression, the illness is often not self-limiting, and carries a significant risk of severe adverse outcomes such as suicide, and there is evidence that medical treatments (whether physical or psychological) impact prognosis.

Terminology

Specific terms—'the five Rs' of response, remission, recovery, relapse, and recurrence—are used by mental health professionals to describe the course of psychiatric disorder. For ordinary clinical practice, the precise definitions are not critical, but they need very careful thought and definition in clinical research. The following descriptions are intended to help the reader to comment on prognosis in specific cases, and to tackle the relevant literature.

Response is some relief of symptoms and some improvement in functioning. The term 'response' implies that this improvement arises from treatment, usually because it is associated in time with that treatment. For example, 'Mr A appears to have *responded* to starting an antidepressant 2 weeks ago', or 'I think that it is unlikely that she will *respond* to the antidepressant, due to her continued heavy drinking'.

Remission is a period of complete relief of symptoms and a return of full functioning. This period of time may be brief. For example, 'Currently Mrs B appears to be in *remission*, with no depressive or anxiety symptoms for 1 month, and she is coping well at work', or 'Mr C's depressive symptoms *remitted* within weeks of him stopping drinking alcohol, but returned within days of him restarting'.

Recovery is a period of complete relief of symptoms and a return of full functioning, which is likely to be longer term. For example, 'Mr D appears to have *recovered* from his recent depressive episode, and has now been symptom free for 6 months'.

Relapse is the return of symptoms, satisfying the diagnostic criteria for the disorder, after a patient has either *responded* or *remitted*, but before *recovery*. For example, 'Ms E was symptom free for 4 weeks, but in the last fortnight she appears to have *relapsed*, with a significant deterioration in her mood, and inability to work', or 'There is a high probability of *relapse*, as Miss F has stopped taking her antidepressant, and her abusive partner has returned to her home after a period of time away'. In the mood disorders, *relapse* is usually conceived as being a return of the original mood episode, rather than the start of a new one.

Recurrence is the return of symptoms, satisfying the diagnostic criteria for the disorder, after the patient has *recovered*. The distinction from *relapse* is therefore temporal. In the mood disorders, recurrence is usually conceived as being a new mood episode. For example, 'Mr G had been well for 1 year after his first depressive episode, but there appears to be *recurrence*: depressive symptoms have returned and he again meets criteria for a depressive episode', or 'Due to the high frequency of mood episodes in recent years, the likelihood of *recurrence* is high'. This term is used by the ICD-10 and draft ICD-11 in the important diagnosis '*recurrent* depressive disorder', in which there are two or more depressive episodes 'separated by at least several months without significant mood disturbance'.

Prognosis and treatment

Inevitably, consideration of the prognosis in a particular case is closely linked to consideration of treatment. In the last example in the previous paragraph, for example, the comment could have continued:

'Due to the high frequency of mood episodes in recent years, the likelihood of *recurrence* is high, but can be reduced significantly by improved compliance over a period of years with a mood stabilizer such as lithium carbonate'. This demonstrates the importance of considering both static and dynamic factors when assessing prognosis:

- *Static factors* are those that cannot be changed—the recent high frequency of mood episodes, for example, or gender, or early onset.
- *Dynamic factors* are those that can be changed—compliance with medicines, for example, or reducing alcohol or substance use, or finding work.

There are two stages to thinking about prognosis and treatment:

- The first is to determine whether any treatment is necessary, by considering the prognosis without treatment. If this is good, then it may well be desirable to pursue a policy of 'active monitoring' (or 'watchful waiting'), watching for signs of deterioration, but without active treatment, therefore avoiding the side effects and risks associated with many treatments. If, on the other hand, prognosis is moderate or poor, then treatment should be considered.
- The second stage is to determine whether treatment will improve prognosis and, by implication, which treatment will be most *effective*, that is, most improve the prognosis (and, furthermore, be *acceptable* to the patient and *feasible* for health services to deliver).

Communicating prognosis

With health professionals

In day-to-day clinical practice, prognosis is usually mentioned only briefly, often by stating simply that the patient's prognosis is 'good', 'moderate', or 'poor'. This is unfortunate: high-quality clinical practice needs a rigorous approach to the assessment and communication of prognostic information, and we would urge you

to practise a more comprehensive method. It is helpful to outline as many of the following as are appropriate in the time available:

- *Overall*, whether the patient's prognosis is good, moderate, or poor.
- Specifically *what* will be good or poor compared to their current situation, and *over what time period*.
- Particular *risks*, if these have not been mentioned elsewhere.
- Your *justification* of those views, citing evidence that is personalized to your particular patient, by combining evidence from the clinical assessment of your specific patient with evidence from textbooks or the scientific literature about groups of patients like yours.
- *What can improve or worsen prognosis* (dynamic factors), for example, starting a treatment, complying with a treatment, stopping drinking alcohol or using substances, finding or returning to work, being admitted to hospital, keeping a regular sleep–wake schedule, or engaging with the mental health team. Notably, these are all aspects that should be mentioned in your treatment plan, with which your prognostic assessment will therefore be closely linked.

With patients

Before starting your discussion, ask the patient what they know about their prognosis—what might happen, how likely are those things to happen, and over what time period, and what can they do to improve their prognosis. Of course, you are likely to need to find more patient-friendly terminology than 'prognosis', unless you are talking to a healthcare professional. From that conversation, assess whether the patient understands the implications of their illness, and the impact that their own actions can have on their prognosis. Overall, form a view on whether the patient is *realistic* about their prognosis, *overpessimistic*, or *overoptimistic*. Your subsequent approach will be different depending on your assessment of patient understanding—for example, you may choose to emphasize the more worrying aspects of their prognosis with patients who are overoptimistic, in an attempt to improve engagement with long-term management; or, you may emphasize the more positive ones with the overpessimistic, in an attempt to enable them to move forward with their life with some confidence. Your aim is for the patient and their carer(s) such as key family members to have a realistic understanding of their prognosis, and, crucially, to understand how their own actions can improve outcomes. In every case, the actions of the patient and of the people around them can help to improve the patient's outcomes. That message of optimism is an important part of being an effective doctor/psychiatrist.

Discussing prognosis can be difficult for patients and their relatives. Oncology and palliative care settings have set the pace in terms of considering the issues, and developing guidelines to assist clinicians in this area. Useful suggestions include to:

- arrange privacy and time;
- develop rapport, and show empathy;
- involve a key family member or close friend, with the patient's permission;
- consider what the patient (and key carer/s) knows and doesn't know;
- consider what the patient (and key carer/s) doesn't want to know;
- take time, and avoid or explain jargon;
- be realistic about uncertainty—your prognostic estimate is just that, and may well have wide 'confidence intervals'/significant uncertainty;
- be aware of the patient's cognitive biases—a depressed patient will tend to see the worst in everything; a manic patient will struggle to see a bad outcome in anything;
- consider the family's/carer's needs, which may be distinct;
- encourage questions and clarification;
- consider the consistency of information from different teams (e.g. mental health/primary care) and different team members;
- record in the case notes what you have discussed;
- write to other health professionals involved in the case, to let them know what you have said;
- don't just share the bad news—emphasize good news, too.

Increased risk of harm to self and others occurs in several mental disorders, and the prediction and assessment of risk has become an important component of psychiatric practice.

Fatal self-harm—or suicide—is the most important risk to assess. At least a brief assessment of suicidal risk should be included in all psychiatric assessments. However, harm to others—both homicide and non-fatal harm—is increased in some mental disorders, and a thorough assessment of the nature, severity, and likelihood of such risks will often form an important part of a psychiatric assessment. When assessing risk, it is useful to consider **static** and **dynamic** risk factors. Static risk factors cannot be changed, whereas dynamic risk factors change over time and include mental disorder.

Generally, the assessment of risk should include:

- the nature of the risk;
- the probability of the risk in the short and longer term;
- whether there are any factors that increase the risk;
- whether there are any factors that decrease the risk;
- whether there are any interventions that may reduce the risk.

A risk management plan will aim to:

- reduce the risk;
- review the risk.

Often, the most appropriate intervention to reduce risk will be to ensure that the patient is offered the most effective treatment for their specific condition. For example, a depressed person with suicidal ideation may be offered a low-toxicity antidepressant and regular follow-up. On the other hand, the management of a new mother with a postpartum psychotic depressive disorder who has thoughts of harming her new child may involve specific intervention to reduce the risk of harm to her baby as well as effective therapy for the depressive disorder.

Suicide

Many patients deliberately take drug overdoses or harm themselves in other ways. Some die (suicide, completed suicide); others survive (attempted suicide, parasuicide, or deliberate self-harm). The characteristics of those who kill themselves and those who harm themselves are rather different, although they overlap.

The main clinical issues are the assessment of suicide risk and the management of deliberate self-harm.

Suicide accounts for about 1 per cent of deaths worldwide. There is a twofold variation in rates between different countries, suggesting considerable influence of cultural factors. It is rare among children and uncommon (but increasing) in adolescents. Rates increase with age and are higher in men than in women. There are three sets of interacting causes: genetics, medical factors, and social factors.

The assessment of suicide risk depends on evaluating:

- the presence of suicidal ideas;
- the presence of psychiatric disorder;
- factors known to be associated with increased risk of suicide.

Referral to specialist mental health services is usually appropriate when the suicidal intentions are strong, associated psychiatric illness is severe, and/or the person lacks social support. If the risk does not seem to require hospital admission, management depends on ensuring good support, telling the patient how to obtain help quickly if needed, and ensuring that all those who need to know are informed.

Most completed suicides are planned and precautions against discovery are often taken. About one in six leaves a **suicide note**. Some notes are pleas for forgiveness. Other notes are accusing or vindictive, drawing attention to failings in relatives or friends. In most cases, some warning of intention is given to relatives or friends, or to doctors. There is a history of deliberate self-harm in between a third and a half of completed suicides. WHO data reports 45% of completed suicides had seen a doctor in the month preceding their death.

An understanding of the epidemiology and causes of suicide is clinically useful for several reasons including:

- as a basis for assessing suicidal risk;
- to help the relatives and others in the aftermath of suicide;
- as a guide to suicide prevention.

Epidemiology

In the UK, the suicide rate has decreased over recent years (Fig. 9.1), and is about 16 per 100,000 per year

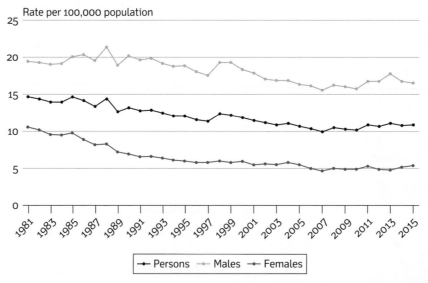

Fig. 9.1 UK suicide rates per 100,000 for males and females over the period 1981–2015.

Reproduced from Office for National Statistics. Contains public sector information licensed under the Open Government Licence v3.0, http://www.nationalarchives.gov.uk/doc/open-government-licence/version/3/.

in males and 6 per 100,000 in females (which is in the lower range of rates reported for developed countries). Suicide accounts for about 1 per cent of all deaths. However, official suicide statistics almost certainly underestimate the numbers of actual suicides because uncertain cases are not counted.

Suicide rates are highest in older people, in men (75 per cent), and those who are divorced or unmarried. In most countries, *drug overdoses* (especially analgesics and antidepressants) account for about two-thirds of suicides among women and about a third of those among men. The remaining deaths are by a variety of *physical means*, namely hanging, shooting, wounding, drowning, jumping from high places, and falling in front of moving vehicles or trains.

Causes of suicide

The large international, regional, and temporal variations in the prevalence of suicide reflect the importance of social causes. These causes interact with individual psychiatric and medical factors (see Box 9.1). Psychiatric disorder is an important cause of suicide; in contrast, it is less important in deliberate self-harm (see Table 9.1). Social factors sometimes influence the

Box 9.1 Associations with suicide

Social

- Old age
- Social isolation (especially living alone)
- Unemployment
- Lack of family and other support
- Stressful events (especially bereavement)
- Publicity about suicides
- Periods of rapid social change or economic stress (population level risk)

Medical

- Depressive disorder
- Alcohol abuse
- Drug abuse
- Schizophrenia
- Personality disorder
- Chronic painful physical illness and epilepsy

Table 9.1 Comparison of those who die by suicide and those who harm themselves

	Suicide	Deliberate self-harm
Age	Older	Younger
Sex	More often male	More often female
Psychiatric disorder	Common, severe	Less common, less severe
Physical illness	Common	Uncommon
Planning	Careful	Impulsive
Method	Lethal	Less dangerous

means chosen for suicide. Thus a case that has attracted attention in a community or received wide publicity in newspapers or on television may be followed by others using the same method.

Psychiatric and medical causes

The great majority of people who die from suicide are suffering from a mental disorder at the time of death.

Depressive disorder. The rate of suicide is increased in patients with depressive disorder, with a lifetime risk of about 15 per cent in severe cases. Depressed patients who commit suicide differ from other depressed patients in being older, more often *single, separated,* or *widowed*, and having made more *previous suicide attempts*.

Schizophrenia has a high risk of suicide, with a lifetime risk of about 10 per cent. The risk is particularly great in younger patients who have retained insight into the serious effect which the illness is likely to have on their lives.

Alcohol abuse also carries a high risk of suicide. The risk is particularly great among (1) older men with a long history of drinking, a current depressive disorder, and previous deliberate self-harm; and (2) people whose drinking has caused physical complications, marital problems, difficulties at work, or arrests for drunkenness offences.

Anorexia nervosa has the highest risk of death of any mental disorder. About half of these deaths are from suicide: 20% of patients with anorexia nervosa make a suicide attempt.

Personality disorder is detected in a third to a half of people who die by suicide. Personality disorder is often associated with other factors that increase the risk of suicide, namely abuse of alcohol or drugs and social isolation.

Drug abuse also carries an increased risk of suicide.

Chronic physical illness is associated with suicide, especially among the elderly.

Causes among special groups

Rational suicide. Suicide is sometimes the rational act of a mentally healthy person. However, even if the decision appears to have been reached rationally, given more time and more information the person may change their intentions. For example, a person with cancer may change a decision to take their life when they learn that there is treatment to relieve pain. Doctors should try to bring about this change of mind, but some rational suicides will take place despite the best treatment.

Physician-assisted suicide has been an increasingly prominent matter of public and medical concern. It raises several important ethical and legal issues including:

- a conflict between the duty to help the patient and the duty not to harm;
- competence of the patient to decide;
- differences between actively promoting death, withholding treatment which might prolong life, and the use of medication which as a side effect may shorten life.

Box 9.2 lists some of the clinical issues that may need to be considered and may need to be discussed with the patient and family.

Children and young adolescents. As noted earlier, suicide is rare among children, and uncommon in adolescents, although rates in older adolescents have increased recently. In adolescence, suicide is associated with unstable home environments, social isolation,

Box 9.2 Physician-assisted suicide: clinical issues

- Need to discuss medical and other opportunities to minimize pain and suffering
- Importance of understanding the patient's and family's views on death
- Importance of treating depression as a cause of the wish to die
- Need to assess the patient's competence and/or review any advance directive
- Need to provide high-quality care and support to patient and family
- Awareness of pressure on patient from others, for instance, those who may benefit financially

and depression, and also with impetuous behaviour and violence.

Doctors. The suicide rate among doctors is greater than that in the general population. The reason is uncertain although several factors have been suggested, such as the ready availability of drugs, increased rates of addiction to alcohol and drugs, the extra stresses of work, reluctance to seek treatment for depressive disorders, and the selection into the medical profession of predisposed personalities.

Suicide pacts. In a suicide pact, two people, usually in a close relationship in which one is dominant and the other is passive, agree that at the same time each will die by suicide. They are uncommon, and must be distinguished from murder followed by suicide (occurring sometimes when the murderer has a severe depressive disorder). When one person survives, a suicide pact has to be distinguished from the aiding of suicide by a person who did not intend to die, and also from an attempt to disguise murder.

The assessment of suicide risk

Every doctor will encounter, at some time, patients who express suicidal intentions, and must be able to assess the risk of suicide (see Box 9.3). This assessment requires:

- evaluation of suicidal intentions;
- assessment of any previous act of deliberate self-harm (see p. 87);

Box 9.3 Risk factors for suicide

Intention

- Evidence of intent to die
- Previous attempts at suicide

Biological factors

- Age
- Male sex
- Family history of suicide

Psychiatric and psychological factors

- Depression
- Schizophrenia
- Personality disorder
- Alcohol and drug dependence
- Impulsive personality traits
- Feelings of hopelessness and helplessness
- Losses or bereavements

Social and demographic factors

- Childhood abuse
- Severe social and interpersonal stressors
- Isolation
- Occupations with easy access to lethal methods

Medical factors

- Chronic, painful illness
- Terminal illness

- detection of psychiatric disorder;
- assessment of other factors associated with an increased risk of suicide;
- assessment of factors associated with a reduced risk;
- in some cases, assessment of associated homicidal ideas.

Evaluation of intentions. Some people fear that asking about *suicidal intentions* will make suicide more likely. It does not, provided that the enquiries are made sympathetically. Indeed, a person who has thought of suicide will feel better understood when the interviewer raises the issue, and this feeling may reduce the risk. The interviewer can begin by asking whether the patient has thought that life is not worth living. This question can lead to more direct ones about thoughts of suicide, specific plans, and preparatory acts such as saving tablets. Table 9.2 shows a useful standard instrument—the Beck Suicide Intent Scale—which combines these and other informative questions.

When suicidal intentions are revealed, they should be taken seriously. *There is no truth in the idea that people who talk of suicide do not enact it*; on the contrary, two-thirds of people who die by suicide have told someone of their intentions. A few people speak repeatedly of suicide so that they are no longer taken seriously, but many of these people eventually kill themselves. Therefore their intentions should be evaluated carefully on every occasion.

Previous deliberate self-harm of any kind is an indicator of a substantially increased risk of suicide. Systematic review evidence suggests that the strongest predictors of completed suicide after deliberate self-harm are ongoing suicidal ideation, chronic physical illness, and male sex. Certain other features of previous self-harm are particularly important predictors of suicide; these are summarized on p. 89 and in Table 9.2.

Detection of psychiatric disorder is an important part of the assessment of suicide risk. If possible, an informant should be interviewed. *Depressive disorder* is highly important, especially when there is severe mood change with hopelessness or delusions. It is important to remember that suicide may occur during recovery from a depressive disorder in patients who, when more severely depressed, had thought of the act but lacked the initiative to carry it out.

Factors that may reduce risk. These include the availability of good support from the family and others to assist with social, practical, and emotional difficulties. Providing the individual with help and instilling a sense of hope is the best method of reducing suicide risk.

Homicidal ideas in suicidal patients. A few severely depressed suicidal patients have homicidal ideas; for example, the idea that it would be an act of mercy to kill the partner or a child, in order to spare that person intolerable suffering. If present, such ideas should be taken extremely seriously since they may be

Table 9.2 Beck Suicide Intent Scale

Circumstances related to suicidal attempt	
1. Isolation	0 Somebody present
	1 Somebody nearby or in contact (as by phone)
	2 No one nearby or in contact
2. Timing	0 Timed so that intervention is probable
	1 Timed so that intervention is not likely
	2 Timed so that intervention is highly unlikely
3. Precautions against discovery and/or intervention	0 No precautions
	1 Passive precautions such as avoiding others but doing nothing to prevent their intervention (alone in a room with unlocked door)
	2 Active precaution such as locked door
4. Acting to gain help during/after attempt	0 Notified potential helper regarding the attempt
	1 Contacted but did not specifically notify potential helper regarding the attempt
	2 Did not contact or notify potential helper
5. Final acts in anticipation of death	0 None
	1 Partial preparation or ideation
	2 Definite plans made (changes in will, giving of gifts, taking out insurance)
6. Degree of planning for suicide attempt	0 No preparation
	1 Minimal preparation
	2 Extensive preparation
7. Suicide note	0 Absence of note
	1 Note written but torn up
	2 Presence of note
8. Overt communication of intent before act	0 None
	1 Equivocal communication
	2 Unequivocal communication
9. Purpose of attempt	0 Mainly to change environment
	1 Components of '0' and '2'
	2 Mainly to remove self from environment

Table 9.2 Continued

Circumstances related to suicidal attempt	
Self-report	
10. Expectations regarding fatality of act	0 Patient thought that death was unlikely
	1 Patient thought that death was possible but not probable
	2 Patient thought that death was probable or certain
11. Conception of method's lethality	0 Patient did less to himself than he thought would be lethal
	1 Patient wasn't sure, or did what he thought might be lethal
	2 Act equalled or exceeded patient's concept of its medical lethality
12. 'Seriousness' of attempt	0 Patient did not consider act to be a serious attempt to end his life
	1 Patient was uncertain whether act was a serious attempt to end his life
	2 Patient considered act to be a serious attempt to end his life
13. Ambivalence towards living	0 Patient did not want to die
	1 Patient did not care whether he lived or died
	2 Patient wanted to die
14. Conception of reversibility	0 Patient thought that death would be unlikely if he received medical attention
	1 Patient was uncertain whether death could be averted by medical attention
	2 Patient was certain of death even if he received medical attention
15. Degree of premeditation	0 None; impulsive
	1 Suicide contemplated for 3 hours or less prior to attempt
	2 Suicide contemplated for more than 3 hours prior to attempt

Reprinted from Beck A T, Resnik H, Lettieriet D, *The Prediction of Suicide*, 1974, Charles Press. In the public domain.

carried into practice. It is especially important to be aware of these dangers when assessing a mother of small children.

Management of a patient at risk of suicide

The risk of suicide should be considered in any patient who is depressed or whose behaviour or talk gives any suggestion of the possibility of self-harm. In hospital inpatient or emergency departments, evidence of suicidal intent should normally lead to obtaining advice from a specialist. However, other medical staff need to be aware of the general principles of assessment, especially with patients who are reluctant to stay and who are medically fit. Box 9.4 summarizes reasons for referral.

The main principles of treatment are as follows:

1 **Prevention of harm.** The obvious first requirement is to prevent the patient from self-harm by preventing access to methods of harm, and appropriately close observation. Most patients at serious suicidal risk require *admission to hospital*. The first requirement is the safety of the patient. Achieving this requires

Box 9.4 Referral to a psychiatrist of patients at risk of suicide

In primary care, referral to a psychiatrist is usually appropriate when:

- suicidal intentions are clearly expressed;
- there is any change of presentation in a patient who has previous expressed suicidal ideas or repeatedly self-harmed;
- associated psychiatric illness is severe;
- the person lacks social support.

In the UK, there is a national guideline which recommends that all patients attending the emergency department with suicidal thoughts are referred to a psychiatrist and assessed within 4 hours.

an adequate number of vigilant nursing staff, an agreed assessment of the level of risk, and good communication between staff. If the risk is very great, nursing may need to be continuous so that the patient is never alone. If *outpatient treatment* is chosen, it is usually when the patient lives with reliable relatives, who wish to care for the patient, understand their responsibilities, and are able to fulfil them. The patient and relatives should be told how to obtain help quickly if the strength of suicidal ideas increases, for example, an emergency telephone number. Frustrated attempts to find help can make suicide more likely. If hospital treatment is essential but the patient refuses it, compulsory admission will be necessary.

2 **Treatment of any associated mental illness.** This should be initiated without delay.

3 **Reviving hope.** However determined the patient is to die, there is usually some remaining wish to live. These positive feelings can be encouraged and the patient helped towards a more positive view of the future. One way to begin this process is to show concern for the problems.

4 **Problem-solving.** Initially overwhelming problems can usually be improved if they are dealt with one by one.

A number of patients remain at *long-term suicidal risk* despite specialist assessment that there are no

indications that hospital treatment would be of benefit. An example would be a patient with long-standing problems who has had intensive psychiatric and social help without benefit, and for whom it is evident that further hospital admission would do nothing to help with the long-term problems in everyday life. Such a decision requires a particularly thorough knowledge of the patient and their problems, and should generally be made by a psychiatrist in conjunction with the general practitioner.

Help after a suicide

When a person has died by suicide, help is required by surviving relatives and friends who may need to deal with feelings of loss, guilt, or anger. They should have a full explanation of the nature and reasons for medical and other actions to assess the suicidal risk, to treat the causes, and prevent harm. They should also have an opportunity to discuss their own feelings, including guilt that if they had behaved differently the suicide could have been prevented. Those most directly involved in the previous care of the dead person should offer to meet the relatives as soon after the suicide as possible and to meet again at a later stage if the family and friends believe it would be helpful. The relatives' distress may be considerable and may be expressed indirectly in complaints about medical care. Some relatives suffer from long-standing or psychiatric or other problems which deserve treatment in their own right.

The doctor should also support other professional staff who had been closely involved with the patient. After suicide, the case should be reviewed carefully to determine whether useful lessons can be learnt about future clinical practice. This review should not be conducted as a search for a person at fault; some patients die by suicide however carefully the correct procedures have been followed.

Suicide prevention

There are two main approaches to prevention, namely *early recognition and help for those at risk* and *modification of predisposing social factors*.

- **Identifying high-risk patients.** Many people who commit suicide have contacted their doctors shortly beforehand, and many of these have a psychiatric disorder, or alcohol dependence. Doctors can identify at least some of these patients as at high risk, and offer help.

- **Supporting those at risk.** This is the responsibility of all healthcare agencies who may come into contact with the patient. Organizations such as Samaritans give emergency 24-hour support to people who feel lonely and hopeless and express suicidal ideas, but it has not been shown convincingly that this support reduces suicide. In addition, it is possible that there are opportunities for modification of predisposing social factors.

- **Reducing the means** may help to reduce suicide (e.g. providing safety rails at high places, reducing the packet size of over-the-counter analgesics, and cautious prescribing). However, people determined to commit suicide can find other means.

- **Education** might be provided for teenagers about the dangers of drug overdosage and about ways of coping with emotional problems. However, there is little evidence that such education is effective.

- **Public health or social and economic policy.** Isolation and other social factors which increase the risk of suicide cannot be modified by the medical profession. They require public policy decisions.

Deliberate self-harm

Deliberate self-harm is not usually failed suicide. Only about a quarter of those who have deliberately harmed themselves say they wished to die; most say the act was impulsive rather than premeditated (see Fig. 9.2). The rest find it difficult to explain the reasons or say that:

- they were *seeking unconsciousness* as a temporary escape or relief from their problems;

- they were trying to *influence another person* to change their behaviour (e.g. to make a partner feel guilty about threatening to end the relationship);

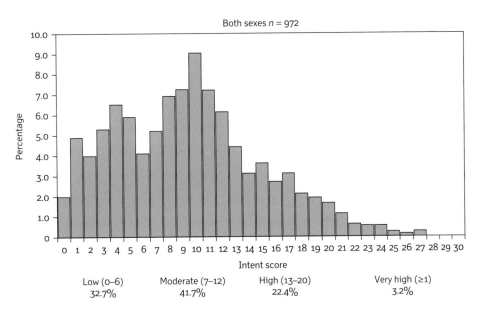

Fig. 9.2 Beck scores in deliberate self-harm attenders in 2001.
Courtesy of Professor K. E. Hawton, Oxford University.

- they are *uncertain* whether or not they intended to die—they were 'leaving it to fate';
- they were *seeking help*.

Epidemiology

Deliberate self-harm is common and rates have risen progressively over the last 30 years. Deliberate self-harm is more common among:

- **younger adults** (see Fig. 9.3): the rates decline sharply during adult life (they are also very low in children under the age of 12 years);
- **young women**, particularly those aged 15–20 years;
- **people of low socioeconomic status**;
- **divorced individuals, teenage wives, and younger single adults**;

- individuals with personality disorders, especially emotionally unstable or histrionic traits.

Deliberate self-harm is commonest among younger people. **Predisposing factors** include childhood difficulties, adverse social circumstances, and poor health. **Precipitating factors** include stressful life events, such as quarrels with spouses or others in close relationships. Only a minority have psychiatric disorder. The motives are complex and often uncertain. Frequently there is no particular wish to die.

Up to a quarter of people who harm themselves do so again in the following year, and the risk of suicide during the year is about 1–2 per cent, a hundred times the risk in the general population.

Assessment must include:

- the risk of suicide;

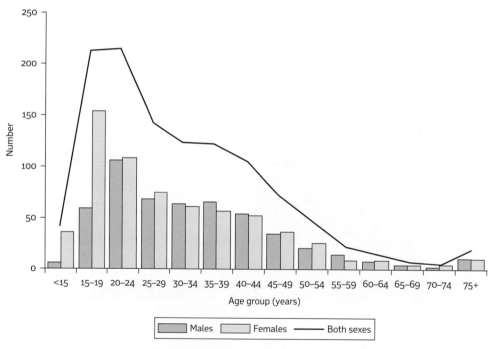

Fig. 9.3 The age groups of deliberate self-harm patients by sex in 2001.
Courtesy of Professor K. E. Hawton, Oxford University.

- the risk of further deliberate self-harm;
- current medical and social problems.

Those with severe mental disorder may require admission, and others need continuing help from a mental health service or GP. About a quarter require no special treatment.

Methods of deliberate self-harm

Drug overdosage. In the UK, about 75 per cent of the cases of deliberate self-harm treated by general hospitals involve drug overdose. The drugs taken most commonly in overdose are **anxiolytics**, **non-opiate analgesics**, such as salicylates and paracetamol, and **antidepressants**. Paracetamol is particularly dangerous because it damages the liver and may lead to delayed death, sometimes in patients who had not taken the drugs with the intention of dying.

Antidepressants are taken in about a fifth of cases. Of these drugs, tricyclics are particularly hazardous in overdosage since they may cause cardiac arrhythmias or convulsions. Despite these and other dangers, most deliberate drug overdoses do not present a serious threat to life.

The use of alcohol. About half of the men and a quarter of the women who harm themselves have taken alcohol within 6 hours before the act. This often precipitates the act by reducing self-restraint. Its effects interact with those of the drugs.

Self-injury. In the UK, between 15 and 20 per cent of all cases of deliberate self-harm treated in general hospitals are self-inflicted injuries. Most of these injuries are lacerations, usually of the forearm or wrist. Most patients who cut themselves are young, have low self-esteem, impulsive or aggressive behaviour, unstable moods, difficulty in interpersonal relationships, and often problems of alcohol or drug abuse. Usually, the self-laceration follows a period of increasing tension and irritability which is relieved by the self-injury. The cuts are usually multiple and superficial, often made with a razor blade or a piece of glass.

Less frequent and medically more serious forms of self-injury include deeper lacerations, jumping from heights or in front of a moving train or motor vehicle, shooting, and drowning. These highly dangerous acts occur mainly among people who intended to die but have survived.

Causes

Deliberate self-harm is usually the result of multiple social and personal factors (see Box 9.5), including national and local attitudes. Overall, rates appear to be affected by awareness of the occurrence and methods of self-harm in a population (e.g. television and press reports and local knowledge of suicide and attempted suicide in the neighbourhood). Psychiatric disorder is less important than in suicide.

Association of deliberate self-harm with psychiatric disorder

Although many patients who harm themselves are anxious or depressed, relatively few have a psychiatric disorder other than an acute stress reaction, adjustment disorder, or personality disorder. The latter is

---

Box 9.5 Associations with deliberate self-harm

Historical factors

- Early parental loss
- Parental neglect or abuse
- Lack of emotional attachment to parents in early childhood

Current factors

- Psychiatric disorder (mood disorders, adjustment disorder)
- Personality disorder or traits (especially emotionally unstable, histrionic)
- Alcohol dependence
- Unstable relationship(s)
- Long-term social problems: family, employment, financial
- Poor physical health

Precipitating social factors

- Arguments with family members, especially threats of rejection by spouses or sexual partners
- Acute financial crises (e.g. redundancy)

found in about a third to a half of self-harm patients, and dependence on alcohol is also frequent. (In contrast, psychiatric disorder is common among patients who die by suicide; see p. 81.)

The differences between factors associated with suicide and deliberate self-harm are summarized in Table 9.1.

Outcome

Since deliberate self-harm results from long-term, adverse social factors and is associated with personality disorder, it is not surprising that a significant proportion of subjects have a poor overall outcome in terms of personal and social adjustment. More specifically, outcome is assessed in terms of repetition of self-harm and of suicide. Between 15 and 25 per cent of people who harm themselves do so again in the following year and 1–2 per cent commit suicide. Of those who harm themselves again:

- some repeat the act only once;
- some repeat it several times within a period in which there are continuing severe stressful events;
- a few repeat it many times over a long period as a habitual response to minor stressors.

The factors associated with repetition of deliberate self-harm are shown in Box 9.6.

Box 9.6 Factors that predict the repetition of deliberate self-harm

- Previous deliberate self-harm before the current episode
- Previous psychiatric treatment
- Alcohol or drug abuse
- Personality disorder
- Criminal record
- History of violence
- Low social class
- Unemployment
- Age 25–54 years
- Single, divorced, or separated

Box 9.7 Factors predicting suicide after deliberate self-harm

Evidence of intent

- Evidence of serious intent (see Box 9.5)
- Continuing wish to die
- Previous acts of deliberate self-harm

Psychiatric disorder

- Depressive disorder
- Alcoholism or drug abuse
- Antisocial personality disorder

Social and demographic

- Social isolation
- Unemployment
- Older age group
- Male sex

People who have deliberately harmed themselves have a much increased risk of later suicide. In the year after the self-harm, the risk of suicide is about 1–2 per cent, that is, about 100 times the risk in the general population. The risk factors for suicide after deliberate self-harm are shown in Box 9.7.

It is important to note that a *non-dangerous method of self-harm does not necessarily indicate a low risk of subsequent suicide* (although the risk is higher when a violent or dangerous method has been used).

Assessment

Every act of deliberate self-harm should be assessed thoroughly. For many patients seen in primary care, the physical consequences of the act and concern about the risk of repetition will lead to hospital referral. In other cases, referral may not be necessary, for instance, when the act was not reported until sometime later, when the results are clearly not medical serious, where suicidal intent was low, and where the patient and family are known to the doctor.

All deliberate self-harm patients seen in hospital emergency departments should have a psychiatric and social assessment (Fig. 9.4). This assessment can be carried out by a psychiatrist, by general medical staff,

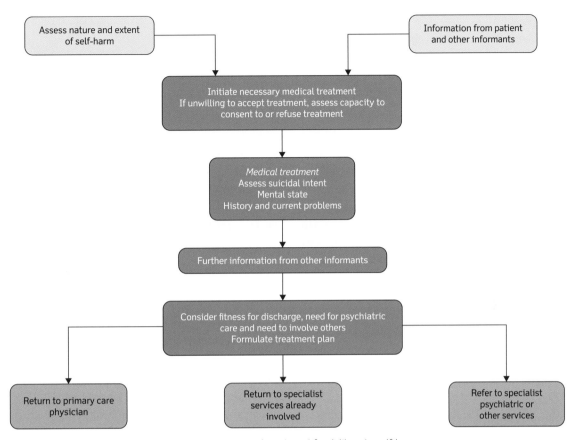

Fig. 9.4 Action that should be taken in the emergency department for deliberate self-harmers.

by psychiatric nurses or social workers with appropriate special training, or by a psychiatrist. All patients found on this assessment to be suffering from psychiatric disorder or with a high risk of further self-harm should be seen by a psychiatrist. Since many patients who are medically fit do not wish to stay for specialist assessment, it is essential that all emergency department medical staff are competent to assess risk.

Steps in assessment

The assessment should be carried out in a way that encourages patients to undertake a constructive review of their problems and of the ways they can deal with them. If patients can then resolve their problems in this way, they may be able to do so again in the future instead of resorting once more to self-harm.

When to assess. When patients have recovered sufficiently from the physical effects of the self-harm

they should be interviewed, if possible, where the discussion will not be overheard or interrupted. After a drug overdose, the first step is to determine whether consciousness is impaired. If so, the interview should be delayed until the patient has recovered further and can concentrate on the questions.

Sources of information. Information should be obtained also from relatives or friends, the GP, and any other person (such as a social worker) already involved in the patient's care. Such information frequently adds significantly to the account given by the patient. The following issues should be considered.

1 **What were the patient's intentions before and at the time of the attempt?** Patients whose behaviour suggests that they intended to die as a result of the act of self-harm are at greater risk of a subsequent fatal act of self-harm. Intent is assessed by considering the following.

- Was the act *planned* or carried out on impulse?
- Were *precautions* taken against being found?
- Did the patient seek *help after the act*?
- *Was the method dangerous?* Not only should the objective risk be assessed, but also the risk anticipated by the patient, which may be different (e.g. if they believed that they had taken a lethal dose of a drug even though they had not).
- *Was there a 'final act'* such as writing a suicide note or making a will?

2 **Does the patient now wish to die?** The interviewer should ask directly whether the patient is relieved to have recovered or wishes to die. If the act suggested serious suicidal intent, but the patient denies such intent, the interviewer should try to find out by tactful but thorough questioning whether there has been a genuine change of resolve.

3 **What are the current problems?** Many patients will have experienced a mounting series of difficulties in the weeks or months leading up to the act of self-harm. Some of these difficulties may have been resolved by the time the patient is interviewed, but if serious problems remain, the risk of a fatal repetition is greater. This risk is particularly great if the problems are of loneliness or ill health. Possible problems should be reviewed systematically, covering *intimate relationships* with the spouse or another person; *relations with children and other relatives; employment, finance,* and *housing; legal problems; social isolation; bereavement;* and *other losses.*

4 **Is there psychiatric disorder?** This question is answered with information obtained from the history, from a brief but systematic examination of the mental state, and also from other informants and from medical notes.

5 **What are the patient's resources?** These include the capacity to solve problems, material resources, and the help that others may provide. The best guide to future ability to solve problems is the past record of dealing with difficulties such as the loss of a job, or a broken relationship. The availability of help should be assessed by asking about the patient's friends and relatives, and about support available from medical services, social workers, or voluntary agencies.

6 **Is treatment required and will the patient agree to it?** Management aims to:
- treat any psychiatric disorder;
- manage high suicide risk;
- enable the patient to *resolve difficulties* that led to the act of self-harm;
- *deal with future crises* without resorting to self-harm.

Of the patients referred to hospital for treatment of deliberate self-harm:

1 about one in ten need immediate inpatient psychiatric treatment, usually for a depressive disorder or alcohol dependency, or for a period of respite from overwhelming stressors;

2 about two-thirds need care from a psychiatric outpatient team or from the primary practitioner (but many do not accept this help);

3 about a quarter require no special treatment because their self-harm was a response to temporary difficulties and carried little risk of repetition.

Management

Underlying psychiatric disorder should be treated along usual guidelines. For patients who repeatedly self-harm, problem-solving techniques, dialectical behaviour therapy, and mindfulness-based CBT are helpful interventions.

When there are interpersonal problems, better outcomes are seen if there is a family component to treatment and multiple sessions are offered.

The results of treatment

Successful treatment of a depressive or other psychiatric disorder reduces the risk of subsequent self-harm. There is less strong evidence that problem-solving and other psychological methods reduce repetition, although they do reduce personal and social problems. This lack of strong evidence may be due, in part, to the methodological difficulties of randomized trials in this heterogeneous population. Particular types of psychological or social problem have been shown to benefit from specific treatments, such as couple therapy for problems between couples, problem-solving for practical and everyday difficulties, and CBT for long-standing personal difficulties.

Management of special groups

Certain subgroups of patients pose special management problems. In most cases, specialist advice should be obtained.

Mothers of young children. Because there is an association between deliberate self-harm and child abuse, it is important to ask any mother with young children about her feelings towards the children, and to enquire from other informants, as well as the patient, about their welfare. If there is a possibility of child abuse or neglect, appropriate assessment action should be carried out (see p. 192). There is also an association between depression and infanticide.

Children and adolescents. Deliberate self-harm is uncommon among young children, but becomes increasingly frequent after the age of 12, especially among girls. The most common method is drug overdosage; in only a few cases is there a threat to life. Self-injury also occurs, more often among boys than girls.

The motivation for self-harm in young children is difficult to determine, but it is more often to communicate distress or escape from stress than to die. Deliberate self-harm in children and adolescents is associated with unstable home environments, family psychiatric disorder, and child abuse. It is often precipitated by difficulties with parents, boyfriends or girlfriends, or schoolwork.

Most children and adolescents do not repeat an act of deliberate self-harm, but an important minority do so, usually in association with severe psychosocial problems. These repeated acts of deliberate self-harm carry a significant risk of suicide. Children or adolescents who harm themselves should be assessed by a child psychiatrist. Treatment is not only of the young person but also of the family.

Patients who refuse assessment and treatment

In most countries, there is a legal power to detain those who require potentially life-saving treatment and whose competence or capacity to take an informed decision about discharge is likely to be impaired by their mental state. The doctor should obtain as much information about mental state and suicidal risk as time allows. The patient should only be allowed to leave hospital when serious suicidal risk has been excluded (Box 9.8).

In taking decisions about emergency treatment, the doctor is likely to be helped by relatives, inpatient medical notes, and by telephoning the primary care doctor and any other doctor, social worker, or person

---

Box 9.8 Patients who harm themselves and refuse treatment

- There are wide differences in national procedures, practice, and legislation.
- The patient who has harmed himself and is alert and conscious should be presumed to be competent to refuse medical advice and treatment unless there is evidence to the contrary.
- The most senior experienced doctor available should be prepared to discuss the need for treatment, the alternatives, and the patient's anxieties. It is often appropriate to involve relatives. Calm, sympathetic discussion is often effective in enabling the patient to decide to consent to treatment.

- Capacity should be assessed (see p. 128), preferably by a psychiatrist.
- If the patient is competent and continues to refuse consent, the consequences should be clearly outlined to the patient and the discussion fully recorded. The patient should be allowed to go, but encouraged to return. Where possible, an alternative plan should be agreed with the patient and, if possible, relatives or friends. If the patient is assessed as being incompetent, then the reasons should be recorded fully. Emergency treatment should proceed and a compulsory order under mental health legislation should be sought.

who has been involved with the patient in the past. It is essential to write detailed notes and to be aware of the legal requirements about both emergency treatment and confidentiality.

Frequent repeaters. Some people take overdoses repeatedly, often at times of stress in circumstances that suggest that the behaviour is to reduce tension or gain attention. These people usually have a personality disorder and many insoluble social problems. Although sometimes directed towards gaining attention, repeated self-harm may cause relatives to become unsympathetic or hostile, and these feelings may be shared by professional staff as their repeated efforts at help are seen to fail. Usually, little can be done to change the pattern of behaviour. Neither counselling nor intensive psychotherapy is effective, and management is limited to providing support. Sometimes a change in life circumstances is followed by improvement, but unless this happens the risk of death by suicide is high.

Deliberate self-laceration. It is difficult to help people who lacerate themselves repeatedly. They often have low self-esteem and experience extreme tension. They also often have difficulty in recognizing feelings and expressing themselves in words. Efforts should be made to increase self-esteem and to find an alternative, simple way of relieving tension, for example, by taking exercise. Anxiolytic drugs are seldom helpful and may produce disinhibition.

Risk to others

The assessment of risk to others is an important part of clinical practice. It is, however, important to get the magnitude of the risk to others into perspective. Although several mental disorders are associated with increased risk of violence to others, the vast majority of violent crime is committed by people who are not mentally unwell. Furthermore, people with mental disorders are much more likely to be victims of crime than perpetrators.

Assessment of risk to others

Several psychiatric disorders are known to be associated with an increased risk of violence to others including:

- substance abuse: relative risk (RR) compared with general population 8;
- schizophrenia: RR approximately 5;
- bipolar disorder: RR approximately 5.

The risks associated with these disorders interact—thus the RR of schizophrenia with substance abuse co-morbidity is around 22.

Violence may result directly from the psychopathology of the disorder itself. For example, hallucinatory voices may command the patient to act in a specific way—which may be aggressive or homicidal. It may also arise from the combination of frustrations, difficulties, and disabilities that result from chronic mental disorder. Furthermore, there are a number of specific clinical situations which are known to be high risk in psychiatry including:

- morbid jealousy (see p. 308);
- misidentification syndromes;
- depressive disorder with suicidal ideation in mothers of small children;
- stalking.

The clinical prediction of risk to others has become a major focus of interest in recent years and extensive risk assessment tools have been developed. A commonly used example is the Psychopathy Checklist–Revised, which is used to measure psychopathic attributes and has reasonable predictive characteristics in some settings. The main difficulty with the general application of these tools to low-risk situations is that the performance remains limited and both the positive and negative predictive values of an assessment are low. This means that very few of those patients assessed as high risk will be violent, and most cases of violence will occur in those patients who are judged low risk. This is simply an epidemiological fact due to the limitations of the prediction and the low absolute risk of a violent event.

Nonetheless, there are two things always worth considering. First, it appears that *risk estimates are more accurate in the short term* and it is always worth considering the likelihood of immediate harm to others. Secondly, the *past is the best predictor of the future* and so patients with a past history of violence to others should be considered at relatively high risk of reoffending.

All assessments should be clearly recorded in the clinical notes.

Management of risk to others

The goal of managing risk to others is to do all that can be reasonably done to reduce the risk of harm. Psychiatric disorder should be diagnosed and treated, if necessary in hospital using compulsory detention. If there is clear evidence of harm to a particular person, consider warning them—this may mean compromising confidentiality.

Further reading

Useful general resources on suicide and deliberate-self harm

Mullen PE, Ogloff JRP. Assessing and managing the risks of violence towards others. In: Gelder MG, Andreasen NC, López-Ibor JJ, Geddes JR, eds. *New Oxford Textbook of Psychiatry*. 2nd ed. Oxford: Oxford University Press; 2012:1991–2002.

Samaritans. Suicide statistics report 2016: including data for 2012–2014. Published May 2016. https://www.samaritans.org/sites/default/files/kcfinder/files/Samaritans%20suicide%20statistics%20report%202016.pdf

Turecki G, Brent D. Suicide and suicidal behaviour. *The Lancet* 2016;387:1227–1239.

UK guidelines

National Institute for Health and Care Excellence. Self-harm in over 8s: long-term management. Clinical guideline [CG133]. Published November 2011. https://www.nice.org.uk/guidance/cg133.

National Institute for Health and Care Excellence. Self-harm in over 8s: short-term management and prevention of recurrence. Clinical guideline [CG16]. Published July 2004, updated November 2011. https://www.nice.org.uk/guidance/cg16/chapter/Update-information.

Royal College of Psychiatrists. Managing self-harm in young people (College Report CR192). Published October 2014. http://www.rcpsych.ac.uk/usefulresources/publications/collegereports/cr/cr192.aspx.

10 Communicating your findings

The first part of this chapter offers guidance on how to explain to patients and their carers the results of your assessment. The second part of this chapter offers guidance on communicating with other healthcare professionals, which is a vital part of modern healthcare: no longer can one nurse or one doctor, working in geographical and professional isolation, seek to deliver effective health interventions to a population. Instead, healthcare is delivered in complex systems, integrating primary, secondary, and tertiary care; different medical specialties; and different disciplines, such as doctors, nurses, psychologists, and occupational and physiotherapists.

Communicating with the patient and their relatives

Confidentiality

Interviewers should be aware of the ethical and legal principles that govern the giving of information to people other than the patient. These principles are summarized in Box 10.1. Sometimes a relative or another person telephones the interviewer to ask for information about the patient. In general, the patient should be told of the request, and asked whether or not they are happy to give their permission. The clinician should never allow a conspiratorial atmosphere to develop in which he or she conceals from the patient conversations with family, friends, or others.

Explaining the diagnosis and management plan

Patients and relatives need to know more than the diagnosis and the basic facts about treatment. It is useful to begin by finding out what they know already, and what help they are expecting. This information makes it easier to meet their requirements, help with their concerns, and explain the treatment plan. It is useful to keep in mind the list of frequently asked questions shown in Box 10.2. The management plan should be explained using the usual principles of patient communication such as:

- delivering information in an unhurried way;
- avoiding jargon;

Box 10.1 Ethical issues of confidentiality

General rule

Confidentiality is vital in psychiatry because patients often reveal highly personal information, and they need to know that it will be held and used in confidence, for their benefit. Doctors have a general duty to maintain confidentiality unless the patient gives informed consent to disclosure. In the UK, the General Medical Council (GMC, 2017) gives excellent guidance on this matter in 'Confidentiality: good practice in handling patient information', which is available to download online.

Exceptions to the rule

This general duty may be overridden in four circumstances:

* The patient consents, either implicitly (e.g. in relation to their own care) or explicitly
* The patient lacks the capacity to consent, and the disclosure is for their benefit
* The disclosure is in the public interest (e.g. serious crime, serious communicable disease)
* The disclosure is required by law or is permitted by law (e.g. in response to a court order)

Further details are given in the GMC guidance. Whenever an individual healthcare practitioner is uncertain about disclosure, they should consult the guidance and discuss within their own clinical team, and also consider discussion with their employer's Caldicott guardian and/or their own medicolegal representative.

Confidentiality and the treatment team

Psychiatric treatment often involves not only the interviewer but also other members of a treatment team. To do their job effectively, these members need at least a part of the information given by the patient to the interviewer. Interviewers should explain the need to share information and seek the patient's agreement to this way of working. The other members of the team must, of course, respect the confidence of the information. The sharing of information with other members of the team for the purpose of providing best treatment is not generally viewed by the law as a breach of confidence. Electronic patient records, and the increasing recognition that high-quality patient care requires prompt access to patient data across a distributed health service, present new challenges to the management of patient confidentiality.

Consent to obtaining further information

Generally, patients' consent should be obtained before eliciting information from other people. The exception to this rule is when patients who are unable to give an account of themselves are unable to give consent to seeking information from others, and the information requested would be considered to be in their best interests. The same considerations apply when information is given to relatives or others, concerning a patient who is unable to give consent. In such cases, where the patient lacks capacity, the professional and their team must always be guided by the best interests of the patient, and must think carefully about what those are.

* checking from time to time that the patient has understood;
* involving a relative/carer whenever possible and permitted by the patient;
* encouraging questions;
* summarizing the plan in writing (e.g. in a subsequent letter).

If, after a full discussion, the patient does not accept some part of the plan, or the relatives do not accept the role proposed for them, a compromise should be negotiated. It is now usual to copy the assessment letter to the patient, so that they have

a written record of what has been decided, and so that they can be more aware of their care and more active in it. Crucially, if this is the case, that letter needs to be written with the patient's understanding in mind.

Communicating with healthcare professionals

It is vital that every healthcare practitioner is able to *transmit* and *record* information about patients in a way that is understandable by others, and is equally able to *receive* information from others about shared patients. We would urge all trainee

Box 10.2 Communicating with patients and relatives

When giving information to patients and their relatives, it is useful to keep in mind relevant questions from the following list.

The diagnosis

- What is the diagnosis – if it is uncertain, what are the possibilities?
- Is further information or special investigation required?
- What may have caused the condition?
- What are the implications of the diagnosis for this patient's life?

The care plan

- What is the plan, and how far is it likely to help the patient and the family?
- What can the patient do to help themselves?
- What can the family do to help the patient?
- Can symptoms be monitored, to determine response to treatment and stay alert for early warning signs of relapse? If so, which symptoms, and how?
- What can health services do to help the patient?
- If medication is included:
  - What is its name, and why has it been chosen?
  - What is the dosage schedule?
  - What are the benefits, and when might they be seen?
  - What are the side effects, and will they settle down with time (e.g. Li^+ side effects at normal serum level)?

- Are there any possible toxic effects, and what should be done if they are noted (e.g. Li^+ toxic effects at high serum level)?
- Has the patient any concerns (e.g. that 'antidepressants are addictive'—they're not)?
- How long is the planned course of treatment?
- If psychological treatment is included:
  - What is involved, and who is involved?
  - How often will it take place, and how long will it last?
  - Where will it take place?
  - When will it start? If there is a waiting list, what can the patient do to cope/prepare, in the meantime?
  - When should improvement be expected?

Who does what?

- Will the GP carry out the treatment alone, or will another person be involved (e.g. practice nurse, consultant psychiatrist, member of community mental health team)?
- If others are involved, what is/are their role(s)? And how are they contactable?

Emergencies

- Are they likely, how can they be avoided, and if one occurs, what should be done?
- Are there possible warning signs of a crisis/relapse? If these emerge, what's the plan?
- Who should be approached in an emergency, and how can they be found urgently?

---

healthcare practitioners to focus considerable effort on developing their skills to communicate concisely, accurately, and clearly with their colleagues. This is an important area of research in fields where 'critical incidents' are potentially of high consequence, such as in aviation, the military, and healthcare. We would urge every reader to find out more by reading the influential article 'The human factor: the critical importance of effective teamwork and communication in providing safe care' (Leonard et al. 2004), in which it is stated that:

A large and ever present cultural barrier [to the delivery of high-quality, safe patient care] is the deeply embedded belief that quality of care and error free clinical performance are the result of being well trained and trying hard. In this paradigm, inevitable mistakes are viewed as episodes of personal failure, with the predictable result that these events are minimised and not openly discussed. Human factors science tells us that the inherent limitations of human memory, effects of stress and fatigue, the risks associated

with distractions and interruptions, and limited ability to multitask ensure that even skilled, experienced providers will make mistakes. As such, effective communication that creates a well understood plan of care greatly reduces the chances of inevitable errors becoming consequential and injuring patients.

Structure and content of the case presentation

Psychiatry is a medical specialty, and the presentation of the psychiatric assessment is structured in a similar way to that in medicine and surgery, with a brief **introduction** to set the context, followed by a description of the **history**, the **examination**, and any **investigations** carried out to date (Table 10.1). There are three important ways in which the presentation of the psychiatric assessment may differ from that seen elsewhere:

- First, the physical examination is supplemented by the mental examination or, as it is usually called, the *mental state examination* (MSE).

- Second, the most important investigation is to obtain a *corroborative history*, to corroborate the patient's report.

- Finally, some psychiatrists will present the background history *before* the history of the presenting complaints, which is the opposite of usual practice in medicine and surgery. This alternative approach may help the listener to understand the temporal relationship of events, as a more narrative approach is possible. Think of the assessment as moving through the distant past (background history), to the recent past (history of presenting problems), and finally to the present (mental and physical examination). The assessment therefore combines *longitudinal* data about the past (history) and *cross-sectional* data about the present (examination).

As you describe relevant features from your assessment, make sure that you mention them at the appropriate stage. For example, 'The patient suffered from a depressive episode about ten years ago ...' (*background history*: past psychiatric

Table 10.1 The presentation of the psychiatric assessment

Introduction

History
- Background
- Of presenting problems

Examination
- Mental state
- Physical

Investigations
- Corroborative history
- Near-patient tests
- Other investigations

Diagnosis
- Preferred psychiatric diagnosis
- Differential psychiatric diagnosis
- Relevant physical diagnoses
- Social problems
- Extent of functional impairment

Aetiology
- Predisposing factors
- Precipitating factors
- Perpetuating factors

Prognosis
- Short term
- Long term

Risks
- To self
- To others

Management
- Short term and long term
- General, physical, psychological, and social aspects

history), 'has suffered the onset of low mood and other depressive symptoms including hopelessness in recent weeks ...' (*history of presenting problems*), and 'appeared depressed today, and reported feeling hopeless with some thoughts of ending his life' (*mental state examination*: appearance and behaviour, mood, and thought content).

Diagnosis is considered next:

- First, the *preferred diagnosis* is presented, together with evidence for it and against it; clearly the former will outweigh the latter.

- Then *alternative mental diagnoses* are presented, again alongside evidence for and against each. To obtain a full, biopsychosocial, picture of the patient's clinical condition, several other aspects also need to be detailed. These include the presence, nature, and extent of any *physical disorder(s),* and the presence, nature, and extent of any *social problem(s).*

- Finally, the extent of *functional impairment* arising from physical, psychological, and social problems should be assessed, either using a formal scale such as the Global Assessment of Functioning, or by simply recording 'mild', 'moderate' or 'severe' functional impairment.

Do remember that the effective practice of medicine is about making decisions. In relation to diagnosis, the decisions are: (1) which diagnosis will you prioritize? (your preferred diagnosis); (2) which other diagnoses will you consider?; and (3) which diagnoses will you exclude as not even worthy of mentioning? Don't avoid making decisions by having a long list of possible diagnoses—one preferred and three or a maximum of four alternatives should be ample. If you are struggling with this, consider whether each possible diagnosis is (1) 'likely' vs 'not likely' and (2) 'important' vs 'not important'. If a possible diagnosis is neither likely nor important, then exclude it.

The order of the following elements of the assessment varies, depending on local traditions and preferences. There is no 'correct' order, but it is helpful to individual practitioners if they practise delivering summaries in a consistent way, and it is helpful for all members of the same mental health team to share the same approach.

Aetiology is described next, after diagnosis. Its division into predisposing, precipitating, and perpetuating factors has been addressed in Chapter 7. In order for the case presentation to be coherent, it is important that key conclusions about aetiology and, especially, about perpetuating factors, map onto and are echoed in the management plan.

Prognosis is described next, and has been described in Chapter 8. General comments should be included on prognosis in the short term (recovery from this episode) and longer term (risk of further episodes), alongside comments on what will impact prognosis, for better (e.g. adherence to medication, support from family members) or worse (e.g. further marital infidelity).

Risks are described next, and have been considered in Chapter 9. It is important to consider the full range of risks, including risks to self and others, and those risks that are very often relevant but are sometimes neglected, such as the risk of driving, occupational risks, or risks to dependents such as children or elderly relatives.

Finally, **management** is described. The management of particular disorders is described in subsequent chapters on clinical syndromes. The management plan should address the required:

- *General* aspects of treatment, such as inpatient or outpatient care; support from family, or support from specific professionals; symptom monitoring, and actions to take if there are signs of relapse or in an emergency.

- *Physical* aspects of treatment, such as abstinence from alcohol and illicit drugs; medicines such as antidepressants; exercise; and specific treatments such as ECT.

- *Psychological* aspects of treatment, such as educating the patient and their relative(s) about their illness and how to manage it; self-help psychological treatments; and formal psychological treatments such as CBT, and how such treatments might be delivered (e.g. individual or group).

- *Social* aspects of treatment, such as a phased return to work, with consultation with the employer's occupational health department; involvement in voluntary activities that can help to restore a sense of worth and purpose; or day hospital attendance that can help to bring structure to the patient's day.

The management plan should also consider *short-term* aspects of treatment, which are usually those focused on achieving remission and subsequently recovery from the current episode, and *longer-term* aspects of treatment, which are focused on maintaining recovery and reducing the likelihood of recurrence.

Flexibility in your case presentation

Psychiatric assessment can involve the collection and integration of a great deal of information. It is rarely appropriate to present all of this information to colleagues. We would urge readers to be able to deliver several different levels of case presentation, depending on the circumstances, as follows:

Long case presentation. Occasionally, it is helpful to present the bulk of the information that is known about a particular patient. However, this is a lengthy process, taking perhaps 15 minutes. There must therefore be a clear rationale for it, such as when a patient has not responded to treatment after some time, and the case is being thoroughly reviewed to determine whether an important factor has been missed. Even then, prioritization will be important.

Short case presentation. This is the usual way in which a case will be presented. The results of the assessment are summarized, in a standardized way, so that they can be presented in less than 5 minutes. An example is shown in Box 10.3. This approach is often called '*formulation*', but we are not keen on this term, because it is not in common use outside mental health settings, and may therefore mystify observers of psychiatric practice in a way that is unnecessary and unhelpful.

Brief summary. This is a very brief summary of a case, taking 1 minute or less, presenting only the most salient features, and often focused on key problems. This is commonly used when introducing a patient on a ward round, for example, so that all those in attendance are aware of the context, are orientated to the case, and can contribute appropriately. A brief summary before each patient is discussed is a courteous, considerate, and helpful approach when students are present.

Prioritizing. In our experience, students are often very good at collecting large quantities of information and presenting it in an organized and coherent way. However, they are often less good at cutting down that information such that it is usable in ordinary clinical practice. It is vital to practise prioritizing the information that you have: making decisions about what is 'essential' to understanding a case, what is 'important' to understanding a case, and what is 'interesting' but probably not important. This is the same type of process as reducing a very large number of diagnostic possibilities to only three or four—at each stage, there are advantages (increasing focus) and disadvantages (possibility of eliminating the 'real' diagnosis) associated with reducing the size of the list. It is only through practice that you will be able to do this.

Helping the listener to hear what you're saying

It is easy to think that presenting is the hard part, and that listening is easy. However, effective listening is easy only if the presenter helps. The following techniques can be used by the presenter:

- **Pace yourself.** When anxious, or when there is a lot to present, most presenters will speed up, so that they become more difficult to hear, more difficult to follow, and more difficult to understand. Quicker isn't necessarily better! A more measured, considered pace allows the listener to keep up, and to consider the information presented.

- **Use pauses as punctuation.** In written communication, we use commas, full stops, and paragraph breaks to indicate the beginning and end of clauses and sentences, and to provide emphasis. In verbal communication, these cues are absent and, instead, verbal and non-verbal cues must be deployed. A powerful cue is the pause. It alerts the listener to a change, and arouses their interest. A pause can be particularly powerful when used just before a signpost.

- **Signpost.** This is exactly what it says on the tin— a verbal signpost to what is coming next. So, for example, the presenter finishes talking about the findings on examination, pauses for a second or

Box 10.3 Example of a short case presentation

Mrs AB is a 30-year-old married woman who has been feeling increasingly depressed for 6 weeks and is now unable to cope adequately with the care of her children.

Regarding **diagnosis**, my *preferred diagnosis* is of a depressive episode, of moderate severity. Mrs AB has several typical symptoms of a depressive episode: she wakes unusually early, feels worse in the morning than in the evening, and has lost her appetite and libido. She blames herself unreasonably, feels guilty, and does not think that she can recover, though she has no ideas of suicide or of harming the children. Her functioning is impaired to a moderate degree. None of the findings are incompatible with this diagnosis.

There are three *other diagnoses* that I have considered but excluded at this stage.

The first is adjustment disorder. Although Mrs AB has experienced several stressful events, including her husband's recent infidelity, the presence of clear symptoms of a depressive disorder and their duration overrule the diagnosis of adjustment disorder.

The second is personality disorder. There is no evidence for personality disorder. Mrs AB is normally a resilient, caring, and sociable person who is a good mother.

The third is physical disorder. Mrs AB has no significant past medical history, and there are no new physical symptoms on systematic enquiry.

Regarding **aetiology**, although she has not been depressed before, both her mother and sister have had depressive disorders, so it is possible that she is *predisposed* to develop a depressive disorder. The symptoms were *precipitated* by her husband's infidelity. The disorder may be *maintained* by continuing quarrels with her husband, concerns about her mother's health, and active negative cognitive biases.

Regarding **risk**, suicide risk and risk of harm to the children are currently both low, but need monitoring.

Regarding **prognosis**, provided that the marital problems and her mother's health improve, Mrs AB should recover. The possible predisposing factors indicate that she may develop further depressive disorder.

Regarding **management**, Mrs AB does not currently need inpatient care, but her mental state will need monitoring by the primary care team, especially with a view to risk of suicide. Her sister has offered to provide short-term help with the care of the children and Mrs AB is normally a good mother and should be able to take full care of her children when her condition improves. An SSRI antidepressant is appropriate. SSRIs occasionally cause increased agitation during the first few days of treatment, and Mrs AB will need to be warned of this, and of other common side effects. To prevent relapse, medication should be continued for about 6 months and, again, it is important that Mrs AB is aware of this. Her husband regrets his infidelity and is now supportive. If problems continue in their relationship, marital counselling through Relate or a similar organization will be appropriate. This management plan should be reviewed in 1 week, and regularly thereafter.

two to alert the listener, and says 'on investigation', to orientate them to what is about to be said.

- **Summarize.** It's easy to get bogged down in a wealth of detail. Summarize whenever possible—the listener can always ask for more detail or for clarification. So, for example, rather than reading a long list of individual biological symptoms of depression, simply state that the patient reported several biological symptoms.

- **Think rather than read.** Case presentations generally make sense when we are forced to think about what we are saying, rather than reading what we are saying. In other words, don't focus on the patient's case notes or your presentation notes; instead, think about your *key messages*, and refer to your notes for clarification only if needed.

- **Attend to your listeners.** Look up rather than down, and look at them in turn. If you are presenting in front of the patient, be sure to attend to the patient as well, especially when relating particularly sensitive or emotional aspects of their case; show that you are on their side, and that you understand their predicament.

- **Have an obvious ending.** It can be unclear when someone has finished talking. Avoid this uncertainty by making it clear, with non-verbal and verbal cues.

Communicating in writing with healthcare professionals

Communication is either *verbal* (such as on ward rounds, or on the telephone) or *written* (such as referral letters, assessment letters, psychiatric notes, or general hospital notes). In each of these situations, a problem list can be helpful for prioritizing care and facilitating communication.

Problem lists

A problem list is a useful way of summarizing any case other than the very simplest. It is particularly useful in cases with both medical and psychiatric aspects, and is therefore suitable for use in primary care and in general hospital medical practice. The problem list makes the active problems and components of management clear to anyone who sees the patient when their usual healthcare professional is not available.

A summary of a case is shown in Case study box 10.1, together with its associated problem list. Importantly, the problem list also incorporates a list of what will be done, and by whom, and when the status of that problem will be reviewed.

Letters of referral to psychiatrists

A referral letter should make it clear to the recipient why the patient is being referred, and how the referrer would like to be helped by this referral. For example, 'The patient's depressive illness has not responded to citalopram 20 mg, rising to 40 mg daily, despite good compliance during a period of 6 weeks, and I would welcome your advice on further pharmacological management'. The letter should be concise, but should also include as a minimum:

- the *course and development* of the disorder, with the dates at which problems began or changed;
- the *mental state* at the time of writing;
- any *behaviour or problem that may be concealed or denied* by the patient when interviewed by the psychiatrist (e.g. excessive use of alcohol, bingeing/vomiting/laxative abuse) or not recognized by the patient (e.g. lapses of memory);
- relevant points in the *medical history,* and current *medications*;
- details of any *treatment*, together with a note of the therapeutic response and side effects;

CASE STUDY BOX 10.1

Making a problem list

A 54-year-old woman consulted her GP because of mixed anxiety and depressive symptoms. The diagnosis was depressive disorder, and the immediate cause appeared to be the stress of caring for her elderly, debilitated mother (also the GP's patient), whose condition had worsened in the last 2 months. Important contributory factors were menorrhagia and chronic agoraphobia, which prevented the patient from visiting friends and relatives. The immediate plan was to treat the patient's depressive disorder with an SSRI, and to obtain respite care for her mother. In the longer term, the agoraphobia would be treated with behaviour therapy, and a gynaecological opinion would be obtained about the menorrhagia.

Problem list

Problem	Action	Agent	Review
Anxiety and depression	Citalopram 20 mg (an SSRI) in the morning	GP	Check response weekly for 3 weeks then review
Caring for elderly mother	Obtain respite care for mother	Geriatrician/ elderly care social worker	3 weeks
Chronic agoraphobia	Behaviour therapy	Clinical psychologist	3 months
Menorrhagia	Gynaecological opinion	GP	1 month

- *family relationships*, including marital problems and difficulties between parents and children;
- *personality* as known to the referring doctor from previous contacts with the patient.

Assessment letters from psychiatrists

It is important that assessment letters from mental health professionals to non-specialists:

- are *brief*;
- *focus* on the issues that triggered the referral or presentation;
- *avoid psychiatric jargon*, unless it is explained;
- *make it clear what treatment is proposed*, and who will be responsible for delivering that treatment;
- *make it clear if and when the patient will be seen again* by psychiatric services, and for what purpose.

Unfortunately, assessment letters are often used not only to *communicate* with the referrer, but also to *record* the much more extensive information that forms the background history, history of presenting complaint, and examination. While this may assist the person who has conducted the assessment, it is rarely helpful either to the referrer or to the patient: the more copious the information included, the more likely is the 'action list' for the referring doctor and the patient to be lost or ignored. *Less is more!*

Finally, many such letters are now routinely copied to the patient and they should, therefore, be written with the patient in mind.

Recording in psychiatric case notes

Good case notes are important in psychiatry, as in other branches of medicine, for both clinical and medicolegal reasons. Case notes are not only an aide-memoire for the writer but are also an essential source of information for any other person called to help the patient in an emergency. The results of the assessment

and the progress notes should be recorded with this purpose in mind. Since patients may ask to read their notes, any information that informants have refused to make available to the patient should be recorded distinctly and separately.

A **life chart** can be a useful way of summarizing information in the case notes, which are often unwieldy in patients with long histories of mental disorder. A life chart summarizes life events, both 'good' and 'bad', alongside the occurrence of episodes of medical and psychiatric illness. The chart has five columns: the year, patient's age, life events, physical illness, and psychiatric disorder. The example in Table 10.2 is of a woman with a depressive disorder. She has had two episodes of emotional disorder in childhood (bed-wetting and school refusal), a third at the age of 18 (adjustment disorder), and a depressive disorder at age 34. The chart shows that the episodes of emotional disturbance were related in time to separations (starting school and going to university) and loss (the deaths of her grandmother and mother). The present illness is related in time to the death of her husband. None of the episodes were related to physical illness or childbirth.

Recording in general hospital case notes

When patients on general hospital wards are seen by mental health professionals, it is important that written communication in the notes has the same characteristics as assessment letters to non-specialists (mentioned previously) and, in addition:

- is, whenever possible, supplemented by a conversation with the person who made the referral to psychiatric services;
- is 'topped' by a clear heading indicating that this is a summary of a mental health assessment;
- is 'tailed' by a clear record of the name, status, and contact details of the person who has conducted the assessment, so that the general hospital team can make contact again should the need arise.

Table 10.2 Example of a life chart

Year	Age (years)	Events	Physical illness	Psychiatric illness
1967	Born			
1968	1			
1969	2			
1970	3			
1971	4			
1972	5	Started school	Bed-wetting	
1973	6			
1974	7			
1975	8			
1976	9			
1977	10	Grandmother died		School refusal
1978	11			
1979	12			
1980	13	Father's illness	Unexplained abdominal pain	
1981	14			
1982	15			
1983	16			
1984	17			
1985	18	Started at university		Adjustment disorder
1986	19			
1987	20			
1988	21			
1989	22	Married		
1990	23			

Table 10.2 Continued

Year	Age (years)	Events	Physical illness	Psychiatric illness
1991	24	First child born		
1992	25			
1993	26	Second child born		
1994	27			
1995	28			
1996	29		Cone biopsy	
1997	30			
1998	31			
1999	32			
2000	33			
2001	34	Mother died		Depressive episode
2002	35			
2003	36	Intestinal obstruction		
2004	37			
2005	38			
2006	39	Husband's illness		Depressive episode
2007	40			
2008	41	Son started university		Depressive episode
2009	42			
	43			
2010	44	Husband died		Adjustment disorder
2011	45			Depressive episode

Further reading

Leonard M, Graham S, Bonacum D. The human factor: the critical importance of effective teamwork and communication in providing safe care. *Quality & Safety in Health Care* 2004;13(Suppl 1):i85–i90.

Part 3 Management

3 Management

11 General aspects of care: settings of care

Current mental healthcare services in most of the developed world are unrecognizable compared with those of the mid twentieth century. There has been a major shift from long-term institutional to community care. This chapter describes current approaches to providing mental health services, particularly for people between the ages of 18 and 65 (services for children are discussed in Chapter 17, and services for the elderly in Chapter 18). It is important for all doctors to have a basic understanding of the structure of services for three main reasons:

1 It will help you to get the most out of clinical rotations in psychiatry, either at undergraduate or postgraduate level.

2 All clinicians need to know when and how to refer their patient to appropriate services.

3 Patients being treated by other medical specialties may have psychiatric co-morbidities. Effective management and liaison with mental health services requires a working knowledge of common conditions and their treatment.

Mental health services are organized in different ways from country to country. This chapter describes mainly the provision of services in the UK, but the principles apply generally.

Epidemiology: the need for mental healthcare services

To understand the range of psychiatric services that are required for a specific community it is necessary to know:

1 the frequency of mental disorders in the population;

2 the severity of these conditions and the impact they have upon a person's ability to function;

3 how patients with these disorders come into contact with the health services;

4 what type of services people engage with and find effective.

The local prevalence of mental disorders will vary, but approximate estimates can be obtained from national surveys (Table 11.1). Approximately 20 per cent of adults and 10 per cent of children experience a mental health problem in any given year.

Table 11.1 Epidemiology of mental disorders in the USA

Condition	Prevalence (% population)
Any mental health disorder	18.1
All mood disorders	9.5
Unipolar depression	6.7
Post-traumatic stress disorder	3.5
Anorexia nervosa	0.6 (females)
Bipolar disorder	2.6
Schizophrenia	1.1
Obsessive–compulsive disorder	1.0
ADHD	4.1
Autism	0.01
Alzheimer's disease	10% of over-65s
Any personality disorder	9.1

Source data from the US National Institute for Mental Health (2014), www.nimh.nih.org.

A more detailed discussion of the epidemiology of mental health as a whole can be found in Chapter 2, p. 5, and for specific disorders in their individual chapters.

The principles of providing mental healthcare

The basic principles of the provision of mental health services are the same as for any other health service. Services should be accessible, comprehensive, appropriate to the needs of the community, offer up-to-date treatments, effective, and economical. Patients should be offered a choice in the treatment they receive, although the caveat to this is when an individual is being treated under the Mental Health Act.

What makes mentally ill people seek help?

Not everyone with a psychiatric disorder seeks medical advice. Some people with minor emotional reactions to stress obtain help from family and friends, religious groups, or voluntary agencies. Online message boards and chat sites have become a huge source of support for many people with mental illness. The majority of people with problems of substance abuse do not seek help of any kind. Nevertheless, in the UK, about nine in ten people with a mental disorder attend a GP, although many do not complain directly of psychological symptoms. Whether a person with *clinically significant psychiatric disorder* consults a GP depends on several factors (Box 11.1). Mental disorders are stigmatized and poorly understood in society.

It is commonly believed that patients are more likely to make use of, and to benefit from, services that take fully into account the views of those who use them. For this reason, patients are encouraged to be involved in all stages of service development.

Box 11.1 Factors influencing a person's decision to seek medical advice

- Severity and duration of the disorder
- The person's attitude to psychiatric disorder—some people feel ashamed and embarrassed to ask for help
- Attitudes and knowledge of family and friends
- The person's knowledge about possible help—if he does not know that help can be provided, he may not seek it
- The person's perception of the doctor's attitude to psychiatric disorder—if the doctor is viewed as unsympathetic, the person is less likely to ask for help
- The person's previous experiences of mental healthcare services
- Financial issues (this is more or less relevant, depending on the type of healthcare system in a particular country)

The structure of mental healthcare services

A very simplified example diagram of the structure of services is shown in Fig. 11.1. The majority of patients seen in secondary care psychiatric services are referred from primary care, although a few may be seen as emergencies or referrals from other specialties. Only about 50 per cent of those presenting to primary care with psychiatric symptoms need any intervention and many fewer a referral to mental health services.

The role of primary care

Although in the UK primary care is very separate from secondary services, it is an essential part of psychiatric service provision. GPs detect most mental illness, treat the majority of patients without the need for specialist input, and if referrals are made, act as a liaison between different agencies.

Many patients presenting to primary care with psychological or somatic manifestations of mental disorder are suffering from anxiety and/or depression. Identifying these patients effectively involves:

1 always considering the *possibility of mental disorder* in consultations;

2 having good *interviewing skills*. The key skills are the ability to gain the patient's confidence and the ability to identify any psychological factors that are contributing to physical symptoms.

GPs can improve their ability to detect common psychiatric disorders, by using screening questions or questionnaires, for example, the two-question screening for depression, or the SCOFF questions for eating disorders.

Once a psychiatric disorder has been identified, it is usually treated by GPs themselves. This includes most adjustment, anxiety, and less severe mood disorders. GPs refer about 5–10 per cent of patients with psychiatric disorders to secondary care, especially those with severe mood disorders, psychosis, eating disorders, and other disorders when severe and persistent. The decision to refer to a psychiatrist is determined by several factors (Box 11.2). In the UK, the common point of referral for the majority of psychiatric diagnoses is the **community mental health team (CMHT)**.

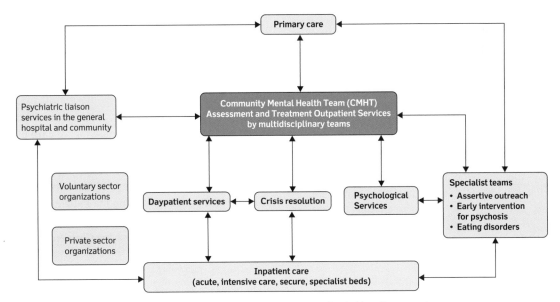

Fig. 11.1 A simplified structure of mental healthcare services in a state-funded healthcare system.

Box 11.2 Factors influencing a general practitioner's decision to refer to the specialist psychiatric services

- Uncertainty about diagnosis
- Failure to respond to treatment in primary care
- Severe condition needing hospital admission
- Safety of the patient, family, and community
- Need for treatment that is unavailable in primary care
- Willingness of the patient to see a psychiatrist
- Accessibility of psychiatric services, how far the patient has to travel, and how promptly patients are seen by the psychiatrist
- Local or national guidelines regarding referrals

In the UK, almost all GP surgeries now have access to counsellors and/or clinical psychologists. This has allowed basic psychological therapies (e.g. CBT for depression or obsessive–compulsive disorder, bereavement counselling) to be delivered in primary care. Polyclinics or **community mental health clinics**, which are centres in which several GP surgeries pool their mental health resources, are becoming an increasing source of treatment in the community.

Specialist mental healthcare services

Psychiatric disorders vary substantially in severity and services must take this into account. Many countries (especially those with state-funded or nationalized healthcare) have adopted a tiered system with a common entry for assessment. The aim is to provide the least intense treatment appropriate for the patient, focusing on community care. A good summary of historical changes in mental health service provision can be found under 'Further reading'. The main components of adult psychiatric services are seen in Fig. 11.1.

Community mental health teams

The CMHT model was developed with the following aims:

1 To provide a single point of referral for primary care or referrals from hospital specialties.

2 To avoid unnecessary admission to hospital by providing intensive treatments in the community.

3 To include a multidisciplinary team, providing a coordinated care package for each patient.

4 To provide services as close as possible to the patient's home.

5 To provide continuity of care for patients with chronic psychiatric disorders.

In the UK, a CMHT usually covers a geographical area including 20,000–50,000 people, of whom 200–250 will be on the caseload at any given time. The multidisciplinary team typically consists of 12–20 people, including psychiatrists, clinical psychologists, social workers, mental health nurses, and occupational therapists (Table 11.2). The CMHT is often split into a team whose role it is to assess new patients and undertake short-term interventions and a 'treatment' team who look after longer-term patients.

It is usual for a routine referral to be assessed within 4 weeks, an urgent referral within 1 week, and an emergency to be seen the same day.

The model of community care favoured in the UK is **case management**. For every patient, a **care coordinator** is identified, who may be any member of the multidisciplinary team but is most frequently a community psychiatric nurse. It is their responsibility to make sure that the patient's needs are met and clinical status is regularly assessed. When a patient is initially referred to the service, a psychiatrist will assess them. They will make a diagnosis, discuss the case with the team, and together decide on the best form of management. A formal **care plan** is then drawn up, in which members of the team are assigned specific tasks to carry out. An example of a care plan is shown in Box 11.3: this is distributed to all concerned parties, including the patient and their GP. The team meet regularly and review the care plan. This way of working is known as the **Care Programme Approach (CPA)**.

The key to the CMHT approach is *effective collaboration between all those involved in care*. Team members should communicate effectively with each other and with the patients, relatives, carers, and third parties, such as social services or the GP. One major

Table 11.2 Mental health professionals in a community mental health team

Profession	Role
Psychiatrist	The clinical leader with responsibility for psychiatric assessments, treatment, and Mental Health Act work. May be involved in outpatient, inpatient, and/or day patient care. Supervises junior psychiatrists and may have teaching roles
Community psychiatric nurse (CPN)	Acts as care coordinator for patients with chronic mental disorders, monitors medication and side effects, and provides some psychological treatments
Clinical psychologist	Performs psychological assessments and provides a full range of psychological treatments
Occupational therapist	Performs functional assessments, provides social skills training, some psychological treatments, and assists the patient in finding employment
Social worker	Performs social and Mental Health Act assessments and assists the patient in meeting accommodation and financial needs. May also provide some psychological treatments

Box 11.3 An example Care Programme Approach Review

Name of patient: John Smith

Address: 42 West Street

CMHT: North East City

Diagnoses: 1. Bipolar disorder I

2. ....

GP: Dr Robinson

Mobile number: 0000000000

Care coordinator: Jane (social worker)

Team members present at meeting: Dr Brown, Sarah (CPN), Katie, Jane, Martin, and two medical students.

Problem	Intervention	Team member allocation
1. Mania	• Take regular medications (olanzapine and lithium) • Attend outpatient appointments • Be at home when team members visit	Dr Brown (psychiatrist)
2. Too much spare time	• Activity planning • Attend day centre • When stable, look for a part-time course in photography	Sarah (CPN) Katie (occupational therapist)
3. Fighting with family	• Attend early intervention training course with parents • Phone daughter's mother weekly	Dr Brown to organize Sarah (CPN)
4. Money	• Complete and send off social benefit forms • Complete free school meals form for daughter	Jane (social worker)
5. Avoiding relapse	• Medication adherence • Attend CBT for bipolar disorder • When stable, attend local support group • Phone Jane when feeling unwell	Martin (psychologist)

Risks considered? Yes—self neglect

Date of next review: 01/06/2019 at 4 pm

Signature of care coordinator:

Signature of patient:

advantage of this approach is that as a patient moves between care settings (e.g. outpatient clinic to inpatient), the care coordinator remains the same.

Outpatient clinics

Psychiatric outpatient clinics are an efficient way of providing psychiatric assessment and treatment. They provide the majority of specialist mental healthcare services; most patients do not need more intensive treatment. They are suitable for stable patients, or those whose mental illness is not severe enough to put themselves or others in danger. Patients are typically seen by a psychiatrist, CPN, or psychologist. The frequency of appointments is variable; CBT is usually delivered weekly by clinical psychologists, but a psychiatrist reviewing a stable patient may only see them every 3 months.

Day hospitals

Day hospitals—called **partial hospitalization** in some countries—provide a step between the outpatient clinic and inpatient care. They usually run 5 days a week, from 8 am–4 pm (or equivalent), but there has been a move to provide evening sessions (6–10 pm) to cater for those in education or employment. Day hospitals are usually based in a psychiatric hospital, and provide treatment for patients who need intensive care but can sleep safely at home. An example might be of a patient whose depression has not responded to an antidepressant and outpatient CBT, is not suicidal, but is struggling to motivate themselves to do daytime activities. Day hospitals provide supervised drug treatment, a range of psychological treatments (in group and individual formats), occupational therapy, art/music therapy, and support from peers (Table 11.3). Day treatment is suitable for patients with mood disorders, psychosis, anxiety disorders, dementia, and personality disorders. Eating disorders lend themselves particularly well to day treatment, but this is usually delivered in a specialist unit. Day hospitals can shorten the length of inpatient stay or avoid admission altogether for some patients.

Table 11.3 An example of a mood disorders day hospital timetable

Time	Activity
8.45–9.30	Arrival and morning review group
	(Group discussion of how their evening/weekend went)
9.30–10.30	Therapy group
	(e.g. CBT for mood disorders, art therapy, creative writing)
10.30–11.00	Coffee break and free time
11.00–12.00	Individual therapy
12.00–13.00	Lunch and free time
13.00–14.00	Community group
	(Discussion of issues pertaining to life in the group)
14.00–15.00 Tues–Fri	Therapy group
15.00–16.00	Evening planning and home
14.00–17.00 Mondays only	Ward round, CPA reviews 20–30-minute slots per patient

Crisis resolution

The crisis resolution (or **home treatment**) team aim to provide a rapid response and accessibility to intensive psychiatric services. Their aim is to keep patients who would otherwise be admitted to hospital in the community. The team usually consists of specially trained community psychiatric nurses, social workers, and, occasionally, psychiatrists. The team aim to see all the referrals within 24 hours. They have a small number of patients at a time, visiting each one to three times daily, and providing 24-hour phone support for the patient and their family. The crisis team is particularly useful for patients with severe mood depression, anxiety disorders, or schizophrenia. An adolescent version focusing on managing eating disorders in the community has been very successful.

Assertive outreach

Assertive outreach (called **assertive community treatment** or **intensive case management** in some countries) is another method of reducing hospitalization, but has been designed especially for patients with chronic psychoses. It focuses on those patients who are difficult to engage, non-compliant with medications, and have frequent relapses. The service works on a proactive basis—they do not wait for patients to attend appointments but visit them at home regularly, trying to enhance motivation and compliance with treatment. Community psychiatric nurses and social workers take the main role, not only doing home visits but also taking patients out shopping, to the cinema, to job interviews, or to GP appointments. Various meta-analyses have demonstrated these services to be clinically and economically effective (see 'Further reading').

Inpatient facilities

Although every effort has been made to treat as many patients in the community as possible, there are situations where hospitalization is the safest option. All specialist psychiatric services require an inpatient unit, capable of treating patients with severe mental disorders (voluntarily or involuntarily), and able to admit patients promptly in an emergency. Admission to hospital is needed when:

- patients need a level of assessment that cannot be provided elsewhere;
- patients need a treatment only available in hospital;
- patients have insufficient social support;
- patients might put themselves or other people at risk;
- arrangements for care outside hospital break down.

Psychiatric inpatient units may be grouped together in a single psychiatric hospital or be accommodated in general hospitals. Units in specialist hospitals have the advantage that a wider range of treatments can be made available (e.g. specialized occupational and rehabilitation facilities). Units in a general hospital have the advantages of reduced stigma, early liaison with other specialties, and, usually, closeness to the patient's home. There are four main types of adult inpatient wards in most countries:

1 **Acute psychiatric wards.** These are the mainstay of inpatient beds, and provide short-term care for conditions such as acute psychosis, mania, and severe depression with suicidal intent. They provide 24-hour nursing care and observation (Box 11.4), and typically run a therapeutic

Box 11.4 Levels of observation on a psychiatric ward

Observations refer to the level of monitoring that patients receive on a psychiatric ward, and are usually undertaken by nursing staff. They are designed to keep each patient safe, preventing primarily self-harm and suicide attempts, but also aggressive or disruptive behaviour. Observations can be individually tailored—for example, to help reduce behaviours such as vomiting after meals in bulimia nervosa or hand washing in obsessive–compulsive disorder. A decision will be made during the admission assessment or interview as to which level to start at, and this will be regularly reviewed (often daily) by staff.

Level	Frequency of observation
1	Constant observation: within sight and constant close proximity to staff at all times
	'At arm's length'
2	Constant observation: within sight of staff at all times
3	Observations at defined time intervals
	Typically 15 minutes, but can be 5, 10, or 30 minutes
4	Hourly observations

programme similar to that in day hospitals, but full-time. The average inpatient stay in the UK is 6 weeks but in the USA it is only 8 days. Patients may be admitted under mental health legislation or be there voluntarily.

2 **Psychiatric intensive care units.** These are low-security units, or locked sections of the general psychiatric hospital, usually only catering for a few patients at a time. They have one-to-one nursing and manage acutely disturbed patients under the mental health act who cannot be safely treated on an open ward.

3 **Specialist inpatient units.** These provide specialist care for particular conditions—the majority cater for alcohol/drug problems or eating disorders. The advantage of these wards is that they have a specialist team who intensely focus on the behavioural problems that the patients have, away from the challenging environment of the acute psychiatric ward. In set-up they are similar to acute wards, with 24-hour nursing care and highly structured timetables providing therapy and activities.

4 **Medium- and high-secure units.** These provide a secure environment for the treatment of patients with mental disorders who have committed crimes and/or are deemed to be a danger to the public. Patients are admitted from prisons, the courts, or less secure units. High-security hospitals usually treat patients indefinitely, but the medium-secure units aim to rehabilitate the patient to move back into the community in a number of years.

In the past, patients often remained in inpatient units long after the acute stage of illness had passed; when recovery was incomplete, some patients remained for many years. Now patients with residual problems are usually discharged from hospital for continuing community care. The advantage of remaining in hospital ('asylum') is easier provision of accommodation, treatment, rehabilitation, and protection; the disadvantage of a prolonged stay in hospital can be the extra handicap of institutionalization. If community care can meet patients' needs it is generally preferred by patients and their carers. However, when patients are discharged from hospital without adequate provision for their needs for accommodation and treatment, community care can be worse for the patient than long-term care in hospital. The **stepped model of care** is used to try and safeguard against this happening. For patients who have received intense treatments (i.e. inpatient or day-patient care), they are stepped down to the next level prior to discharge. Typically, a patient will be discharged from the ward, but attend the day hospital for some time. For patients being treated in units a long way from home, or who do not have access to a day hospital, periods of leave are granted while still an inpatient.

Early intervention

It is well recognized that early intervention and treatment of patients with psychosis improve outcome. Early intervention teams have three main roles:

1 To identify and monitor high-risk patients.

2 To raise awareness of psychoses in the wider community.

3 Ongoing patient care.

Frequently, early intervention and family education can avoid hospital admission and reduce the morbidity associated with psychosis.

Liaison with other medical services

Liaison psychiatry (or **consultation psychiatry**) is the specialty of treating mental health disorders in the general hospital population. This includes pre-existing psychiatric conditions and new diagnoses which may be related to physical health problems. The role of the liaison service is to:

● assess patients with new psychiatric symptoms;

● manage pre-existing mental health problems;

- manage behavioural disturbance;

- provide advice on treatments, especially medications;

- assess and manage patients presenting with deliberate self-harm;

- assist with management of patients under the care of the mental health teams, but who need treatment in the general hospital;

- provide a link between the acute hospital and the CMHT.

As well as the dedicated liaison service, there are other links to medical specialties which are essential to providing a comprehensive mental health service. A good example is the link between an eating disorders unit and the local gastroenterology/acute medical department. Patients may need admission for hypokalaemia, dehydration, or nasogastric feeding.

Culturally specific approaches to treatment

It is important to recognize that patients from varying cultural and religious groups have markedly different beliefs surrounding mental illness. In many cultures, mental illness as an entity is not recognized, and this can make cooperation with treatment (especially from the wider family and community) very challenging. Specialist help may be needed to overcome problems of denial, and a patient advocate or professional with knowledge of the relevant culture can be an invaluable member of the team. Specialist interpreters should be used to ensure a full history is obtained. Many people of African origin rarely experience the typical psychological symptoms of depression or anxiety, instead presenting with somatic symptoms (e.g. pain). Always keep an open mind.

There are situations where patients, especially women, may not be free to visit a doctor or attend appointments without their family (usually husband) present. This can make regular follow-up and patient confidentiality very difficult. It is usually necessary for these patients to be visited at home, with appropriately trained staff present.

Some treatments are more efficacious in particular ethnic groups, and psychiatrists should be aware of that. Large, randomized controlled trials (RCTs) of medications frequently include a subgroup analysis of efficacy in different ethnic groups; for example, it has been reported that antipsychotics for psychosis are more effective in black Africans than in Caucasian males. Psychological therapies are also more effective in some cultures, but this seems to have more to do with acceptance of mental illness than inherent physiological differences.

The role of the voluntary and private sectors

In most countries, there are voluntary organizations that provide a variety of services for those with mental health problems. Some examples include:

- Alcoholics Anonymous;

- Cruse (a UK charity providing bereavement counselling and services);

- Mind (a UK national mental health charity providing accommodation, employment, and advice);

- Relate (provides marriage guidance counselling);

- National Alliance for Mental Health (USA);

- Malaysian Mental Health Foundation (Malaysia).

In a state-funded health service, there are always limitations on the care that can be provided. In the UK, there is a growing private sector providing specialist treatment for most psychiatric conditions, and in many countries all care is accessible only by those with insurance or capital. This includes office-based outpatient psychiatrists and psychologists, and day/inpatient units. The private sector also targets those areas which have been less provided for by national services, for example, adolescent inpatient care, eating disorders, and alcohol and drug problems.

Accommodation and employment

The vast majority of those with a mental health disorder live with their families, in owned or rented accommodation, and can care for themselves. However, some others need more help, and can benefit from specialized accommodation. This is provided from a variety of sources, including the voluntary sector, social services, health services, or private companies. There are four main types of assisted accommodation:

1 **Group homes.** Some relatively independent patients are able to live in group homes, which are houses in which four or five patients live together. These houses are often owned by a charitable organization. Patients perform all the essential tasks of running the house together, even though separately they could do only some of them.

2 **Day staffed accommodation.** Patients with greater handicaps can live in accommodation where members of staff are present throughout the day to provide support. These are usually not nursing staff, but trained individuals who help with activities of daily living and encourage medication compliance.

3 **Night staffed accommodation.** These houses are staffed 24 hours a day, ensuring greater supervision and assistance.

4 **Twenty-four-hour medically staffed homes.** This form of accommodation is usually in the private sector, and is for those patients with long-term, uncontrolled, severe mental illness. It includes those with severe and profound learning disabilities. There is specialist nursing care on hand, and they are run more in the style of a nursing home for older adults.

Provision of appropriate occupation

Some patients with chronic psychiatric disorder can undertake normal employment or, if beyond retirement age, can take part in the same activities as healthy people of similar age. Other patients require **sheltered work**, in which they can work productively, but more slowly or with extra assistance than would be possible elsewhere. Patients who remain unwell need **occupational therapy** to avoid boredom, under-stimulation, and lack of social contacts. Many voluntary organizations run centres with regular activities (e.g. art, photography, sport, and cookery) or more specialized schemes (e.g. gardening) which are very beneficial.

Adequate support for carers

Family and friends are the main carers of most patients living outside hospital. It is their role to encourage suitable behaviours, provide psychological support, and encourage adherence with treatment. They have to tolerate unusual and challenging behaviour. Prolonged involvement in care is stressful, and the impact of mental illness on both carers and the extended family should not be underestimated. The welfare of carers should be considered within a patient's care plan, and support provided. As for patients, there are many online resources and local support groups which carers find invaluable. Many inpatient and day-patient units run carers groups, in which families/carers can come together to discuss the challenges of living with someone with psychiatric problems.

Involvement of the patient in service provision

All patients who have the capacity to make decisions for themselves should be included in the decision-making processes surrounding their care. This includes agreeing to referrals, which professionals they see, and the type of treatments they receive. The situation for those being treated under the Mental Health Act is slightly different, but efforts should always be made to help the patient to agree to treatment. However, a busy, complicated health service can be difficult for patients to negotiate (especially if acutely unwell), or they may have problems or complaints to make about the service. In the UK, the **Patient Advice and Liaison Service (PALS)** has been created to provide information to patients and deal with complaints. Most other countries have similar schemes, with privately run hospitals managing their own internal complaints. The aims of PALS are to:

- provide patients with information about available services;
- help resolve concerns and problems;
- provide information about making complaints;
- provide a link to agencies and supportive groups outside the health service;
- improve services by listening to patient experiences and views;
- give feedback to health trusts about the positive and negative aspects of the services they provide, from the patient's perspective.

All patients also have access to patient advocates, some of whom are linked to PALS, but mostly are from charitable organizations, who provide an independent liaison between the patient and health services. These can be especially helpful when patients are being treated non-voluntarily.

Many hospital foundation trusts in the UK now run schemes by which any member of the public can become a member of the trust. The idea is that this group will represent all areas of society, and will provide a voice for patients within the structure of the trust. Members can share their experiences, sit on advisory panels, and even become non-executive members of the board of directors.

Further reading

Dieterich M, Irving CB, Bergman H, Khokhar MA, Park B, Marshall M. Intensive case management for severe mental illness. *Cochrane Database of Systematic Reviews* 2017;1:CD007906.

Gilbert HP, Peck E. *Service Transformation: Lessons from Mental Health*. London: The King's Fund; 2014. [Includes a historical summary of changes in mental health service structure.]

Marshall M, Rathbone J. Early intervention for psychosis. *Cochrane Database of Systematic Reviews* 2011;6:CD004718.

Mind (UK). http://www.mind.org.uk/. [The UK national charity for mental health. This website has a lot of useful links to other voluntary organizations providing mental healthcare.]

Muijen M, McCulloch A. Public policy and mental health. In: Gelder MG, Andreasen NC, López-Ibor JJ, Geddes JR, eds. *New Oxford Textbook of Psychiatry*. 2nd ed. Oxford: Oxford University Press; 2012:1425–1431.

National Institute for Mental Health (USA). Mental health information. Statistics. https://www.nimh.nih.gov/health/statistics/index.shtml.

World Health Organization. The WHO website provides copious reading material on all aspects of mental health epidemiology, including a searchable database of psychiatric service provision for all countries. http://www.who.int/topics/mental_health/en/.

12 Psychiatry and the law

Psychiatry and civil law

The interface between psychiatry and the law

In most of medicine, legal situations are rarely encountered, typically related to complaints or complex ethical issues. Unusually, psychiatry is closely connected with the law, with most psychiatrists dealing with legal issues on a daily basis. There are three main areas of law which are relevant to psychiatry:

1 Civil law relating to the involuntary admission and treatment of patients with mental disorders (in the UK, this is outlined in the **Mental Health Act (MHA) 2007**).

2 Civil law concerning issues of consent, capacity, and deprivation of liberty (**Mental Capacity Act 2005 including Deprivation of Liberty Safeguarding (DoLS)**).

3 Criminal law as it relates to individuals with mental disorders.

There are various reasons why knowledge of mental health legislation is helpful to all clinicians:

- Laws and official guidelines provide backing to some aspects of ethical decision-making within medicine.

- The law regulates the circumstances under which treatment can be given without patients' consent. All doctors may encounter situations in which patients refuse essential treatment, and may have to decide whether to invoke powers of compulsory admission and/or best interest treatments.

- Doctors may be asked for reports used in legal decisions, such as the capacity to make a will or claims for compensation for injury. They may be asked for reports that set out the relationship between any psychiatric disorder and criminal behaviour.

- A minority of patients behave in ways that break the law. Doctors need to understand legal issues as part of their management of care.

- Victims of crime may suffer immediate and long-term psychological or physical consequences.

This chapter will describe the main principles of mental health legislation with particular reference to UK law. While some of the detail discussed (e.g. particular definitions or legislative act numbers) may not be relevant to international readers, legal frameworks across the globe are broadly similar. Information of mental health legislation in most countries is now easily available online. The latter part of the chapter will provide an overview of the relationship between mental disorders and crime.

The Mental Health Acts 1983 and 2007

In the UK, the key legislation covering involuntary admission and treatment of individuals with mental health problems is the MHA 1983, and its amendments in the MHA 2007. These laws have three purposes:

1 **To ensure essential treatment** is provided for patients with mental disorders who do not recognize that they are ill, and refuse treatment. Three criteria are used to decide whether treatment is essential: the safety of the patient, the safety of others, and the need to prevent deterioration in health that would lead to one of the former categories.

2 **To protect other people**—for example, from the violent impulses of a paranoid patient.

3 **To protect individuals from wrongful detention.**

Mental health laws tend to provide legislation covering all of the areas shown in Box 12.1.

Box 12.1 What is included in mental health legislation?

- Definition of mental disorder
- Procedures for the assessment of patients with mental disorders who may need involuntary admission and treatment
- Urgent admission procedures for patient with mental disorders who are not in hospital
- Criteria for and procedures of providing involuntary treatment
- Emergency treatment by doctors (psychiatrists or generalists)
- Emergency procedures for compulsory detention of patients already in hospital (general or psychiatric)
- Police powers to detain for medical assessment
- Criminal or forensic detainment and treatment
- Safeguards: patient advocacy and mental health tribunals
- Discharge and follow-up community treatment
- Capacity and consent (*in the UK, covered by the Mental Capacity Act*)

Definition of mental disorder

Under the MHA 2007, mental disorder is defined as **any disorder or disability of the mind**. The four categories of mental disorder originally described in the MHA 1983 are no longer included. The only exclusion criterion is that dependence on alcohol or drugs alone is not considered to be a mental disorder. Similarly, a person with a learning disability is not considered to be suffering from a mental disorder simply as a result of that disability unless it is *associated with abnormally aggressive or seriously irresponsible conduct*.

Professional roles within the MHA 2007

In order to understand the conditions by which the various parts of the MHA can be instigated, various pieces of terminology need to be explained. Many of them have been redefined between the MHA 1983 and MHA 2007 in order to allow a broader range of health professionals to carry out parts of the act.

- An Approved Mental Health Professional (AMHP) may be any mental health professional (e.g. social worker, nurse, or psychologist) who has undergone specific training in assessing and dealing with patients with mental disorder. They can apply for patients to be assessed or treated under sections of the MHA.

- The term Approved Clinician (AC) is a mental health professional who has been trained to carry out certain duties under the MHA.

- The term Responsible Clinician (RC) has replaced the Responsible Medical Officer (RMO) and is the person with overall responsibility for a patient's care while under the MHA. An AC can act as an RC.

- A 'Section 12 Approved Doctor' (usually a consultant psychiatrist or senior registrar) is a doctor with special expertise in the diagnosis and treatment of mental disorders. Two doctors, at least one with Section 12 approval, are required to make recommendations for use of the MHA under Sections 2 and 3.

- The nearest relative (NR) of a patient is a family member who has rights to apply for a patient to be assessed under the MHA, object to its use, or request to discharge a section.

Commonly used sections of the MHA 2007

The most commonly used sections of the MHA in England and Wales are summarized in Table 12.1; abbreviations are as outlined in the preceding text. At any one time, approximately 10–15 per cent of psychiatric inpatients in the UK are admitted under the MHA; the majority of patients are therefore admitted voluntarily—this comes as a surprise to many people.

Section 2

When psychiatrists are asked to go out into the community to do an MHA assessment, it is usually with a view to admitting the patient under Section 2 of the MHA. Section 2 allows detention of the patient for up to 28 days for assessment of their mental disorder. At the end of this time, the section must either be converted to a treatment order (Section 3) or the patient discharged; it cannot be renewed. Application for a Section 2 is made by an AMHP, and two doctors (one

of whom must be Section 12 approved) are needed to recommend use of the section. The criteria that the patient must fulfil to be held under a Section 2 are as follows:

- *The person must be suffering from a mental disorder of a nature or degree that warrants their detention in hospital for assessment* and
- *The person ought to be detained in the interests of their own health or safety or with a view to the protection of others.*

The word **nature** refers to the exact mental disorder from which the patient is suffering, and **degree** refers to the current manifestation and severity of the disorder.

Section 3

Section 3 is a treatment order up to 6 months, after which it may be renewed for another 6 months, and then after that for a year at a time. If a patient is deemed well enough to no longer require involuntary treatment, the section may be discharged at any time. As with Section 2, an AMHP must make an application

Table 12.1 Mental Health Act 2007 for England and Wales

Section number	Order	Duration (maximum)	Application	Authorization
2	Assessment order	28 days	AMHP	Two doctors (at least one Section 12 approved)
3	Treatment order	6 months	AMHP	Two doctors (at least one Section 12 approved)
4	Emergency order	72 hours	NR or AMHP	One doctor
5(2)	Holding order for patient already in hospital	72 hours	Not needed	One doctor or RC
5(4)	Holding order for an informal psychiatric inpatient	6 hours	Not needed	One registered mental health nurse or AMHP
136	Police order to remove a person to a place of safety	72 hours	Not needed	Police officer

for use of the section, and two doctors (one Section 12 approved), who must have seen the patient within 24 hours, recommend its use for the patient. The criteria are as for Section 2, plus one additional criterion which is a new addition to the law from 2007. This is that there must be *appropriate medical treatment available* for the mental disorder from which the patient is suffering. This can include nursing, psychological interventions, provision of new skills, rehabilitation and care, as well as traditional medical treatments.

Section 4

Section 4 allows the emergency admission of patients not already in hospital for whom waiting for the paperwork or personnel to complete Section 2 would cause a dangerous delay. An application from an NR or AMHP is made on recommendation from one doctor, who does not need to be Section 12 approved. It is usually converted to a Section 2 upon arriving at hospital. Section 4 can last up to 72 hours, and is non-renewable.

Section 5(2)

This section provides a means of detaining a patient who is already in hospital; this includes general and psychiatric hospitals, but not the emergency room. Any doctor can detain a patient for up to 72 hours, during which time they should liaise with a psychiatrist to plan for admission under Section 2.

Section 5(4)

Popularly known as the 'nurses' holding power', Section 5(4) allows a registered psychiatric nurse or AMHP to detain an informal patient for up to 6 hours. This is used when an informal patient is attempting to discharge against medical advice and/or might cause serious harm to themselves or others (e.g. commit suicide). The 6 hours allows adequate time to organize assessment for a Section 2.

Section 136

This section allows police officers to remove a person believed to be suffering from a mental disorder from a public place and take them to a place of safety.

This is usually the local psychiatric ward/hospital, a designated room in the police station, or an emergency room. Once there, a doctor and AMHP must assess the patient; 90 per cent are then detained under Section 2 or 3.

Other sections of the MHA 2007

Some less commonly used sections include the following:

- **Section 7 (guardianship).** A guardian is appointed in the interests of the patient's welfare and/or to protect other people. The guardian can require the patient to live in a particular place, attend appointments, and allow authorized persons to visit. Application is by an AMHP or NR and needs two medical recommendations.

- **Section 17.** This section permits patients being treated under Section 3 to go on leave from hospital while still under the section. It requires the RC to agree and sign the section.

- **Section 17A-G (compulsory treatment order, CTO).** This requires a patient discharged from inpatient care to attend for/comply with treatment in the community (e.g. attend for depot antipsychotic doses or therapy). There is also a power to recall the patient to hospital if they do not comply with restrictions.

- **Section 117 (aftercare).** This is a legal requirement that all patients detained on longer-term sections (3, 37, 47, or 48) are provided with formal aftercare. All patients must have regular reviews of health and social needs, an agreed care plan, an allocated health worker, and regular progress reviews.

- **Sections 35 and 26 (criminal pre-trial orders).** These are allied to Sections 2 and 3, but are for individuals with a mental disorder that warrants treatment in hospital but who are awaiting trial for a serious crime. The patient will then be held in a secure hospital rather than a prison.

- **Section 37 (criminal post-trial order).** This applies to patients who have a mental disorder that warrants treatment in hospital, but who have already been convicted of an offence punishable with imprisonment by the courts. There does not need to be a link between the offence and illness. The procedure is then as for Section 3.

Safeguarding patients

Individuals with mental health disorders are by definition a vulnerable group, and those who are acutely unwell are at high risk of exploitation by others. In order to ensure that patients are not wrongfully detained, or kept under a MHA section for longer than necessary, the law contains various safeguards.

Appeals against detention

An important safeguard against misuse of the power to detain is a system of independent review. In England and Wales, all patients detained under a Section 2, 3, or CTO must be referred to a **Mental Health Review Tribunal (MHRT)**, at the latest by 6 months from the date the initial MHA application was made, unless the patient has already applied themselves. A patient can also ask for a hearing at any time. In the USA, these proceedings are very similar, and are called 'commitment hearings'. The review panel consists of three people:

1 A legal member—chairs the panel, usually a lawyer with experience of mental health cases.

2 A doctor—typically an independent consultant psychiatrist, who must have examined the patient before the tribunal takes place.

3 A lay member—this is a member of the public who has volunteered to sit on these panels. The majority have practical experience of working in social or mental health.

The tribunal happens in a designated room within the hospital, and the patient, their NR, the patient's legal representative, and members of the clinical treatment team may all attend. The panel questions the patient about why they feel they do not need to be in hospital any longer and the team for evidence to the contrary. If the panel decides the criteria for discharge have been met, the section is lifted and the patient must be discharged. The reality is that the majority of decisions recommend that the patient needs further involuntary treatment.

Advocacy

Advocacy ensures patients do not face discrimination or unfairness due to their mental health problems. It provides the patient with a voice to express their views and defend their rights. An advocate is an independent person who represents the patient's wishes non-judgementally, and without putting forward their own opinion. While advocacy has been widely available throughout the UK for some years, the 2007 amendments to the MHA 1983 placed a duty on local authorities to provide an independent advocate for patients detained involuntarily. They typically help the patient understand the process of what is happening to them (e.g. explaining the law), help them to complete paperwork (e.g. preparing for a MHRT), and stand up for their rights (e.g. to have vegetarian food provided in hospital).

Other relevant parts of the MHA 2007

Consent to certain treatments

Generally, the legal authority to detain a patient carries with it the authority to give basic treatment even without the patient's consent (e.g. intramuscular sedation). Under a Section 3, medications can be given for up to 3 months of detention. After this time, either the patient has to consent or an independent doctor must provide a second opinion to confirm that the treatment is still in the patient's best interests.

ECT has specific guidance relating to its usage. ECT may not be given to a refusing patient who has the capacity to refuse it, and may only be given to an incapacitated patient where it does not conflict with any advance directive, decision of their NR, or decision of the courts. The only exception to this is emergency (life-threatening) situations, in which the RC can authorize up to two ECT treatments for patients detained under Section 3.

Treating physical illness

The MHA 1983/2007 relates only to the treatment of mental disorders, not physical disorders. It does not permit the treatment of any physical co-morbidity that a detained psychiatric patient may have. There are only two exceptions to this rule:

1 Enforced refeeding of a severely emaciated patient suffering from anorexia nervosa. This is allowed because anorexia nervosa is a mental disorder, and refeeding constitutes a necessary first stage of its treatment sequelae.

2 Treatment of physical sequelae of an attempted suicide, which was a direct result of an underlying mental disorder.

Patients with co-morbid physical conditions, who are deemed not to have capacity, may need treatment under the Mental Capacity Act 2005.

Age-appropriate services

The law now requires that for patients aged under 18 who are admitted to hospital, an environment suitable to their needs is provided. In practical terms, this is supposed to prevent the treatment of adolescents on adult wards. It is no longer the case that if a child aged 16 or 17 refuses hospital admission, their parents can consent for them—a MHA assessment should be requested.

Laws concerning capacity and consent to treatment

Across medicine it is essential that a patient's consent is gained before a health practitioner treats them; without consent, this treatment is an assault. **Consent must be informed, given voluntarily without undue influence, and be given by the patient.** It is good practice to document consent. There are a variety of different groups of people within society who may not be in a position to make decisions for themselves, and various other (often emergency) situations in which gaining consent can be problematic. Some of these are shown in Box 12.2.

The Mental Capacity Act 2005

In the UK, the MCA 2005 provides the first definite legislation to protect vulnerable individuals who are deemed not to have capacity to make their own decisions. The act provides the means to assess whether or not an individual has capacity, and, if not, how those caring for them can make decisions in their best interests. It applies to people aged 16 or over, as those

Box 12.2 Situations in which problems of consent to treatment are likely to arise

- Emergency life-threatening situations
- Increasing or severe cognitive impairment
- Mental disorder impairing ability to give informed consent to treatment of a physical disorder
- Unwilling or unable to give consent to treatment of a major mental disorder
- Children
- People with a learning disability

below the age of 16 can have consent given by their parents. The act is underpinned by five principles:

1 An adult is assumed to have capacity unless it is established that they lack capacity.

2 A person is not to be treated as unable to make a decision unless all practicable steps to help them to do so have been taken without success.

3 A person is not to be treated as unable to make a decision merely because they make an unwise decision.

4 Anything done for, or on behalf of, the person must be in their best interests.

5 Anything done for, or on behalf of, the person should be the least restrictive option with respect to their basic rights and freedoms.

Assessing capacity

The MCA 2005 sets out a clear two-stage test for assessing whether a person lacks capacity to make a particular decision at a particular time:

1 **Does the individual concerned have an impairment of the mind or brain, or a disturbance of mental function?** This may be as a result of a condition, illness, or external factors such as alcohol or drug use.

2 **Does the impairment or disturbance mean the individual is unable to make a specific decision when they need to?** Individuals can lack capacity to make some decisions but have capacity to make others, or their capacity may fluctuate over time.

To have capacity to make a decision, a person must:

- **understand** the information relevant to the decision;
- **retain** that information;
- use or **weigh up** the information in order to make a decision;
- and be able to **communicate** their decision to others.

If it is decided that the person does not have capacity to make the particular decision, the rest of the act applies.

Best interests

Everything that is done for the patient who lacks capacity must be in their best interests. The act contains a checklist of factors which must be worked through to make a best interests decision. All patients have the right to make a written statement, which must be considered, as must the feelings of family and carers.

Acts in connection with care or treatment

The act offers statutory protection from prosecution where a person is performing an act in connection with care or treatment of someone who lacks capacity. For example, if a doctor was to decide that examining a patient was in their best interests, it would not be assault to do so. Individuals who neglect or ill-treat a person who lacks capacity can be imprisoned for up to 5 years.

Advance decisions to refuse treatment

The act makes it possible to make an advance decision to refuse treatment should a person lack capacity in the future. Advance decisions can only be made by adults with capacity. Any treatment may be refused, except for those needed to keep them comfortable (e.g. warmth, offering food and water by mouth).

Lasting power of attorney

This allows a person to appoint an attorney to act on their behalf if they should lose capacity in the future. The lasting power of attorney (LPA) can then make financial, property, health, and welfare decisions for them. There is a formal legal protocol to register an attorney.

Safeguards

A number of safeguards have been put in place to ensure that individuals lacking capacity are treated in the rightful manner. These include a court of protection, a public guardian (who is responsible for creating all LPAs), and independent mental capacity advocates (IMCAs). The latter are individuals appointed to speak for a person who lacks capacity and has no one to speak for them.

Deprivation of Liberty Safeguarding

People should always be cared for without limiting their freedom, but this is not always possible to ensure safety. DoLS, a subsection of MCA, ensures patients lacking capacity that are being deprived of their freedom in order to provide safe care are appropriately protected. A common example is the wandering care home patient with Alzheimer's disease. To deprive an individual of a specific liberty the authority with caring responsibility (e.g. a hospital trust, care home manager) must apply to the court of protection for permission to do this under DoLS legislation. It will be assessed if the deprivation is in the patient's best interests and a reasonable response to the situation. Exclusions include eligibility for detention under the MHA, advance directives, and conflicts with decisions made by an appointed LPA.

Other aspects of civil law relevant to psychiatry

Making a will

Doctors are sometimes asked to advise whether a patient is capable of making a will—that is, whether he has 'testamentary capacity'. The requirements are that the person:

- understands what a will is;
- knows the nature and extent of his property (although not in detail);

- knows who his close relatives are and can assess their claims to his property;
- does not have any mental abnormality that might distort his judgement (e.g. delusions about the actions of his relatives).

Most patients with mental disorder are wholly capable of making a will.

Fitness to drive

Questions about fitness to drive arise quite often in relation to psychiatric disorder. Patients may drive recklessly if they are manic, depressed and suicidal, or aggressive, or if they abuse alcohol or drugs. Concentration on driving may be impaired by a psychiatric disorder, or by the sedative medications. The issue should be considered in all cases in which a patient drives a motor vehicle. Advice to stop driving should be given if necessary and the patient reminded of their duty to report illnesses to the licensing authority. In the UK, the Driver and Vehicle Licensing Agency publishes a guide for clinicians as to which conditions should be reported, and with which the patient's driving licence is invalid. Examples include mania, acute psychosis, and severe depression with suicidal ideation.

Compensation for personal injury

Doctors are often asked to write medical reports about disability following accidents and in relation to claims of medical negligence. Such reports are concerned mainly with the nature and outlook of physical disability, but they should include any psychiatric consequences directly attributable to the trauma or induced by the physical disability. The conclusions should summarize the psychological and social consequences of the trauma and the extent to which they appear to be attributable to it.

In many cases there is evidence that there were psychological problems before the event, and it is important to decide how far the psychological and social changes found afterwards represent a continuation of these previous difficulties. Evidence from a close relative or other informant, interviewed separately, should be obtained whenever possible.

Psychiatry and criminal law

Forensic psychiatry is concerned with the assessment and treatment of people with mental health conditions who break the law and/or pose a significant risk to the public. Legally, there are two UK concepts relevant to mentally disordered offenders:

1 **The defence of insanity** can be used as a defence against any crime of which the defendant is charged. In order to 'qualify' for insanity, the defence must prove not only that the defendant had a disease of the mind at the time of the offence, but also that this led to a defect of reason. This leads to the supposition that the defendant did not know that what they were doing was wrong at the time. The defendant is then acquitted on grounds of insanity.

2 **Diminished responsibility** is a defence that can only be used for a charge of homicide. If the defence convinces the jury that due to their underlying mental illness the defendant is not fully to blame for their crime, the charge may be reduced to manslaughter.

This section provides a brief overview of the links between mental disorders and crime, and the structure of forensic psychiatry (see also 'Further reading' on p. 127).

Current patterns of crime

The prevalence and pattern of criminal offending changes over time, as does the culture around reporting and defining criminal activities. Typically, the public tend to overestimate both the number of and severity of crimes committed in their neighbourhood. In the UK, crime has been steadily reducing for the past three decades, most recently by 5–7 per cent per annum. Fig. 12.1 gives an overview of current UK crime patterns.

Risk factors for criminal offending

Although this chapter is mainly concerned with the links between mental disorders and crime, it is worth

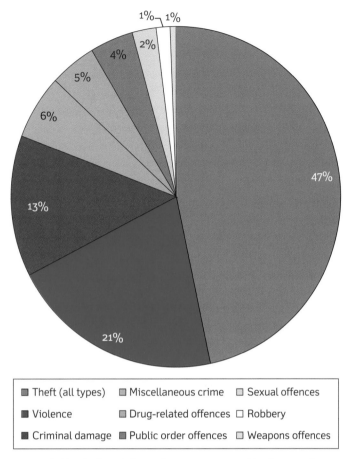

Fig. 12.1 Types of crime as recorded by the British Crime Survey 2014–2015. Numbers are the proportion as a percentage of total crime recorded.

Reproduced by permission of the Home Office. Contains public sector information licensed under the Open Government Licence v3.0, http://www.nationalarchives.gov.uk/doc/open-government-licence/version/3/.

considering the general risk factors for criminal offending, as there is considerable overlap. Box 12.3 demonstrates that family and social factors are particularly important.

Mental disorders and crime

Contrary to public perception, few psychiatric patients break the law, and when they do, it is usually in minor ways. Although serious violent offences by psychiatric patients receive much publicity, they are extremely infrequent. However, when treating mentally unwell patients, threats of violence to self or to others should

be taken seriously, as should the possibility of unintended harm resulting from disinhibited, reckless, or ill-considered behaviour.

There is a small but significant association between mental disorder and violence; 5 per cent of UK violent crimes are committed by an individual with a severe psychiatric illness. The prevalence of violent behaviour in different groups is as follows:

- General population without mental disorder: 2 per cent.
- All psychiatric outpatients: 5 per cent.
- Individuals with a *major* mental illness: 7 per cent.

Box 12.3 Risk factors for criminal offending

Biological
- Male sex
- Low IQ
- Age (peak 10–25 years)
- Genetics: in monozygotic twins, concordance for committing crime is 80 per cent
- Ethnicity (Afro-Caribbeans > Caucasians > Asians)
- Hyperactivity and impulsivity
- Teenage mother

Psychological
- Personality traits: lack of empathy
- Poor parental supervision and poor attachment
- Harsh discipline in childhood
- Aggression, violence, or criminal activity within the family
- Parental conflict
- Separation from biological parents before 10 years of age

Social
- Larger family size
- Lower socioeconomic status
- Poor housing
- Unemployment
- Peer influences and gang culture
- Spouse or partner is an offender
- Inner-city living
- Alcohol and substance abuse

Box 12.4 Risk factors for violent behaviour in patients with mental disorders

- Major psychoses (especially if associated with the following):
  - Paranoia
  - Command hallucinations
  - Passivity phenomena
- Puerperal psychosis—increased risk to the child
- Delusional disorders (especially delusional jealousy towards a partner)
- Severe depression (increased risk of infanticide and arson, but not most other crimes)
- Antisocial, impulsive, or narcissistic personality traits (increases risk by 16-fold)
- Poor impulse control
- Co-morbid use of alcohol or substances
- Prior history of conduct disorder
- Poor insight into illness or behaviour

It is widely appreciated that mental disorders are massively over-represented among prison populations, and several large meta-analyses have been undertaken which confirm this (see Table 12.2). The prevalence of psychosis and major depression appears to be at least twice as high as in the general population, and the prevalence of personality disorders about ten times as high. At the time of writing,

- Individuals with a substance abuse disorder: 20 per cent.

There are a few specific risk factors associated with violent behaviour: these are shown in Box 12.4. Remember that no matter what the underlying diagnosis is, **a past history of violent behaviour is the greatest predictor of future behaviour**, and that all the general risk factors in Box 12.3 are relevant. It is worth noting that while manic patients are at high risk of disinhibited behaviour, reckless spending/driving, and agitation, violence towards others or property is rare.

Table 12.2 Prevalence of mental disorders among prison inmates

Diagnosis	Males (%)	Females (%)
Psychosis	3.7	4
Major depression	10	12
Personality disorder	65	42
Antisocial personality disorder	47	21

Reprinted from *The Lancet*, 359, Fazel S and Danesh J, Serious mental disorders in 23 000 prisoners: a systematic review of 62 surveys, pp. 545–550. Copyright (2002) with permission from Elsevier.

approximately 5 per cent of the UK prison population were mentally disordered offenders detained in specialist secure psychiatric hospitals.

Associations between specific psychiatric disorders and types of offence

It is difficult to directly link specific psychiatric diagnoses with particular offences. Mental disorders have great clinical heterogeneity and this is represented in the variety of offences that may be committed. Tables 12.3 and 12.4 and Box 12.5 provide a brief overview of some associations between crime and specific clinical diagnoses.

The role of doctors

There are a variety of criminal legal issues with which doctors may be involved (Box 12.6), most commonly by providing a factual medical report. It is an important ethical principle that both doctors and those they are assessing are clear that *acting for a third party*, such as a court, involves different obligations and responsibilities to usual clinical practice, where

Table 12.3 Associations between specific psychiatric disorders and types of offence

Condition	Risk of offending	Clinical associations
Schizophrenia	• Overall crime is usually minor • 2–4-fold increase in violence in men • 6–8-fold increase in violence in women	Persecutory delusions Command hallucinations Passivity phenomena Alcohol and substances
Delusional disorders	• Over-represented in secure psychiatric hospitals but objective risk of crime is low • Increase risk of violence, stalking, and homicide • 60% of violence is towards a partner	Delusional jealousy or love Misidentification delusions
Depression	• Very low risk • Weak association with shoplifting (esp. women) • Violence is very rare	Nihilistic delusions Socioeconomic problems
Mania	• Petty crime is frequent • Indecent exposure, driving offences, disrupting the peace, minor theft are commonest • Violence is very rare	Disinhibition
Personality disorders	• Strong associations with violence and sexual crime • 2/3 prison inmates • Up to 50% of homicide perpetrators fit criteria	Antisocial, paranoid, and borderline traits Co-morbid substance misuse increases risk 16-fold
Substance abuse	• Strong association with all types of offending • Most common are thefts • Alcohol responsible for 1/3 traffic-related deaths • Plays role in 40% UK murders	
Learning disabilities and autistic spectrum disorders	• Extremely low risk	Individual usually lacks understanding of the implications of their actions

Table 12.4 The association between psychopathology and specific crimes

Type of crime	Associations with mental health
Homicide	<ul><li>10% committed by patients in touch with mental health services (UK), lower proportion in countries with higher baseline homicide rates</li><li>3% of murderers have had admissions under the MHA</li><li>In 80% of all homicides the victim is known to the perpetrator</li><li>5–10% of convictions are reduced to manslaughter due to a plea of diminished responsibility, or acquitted on grounds of insanity</li></ul>
Infanticide *The killing of a child below the age of 12 months by the mother*	<ul><li>First 24 hours of life: strongly associated with young, distressed mothers with poor social support</li><li>From day 2: mother usually has puerperal psychosis, postnatal depression, or another form of psychosis</li><li>High risk of maternal suicide after the infanticide</li></ul>
Family violence	<ul><li>10% of women experience some form of domestic violence</li><li>Strong associations with alcohol, personality disorders, and sexual jealousy</li><li>Have a low threshold for providing safe accommodation for victims and their children</li></ul>
Sexual offences (Box 12.5) *Sex offender: an individual whose sexual behaviour contravenes the law*	<ul><li>>98% of victims of sexual offences report the perpetrator was male</li><li>Severe mental disorders are very rare but personality disorders are over-represented</li><li>More minor sexual offences may be associated with learning disabilities (e.g. voyeurism)</li></ul>
Shoplifting	Associations with:<ul><li>alcohol and substance misuse (lack of money)</li><li>psychosis (lack of money or loss of touch with reality)</li><li>dementia (forget to pay)</li><li>depression (middle-aged women)</li><li>eating disorders (food)</li></ul>
Arson	<ul><li>Majority of arsonists are male; few have psychiatric conditions</li></ul>
Gambling-related offences	<ul><li>Large debts are associated with theft and fraud</li><li>Pathological gambling may be treated like an addiction</li></ul>

the relationship is between the doctor and the patient. Box 12.7 provides some guidance on the writing of a medical report for the courts.

Treatment of mentally disordered offenders

The fundamental aspect of treating mentally disordered offenders is that the principles remain the same as for any other patient. However, it may need to be undertaken in a more secure environment. Forensic psychiatrists tend to treat these patients, be they in prison, a (low-, medium-, or high-) secure psychiatric hospital, or in the community.

The prison psychiatrist

As discussed, at least two-thirds of the prison population have psychiatric disorders. The majority of forensic psychiatrists work in 'normal' prisons, and only a few in secure psychiatric hospitals. There are four main

Box 12.5 An overview of sexual offences

(Further information on UK-specific law can be found at https:// www.legislation.gov.uk.)

Indecent exposure. Indecent exposure of the genitalia is mainly an offence of men between 25 and 35 years of age. The offence is usually a result of the psychiatric disorder known as **exhibitionism**, although in a minority exposure is a prelude to a sexual assault or disinhibition caused by alcohol or drug intoxication.

Voyeurism. This is the sexual interest of watching people engaged in intimate activities (e.g. undressing, having sex). The perpetrators are commonly known as 'peeping Toms'.

Rape. This is when a male penetrates with his penis the vagina, anus, or mouth of a female or male without their consent. Few rapists have a psychiatric disorder.

Sexual assault. When any male or female intentionally touches another person sexually without his or her consent.

Sexual offences against people with mental health conditions. Any sexual activity undertaken with an individual who does not have capacity due to a mental disorder.

Child sexual abuse. When a child is forced or persuaded to undertake any sexual activities. This does not have to be physical and includes online activities (see also p. 192). An adult who commits sexual offences against children is known as a paedophile, the majority of which are male.

Incest. Incest is sexual activity between members of the same family. When incest has been discovered, the family needs much specialist support to deal with guilt and recriminations.

situations in which a psychiatrist may be asked to see a prisoner:

1 To provide a court report before a trial (for prisoners on 'remand').
2 To assess a patient in prison for a new or ongoing problem.
3 To provide treatment for prisoners.
4 To provide a report for the parole board.

Prisoners should be assessed as for any other patient, and offered the same range of treatments as would be available in the community.

Secure psychiatric hospitals

Patients may be admitted to secure psychiatric hospitals from the courts, prisons, or less secure hospitals. The majority of mentally disordered offenders

Box 12.6 The role of doctors in relation to crime

- Assessment of offenders who may have a mental disorder.
- Advice to the police when they are deciding whether to proceed with charges against mentally disordered offenders.
- Fitness to plead. To be fit to plead, a person must be able to understand the nature of the charge and the difference between a plea of guilty and a plea of not guilty, instruct lawyers, know they may challenge jurors, and follow evidence presented in court. A person can suffer from severe mental disorder and still be fit to plead. A person judged

unfit to plead is not tried but detained in a hospital until fit to plead, at which time (if it comes) the case is tried.
- Assessment of responsibility; providing evidence and/or an opinion as to whether the defence of insanity or diminished responsibility is appropriate.
- Giving evidence in court, or writing a formal report for the criminal court.
- Treatment of offenders while in custody or prison, in hospital, or in the community.
- Providing risk assessments of offenders anywhere within the criminal legal system.

Box 12.7 Preparing a medical report for criminal proceedings

When a doctor is asked for a written medical report on a person it is sensible to (as far as possible) avoid technical language, explain any technical terms that are essential, and not use jargon. The report should be concise, have a clear structure, and be limited to matters relevant to the reason for the report. The following headings are recommended:

1 The doctor's particulars: full name, qualifications, and present appointment.

2 When the interview was conducted and whether any third person was present.

3 Sources of information, including any documents that have been examined.

4 Relevant points from the family and personal history of the defendant.

5 The accused person's account of the events of the alleged offence, whether they admit to the offence or have another explanation of the events, and if they admit to it, their attitude and expressed degree of remorse.

6 Other relevant behaviour such as the abuse of substances, interpersonal relationships, general social competence, and personality traits or behaviour indicating ability to tolerate frustration.

7 Mental state at the time of the assessment, mentioning only positive findings or specifically relevant negative ones.

8 A decision as to whether or not the person has a mental disorder as defined by the MHA and what the specific diagnosis is.

9 Mental state at the time of the alleged offence. As explained earlier, this question is highly important in law but difficult to answer on medical evidence. A judgement is made from the present mental state, diagnosis, the accused person's account, and accounts from any witnesses. If the person has a chronic mental illness (such as dementia), it is easier to infer their mental state at the time of the alleged offence than it is if they had a depressive disorder, which could have been more or less severe at the former time than it was at the assessment. To add to the difficulty, the court does not simply require a general statement about the mental state at the time, but a specific judgement about the accused person's intentions.

10 Fitness to plead is referred to when this is relevant.

11 Assessment of criminal responsibility. For most offences, a person is not regarded as culpable unless they were able to choose whether or not to perform the unlawful action, and unless they were able to control their behaviour at the time. Again, a judgement has to be made on the available evidence, and may not be clear cut. This is especially important in cases where a defence of insanity or diminished responsibility is being made.

12 Advice on further treatment and an appropriate setting for this. It is not the doctor's role to advise the court about sentencing, although sometimes it is helpful to indicate the likely psychiatric consequences of different forms of sentence that might be considered by the court (e.g. custodial vs non-custodial).

---

are sentenced to undertake a prison sentence in the mainstream system or compulsory treatment in the community. However, when there is a continuing risk to other people of aggression, arson, or sexual offences, treatment is arranged in a unit providing greater security to ensure the protection of society.

There are several parts of the MHA 1983/2007 which provide specific legislation for mentally disordered offenders.

• Sections 35 and 36 are equivalent to Sections 2 and 3 in civil law, and are used for patients awaiting trial ('on remand') for a serious crime. They are an alternative to sending the patient to prison while awaiting trial.

• Section 37 is a treatment order (similar to Section 3) which can be used for mentally disordered offenders who have been convicted of a serious crime and sentenced to imprisonment. After 6 months, the patient may request an MHRT in the usual way, but if the patient is found to have recovered from the mental disorder they are transferred to prison rather than discharged home.

• Patients who pose an extremely high risk to others may have a Section 41 added to their Section 37. This imposes further restrictions, most importantly that only the Home Secretary can decide that the person can leave hospital.

- Section 47 allows for prisoners to be transferred from a prison to a psychiatric hospital for treatment.

In the UK, there are three tiers of secure psychiatric hospitals; high-, medium-, and low-security facilities. There are five high-security hospitals in the UK:

1 England: special hospitals at Broadmoor, Rampton, and Ashworth.

2 Scotland: the state hospital at Carstairs.

3 Northern Ireland: the central mental hospital at Dundrum.

These facilities take patients who pose *grave imminent danger to the public*, and are extremely secure. The majority of patients are suffering from mental disorders but some may have personality disorders. The ratio of staff to patients is very high, both clinicians and security personnel. The average stay in Broadmoor is 8 years, and contrary to popular belief, most patients who receive treatment in a high-security facility are eventually rehabilitated sufficiently to move back into the community. The emphasis is on in-depth therapy, rehabilitation, and building new skills as well as using conventional psychotropics. On discharge, patients typically move to a medium-secure hospital.

Medium-secure facilities fall somewhere between the 'escape-proof' secure facilities and locked wards. The majority of patients in these facilities move there due to behaviour that is unmanageable in lower-security environments. The length of stay is much shorter—2 years on average—and then most patients are well enough to return to a less restrictive environment. There are several facilities in the UK that admit adolescents needing a medium level of security.

Low-security units are mainly based in large general psychiatric hospitals or on the same site as a medium-secure facility. They are essentially locked wards, with similar security to that which is provided in intensive care units for patients who have not offended. Most patients are admitted for a relatively short time, until their illness is under better control and they are able to return to a non-secure environment.

Community treatment

As in the rest of psychiatry, treating a mentally disordered offender has two parts: managing the acute psychiatric disturbance and then rehabilitating the patient to life in the community. Once a mentally disordered offender is deemed fit for discharge from hospital, and has completed their mandatory sentence, it is essential they receive appropriate community follow-up under section 117. This is provided in a similar way to that in the general services, but input is needed to both maintain a stable mental state and reduce the risk of reoffending. Patients require help finding somewhere to live, employment, hobbies, financial assistance, and reintegration with family. The latter can be extremely difficult, and family therapy plays a vital role.

Further reading

Department of Health and Social Care. Code of practice: Mental Health Act 1983. Published 15 January 2015, updated 31 October 2017. https://www.gov.uk/government/publications/code-of-practice-mental-health-act-1983. [Guide to updated 2015 guidance for clinicians in using the MHA.]

Driver and Vehicle Licensing Agency (DVLA). Assessing fitness to drive: a guide for medical professionals. https://www.gov.uk/government/publications/at-a-glance. [DVLA guidance on driving with medical conditions.]

Office of the Public Guardian. Mental Capacity Act: making decisions. Published 30 September 2014, updated 22 October 2014. https://www.gov.uk/government/collections/mental-capacity-act-making-decisions. [Information about the Mental Capacity Act 2005.]

Royal College of Psychiatrists. http://www.rcpsych.ac.uk/usefulresources/publications/seminarsseries/practicalforensicpsychiatry.aspx. [A good series of seminars covering basic forensic psychiatry from the Royal College of Psychiatrists.]

Social Care Institute for Excellence. Deprivation of Liberty Safeguards (DoLS) at a glance. Published May 2015, reviewed June 2017. http://www.scie.org.uk/publications/ataglance/ataglance43.asp. [A useful resource summarizing DoLS legislation.]

13 Drugs and other physical treatments

This chapter is about the use of drugs and electroconvulsive therapy (ECT). Stimulants for ADHD are covered in Chapter 32, and psychological treatments in Chapter 14. This is a convenient way of dividing the subject matter of a book, but in practice these *physical treatments should always be combined with psychological treatment*, unless the patient chooses not to undertake this.

The account in this chapter is concerned with practical therapeutics rather than basic pharmacology, and it will be assumed that the reader has studied the basic pharmacology of the principal types of drug used in psychiatric disorders (readers who do not have this knowledge should consult a textbook, see, for example, 'Further reading'). Nevertheless, a few important points about the actions of psychotropic drugs will be considered, before describing the specific groups of drugs (see Science box 13.1).

General considerations

Pharmacokinetics of psychotropic drugs

To be effective, psychotropic drugs must reach the brain in adequate amounts. How far they do this depends on their absorption, metabolism, excretion, and passage across the blood–brain barrier.

Absorption

Most psychotropic drugs are absorbed readily from the gut, but absorption can be reduced by intestinal hurry or a malabsorption syndrome. Absorption can be slowed down by use of enteric coatings on capsules, should the clinician wish for a drug to be delivered over a longer period of time.

Metabolism

Most psychotropic drugs are metabolized partially in the liver on their way from the intestine via the portal system to the systemic circulation. The amount of this so-called **first-pass metabolism** differs from one person to another, and it is altered by certain drugs, taken at the same time, which induce liver enzymes (e.g. carbamazepine) or inhibit them (e.g. MAOIs). Although first-pass metabolism reduces the amount of the original drug reaching the brain, the metabolites of some drugs have their own therapeutic effects. As many psychotropic drugs have active metabolites, the *measurement of plasma concentrations of the parent drug is generally a poor guide to treatment*. Such

---

SCIENCE BOX 13.1

Drug discovery in psychiatry

The first generation of effective drugs for mental disorders were, in the main, identified by acute clinical observation of the effects of drugs that were originally developed for different purposes. Thus, the monoamine oxidase inhibitors (MAOIs) were originally investigated as antituberculosis agents, chlorpromazine began life as an antihistamine, and the effectiveness of lithium was discovered when it was used to increase the solubility of uric acid, which had been hypothesized to cause mania.

Second-generation drugs tended to be refined, more selective versions of first-generation drugs. So, for example, selective serotonin reuptake inhibitors (SSRIs) were developed to target the 5-hydroxytryptamine (5-HT) system and, by avoiding the broader effects of tricyclic drugs, caused less side effects and toxicity. Second-generation antipsychotics were designed to replicate the dopamine-blocking effects of first-generation antipsychotics without causing motor side effects.

By the early 2000s, a large number of 'me-too' compounds had been developed in the major areas of antidepressants and antipsychotics, but there were no major breakthroughs in treatment to lead to fundamental control of mental disorders. Rational development was inhibited by the slow pace of increasing knowledge on the basic mechanisms of the disorders.

At the time of writing, the difficulty of discovering new drugs has led to the withdrawal of several major drug manufacturers from active drug development in psychiatry. We hope (and predict), however, that this will act as a spur to the international academic community to take up the challenge to fill the black hole left by the withdrawal of industry. A key challenge will be the development of reliable experimental models of psychiatric disorders to allow the efficient development of promising agents. Perhaps the next step will be to aim to repeat the successes of the early pioneers by investigating existing agents for potential benefits.

---

measurement is *used routinely only with lithium carbonate*, which has no metabolites and undergoes no hepatic metabolism (see p. 147).

Distribution

In plasma, psychotropic drugs are bound largely to protein. Because they are lipophilic, they pass easily across the blood–brain barrier. For the same reason, they enter into **fat stores** from which they are released slowly, often for many weeks after the patient has ceased to take the drug. They also pass into **breast milk**—an important point when a breastfeeding mother is treated.

Excretion

Psychotropic drugs and their metabolites are excreted through the kidneys, so smaller doses should be given when renal function is impaired. Lithium is unique among the psychotropic drugs in being filtered passively in the glomerulus and then partly reabsorbed in the tubules by the mechanism that absorbs sodium. The two ions compete for reabsorption so that when sodium levels fall, lithium absorption rises and lithium concentrations increase—potentially to a toxic level.

Drug interactions

When two drugs are given together, one may either interfere with the other, or enhance its therapeutic or unwanted effects. Interactions can take place during absorption, metabolism, or excretion, or at the cellular level. For psychotropic drugs, most pharmacokinetic interactions are at the stage of liver metabolism, the important exception being lithium, for which interference is at the stage of renal excretion. An important pharmacodynamic interaction is the antagonism between tricyclics and some antihypertensive drugs. When prescribing a psychotropic and another drug it is good practice to consult the Summaries of Product Characteristics (SPCs, online at http://www.medicines.org.uk) or a work of reference such as the *British National Formulary* (*BNF*) to determine whether the drugs interact.

Drug withdrawal

When some drugs are given for a long period, the tissues adjust to their presence and when the drug is withdrawn there is a temporary disturbance of function until a new adjustment is reached. This disturbance appears clinically as a withdrawal syndrome. Among psychotropic drugs, anxiolytics and hypnotics are most likely to induce this effect (see p. 132).

General advice about prescribing psychotropic drugs

Use well-tried drugs. When there is a choice of equally effective drugs (as is often the case in psychiatry), it is generally good practice to use the drugs whose side effects and long-term effects are understood better. Also, well-tried drugs are generally less expensive than new ones. Clinicians should become familiar with a few drugs of each of the main types—antidepressants, antipsychotics, and so on. In this way, they will become used to adjusting dosage and recognizing side effects.

Change drugs only for a good reason. If there is no therapeutic response to an established drug given in adequate dosage for a sustained period, it is unlikely that there will be a better response to another from the same therapeutic group. The main reason for changing medication is that side effects have prevented adequate dosage. It is then appropriate to change to a drug with a different pattern of side effects—for example, from an antidepressant with strong anticholinergic effects to another with weaker ones.

Combine drugs only for specific indications. Generally, drug combinations should be avoided (see 'Drug interactions'). However, some drug combinations are of proven value for specific purposes, for example, lithium and antidepressant for drug-resistant depressive disorder (see p. 147), or lithium and valproate for preventing relapse in bipolar disorder. Usually, drug combinations are initiated by a specialist because the adverse effects of such combinations can be more hazardous than those of a single drug. However, GPs may be asked to continue prescribing.

Adjust dosage carefully. Dose ranges for some commonly used drugs are indicated later in this chapter; others will be found in the SPC or *BNF*. Within these ranges, the correct dose for an individual patient is decided from the severity of the symptoms, the patient's age and weight, and any factors that may affect drug metabolism or excretion. For elderly patients, start at half the normal dose and increase slowly in small increments.

Plan the interval between doses. Less frequent administration has the advantage that patients are more likely to be reliable in taking drugs. The duration of action of most psychotropic drugs is such that they can be taken once or twice a day while maintaining a therapeutic plasma concentration between doses.

Decide the duration of treatment. The duration depends on the risk of dependency and the nature of the disorder. In general, anxiolytic and hypnotic drugs should be given for a short time—a few days to 2 or 3 weeks—because of the risk of dependency. Antidepressants and antipsychotics are given for a long time—months to years—because of the risk of relapse.

Advise patients. Before giving a first prescription for a drug, the doctor should explain several points:

1 The likely **initial effects** of the drug (e.g. drowsiness or dry mouth).

2 The **delay** before therapeutic effects appear (about 2 weeks with antidepressants).

3 The likely **first signs of improvement** (e.g. improved sleep after starting an antidepressant).

4 **Common side effects** (e.g. fine tremor with lithium).

5 Any **serious effects** that should be reported immediately by the patient (e.g. coarse tremor after taking lithium).

6 Any **restrictions** while the drug is taken (e.g. not driving or operating machinery if the drugs reduce alertness).

7 **How long** the patient will need to take the drug: for anxiolytics, the patient is discouraged from taking them for too long; for antidepressants or antipsychotics, the patient is encouraged to continue taking the drug after symptoms have been controlled.

Adherence to treatment

Many patients do not take the drugs prescribed for them. Their unused drugs are a danger to children and a potential source of deliberate self-poisoning. Other patients take more than the prescribed dose, especially of hypnotic or anxiolytic drugs. It is important to check that repeat prescriptions are not being requested before the correct day. (Adherence to prescribed treatment is referred to as **compliance**, and the agreement between doctor and patient on a course of treatment is sometimes called **concordance**.)

To adhere to prescribed treatment, a patient must be:

1 **convinced of the need to take the drug.**
Psychotic or seriously depressed patients may not be convinced that they are ill, or may not wish to recover. Those with a learning disability or dementia may not understand the doctor's explanation. Deluded patients may distrust their doctors;

2 **free from fears or concerns about its dangers.**
Some patients fear that antidepressant drugs will cause addiction; some fear unpleasant or dangerous side effects;

3 **able to remember to take it.** Patients with memory impairment may forget to take medication, or take the dose twice.

Time spent at the start of treatment in discussing reasons for drug treatment and the patient's concerns, and explaining the beneficial and likely adverse effects of the drugs, increases adherence. Adherence should be checked at subsequent visits and, if necessary, the discussion should be repeated and extended to include any fresh concerns of the patient.

What to do if there is no therapeutic response

The first step is to find out whether the patient has taken the drug in the correct dose. If not, the points described earlier under 'Adherence' should be considered. If the prescribed dose has been taken, the diagnosis should be reviewed: if it is confirmed, an increase of dosage should be considered. Only when these steps have been gone through should the original drug be changed.

Review of drugs used in psychiatry

Psychotropic drugs are those which have effects mainly on mental symptoms. They are divided into groups according to their principal actions. Several have secondary actions used for other purposes. For example, antidepressants are frequently used to treat anxiety (Table 13.1).

The main groups of drugs will be reviewed in turn. For each group, an account will be given of important points concerning therapeutic effects, the compounds in most frequent use, side effects, toxic effects, and contraindications. General advice will also be given about the use of each group of drugs, but *specific applications to the treatment of individual disorders will be found in the chapters dealing with these conditions*. Drugs with a use limited to the treatment of a single disorder (e.g. disulfiram for alcohol problems) are discussed solely in the chapters dealing with the relevant clinical syndromes.

Anxiolytic drugs

Anxiolytic drugs reduce anxiety, and in larger doses produce drowsiness (they are **sedatives**) and sleep (they are also **hypnotics**). (Hypnotics are discussed on p. 135.) These drugs are prescribed widely, and sometimes unnecessarily for patients who would improve without them. The first-line treatment for anxiety should be psychological approaches such as relaxation, mindfulness, or CBT-based techniques. Anxiolytics are used most appropriately to reduce severe anxiety. They should be prescribed for a short time, usually a few days, and seldom for more than 2–3 weeks. Longer courses of treatment may lead to tolerance and dependence.

Buspirone (see separate topic later in this section) seems to be an exception to the general

Table 13.1 Psychotropic drugs

Type	Indications	Classes of drug
Anxiolytic Sometimes referred to as 'minor tranquilizers' in older texts	Anxiety disorders	Benzodiazepines (short term) Buspirone SSRIs
Hypnotics	Sleep disturbances	Z-drugs Benzodiazepines
Antipsychotics Sometimes typical antipsychotics are referred to as 'major tranquilizers' or 'neuroleptics'	Psychosis	Typical antipsychotics Atypical antipsychotics
	Mania	Atypical antipsychotics
Antidepressant	Depressive disorders	SSRIs SNRIs Mirtazapine Tricyclics MAOIs
	Chronic anxiety	SSRIs, mirtazapine
	Obsessive–compulsive disorder	SSRIs, clomipramine
	Nocturnal enuresis	SNRIs
Mood stabilizer	To prevent recurrent mood disorder	Lithium
		Carbamazepine
		Valproate
		Lamotrigine
Psychostimulant	Narcolepsy	Amphetamines
	ADHD	Methylphenidate, dexamphetamine, atomoxetine
Cognitive enhancers	Dementia	Donepezil
		Rivastigmine
		Galantamine

MAOIs, monoamine oxidase inhibitors; SNRIs, serotonin and noradrenaline reuptake inhibitors; SSRIs, selective serotonin reuptake inhibitors.

rule that anxiolytics produce dependency, but its anxiolytic effect develops more slowly and is less intense than that of the benzodiazepines. The drugs called anxiolytics are not the only ones that reduce anxiety. Antidepressant and antipsychotic drugs also have anxiolytic properties. Since they do not induce dependence, they are sometimes used to treat chronic anxiety. Beta-adrenergic agonists are

Box 13.1 Drugs used to treat anxiety

Primary anxiolytics

- Benzodiazepines
- Buspirone

Other drugs with anxiolytic properties

- Beta-adrenergic antagonists (short-term action)
- Some antidepressants
- Some antipsychotics
- Pregabalin

used to control some of the somatic symptoms of anxiety (Box 13.1).

Benzodiazepines

These bind to the benzodiazepine receptor site on gamma-aminobutyric acid type A (GABA$_A$) receptors and thereby potentiate inhibitory transmission. As well as anxiolytic, sedative, and hypnotic effects, benzodiazepines have muscle relaxant and anticonvulsant properties. They are also the first-line treatment for catatonia. Benzodiazepines are rapidly absorbed and metabolized into a large number of compounds, many of which have their own therapeutic effects.

Compounds in frequent use. The many benzodiazepines are divided into short- and long-acting drugs (Table 13.2). Short-acting drugs are useful for their brief clinical effect, free from hangover. Their disadvantage is that they are more likely than long-acting drugs to cause dependence.

Side effects are mainly headache and *drowsiness*, with ataxia at larger doses (especially in the elderly). These effects, which may *impair driving skills* and the operation of machinery, are potentiated by alcohol. Patients should be warned about both these potential hazards. Like alcohol, benzodiazepines can *release aggression* by reducing inhibitions in people with a tendency to this kind of behaviour. This should be remembered, for example, when prescribing for women judged to be at risk of child abuse, or anyone with a history of impulsive aggressive behaviour.

Table 13.2 Long- and short-acting benzodiazepines

Group	Approximate duration of action	Examples
Short acting	<12 hours	Lorazepam
		Temazepam
		Oxazepam
		Triazolam
Long acting	>24 hours	Diazepam
		Nitrazepam
		Flurazepam
		Chlordiazepoxide
		Clobazam
		Clorazepate
		Alprazolam

Paradoxical disinhibition is a curious phenomenon seen in less than 1 per cent of people who take a benzodiazepine. The patient becomes aggressive, impulsive, hyperactive, and may engage in risky activities. Disinhibition is most common at the extremes of age or in those with learning disabilities or neurological conditions. The patient's notes should be clearly marked so that benzodiazepines are avoided in the future.

Toxic effects are few, and most patients recover even from large overdoses which produce sedation and drowsiness. Benzodiazepine effects can be reversed with the benzodiazepine receptor antagonist flumazenil. There is no convincing evidence of teratogenic effects; nevertheless, these drugs should be avoided in the first trimester of pregnancy unless there is a strong indication for their use.

Withdrawal effects occur after benzodiazepines have been prescribed for more than a few weeks; they have been reported in at least half the patients taking the drugs for more than 6 months. The frequency depends on the dose and the type of drug. The withdrawal syndrome is shown in Box 13.2. Seizures occur infrequently after rapid withdrawal from large doses. The

Box 13.2 Benzodiazepine withdrawal syndrome

- Apprehension and anxiety
- Flu-like symptoms
- Insomnia
- Tremor
- Heightened sensitivity to stimuli
- Muscle twitching
- Seizures (rarely)

obvious similarity between benzodiazepine withdrawal symptoms and those of an anxiety disorder makes it difficult, in practice, to decide whether they arise from withdrawal of the drug or the continuous presence of the anxiety disorder for which treatment was initiated. A helpful point is that withdrawal symptoms generally begin 2–3 days after withdrawing a short-acting drug, or 7 days after stopping a long-acting one, and diminish again after 3–10 days. Anxiety symptoms often start sooner and persist for longer. Withdrawal symptoms are less likely if the drug is withdrawn gradually over several weeks. (For the treatment of benzodiazepine dependence, see p. 452.)

Buspirone

This anxiolytic, which is an azapirone, has no affinity for benzodiazepine receptors but acts as a partial agonist at $5-HT_{1A}$ receptors and reduces 5-HT transmission. It does not cause sedation but has side effects of headache, nausea, and light-headedness. It does not appear to lead to tolerance and dependence. Its action is slower than that of benzodiazepines and less powerful, but can be a useful adjunct to an antidepressant.

Beta-adrenergic antagonists

These drugs do not have general anxiolytic effects but can relieve palpitation and tremor. They are used occasionally when these are the main symptoms of a chronic anxiety disorder. An appropriate drug is **propranolol** in a starting dose of 40 mg daily increased gradually to 40 mg three times a day. The several **contraindications** limit the use of these drugs. These are *asthma*

or a history of *bronchospasm*, or *obstructive airways disease*; incipient *cardiac failure* or *heart block*; *systolic blood pressure below 90 mmHg; a pulse rate less than 60 per minute*; metabolic acidosis, for example in *diabetes*; and after prolonged fasting, as in *anorexia nervosa*. Other contraindications and precautions are listed in the manufacturer's literature. There are **interactions** with some drugs that increase the adverse effects of beta-blockers. Before prescribing these drugs, it is important to find out what other drugs the patient is taking, and consult a work of reference about possible interactions.

General advice about use of anxiolytics

- **Use sparingly.** Usually, attention to life problems, an opportunity to talk about feelings, and reassurance are enough to reduce anxiety to tolerable levels.

- **Brief treatment.** Benzodiazepines should seldom be given for more than 3 weeks.

- **Withdraw drugs gradually** to reduce withdrawal effects. When the drug is stopped, patients should be warned that they may feel more tense for a few days.

- **Short- or long-acting drug.** If anxiety is intermittent, a short-acting compound is used; if anxiety lasts throughout the day, a long-acting drug is appropriate.

- **Consider an alternative.** As explained in the section on anxiety disorders (see p. 329), some antidepressant and antipsychotic drugs have secondary anxiolytic effects and are useful alternatives to benzodiazepines.

Hypnotic drugs

An ideal hypnotic would increase the length and quality of sleep without changing sleep structure, have no residual effects the next day, and cause no dependence and no withdrawal syndrome. No hypnotic drug meets these criteria, and most alter the structure of sleep: rapid eye movement sleep is suppressed while they are being taken and resumes once they have been stopped.

Before starting a hypnotic, the patient should be educated on good sleep hygiene and given a chance to put this into practice. For many patients, if they are starting an antidepressant then the improvement in their mood will improve their sleep and the hypnotic may not be required.

Benzodiazepines are the most frequently used hypnotic drugs. A short-acting drug such as temazepam is suitable for cases of initial insomnia and less likely to cause effects the next day than long-acting compounds such as nitrazepam. These hangover effects can be hazardous for people who drive motor vehicles or operate machines.

Non-benzodiazepine drugs acting on GABA receptors. These drugs include **zopiclone**, **zolpidem**, and **zaleplon**, which bind selectively to omega-1 benzodiazepine sites on GABA receptors but not to the omega-2 sites involved in cognitive functions, including memory. They are short-acting and have theoretical advantages over benzodiazepines, although these have not been clearly shown to be clinically significant in patients with insomnia.

Patients should be warned that **alcohol** potentiates the effects of hypnotic drugs, sometimes causing dangerous respiratory depression. This effect is particularly likely to occur with chlormethiazole and barbiturates, which should not be prescribed to people taking excessive amounts of alcohol, except under careful supervision in the management of withdrawal (see p. 438).

Hypnotic drugs are prescribed too frequently and for too long. Some patients are started on long periods of dependency on hypnotics by the prescribing of night sedation in hospital. These drugs should be prescribed only when there is a real need, and should be stopped before the patient goes home. (The management of insomnia is discussed on p. XXX.)

Prescribing for special groups

For *children* the prescription of hypnotics is not justified except occasionally for the treatment of night terrors or somnambulism. For *the elderly*, hypnotics should be prescribed with particular care since they may become confused and thereby risk injury.

Antipsychotic drugs

Antipsychotic drugs reduce psychomotor excitement, hallucinations, and delusions occurring in schizophrenia, mania, and organic psychoses. Antipsychotic drugs block dopamine D_2 receptors to varying degrees. The degree to which they do so may account for their therapeutic effects, and certainly explains the propensity of individual drugs to cause extrapyramidal side effects. Several drugs, particularly the newer 'atypical' antipsychotics, are also $5\text{-}HT_{2A}$ receptor antagonists and this may explain their different clinical effects. Antipsychotic drugs also block noradrenergic and cholinergic receptors to varying degrees, and these actions account for some of their many side effects.

Antipsychotic drugs are well absorbed and partly metabolized in the liver into numerous metabolites, some of which have antipsychotic properties of their own. Because of this metabolism to active compounds, measurements of plasma concentrations of the parent drug are not helpful for the clinician.

Types of antipsychotic drugs available

There are many antipsychotic drugs, with different chemical structures. The following grouping is clinically useful, although it should be recognized that the classification is not based on formal pharmacological class. (See also Table 22.8, p. 305.)

First-generation (also known as 'typical' or 'conventional') antipsychotic drugs (FGAs) bind strongly to postsynaptic dopamine D_2 receptors. This action seems to account for their therapeutic effect but also their propensity to cause movement disorders (see p. 137).

Second-generation (also known as 'atypical') antipsychotic drugs (SGAs) vary in the extent to which they bind to dopamine D_2/D_4, $5\text{-}HT_2$, alpha$_1$-adrenergic, and muscarinic receptors. It is thought that the balance between the D_2 and $5\text{-}HT_2$ antagonism may account for their therapeutic actions. SGAs are less likely to cause movement disorders than the typical antipsychotics and do not cause hyperprolactinaemia. SGAs include **clozapine**, **olanzapine**, **risperidone**, **quetiapine**, **lurasidone**, and **ziprasidone**.

Clozapine was the first SGA and it binds only weakly to D_2 receptors and has a higher affinity for D_4 receptors. It also binds to histamine H_1, 5-HT_2, alpha$_1$-adrenergic, and muscarinic receptors. At the time of writing, clozapine is the only antipsychotic which has been demonstrated to be effective in patients who are unresponsive to adequate trials of at least two antipsychotics, one of which must have been a FGA. Clozapine does not cause extrapyramidal side effects, but it causes neutropenia in 2–3 per cent of patients, which progresses to agranulocytosis in 0.3 per cent of patients. For this reason, it is used only when other drugs have failed, and then with regular blood tests, and an explanation of the risks and benefits.

Dopamine system stabilizers. One current target for new drug development is the production of molecules that 'stabilize' the dopaminergic system. These drugs are partial agonists and can increase dopamine transmission in D_2 receptors when it is low and lower it when high. Thus, it may be possible to achieve relief of psychotic symptoms without inducing parkinsonism. **Aripiprazole** is the prototype of this class of drugs, although older drugs such as sulpiride and amisulpride may have some of the same characteristics.

Slow-release depot preparations are given by injection to patients who improve with drugs but cannot be relied on to take them regularly by mouth. These preparations are esters of the antipsychotic drug, usually in an oily medium. Examples include fluphenazine decanoate, flupentixol decanoate, risperidone, and olanzapine. Their action is much longer than that of the parent drug, usually 2–4 weeks after a single intramuscular dose. Because their action is prolonged, a small test dose is given before the full dose is used. Depot preparations are particularly useful when there are difficulties with compliance.

Adverse effects

The numerous adverse effects of antipsychotic drugs are related mainly to the antidopaminergic, antiadrenergic, and anticholinergic effects of the drugs (Table 13.3). They are common even at therapeutic doses and so are described in some detail. When

prescribing, the general account given here should be supplemented with that found in the SPC or *BNF*.

Antidopaminergic effects give rise to four kinds of **extrapyramidal** symptoms and signs (Table 13.4). These effects often appear at therapeutic doses and are most frequent with conventional antipsychotic drugs:

1 **Acute dystonia** occurs soon after the treatment begins. It is most frequent with butyrophenones and phenothiazines with a piperazine side chain. The clinical features are shown in Box 13.3. The term **oculogyric crisis** is sometimes used to denote the combination of ocular muscle spasm and opisthotonus. The clinical picture is dramatic and sometimes mistaken for histrionic behaviour. Acute dystonia can be controlled by an anticholinergic drug such as procyclidine, given carefully by intramuscular injection following the manufacturer's advice about dosage.

2 **Akathisia** is an unpleasant feeling of physical restlessness and a need to move, leading to inability to keep still. It starts usually in the first 2 weeks of treatment but can be delayed for several months. The symptoms are not controlled reliably by antiparkinsonian drugs but generally disappear if the dose is reduced.

3 **Parkinsonian effects** are the most frequent of the extrapyramidal side effects. They are listed in Box 13.4. The syndrome often takes a few weeks to appear. Parkinsonism can sometimes be controlled by lowering the dose. If this cannot be done without losing the therapeutic effect, an antiparkinsonian drug can be prescribed. With continued treatment, parkinsonian effects may diminish even though the dose of the antipsychotic stays the same. It is appropriate to check at intervals that the antiparkinsonian drug is still required, since these compounds may increase the risk of tardive dyskinesia.

4 **Tardive dyskinesia** is so called because it is characteristically a late complication of antipsychotic treatment. The clinical features are shown in Box 13.5. The condition may be due to supersensitivity of dopamine receptors

Table 13.3 Unwanted effects of first-generation antipsychotic drugs

Effect	Drugs most associated with this effect
Antidopaminergic effects	
Acute dystonia	FGAs
Akathisia	
Parkinsonism	
Tardive dyskinesia	
Antiadrenergic effects	
Postural hypotension[a]—more common after intramusular injection	FGAs
Nasal congestion	
Inhibition of ejaculation	
Anticholinergic effects	
Dry mouth	FGAs
Reduced sweating	Clozapine
Urinary hesitancy and retention	
Constipation	
Blurred vision	
Precipitation of glaucoma	
Other effects	
Prolonged QTc interval → cardiac arrhythmias	All except aripiprazole
Hypothermia[a]	
Weight gain	FGAs, clozapine, olanzapine
Hyperprolactinaemia (→ amenorrhoea and galactorrhoea)	FGAs, risperidone, amisulpride
Dyslipidaemia and type 2 diabetes	Clozapine, olanzapine
Worsening of epilepsy (some)	FGAs
Photosensitivity (some)	Chlorpromazine and similar drugs
Accumulation of pigment in skin, cornea, and lens (some)	Chlorpromazine
Neuroleptic malignant syndrome	See Box 13.5 and text

[a] These are especially important in the elderly.

Table 13.4 Extrapyramidal effects of antipsychotic drugs

Effect	Usual interval from starting treatment
Acute dystonia	Days
Akathisia	Days to weeks
Parkinsonism	A few weeks
Tardive dyskinesia	Several years

Box 13.3 Clinical features of acute dystonia

- Torticollis
- Tongue protrusion
- Grimacing
- Spasm of ocular muscles
- Opisthotonus

Box 13.4 Clinical features of parkinsonism

- Bradykinesia
- Expressionless face
- Lack of associated movements when walking
- Stooped posture
- Rigidity of muscles
- Coarse pill rolling tremor
- Festinant gait (in severe cases)

Box 13.5 Clinical features of tardive dyskinesia

- Chewing and sucking movements
- Grimacing
- Choreoathetoid movements
- Akathisia

resulting from prolonged dopamine blockade. Tardive dyskinesia occurs in about 5 patients per 100 patients treated with FGAs per year— affecting about 15 per cent of patients on long-term treatment. Since it does not always recover when the antipsychotic drugs are stopped, and responds poorly to treatment, prevention is important. This is attempted by keeping the dose and duration of dosage of antipsychotic drugs to the effective minimum and by limiting the use of antiparkinsonian drugs (see point 3). Usually, the best treatment for tardive dyskinesia is to stop the antipsychotic drug when the state of the mental illness allows this. At first the dyskinesia may worsen, but often it improves after several drug-free months. If the condition does not improve, or if the antipsychotic drug cannot be stopped, an additional drug can be prescribed in an attempt to reduce the dyskinesia. No one drug is uniformly successful and specialist advice should be obtained. (The specialist may try a dopamine receptor antagonist such as sulpiride or a dopamine-depleting agent such as tetrabenazine.)

The neuroleptic malignant syndrome (NMS) is a rare but extremely serious effect of neuroleptic treatment, especially with high-potency compounds. The cause of NMS is unknown. The symptoms, which begin suddenly, usually within the first 10 days of treatment, are summarized in Table 13.5. Treatment is symptomatic. The drug is stopped, the patient cooled, fluid balance maintained, and any infection is treated. There is no drug of proven effectiveness. NMS is a serious condition and about 20 per cent of patients die. If a patient has had NMS, specialist advice should be obtained before any further antipsychotic treatment is prescribed.

Weight gain. Both FGAs and SGAs, but particularly clozapine, olanzapine, and quetiapine, can cause substantial weight gain and this can limit their acceptability to patients. It is important to inform the patient about the possibility of weight gain and to monitor their weight while taking the drugs.

Metabolic effects. There is evidence that several of the atypical drugs, including olanzapine and

Table 13.5 Neuroleptic malignant syndrome

Principal features		
Fluctuating level of consciousness		
Hyperthermia		
Muscular rigidity		
Autonomic disturbance		
Associated symptoms		
Mental symptoms	Fluctuating consciousness	
	Stupor	
Motor symptoms	Increased muscle tone	
	Dysphagia	
	Dyspnoea	
Autonomic symptoms	Hyperpyrexia	
	Unstable blood pressure	
	Tachycardia	
	Excessive sweating	
	Salivation	
	Urinary incontinence	
Laboratory findings	Raised white cell count	
	Raised creatinine phosphokinase (CPK)	
Consequent problems	Pneumonia	
	Cardiovascular collapse	
	Thromboembolism	
	Renal failure	

risperidone, can induce hyperglycaemia and diabetes. They should therefore be used with caution in patients at risk of developing diabetes, and blood sugar should be routinely monitored in such patients. It should be noted that many patients with schizophrenia have risk factors for developing diabetes.

Specific adverse effects of clozapine. About 2–3 per cent of patients taking clozapine develop leucopenia, and this can progress to agranulocytosis. With regular monitoring, leucopenia can be detected early and the drug stopped; usually the white cell count returns to normal. (Monitoring is usually weekly for 18 weeks and fortnightly thereafter.) Clozapine is also associated with:

- excessive salivation;
- severe constipation and gastrointestinal pseudo-obstruction;
- tachycardia;
- myocarditis;
- postural hypotension;
- weight gain and type 2 diabetes;
- seizures (dose related);

Clozapine is sedating and respiratory depression has been reported when it has been combined with benzodiazepines.

Teratogenesis. Although these drugs have not been shown to be teratogenic, they should be used with caution in early pregnancy.

Contraindications. There are several contraindications to the use of antipsychotic drugs. They include myasthenia gravis, Addison's disease, glaucoma, and past or present bone marrow depression. Caution is required when there is liver disease (chlorpromazine should be avoided), renal disease, cardiovascular disorder, parkinsonism, epilepsy, or serious infection. The manufacturer's literature should be consulted for further contraindications to the use of specific drugs.

Choice of drug

Of the many compounds available, appropriate choices include:

- a more sedating drug— olanzapine, chlorpromazine;
- a less sedating drug—aripiprazole, risperidone;
- a drug with fewer extrapyramidal side effects—atypical antipsychotics;
- an intramuscular preparation for rapid calming—olanzapine or haloperidol;

- a depot preparation—risperidone or fluphenazine decanoate;
- for patients resistant to other antipsychotics—clozapine (to be initiated by a specialist).

Antiparkinsonian drugs

Although these drugs have no direct therapeutic use in psychiatry, they are used to control the extrapyramidal side effects of antipsychotic drugs. For this purpose, the anticholinergic compounds used most commonly are benzhexol, benztropine mesylate, procyclidine, and orphenadrine. An injectable preparation of procyclidine is useful for the treatment of acute dystonia (see p. 137).

Although these drugs are used to reduce the side effects of antipsychotic drugs, they have side effects of their own. Their anticholinergic side effects can add to those of the antipsychotic drug to increase constipation, and precipitate glaucoma or retention of urine. Also, they may increase the likelihood of tardive dyskinesia (see p. 137). *Benzhexol and procyclidine have euphoriant effects, and are sometimes abused to obtain this action.*

Antidepressant drugs

Antidepressant drugs have therapeutic effects in depressive illness, but do not elevate mood in healthy people (contrast the effects of stimulants such as amphetamine). There is good evidence that the more severe the depression, the more effective antidepressants are. They are not very effective in mild depression, which is why in many countries non-pharmacological treatments are recommended instead. In moderate depression, about 50–70 per cent of patients will respond positively compared to no treatment at all, with a number needed to treat (NNT) of 3. They are also effective in anxiety disorders.

Drugs with antidepressant properties are divided into classes based upon their pharmacological action. Commonly used classes are shown in Table 13.6. There are some differences in efficacy between the drugs but substantial differences in safety and adverse effects. For this reason, consideration of the latter is crucial when selecting an antidepressant. Clinical guidelines (e.g. from NICE) are based along these lines.

Antidepressant drugs increase the monoamines 5-HT and/or noradrenaline. The development of SSRIs suggested that the antidepressant effects result from increased 5-HT function. Serotonin and noradrenaline reuptake inhibitors (SNRIs) are also better than placebo although they seem to be less effective than SSRIs in indirect meta-analyses. Thus, both 5-HT and noradrenaline may be involved in the mechanism of action of conventional antidepressants although neither is necessary. The antidepressant efficacy of other drugs, such as SGAs and new antidepressants with different pharmacological actions (such as mirtazapine, an alpha$_2$, 5-HT$_2$, and 5-HT$_3$ antagonist or agomelatine, which acts as an agonist at melatonergic MT$_1$ and MT$_2$ receptors and an antagonist at 5-HT$_{2C}$ receptors), demonstrates that innovative approaches to drug development may produce useful results.

Most antidepressants have a long half-life and so can be given once a day. Antidepressants should be withdrawn slowly, because sudden cessation may lead to restlessness, insomnia, anxiety, and nausea. Antidepressant action seems to commence very quickly, although it may be 10–14 days before it is easily detectable clinically.

Specific serotonin reuptake inhibitors (SSRIs)

These drugs selectively inhibit the reuptake of serotonin (5-HT) into presynaptic neurons. Examples are fluoxetine, citalopram, paroxetine, and sertraline. Their antidepressant effect is comparable to that of the tricyclic antidepressant drugs, and because they lack anticholinergic side effects they are safer for patients with prostatism or glaucoma, and when taken in overdose. They are not sedating. These properties have led to SSRIs being the first-line choice for depression and anxiety disorders. Their side effects are listed in Table 13.7. SSRIs may induce suicidal thoughts or behaviour in some patients, particularly younger people. SSRIs should be avoided in children. It is important to monitor all patients who start antidepressant drugs of any kind for the emergence of suicidal thoughts.

Table 13.6 Classes of antidepressant drugs

Class of antidepressant	Examples	Uses	Comment
Specific serotonin reuptake inhibitors (SSRIs)	Fluoxetine Sertraline Citalopram Escitalopram Paroxetine	Depression Anxiety disorders OCD Bulimia nervosa PTSD and other stress-related disorders	First-line choice in majority of circumstances
Serotonin (5-HT) and noradrenaline reuptake inhibitors (SNRIs)	Venlafaxine Duloxetine	Depression Anxiety disorders	Second-line choice or used for augmentation
Tricyclics	Amitriptyline Imipramine Nortriptyline Lofepramine Dosulepin Clomipramine	Depression Anxiety disorders OCD (clomipramine)	Cardiotoxic in overdose
Mirtazapine		Depression	Sedating, so good for sleep disturbance
Monoamine oxidase inhibitors (MAOIs)	Isocarboxazid Phenelzine Tranylcypromine Moclobemide	Depression	Due to dietary restrictions and multiple drug interactions, MAOIs are usually third-line antidepressants NOT to be combined with other serotonergic drugs due to risk of serotonin syndrome
Trazodone		Depression Anxiety	Probably less potent than SSRIs, SNRIs, or tricyclics. Side effects: postural hypotension, dizziness, headache sedation, minor gastrointestinal disturbances
Bupropion		Depression Smoking cessation	Second- or third-line choice. Contraindicated in eating disorders

OCD, obsessive–compulsive disorder; PTSD, post-traumatic stress disorder.

Drug interactions. The combination of SSRIs with **MAOIs** should be avoided since the combination may produce a 5-HT toxicity syndrome (**serotonin syndrome**) with hyperpyrexia, rigidity, myoclonus, coma, and death. **Lithium** and **tryptophan** also increase 5-HT function when given with SSRIs—this combination can be useful clinically but needs to be closely monitored. Combinations of lithium and SSRIs are effective for depressive disorders resistant to other treatment. Other interactions are listed in the manufacturer's literature.

Toxic effects. Overdosage leads to vomiting, tremor, and irritability.

Table 13.7 Side effects of SSRIs

Gastrointestinal	Nausea
	Flatulence
	Diarrhoea
Central nervous system	Insomnia
	Restlessness
	Irritability
	Agitation
	Tremor
	Headache
	(Acute dystonia, rarely)
Sexual	Loss of libido
	Ejaculatory delay
	Anorgasmia
Miscellaneous	Hyponatraemia (especially in the elderly)

Serotonin and noradrenaline reuptake inhibitors (SNRIs)

Venlafaxine blocks 5-HT and noradrenaline reuptake but does not have the anticholinergic effects that characterize tricyclic antidepressants and is not sedative. Side effects resemble those of SSRIs; in full doses it may cause hypotension. Venlafaxine appears to be slightly more effective than SSRIs in comparative trials but less well tolerated than drugs such as sertraline and citalopram. It is a useful second-line drug in those who have not responded or not tolerated an SSRI.

Specific noradrenaline reuptake inhibitors

Several tricyclic antidepressants are relatively specific noradrenaline reuptake inhibitors (e.g. desipramine and lofepramine). Reboxetine is a specific noradrenaline reuptake inhibitor. Meta-analysis shows that it is less effective and less well tolerated than most other antidepressants.

Tricyclic antidepressants

These drugs are so named because their chemical structure has three benzene rings. They have many adverse effects (see next paragraph) and toxic effects on the cardiovascular system. Because of these effects, tricyclics are being replaced for most purposes by SSRIs. However, they are still important because they are of proven effectiveness in severely depressed patients.

Adverse effects. Tricyclic antidepressants have many side effects which can be divided into the groups shown in Table 13.8. Most of the effects are common and those that are infrequent are important, so the list should be known before prescribing. The following points should be noted:

- Difficulty in micturition may lead to retention of urine in patients with prostatic hypertrophy.

Table 13.8 Side effects of tricyclic antidepressants

Anticholinergic effects	Dry mouth
	Constipation
	Impaired visual accommodation
	Difficulty in micturition
	Worsening of glaucoma
	Confusion (especially in the elderly)
Alpha-adrenoceptor blocking effects	Drowsiness
	Postural hypotension
	Sexual dysfunction
Cardiovascular effects	Tachycardia
	Hypotension
	Cardiac conduction deficits
	Cardiac arrhythmia
Other effects	Seizures
	Weight gain

- Cardiac conduction deficits are more frequent in patients with pre-existing heart disease. If it is necessary to prescribe a tricyclic drug to such a patient, a cardiologist's opinion should be sought (it is often possible to choose a drug of another group without this side effect; see 'Choice of antidepressant').

- Seizures are infrequent but important. Antidepressant drugs should be avoided if possible in patients with epilepsy; if their use is essential, the dose of anticonvulsant should be adjusted—usually with the advice of the neurologist treating the case.

- Toxic effects: in overdosage, tricyclic antidepressants can produce serious effects requiring urgent medical treatment. These effects include ventricular fibrillation, conduction disturbances, and low blood pressure; respiratory depression; agitation, twitching, and convulsions; hallucinations, delirium, and coma; and retention of urine and pyrexia.

- Teratogenic effects have not been proved, but antidepressants should be used cautiously in the first trimester of pregnancy and the manufacturer's literature consulted.

Contraindications. These include *agranulocytosis*, severe *liver damage, glaucoma*, and *prostatic hypertrophy*. The drugs should be *used cautiously in epileptic patients* because they are epileptogenic, in the elderly because they cause hypotension, and after myocardial infarction because of their effects on the heart.

Modified tricyclics and related drugs

The chemical structure of the tricyclics has been modified in various ways to produce drugs with fewer side effects. Of the many drugs, two will be mentioned.

1 **Lofepramine** has less strong anticholinergic side effects than amitriptyline and is less sedating; however, it may cause anxiety and insomnia. In overdose it is less cardiotoxic than conventional tricyclics.

2 **Trazodone** also has few anticholinergic effects, but has strong sedating properties.

Mirtazapine

Mirtazapine is a noradrenergic and specific serotonergic antidepressant (NaSSA). It is an effective antidepressant and is increasingly widely prescribed. Mirtazapine blocks alpha$_2$-receptors as well as 5-HT$_2$-receptors. Mirtazapine is highly sedating, making it a useful antidepressant for patients with insomnia or other sleep disturbances. It can be used as a standalone antidepressant or as an adjunct to an SSRI or venlafaxine. Main side effects include:

- sedation (this improves after the first few days);
- weight gain;
- dizziness;
- blood dyscrasias (rare but important).

Monoamine oxidase inhibitors

MAOIs are not used as first-line antidepressant treatment because of their side effects and hazardous interactions with other drugs and foodstuffs (described later in this section). They are usually started by a specialist, but since GPs and hospital doctors may treat patients who are taking MAOIs, their hazardous interactions should be known.

MAOIs inactivate enzymes that metabolize noradrenaline and 5-HT, and this action probably accounts for their therapeutic effects. They also interfere with the metabolism of tyramine, and certain other pressor amines taken medicinally. MAOIs also interfere with the metabolism in the liver of benzodiazepines, tricyclic antidepressants, phenytoin, and antiparkinsonian drugs. When the drug is stopped, these inhibitory effects on enzymes disappear slowly, usually over about 2 weeks, so that the potential for food and drug interactions outlasts the taking of the MAOI. MAOIs with more rapidly reversible actions have been produced. Reversible MAOIs are less likely to give rise to serious interactions with foodstuffs and drugs. The various MAOIs differ little in their therapeutic effects.

Commonly used drugs include phenelzine, isocarboxazid, and tranylcypromine. The latter has an amphetamine-like stimulating effect in addition to its property of inhibiting monoamine oxidase.

This additional effect improves mood in the short term but can cause dependency. Moclobemide is a *reversible* MAOI.

Adverse effects. The common adverse effects of MAOIs are listed in Table 13.9.

Interactions with tyramine in food and drinks. Some foods and drinks contain tyramine, a substance that is normally inactivated in the body by monoamine oxidases. When these enzymes are inhibited by MAOIs, tyramine is not broken down and exerts its effect of releasing noradrenaline, with a consequent pressor effect. (As noted earlier, with most MAOIs the inhibition lasts for about 2 weeks after the drug has been stopped. With the 'reversible' MAOI, moclobemide, inhibition lasts for a shorter time, usually about 24 hours.) If large amounts of tyramine are ingested, blood pressure rises substantially with a so-called **hypertensive crisis** and, occasionally, a cerebral haemorrhage. An important early symptom of such a crisis is a severe, usually throbbing, headache. The main tyramine-containing foods and drinks to be avoided are listed for reference in Box 13.6. About four-fifths of reported interactions between foodstuffs and MAOIs, and nearly all deaths, have followed the consumption of *cheese*. It is important to consult this list and the manufacturer's literature before prescribing MAOIs. Patients should be given a list of foodstuffs and other substances to be avoided (available usually from the manufacturer).

Table 13.9 Side effects of MAOIs

Autonomic	Dry mouth
	Dizziness
	Constipation
	Difficulty in micturition
	Postural hypotension
Central nervous system	Headache
	Tremor
	Paraesthesia
Other	Ankle oedema
	Hepatotoxicity (hydrazines)

Box 13.6 Interactions of MAOIs with drugs and food

Due to inactivation of monoamine oxidase

- Foods and drinks with high tyramine content:
  - Most cheeses
  - Extracts of meat and yeast
  - Smoked or pickled fish
  - Hung poultry or game
  - Some red wines
- Drugs with pressor effects:
  - Adrenaline, noradrenaline
  - Amphetamine, ephedrine
  - Fenfluramine
  - Phenylpropanolamine
  - l-Dopa, dopamine

Due to effects on other enzymes

- Morphine, pethidine
- Procaine, cocaine
- Alcohol
- Barbiturates
- Insulin and oral hypoglycaemics (risk of hypoglycaemia)

Drugs that promote brain 5-HT function

In combination, these lead to a risk of hyperpyrexia, restlessness, muscle twitching, rigidity, convulsions, and coma:

- SSRIs
- Clomipramine
- Imipramine
- Fenfluramine
- l-Tryptophan
- Buspirone

Drug interactions. Patients taking MAOIs should not be given drugs metabolized by enzymes inhibited by MAOIs or those that enhance 5-HT functions (Table 13.9).

Treatment of hypertensive crises. Hypertensive crises are treated by parenteral administration of phentolamine to block alpha-adrenoceptors or calcium channel inhibitors such as nifedipine. Blood pressure should be followed carefully.

Treatment of the 5-HT syndrome. All medication should be stopped and supportive measures given. Drugs with 5-HT antagonist properties may be tried but their benefits have not been proved: propranolol and cyproheptadine are possible choices.

Contraindications to MAOIs

These include liver disease, phaeochromocytoma, congestive cardiac failure, and conditions which require the patient to take any of the drugs that react with MAOIs.

Management

Information for patients. The dangers of interactions with foods and other drugs should be explained carefully, and a warning card should be provided. Patients should be warned not to buy any proprietary drugs except from a qualified pharmacist, to whom the card should always be shown.

Choice of drug. Phenelzine is a suitable choice, starting with 15 mg twice daily and increasing cautiously to 15 mg four times a day. Tranylcypromine, which has amphetamine-like effects as well as MAOI properties, is often effective but as noted previously, some patients become dependent on its stimulant action.

Changing drugs. As noted earlier, if an MAOI is not effective, *at least 2 weeks* must pass between ceasing the MAOI and starting another kind of antidepressant. As MAOIs should be discontinued slowly, the time for changeover is even longer. These periods are shorter for the reversible MAOI, moclobemide (see 'Interactions with tyramine in food and drinks').

Choice of antidepressant

The clinician should become familiar with the use of a small number of drugs from each class in order to choose the best option in different clinical situations:

1 Untreated moderate depression—first-line choice is an SSRI.

2 A sedating antidepressant—mirtazapine.

3 A sedating tricyclic—amitriptyline.

4 A non-sedating antidepressant—SSRIs, venlafaxine.

5 Safest choice in pregnancy—SSRIs.

6 Safest choice in patients with cardiac disease—sertraline.

7 Safest choice if there is concern about overdose—SSRIs (and only prescribe small amounts at a time).

8 An antidepressant with low risk of sexual side effects—mirtazapine.

9 Antidepressants in the elderly—start at a low dose.

Advice to patients

Before prescribing, the following points should be explained and discussed with the patient:

Delayed response. A noticeable therapeutic effect is likely to be delayed for up to 2 or 3 weeks, but side effects will appear sooner. The improvement in symptoms may not be linear over time and there may be temporary setbacks on the road to recovery.

Adverse effects. The common effects should be described, including drowsiness, and a warning given of the dangers of driving a motor vehicle or using machinery even when only slightly drowsy. Patients taking SSRIs may feel irritable or restless. With tricyclics, dry mouth and accommodation difficulties are common side effects.

Effects of alcohol. The effects of alcohol are increased when antidepressants are taken.

Older patients. Older patients should be warned about the effects of postural hypotension and told how to minimize these (e.g. by rising slowly from bed). Effects of tricyclics on bladder function should be explained. Reassurance can be given that most of these effects are likely to decrease with time.

Mood-stabilizing drugs

Drugs that prevent recurrence of bipolar disorder are often called **mood stabilizers**. The term is simply descriptive and does not denote a pharmacological class. The main mood stabilizers are lithium and a number of antiepileptic drugs including sodium valproate, carbamazepine, and lamotrigine. Mood stabilizers may also be effective at treating acute mood episodes. For example, lithium and sodium valproate are used to treat acute mania, and lithium and lamotrigine are used in depressive disorders, especially those occurring in bipolar disorder. Evidence is now emerging that some atypical antidepressants, especially quetiapine, have mood-stabilizing properties. Quetiapine is now being used in some patients with bipolar disorder or mood instability, especially if other mood stabilizers are not tolerated or contraindicated.

Lithium

Pharmacology

It is not known which of lithium's many pharmacological actions explains its therapeutic effects, but its effect in increasing brain 5-HT function may be relevant. Lithium also acts on secondary messenger systems within neurons—in particular it inhibits inositol monophosphatase and glycogen synthase kinase 3 (GSK-3), and current research is investigating these actions as potential approaches to developing new versions of lithium.

Lithium is absorbed and excreted by the kidneys where, like sodium, it is filtered and partly reabsorbed. Lithium concentrations rise, sometimes to dangerous levels, in three circumstances:

1 **Dehydration.** When the proximal tubule absorbs more water, more lithium is reabsorbed.

2 **Sodium depletion.** Lithium is carried by the mechanism that carries sodium, and more lithium is transported when there is less sodium.

3 **Thiazide therapy.** Thiazide diuretics increase the excretion of sodium but not of lithium, and plasma lithium rises.

Dosage and plasma concentrations

GPs are often asked to supervise continuing treatment with lithium started by specialists, and hospital doctors treat these patients for other conditions. Because the therapeutic and toxic doses are close together, it is essential to measure plasma concentrations of lithium regularly during treatment. Measurement is made first after 4–7 days, then weekly for 3 weeks, and then, provided that a satisfactory steady state has been achieved, once every 12 weeks.

The *timing of the measurement* is important. After an oral dose, plasma lithium levels rise by a factor of two or three within about 4 hours and then fall to the steady-state level. Since the steady-state level is important in therapeutics, concentrations are normally measured *12 hours after the last dose*, usually just before the morning dose, which can be delayed if necessary for an hour or two. It is the steady-state level 12 hours after the last dose, not the 'peak', which is the level referred to when discussing the concentrations aimed at in treatment and prophylaxis. If an unexpectedly high concentration is found, the first step is to find out whether the patient has inadvertently taken the morning dose before the blood sample was taken.

The required plasma concentrations are:

- for prophylaxis: 0.5–1.0 mmol/litre, increased occasionally to a maximum of 1.2 mmol/litre;

- for treatment of acute mania: 0.8–1.2 mmol/litre.

Toxic effects begin to appear over 1.5 mmol/litre and may be serious over 2.0 mmol/litre. Although the therapeutic effect is related to the steady-state concentration of lithium, any renal effects caused by the drug (see later in section) may relate to the peak concentrations. For this reason, the drug is often given twice a day. Delayed-release tablets have been introduced for the same reason, but the time course of plasma levels resulting from these tablets is not substantially different from that of standard preparations.

Adverse effects. These effects are listed in Box 13.7. The following points should be noted:

- **Polyuria** can lead to dehydration with the risk of lithium intoxication. Patients should be advised to drink enough water to compensate for the fluid loss.

- **Tremor.** Fine tremor occurs frequently. Most patients adapt to this; for those who do not, propranolol 10 mg three times daily often reduces the symptom. *Coarse tremor is a sign of toxicity.*

Box 13.7 Side effects of lithium

1 Early effects

- Polyuria
- Tremor
- Dry mouth
- Metallic taste
- Weakness and fatigue

2 Later effects

- Fine tremor[a]
- Polyuria and polydipsia (due to nephrogenic diabetes insipidus)
- Thyroid enlargement
- Hypothyroidism
- Impaired concentration
- Weight gain
- Gastrointestinal symptoms
- Sedation
- Impaired memory (see text)
- ECG changes[b]

3 Long-term effects on the kidney (not common, but important)

- Permanent reduction in concentrating ability
- Reduction in glomerular filtration rate → chronic renal failure

[a] Coarse tremor is a sign of toxicity.

[b] T-wave flattening and QRS widening (reversible when drug is stopped).

- **Enlargement of the thyroid** occurs in about 5 per cent of patients taking lithium. The thyroid shrinks again if thyroxine is given while lithium is continued, and it returns to normal a month or two after lithium has been stopped.

- **Hypothyroidism** occurs commonly (up to 20 per cent of women patients) with a compensatory rise in thyroid-stimulating hormone. Tests of thyroid function should be performed every 6 months, and a continuous watch kept for suggestive clinical signs, particularly lethargy and substantial weight gain. If hypothyroidism develops and lithium treatment is still necessary, thyroxine treatment should be added.

- **Impaired memory.** Usually this takes the form of everyday lapses such as forgetting well-known names. The cause is not known.

- **Long-term effects on the kidney.** A few patients develop a persistent impairment of concentrating ability and/or nephrogenic diabetes insipidus due to interference with the effect of antidiuretic hormone. This syndrome does not respond to antidiuretic treatments but usually recovers when the drug is stopped. With long-term treatment (exact timescales unknown as these effects are quite idiosyncratic), some patients may experience a decline in renal function. In most this will not be clinically relevant, but in a few can lead to renal failure. This is especially the case if they have had multiple episodes of lithium toxicity. Provided doses are kept to less than 1.2 mmol/litre, renal damage is rare in patients whose renal function is normal at the start. Nevertheless, it is usual to test renal function every 6 months.

Toxic effects

The toxic effects of lithium (Box 13.8) constitute a serious medical emergency, as they can progress through coma and fits to death. If these symptoms appear, lithium should be stopped at once and a high intake of fluid provided, with extra sodium chloride to stimulate an osmotic diuresis. Lithium is cleared rapidly if renal function is normal but in severe cases renal dialysis may be needed. Most patients recover completely, some die, and a few survive with permanent neurological damage.

Box 13.8 Toxic effects of lithium

- Nausea, vomiting
- Diarrhoea
- Coarse tremor
- Ataxia, dysarthria
- Muscle twitching, hyper-reflexia
- Confusion, coma
- Convulsions
- Renal failure
- Cardiovascular collapse

Teratogenesis

Lithium crosses the placenta, and there are reports of increased rates of **fetal abnormalities**, most affecting the heart. Objectively rates of cardiac malformations (typically 'Ebstein's anomaly') are low at approximately 1/1000. If possible, the drug should be avoided in the first trimester of pregnancy, but the risks to the mother need to be balanced against those to the fetus. Lithium should be stopped a week before delivery or otherwise reduced by half and stopped during labour to be restarted afterwards. However, lithium is **secreted into breast milk** to the extent that plasma lithium concentrations of breastfed infants can be half or more of that in the maternal blood. Therefore, bottle-feeding is usually advisable.

Drug interactions

There are several important interactions between lithium and other drugs. The manufacturer's literature or a book of reference should be consulted whenever lithium treatment is started and a second drug is prescribed for a patient taking lithium. The principal interactions are listed for reference in Box 13.9.

Contraindications

These are not absolute but include *end-stage renal failure* or *recent renal disease, cardiac failure* or *recent myocardial infarction*, and *chronic diarrhoea* sufficient to alter electrolytes. Lithium should not be prescribed if the patient is judged unlikely to observe the precautions required for its safe use.

Management of lithium treatment

Lithium is usually continued for at least 2 years, and often for much longer. In patients taking long-term therapy, the need for the drug should be reviewed every 5 years. Review should take into account any persistence of mild mood fluctuations which suggest the possibility of relapse if treatment is stopped. Continuing medication is more likely to be needed if the patient has previously had several episodes of mood disorder within a short time, or if previous episodes were so severe that even a small risk of recurrence should be avoided. There should be compelling reasons for continuing treatment

Box 13.9 Principal interactions between lithium and other drugs

1 Lithium concentrations may be increased by several drugs, including:
   - *haloperidol*;
   - *thiazide diuretics* (potassium-sparing and loop diuretics seem less likely to increase lithium levels but should be used cautiously);
   - *muscle relaxants*: when a patient on lithium is to have an operation, the anaesthetist should be informed in advance because the effect of muscle relaxants may be potentiated; if possible, lithium should be stopped 48–72 hours before the operation;
   - *non-steroidal anti-inflammatory drugs* (NSAIDs);
   - *some antibiotics*: metronidazole and spectinomycin;
   - *some antihypertensives*: angiotensin-converting enzyme inhibitors and methyldopa.
2 Interaction with antipsychotics:
   - potentiation of extrapyramidal symptoms;
   - occasionally, confusion and delirium.
3 Interaction with specific serotonin reuptake inhibitors (SSRIs):
   - 5-HT syndrome (see p. 142).
4 Later action with ECT may cause a reaction similar to a 5-HT syndrome.

for more than 5 years, although patients have taken lithium safely for much longer periods.

Lithium should be withdrawn gradually over a few weeks; sudden withdrawal may cause irritability, emotional lability, and, occasionally, relapse (more often into mania than depression).

Before starting lithium, a note should be made of any other medication taken by the patient and a *physical examination* including weight and ECG should be done. Glomerular filtration rate, haemoglobin, erythrocyte sedimentation rate, and a full blood count are often performed as well. If indicated, pregnancy tests should be done.

Advice to the patient. The doctor should explain:

1 the common side effects;
2 early toxic effects which would indicate an unduly high blood level of lithium;

3 the need to keep strictly to the dosage prescribed;

4 the arrangements for monitoring blood levels of lithium;

5 the circumstances in which unduly high levels are most likely to arise—low salt diet, unaccustomed severe exercise, gastroenteritis, renal infection, or dehydration secondary to fever;

6 the need to stop the drug and seek medical advice if these conditions arise.

If the patient consents, it is usually appropriate to include another member of the family in these discussions. An explanatory leaflet should be provided, repeating the same points for reference.

Starting lithium prophylaxis. Lithium carbonate is usually given in a single night-time dose. The commonest dose for adults is 800 mg per day, tapered as indicated. The dose is adjusted until a lithium level of 0.5–1.0 mmol/litre is achieved in a sample taken 12 hours after the last dose. The optimal level is usually the highest level within this range tolerated without significant adverse effects. Levels between 1.0 and 1.2 mmol/litre may be used in the treatment of acute mania, but vigilance is required for adverse effects. Steady-state levels are usually achieved 5 days after a dose adjustment.

As treatment continues, lithium estimations should be carried out every 3–6 months or whenever the clinical status of the patient changes. Thyroid and renal function tests should be checked every 12 months. It is important to have a way of reminding the doctor about the times for the next repeat investigation. If two consecutive thyroid function tests a month apart show hypothyroidism, lithium should be stopped or l-thyroxine prescribed. Mild but troublesome polyuria is a reason for attempting a reduction in dose, whereas severe persistent polyuria is an indication for specialist renal investigation. A persistent leucocytosis is not uncommon and is apparently harmless; it reverses soon after the drug is stopped.

While lithium is continued, the doctor must keep in mind the possibility of interactions if new drugs are required by the patient.

Sodium valproate

Pharmacology. Like carbamazepine, sodium valproate was introduced as an anticonvulsant. Later it was found to control acute mania. It is less effective than lithium in preventing recurrence of bipolar disorder, but is used in those who are unable to take lithium for any reason or are already on lithium. The combination of lithium and sodium valproate is the most effective treatment for rapid cycling bipolar disorder. The mechanism of action of valproate is not understood. There are several formulations of valproate which vary in terms of pharmacokinetics but there is no evidence they vary in efficacy. Sodium valproate is the most commonly used formulation in the UK, but valproic acid tends to be favoured in the USA.

Adverse effects. Common adverse effects include:

- sedation;
- tiredness;
- tremor;
- gastrointestinal disturbance (usually resolves);
- reversible hair loss (10 per cent).

Rare but important adverse effects include:

- thrombocytopenia;
- increase in liver functions tests;
- pancreatitis;
- teratogenicity—neural tube defects.

Drug interactions. Valproate displaces highly protein-bound drugs such as other antiepileptic drugs from their protein-binding sites and may therefore increase plasma levels. Valproate inhibits the metabolism of lamotrigine, which must be used at about 50 per cent of the usual dose when prescribed in combination.

Teratogenesis. Valproate is teratogenetic and so must be avoided if possible in women of childbearing potential.

Lamotrigine

Pharmacology. Lamotrigine also is primarily an anticonvulsant. It may be effective in bipolar depression—possibly without inducing mania—and it also prevents depressive (but not manic) relapse in bipolar disorder.

Dosage and plasma concentration. Lamotrigine must be initiated very gradually, initially 25 mg daily for 2 weeks, then 50 mg daily for 2 weeks, and then further gradual increases. The usual dose in bipolar disorder is 100–300 mg daily.

Adverse effects. A rash may occur in 3–5 per cent of patients—the risk can be reduced by using gradual dosing (see previous paragraph). Other side effects include nausea, headache, tremor, and dizziness.

Drug interactions. Lamotrigine levels are increased by valproate. The combination of lamotrigine and carbamazepine may cause neurotoxicity.

Teratogenesis. Lamotrigine has been found to increase rates of cleft palate.

Carbamazepine

Pharmacology. Carbamazepine was introduced as an anticonvulsant. Later it was found to prevent the recurrence of affective disorder. It is effective in some patients who are unresponsive to lithium, and for some with rapidly recurring bipolar disorder. Both the effect in acute mania and the long-term efficacy of carbamazepine are less certain than those of lithium, but it is used successfully both as monotherapy and in combination with lithium in some patients.

Dosage and plasma concentration. Carbamazepine is usually started at 400 mg daily in outpatients but may be increased up to 800–1000 mg or higher in inpatients. The doses used for long-term treatment depend on tolerability and can range from 200 to 1600 mg daily. Monitoring of blood levels is less important than continued clinical vigilance for the emergence of adverse effects.

Adverse effects. Adverse effects may be troublesome if plasma levels are high, and include drowsiness, dizziness, nausea, double vision, and skin rash. A rare but serious side effect is agranulocytosis. A full blood count and liver function tests should be done before commencing treatment.

Drug interactions. Carbamazepine can accelerate the metabolism of some other drugs and of the hormones in the contraceptive pill, reducing its

effectiveness. It is advisable therefore to consider another form of contraception. Drug interactions should be checked in a reference source before prescribing other drugs to a patient taking carbamazepine.

Teratogenesis. Carbamazepine seems to be one of the safest mood stabilizers.

Cognition-enhancing drugs

Anticholinesterase inhibitors

(See also Chapter 26.) These drugs, including donepezil, rivastigmine, and galantamine, increase the function of acetylcholine, which can improve cognitive functioning, and they are used in the treatment of Alzheimer's disease. On average, they have a modest beneficial effect that might persist for a number of months but they do not halt or reverse the disorder. They are recommended for mild to moderate Alzheimer's dementia. Rivastigmine can also be used for moderate dementia in Parkinson's disease. These drugs are used following assessment in a specialist clinic, including tests of cognitive, global, and behavioural functioning and assessment of activities of daily living.

Adverse effects. The main adverse effects of anticholinesterase inhibitors include anorexia, nausea, vomiting, and diarrhoea. This usually remits with continued use. They should be caused with caution in patients with cardiac disease.

Memantine

Memantine is an *N*-methyl-d-aspartate (NMDA)-receptor antagonist. It is used to moderate to severe Alzheimer's disease, or if the anticholinesterase inhibitors have not be tolerated or effective. Adverse effects include agitation, dizziness, and mild gastrointestinal disturbance.

Other physical treatments

Electroconvulsive therapy

ECT is a specialist treatment and the reader requires only a general knowledge of its use; those requiring further information should consult the

Shorter Oxford Textbook of Psychiatry or another specialist text.

In ECT, an electric current is applied to the skull of an anaesthetized patient to produce seizure activity while the consequent motor effects are prevented with a muscle relaxant. The electrodes which deliver the current can be placed with one on each side of the head (**bilateral ECT**) or with both on the same side (**unilateral ECT**). Unilateral placement on the *non-dominant side* results in less memory impairment but may be less effective than bilateral ECT. Bilateral placement is therefore preferred when a rapid response is essential, or when unilateral ECT has not been effective.

The beneficial effect, which depends on the cerebral seizure, not on the motor component, is thought to result from neurotransmitter changes, probably involving 5-HT and noradrenaline transmission. ECT acts more quickly than antidepressant drugs, although the outcome after 3 months is similar.

Indications

The main indications for ECT are the following:

1 **The need for an urgent response:**
   (a) when life is threatened in a severe depressive disorder by refusal to drink or eat or very intense suicidal ideation;
   (b) in puerperal psychiatric disorders when it is important that the mother should resume the care of her baby as quickly as possible.

2 **For a resistant depressive disorder,** following failure to respond to thorough treatment with antidepressant medication.

3 **For resistant psychosis or mania,** following failure to respond to drug treatments.

4 **For two uncommon syndromes:**
   (a) catatonic schizophrenia;
   (b) depressive stupor.

Adverse effects of ECT

ECT has a number of adverse effects. Patients often have a brief period of headache or confusion after the treatment and may experience muscular aches for a couple of days.

A degree of cognitive impairment after treatment is relatively common although this clears rapidly in most patients. The more effective forms of ECT (e.g. higher dose, bilateral) appear to be more likely to cause cognitive problems. Some patients report a persistent loss of autobiographical memories but this has been difficult to show objectively in research studies. Depressive disorder can also lead to cognitive impairment, including memory problems, and it is therefore possible that the disorder itself is responsible. It is probably best to inform the patient that they may experience some short-term problems and that some patients report longer-term problems but that these appear to be uncommon. There are occasional effects from the anaesthetic procedure: the teeth, tongue, or lips may be injured while the airway is introduced and, rarely, muscle relaxants cause prolonged apnoea.

Mortality of ECT

The death rate from ECT is about 4 per 100,000 treatments, closely similar to that of an anaesthetic given for any minor procedure to a similar group of patients. Mortality is greater in patients with cardiovascular disease, and due usually to ventricular fibrillation or myocardial infarction.

Contraindications

The contraindications are those for any anaesthetic procedure and any condition made worse by the changes in blood pressure and cardiac rhythm which occur even in a well-modified fit: serious heart disease, cerebral aneurysm, and raised intracranial pressure. Extra care is required with diabetic patients who take insulin and for patients with sickle cell trait. Although risks rise somewhat in old age, so do the risks of untreated depressive disorder and of drug treatment.

Consent to ECT

Before ECT, a full explanation is given of the procedure and its risks and benefits, before asking for consent. If a patient refuses consent or is unable to give it, for example, because he is in a stupor, and if the procedure is essential, the psychiatrist seeks a second opinion and discusses the situation with relatives (although they cannot consent on behalf of the patient). In the UK and many other countries, there are procedures for authorizing ECT when the patient refuses but it is essential (these are set out in the MHA or corresponding legislation). Patients treated under these provisions seldom question the need for treatment once they have recovered.

The technique

ECT is administered by a psychiatrist, who applies the current, and an anaesthetist and a nurse. The procedure is described in specialist textbooks. ECT is usually given twice a week with a total of 6–12 treatments, according to progress. Response begins usually after two or three treatments; if there has been no response after six to eight treatments, it is unlikely that more ECT will produce useful change.

As some patients relapse after ECT, antidepressants are usually started towards the end of the course to reduce the risk of relapse.

Treatment with bright light

There is some evidence that bright light treatment is effective in seasonal affective disorder (SAD) (see p. 265). When a therapeutic effect appears it is rapid, but relapse is common. Light is administered usually at 6–8 am using a commercially available light box. The intensity of the light is usually about that of a bright spring day. The mode of action is uncertain; the light may correct circadian rhythms, which seem to be phase delayed in seasonal affective disorder.

Prescribing for special groups

Children

Most childhood psychiatric disorders are treated without medication. Many drugs that are licensed for use in adults have not been adequately studied in children. The indications for drug treatment are considered in Chapter 32. When drugs are required, care must be

taken in selecting the appropriate dose. Usually, medication will have been started by a specialist who will advise about continuing treatment.

Elderly patients

These patients are often sensitive to drug side effects and may have impaired renal or hepatic function, so it is important to start with low doses and increase to about half the adult dose in appropriate cases.

Pregnant women

Psychotropic drugs should be avoided if possible during the first trimester of pregnancy because of the risk of teratogenesis. If medication is needed for a woman who could become pregnant, advice is given about contraception. If the patient is already pregnant and medication is essential, the manufacturer's advice should be followed and the risks discussed with the patient. If the patient becomes pregnant while taking a psychotropic drug, the risk of relapse should be weighed against the reported teratogenic risk of the drug. In general, it is safer to use long-established drugs for which there has been ample time to accumulate experience about safety. The following points concern the classes of psychotropic drugs:

- **Anxiolytics** are seldom essential in early pregnancy since psychological treatment is usually an effective alternative.

- **If antidepressants are required,** sertraline, amitriptyline, and imipramine have no convincing evidence of teratogenic effects. There may be mild withdrawal effects in the neonate (usually agitation or twitching) but these resolve in 2–3 days without lasting effects.

- **Antipsychotic drugs.** It is important to discuss contraception with schizophrenic women, and to re-evaluate the need for antipsychotics if the patient becomes pregnant. Olanzapine is the safest first choice.

- **Lithium carbonate** should not be started in pregnancy because its use is associated with an increased rate of cardiac abnormality in the fetus.

Contraception is especially important for women who may become manic, and it is prudent to leave a month between the last dose of lithium and the ending of contraceptive measures. If a patient conceives when taking lithium, there is no absolute indication for termination but the risks should be explained, specialist advice obtained, and the fetus examined by ultrasound. Mothers who are taking lithium at term should, if possible, stop gradually well before delivery. The drug should not be taken during labour. Serum lithium concentration should be measured frequently during labour and the use of diuretics avoided.

- **Valproate** should be used cautiously in women of childbearing potential, and should not be started in pregnancy, because of its teratogenic potential.

Mothers who are breastfeeding

Psychotropic drugs should be prescribed cautiously to women who are breastfeeding because these pass into breast milk and the possibility is not ruled out that they may affect brain development. Benzodiazepines pass readily into breast milk, causing sedation. Most neuroleptics and antidepressants pass rather less readily into the milk; sulpiride, doxepin, and dothiepin are secreted in larger amounts and should be avoided. Lithium carbonate enters milk freely and breastfeeding should be avoided. The advice of a specialist should be obtained, but the safest options to date are sertraline and olanzapine

Patients with concurrent medical illness

Special care is needed in prescribing for patients with medical illness, especially liver and kidney disorders, which may interfere with metabolism and excretion of drugs. Conversely, medical disorders may be exacerbated by the side effects of some psychotropic drugs. For example, cardiac disorder and epilepsy may be affected adversely by some antidepressant drugs (see p. 151), while drugs with anticholinergic side effects exacerbate glaucoma and may provoke retention of urine.

Further reading

McKnight R, Adida M, Budge K, Stockton S, Goodwin GM, Geddes JR. Lithium toxicity profile: a systematic review and meta-analysis. *The Lancet* 2012;379:721–728.

Stahl SM. *Stahl's Essential Psychopharmacology*. 4th ed. Cambridge: Cambridge University Press; 2013. [A comprehensive and very well-illustrated review of psychopharmacology.]

Taylor D, Barnes TRE, Young AH. *Maudsley Prescribing Guidelines in Psychiatry*. 13th ed. Wiley-Blackwell; 2018. [A detailed and practical book useful for prescribing GPs or psychiatrists.]

14 Psychological treatment

Core psychological techniques

Psychological treatment is ubiquitous in medical practice: *all doctors use psychological treatment techniques every day, with every patient*. This is because the words that we use when we speak (or write) to patients have the power to heal (or to harm). This is the essence of the psychological treatments: they are treatments that use the power of words to improve the physical and emotional state of patients.

Carefully chosen words can improve your patient's morale, engage them with self-care, encourage them to adhere to medicines and to attend appointments, and reassure them that the resumption of normal daily activities is permissible and indeed desirable. Ill-chosen words can increase dependency, disability, and distress. All doctors therefore need to be able to use the *core psychological techniques* every day. These techniques (see Box 14.1) are involved in *every* healthcare relationship, whether in psychiatry or other specialties.

- **Develop a therapeutic relationship.** This can improve a patient's adherence to more formal psychological treatment, sustain them through periods of distress, and instil hope. In an appropriate

therapeutic relationship, patients should feel that the professional is concerned about them and takes time for them, but also understand that the relationship is distinct from friendship, and is one that the professional also has with other patients. Occasionally a patient–professional relationship can become too intense so that it impedes progress (see 'Independence versus dependence').

- **Actively listen to your patient's concerns.** Patients feel helped when they describe their problems to a sympathetic person, and many complain that

Box 14.1 Core psychological techniques

- Develop a therapeutic relationship
- Actively listen to your patient's concerns
- Allow the expression of emotion
- Improve morale
- Review and develop personal strengths
- Provide information, explanation, and advice ('psychoeducation')
- Actively endorse, encourage, and facilitate self-help
- Involve, educate, and support carers

doctors do not listen for long enough before they offer advice. To be effective, listening requires adequate time. Patients should feel that they have the doctor's undivided attention and have been understood. Use non-verbal signs of attention. Summarize verbally, and check out understanding of what has been said. Finally, summarize the patient's perspective in clinical letters which are copied to patients.

- **Allow the expression of emotion.** It is a common experience that the expression of strong emotion is followed by a sense of relief. Some patients feel ashamed to reveal their feelings to others and need to be assured that to do this is not a sign of weakness. If a patient or relative cries, offer support by looking concerned, by acknowledging verbally that they are upset (e.g. 'I'm sorry you're upset, it's clearly a difficult time for you'), and by offering a tissue (have some ready on your desk). After an appropriate period of time, aim to improve morale by saying something about the way forward, such as 'Perhaps now would be a good time to start to think about how things can be better for you—how does that sound?'

- **Improve morale.** Patients who have prolonged or recurrent medical or social problems may give up hope of improvement. Low morale, caused in this or other ways, undermines further treatment and rehabilitation. Even if there is no hope of recovery, such as in terminal cancer, it is usually possible to improve morale, for example, by describing how pain and distress can be minimized, and who will be there to help near the end.

- **Review and develop personal strengths.** Medical diagnosis focuses on what is wrong, rather than what is right. However, an effective treatment plan should take into account what abilities and social supports are intact, and help patients reinforce them. This helps overcome the current episode of illness and reduce risk of relapse.

- **Provide information, explanation, and advice.** In mental health settings, this is termed *psychoeducation*, that is, the education of patients (and their carers, if appropriate) about their illness. It is an important part of every patient's management. What is said (or written) needs to be accurate, clear, free from jargon, and relevant to the patient's physical and mental condition. There are five key elements (what, frequency, cause, healthcare, and self-care): see Chapter 20 for more information, in the context of physical disorder. Psychoeducation often involves bibliotherapy (see Box 14.2), and is often considered to be the first level of stepped care (see p. 101).

- **Actively endorse, encourage, and facilitate self-help.** Patients should be helped to achieve an appropriate balance between collaboration with medical treatment and maximal self-sufficiency. It is the patient's illness, and it may be lifelong. It is, therefore, very much in the patient's interest for them to develop the knowledge about their illness, the skills in self-management, and the lifestyle that will help them to get well and stay well. As patients recover and their confidence grows, self-management can and should play an increasing role in their daily care, progressively replacing the input of healthcare professionals.

- **Involve, educate, and support carers.** Carers are partners in the care of the patient, and may play a crucial role in supporting patients through and out of illness. They may also play a crucial role in perpetuating illness, if their attitudes to and beliefs about the illness are unhelpful. For these reasons, involving the carer in some aspects of psychological treatment, with the consent of the patient, can be beneficial. Written materials used during psychological treatment can be shared with carers, for example, or carers can be invited into meetings with patients at which diagnosis and treatment plans are discussed.

Provision of psychological support

For most people facing adverse events (e.g. death of a close relative, or diagnosis of a life-threatening

Box 14.2 Bibliotherapy

This is the use as a treatment by patients of books or booklets, and often comprises level one psychological treatment. A healthcare practitioner should recommend reading material for the patient and, potentially, also their carer(s). Their recommendation should bear in mind the patient's existing level of knowledge, their motivation, and the nature of the problem. Adherence can be increased by the professional:

1 **providing a clear rationale for the self-help approach.**
   'You need to become the expert in managing this problem. I can be here to help and support from time to time, but I can't be there when you most need me.'

2 **actively endorsing a particular resource.**
   'Lots of people with problems like yours find this book useful [show patient the book, from your bookshelf]. It's easy to read, and easy to obtain. I'll give you the details ...'

3 **suggesting reading particular chapters or sections:** in larger texts, some sections may be much more relevant than others.
   'Chapters X and Y are particularly relevant to your problems. Chapter X describes anxiety symptoms and their causes, and Chapter Y describes the beginnings of a self-help approach to managing anxiety.'

4 **making a follow-up appointment,** to review the patient's progress with the self-help approach.
   'I'd like to see you again in 2 weeks' time, when we can see how you've got on with those chapters. Do you have any questions?'

condition) or coping with adverse circumstances (e.g. looking after a disabled child), psychological support is provided informally by their social network including their close and extended family. In other circumstances, it can be provided by statutory bodies (such as social work services) or non-statutory bodies (such as charities and voluntary organizations). Occasionally, however, it will be provided by health services, and it can be an effective and valuable use of healthcare professionals' time.

Psychological support involves the use of the core psychological techniques described earlier to:

- *reduce distress*—during a short episode of self-limiting illness or personal misfortune;

- *support the patient temporarily and instil hope*—until a specific treatment has a beneficial effect (e.g. while waiting for the therapeutic effects of an antidepressant drug);

- *sustain long-term patients*—whose condition cannot be treated, or whose stressful life problems cannot be resolved (e.g. the problems of caring for a disabled child).

Before choosing supportive treatment, the vital question is whether a more structured and active form of psychological or other treatment could bring about change. Supportive sessions generally last for about 15 minutes, though the first session of treatment is often longer. Sessions are often weekly at first but may become less frequent. The length, frequency, and number of sessions should be agreed early, to avoid the development of dependency.

Stepped care

Psychological treatments may be time-consuming, and often need to be delivered by specially trained staff. There are often waiting lists before starting treatment. A 'one-size-fits-all' approach to treatment is inappropriate. Instead, a 'stepped-care approach' is desirable. This means that most patients with a particular disorder will start with 'level one' treatment—simple, quick to provide, and usually inexpensive. If level one treatment fails, the patient moves to level two treatment and, again, if this fails, to level three. Treatment algorithms may dictate that a patient misses out one or more levels if there is a clear clinical need.

In psychological treatments:

- *level one* of this stepped-care approach often involves basic information about the disorder and self-help approaches, delivered by booklet or book ('bibliotherapy'), or the Internet. At this level, there is minimal input by professionals;

- *level two* may involve group treatment (p. 168) or supported computerized delivery of a psychological treatment;

- *level three* may involve individual treatment, that is, face-to-face and one-to-one;

- *finally*, there may be a further level, for the very few treatment resistant patients who need specialist or particularly intensive treatments.

Independence versus dependence

The aim of doctors, other healthcare professionals, and treatments including psychological treatments, is to maximize the patient's functioning and increase their independence, wherever possible. This is why modern management incorporates elements of self-management, and why psycho-education is an essential part of every management plan. However, those aspects of the doctor–patient interaction that can be therapeutic and supportive can also be difficult to give up, and some patients can become too dependent on healthcare professionals.

Dependence is most likely to arise during psychological treatment but it can occur in the course of any treatment. Signs that the relationship is becoming too dependent include, but are not limited to: (1) asking questions about the doctor's personal life; (2) prolonging interviews beyond the agreed time; (3) attempting to contact the doctor for unwarranted reasons; (4) presenting with new or increased problems when reduction in or termination of contact is discussed; and (5) repeatedly bringing gifts.

Dependent patients may also cease to make appropriate efforts to help themselves, may request or demand increased attention, or may make unreasonable demands.

The best strategy is to reduce the risk of dependence, in every patient. Do this by '*planning for the end from the beginning*', that is, discuss, very early, the aim of treatment and the likely duration of treatment. However, if dependence emerges, the following approaches can be helpful:

- Remember how important the relationship is to the patient. Make and keep appointments reliably, letting the patient know when you will be unavailable, for example, due to leave.

- Maintain usual professional boundaries, and behave as a professional rather than as a friend. See Box 14.3 for tips on how to do this.

Box 14.3 Maintaining professional boundaries

- Make sure that you have a 'buffer' between you and the patient, by giving only your secretary's or ward administrator's phone number, rather than your office number, mobile number, or email address.
- Do not fit in additional appointments at the patient's request, unless there is a definite clinical need.
- Maintain the usual rules about touching patients; expressing sympathy and offering a tissue to a crying patient is desirable, but hugging them is not.
- Do not agree to meet the patient 'outside work'.
- Treat the patient as you would any other.
- Keep accurate and contemporaneous notes of all interactions with the patient, whether in person, in phone, by email, or in writing.
- If you sense difficulties, do not avoid seeking early advice from another doctor or healthcare professional—sharing such problems can be very helpful.

- Discuss the perceived difficulties with the patient, alongside a discussion of the way forward, towards independence. Recognize that this transition can be frightening for the patient, but encourage them to believe that this is possible.

Formal psychological treatments

In contrast to the **core psychological techniques** (which every doctor should employ every day), only a few of the **formal psychological treatments** are of direct concern to non-mental-health specialists. These treatments are discrete psychological interventions which are separate to routine clinical care, and for which patients would usually be referred to another healthcare professional, such as a clinical psychologist or specialist nurse, or to a dedicated service—perhaps part of the UK NHS Improving Access to Psychological Treatments (IAPT) programme.

In this chapter, the formal psychological treatments are described under the following headings:

1 **Problem-solving treatment,** which is useful for patients with adjustment disorders, depression, and deliberate-self-harm.

2 **Behavioural treatments and cognitive behavioural treatments,** which are used to alter patterns of behaviour (*behaviour therapy*) and thinking (*cognitive therapy*) that predispose to psychiatric disorders, which can prevent recovery from those disorders, and which can be combined to form a common psychological treatment, *cognitive behaviour therapy* or '*CBT*'.

3 **Dynamic psychotherapy,** which enables patients to recognize unconscious determinants of their behaviour and thereby gain more control over it.

4 **Group treatments,** which are used either as a first step in psychological treatment, when efficiency of delivery is as important as effectiveness, or when the group nature of the intervention may be particularly helpful (e.g. treatment of personality disorders).

5 **Couple and family treatments,** which are used when the core problem appears to be related to the couple's relationship or family interactions.

Terminology

Some terms may cause confusion because they are used with more than one meaning.

- The term **psychotherapy** is sometimes used to mean *all* forms of psychological treatment, often with an additional qualifying term, such as behavioural psychotherapy. Alternatively, the term can be used to refer only to dynamic psychotherapy. We prefer the term psychological *treatment* to psycho*therapy*. However, the term cognitive behaviour(al) therapy is used almost universally, and so we have stuck with that term.

- The term **counselling** refers to a wide range of the less technically complicated psychological treatments ranging from the giving of advice, through sympathetic listening, to structured ways of encouraging problem-solving. By itself, the term does not have a precise meaning and it should be qualified to indicate either the procedures that are used (e.g. problem-solving counselling) or the problem that is being addressed (e.g. bereavement counselling).

Problem-solving treatment

This treatment aims to help patients solve stressful problems and make changes in their lives. It includes the basic supportive processes described earlier together with the approach summarized in Box 14.4. Patients are encouraged to take the lead so that they learn not only a way of resolving the present difficulties but also a strategy for dealing with future problems. It is used for problems requiring:

- **a decision**—for example, whether a pregnancy is to be terminated, or an unhappy marriage ended;

- **adjustment to new circumstances**—such as bereavement, terminal illness, or a move to an

Box 14.4 The problem-solving approach

1 **List current problems.** The patient, with help from the therapist, defines and separates the various aspects of a complex set of problems.
2 **Choose one of the problems to work on.**
3 **List alternative solutions that could solve or reduce the problem.**
4 **Evaluate the alternative solutions and choose the best.** The therapist helps by working with the patient on the pros and cons of each approach.
5 **Try the chosen solution for the first problem.**
6 **Evaluate the results.** If successful, the next problem is acted upon. If unsuccessful, the patient and therapist review results constructively to decide how to increase the chance of success on the next occasion.
7 **Repeat this sequence until all the important problems have been solved.**

unfamiliar environment (e.g. by a student starting university);

- **change from an unsatisfactory way of life to a healthier one**—for example, part of treatment for dependence on alcohol or drugs.

Problem-solving and crisis intervention

When patients are overwhelmed by stressful events or adverse circumstances they are said to be in crisis and help for them is called **crisis intervention**. This approach is prompt, brief, and goal-directed, and includes:

- assessing the risk of suicide and self-harm at each meeting;
- encouraging the patient to express their distress, within a supportive setting;
- encouraging the patient to seek support from friends and family;
- discussing and modifying coping mechanisms; encourage adaptive mechanisms (e.g. phased return

to work/leisure activities, use of distraction) and discourage maladaptive coping mechanisms (e.g. avoidance of thinking about the traumatic event and its consequences, use of alcohol or illicit drugs to numb feelings, use of self-harm to numb feelings);

- providing advice about improving sleep;
- considering, when distress is severe, an anxiolytic/ hypnotic drug (usually a benzodiazepine) for a few days to calm the patient and assist sleep.

Behavioural treatments

These are used to treat symptoms and problems that persist because of behaviours of *the patient* (or other people) that initially lead to improvement but that maintain the problem.

1 **Maintaining behaviours by the patient.** Patients may *avoid* situations that provoke anxiety, for example, flying phobics avoiding plane travel and agoraphobics avoiding busy buses or supermarkets. In the short term, the patient gains, due to the prevention or alleviation of distress, but in the long term they lose, due to avoidance of travelling/shopping.
2 **Maintaining behaviours by other people.** Parents, teachers, or friends may pay more attention to children when they behave badly than when they behave well.

Core behavioural techniques

These include *distraction, relaxation*, and *exposure*.

Distraction

This simple but powerful technique reduces the impact of worrying or depressing thoughts, and is easy to deploy. Options include to:

- *focus attention on some external object*—for example, patients may count blue cars in the street or look intently at an object in the room;

- *use mental exercises*, such as mental arithmetic (e.g. subtract 7s from 100; recite the 13 times table), that require full attention;
- *use day-to-day activities*—if a patient is alone or under-occupied, worrying thoughts can gain the upper hand; if, however, they are busy, at home or at work, on their own or (preferably) with others, their activities will help to distract them.

Relaxation

This technique is also simple and powerful, but patients may need some education on 'how to do it', and need to practise so that it is effective. A common form of relaxation training ('progressive muscular relaxation') has the following steps:

- *Distinguish between tension and relaxation* by tensing a group of muscles and then letting go.
- *Breathe slowly* and regularly.
- *Imagine a restful scene* such as a quiet beach on a warm cloudless day.
- *Relax one muscle group* (e.g. the muscles of the left forearm). Then relax other groups one by one, for example, left upper arm, right forearm, right upper arm, neck and shoulders, face, abdomen, back, left thigh, left calf, right thigh, and right calf.
- *Relax larger muscle groups* (e.g. all the muscles of a limb together) so that complete relaxation is achieved more rapidly.
- *Resume activity gradually.*

The first session may last 30 minutes and each subsequent session about 15 minutes. After about six sessions, most people can relax rapidly. This is time-consuming for professionals to deliver, but relaxation programmes are available to purchase for patients to use at home at a convenient time. There are three steps: (1) the full intervention should be used regularly, with the audio-recording, so that the patient develops confidence and skill; then (2) the patient practises the full intervention without the recording; and (3) finally, the patient shortens the intervention, so that it is a brief, easy-to-use intervention that can be deployed whenever they feel stressed.

Exposure

Exposure to the feared stimulus is a powerful approach that is used mainly for phobic disorders. The basic procedure is to persuade patients to enter, repeatedly, situations that they have previously *avoided*, until, on each occasion, they *habituate* to the *feared stimulus*. This habituation is an *inevitable* consequence of ongoing proximity to the feared situation; anxiety/emotional arousal declines over a period of minutes.

Exposure is usually achieved in real life ('*in vivo*'), but, if this is not practicable (e.g. flying phobia, snake phobia), exposure is possible in the patient's imagination ('*in imagino*'). If you doubt this, close your eyes, and *imagine* the day of your psychiatry exam, in several weeks' time: you wake up, get dressed, cycle to the exam hall, wait to go in while doing some last-minute revision, are called in, and then finally step in to meet the examiners. You are likely to be feeling anxious or very anxious, even though you are not actually there!

Exposure is usually achieved in manageable steps: *graded* exposure, with a behavioural *hierarchy* of difficulty. It is helpful to enlist a relative or friend who can encourage and praise success. The stages of graded exposure are as follows:

- Determine which *situations* are *avoided,* and rate the anxiety experienced (0 = no anxiety, 10 = worst anxiety possible) for each.
- Construct the *hierarchy* by arranging situations in order of anxiety rating, for example, for a supermarket (agora-)phobic, the hierarchy might comprise: local shop with no other customers (3/10); local shop when it is crowded (5/10); supermarket with no queues at the checkouts (7/10); and supermarket at a busy time, with long queues impairing 'escape' (10/10).
- *Teach relaxation* so that it can be used to reduce anxiety during exposure.

- Persuade the patient to (1) *enter a situation* at the bottom of the hierarchy, (2) *monitor* their anxiety regularly, and (3) stay until anxiety has gone or almost gone: it is important that the patient has habituated before the patient leaves the situation. Repeat the procedure until the situation at the bottom of the hierarchy can be experienced without anxiety.
- Repeat with the next situation up the hierarchy, whose predicted anxiety level is likely to have reduced a little following this early success, for example, the rating for a local shop when it is crowded might have reduced from 5/10 to 3/10. Then repeat until the top of the hierarchy is reached.

Occasionally, an abbreviated approach—*flooding*—is used, in which the lower levels of the hierarchy are bypassed, and the initial (perhaps only) exposure is to a situation at or near the top of the hierarchy.

Exposure with response prevention is used to treat obsessional rituals. So, for example, in a patient with OCD with extensive cleaning rituals in response to a fear of contamination, *exposure* to the feared stimulus (i.e. dirt) leads to a rapid rise in anxiety/arousal, due to cognitions such as 'I will get infected and die of an awful disease'. The behavioural responses to exposure might include (1) head to the shower, (2) remove all clothes, (3) scrub contacted skin with disinfectant, and (4) carefully (don't touch the dirt!) put clothes in washing machine on a high temperature wash to kill all known bugs. These *responses* are, in effect, a form of *avoidance* of the feared outcomes (infection, disease, death) from *exposure* to the *feared stimulus* (dirt). The responses lead to a rapid reduction in arousal/anxiety, and the rituals are therefore self-reinforcing.

Behavioural treatment comprises (1) *exposure* to the feared stimulus, for example, clean the inside of a very unpleasant wheelie bin with a small brush, ensuring that nasty, green, smelly stuff ends up on clothes and skin, triggering high emotional arousal; followed by (2) *prevention of behavioural responses* (hence, together, '*exposure with response prevention*'). No behavioural responses are allowed and, eventually, after a period of several minutes, the arousal level starts to fall, as the patient *habituates* to the feared stimulus (dirt). As arousal levels fall, there are associated cognitive changes: the meaning of the dirt changes from 'disease-laden dangerous horribleness' to, well, just 'dirt'.

Other behavioural techniques

Thought stopping is used to treat obsessional thoughts occurring without obsessional rituals (and therefore not treatable by response prevention). A sudden, intrusive stimulus is used to interrupt the thoughts; for example, the mildly painful effect of snapping an elastic band worn around the wrist. When treatment is successful, patients become able to interrupt the thoughts without the aid of the distracting stimulus.

Self-control techniques are used to increase control over behaviours such as excessive eating or smoking. The treatment may be used alone or as part of a wider treatment, such as in CBT for bulimia nervosa. The treatment has two stages: (1) *self-monitoring* is the keeping of daily records of the problem behaviour and of its circumstances. For example, a patient who binge eats would record what is eaten, when it is eaten, and any associations between eating and stressful events or mood. Record-keeping is itself a powerful aid to self-control, because many patients have previously avoided facing the true extent of their problems. 2) *Self-reinforcement* is the rewarding of oneself when a goal has been achieved successfully, to maintain motivation. For example, a woman who has reached a target of no binges in a 7-day period might have a weekend away with her partner.

Contingency management is used to control abnormal behaviour that is being reinforced by other people; for example, by parents who attend more to a child during temper tantrums than at other times. The treatment has two aims: (1) to identify and reduce the reinforcers of the abnormal behaviour, and (2) to find ways of rewarding desirable behaviour. Praise and encouragement are the usual rewards but they may be augmented by material rewards such as points or stars. This behavioural approach includes the following:

1 **The behaviour to be changed is recorded** by the patient or another person (e.g. a parent might record the date/time/nature of a child's temper tantrums).

2 **Triggers (antecedents) are identified.** These immediately precede the behaviour (e.g. the temper tantrums occur after the mother pays attention to a younger sibling).

3 **Reinforcers (consequences) are identified.** These immediately follow the behaviour (e.g. extra attention is given to the child after behaving badly). Sometimes these first three elements are summarized as 'ABC' or 'antecedents—behaviours—consequences'.

4 The **undesirable behaviour is ignored** as far as practicable, and **appropriate behaviour is rewarded** (e.g. the parent would attend to the child when behaving well).

5 Parents or others **monitor progress** by continuing to record the frequency of the relevant behaviour.

Cognitive behaviour therapy

CBT (or simply 'cognitive therapy') is the predominant psychological treatment in the UK. This is due to its extensive evidence base of RCTs demonstrating its effectiveness in (1) the treatment of a range of *psychiatric* disorders, including anxiety, depression, eating disorders, and potentially also psychosis; (2) improving coping and other important outcomes in a range of *physical* disorders; and (3) improving coping in *carers* of patients with psychiatric or physical disorder. It is therefore important to have an understanding of its principles, and of some practicalities.

CBT is used to treat physical symptoms, psychological symptoms, and abnormal behaviours that persist because of the way that patients *think* about them. The person's *thoughts and beliefs*, that is, their *cognitions*, are the focus of assessment via the cognitive behavioural model and of treatment via CBT. For example, an agoraphobic experiencing intense anxiety as they approach a busy supermarket may believe that their palpitations, occurring as part of the 'fight or flight' anxiety response, are evidence of an impending heart attack. Their beliefs about their physical vulnerability are therefore important *maintaining factors* in their phobic disorder.

CBT incorporates and merges important behavioural and cognitive techniques. An agoraphobic may be *exposed* to their feared stimulus (e.g. busy supermarket). This might be beneficial alone, by reducing avoidance, but it will also trigger physical symptoms (palpitations) and associated *negative automatic thoughts* (e.g. 'I'm having a heart attack'). These can be used as the basis for simple cognitive interventions, using a *dysfunctional thought record* (e.g. Table 14.1), which can help the patient to regain control over their anxious thoughts. This increase in self-perception of control makes further exposure easier.

CBT therapists can help the patient to identify and understand the varied forms of *avoidance* in their life, which are maintained by their *beliefs* about their vulnerabilities (in this case cardiac). Avoidance includes *overt* avoidance, such as avoiding busy shops, and also *covert* avoidance, known as '*safety behaviours*'. These are personal ways of reducing the perception of threat, such as always carrying a mobile phone in case of the need to summon urgent assistance, or hanging on very tightly to a supermarket trolley to avoid the perceived risk of collapse.

Principles of CBT

- The focus of the patient and therapist is on understanding and managing *maladaptive thinking and behaviour*.

- The treatment is *structured*: the series of (typically 10 to 15) sessions has a beginning, a middle, and an end; and each session has a beginning (review of previous session, and plan for this session), a middle, and an end (planning of homework and arranging next session).

- The treatment is *collaborative*: the patient is treated as an active and expert partner in care.

- The treatment is *scientific* and *empirical*—it is based on the patient testing out their own reality for

Table 14.1 Examples of CBT symptom diaries (dysfunctional thought records)

A. A diary to record anxiety

Date/time	The situation in which you felt anxious	Symptoms	Rating of anxiety (0–10)	What you were thinking	What you did
12/6/18 4 pm	In a queue at the supermarket	Palpitations and dizziness	8	I am going to die	Ran away from the queue
13/6/18 10 am	In town centre	Palpitations and sweating	5	I must relax	Stood still. Tried to relax

B. A diary to record an eating disorder

Date/time	The problem	The situation at the time	What you were thinking before	What you did
18/7/18 7 pm	Ate a whole loaf of bread with butter and jam	Feeling despondent after being criticized at work	Everything I do goes wrong	Made myself vomit
19/7/18 1 pm	Bought 3 bars of chocolate and a cake	Angry with my friend	No one respects me	Sat alone and ate it all

themselves, rather than relying on 'truth' spoken by the therapist.

- Patients undertake '*homework*' between the sessions of treatment, practising and evaluating new ways of thinking and behaving.

- Symptoms, cognitions, and associated behaviours are monitored by recording them, as soon as possible after they have occurred, in a *diary* or *dysfunctional thought record*. This records (1) symptoms, (2) thoughts and events (including behaviours) that precede and possibly provoke the symptoms, and (3) thoughts and events (including behaviours) that follow and possibly reinforce the symptoms (Table 14.1).

- *Maladaptive thinking is challenged* by pointing out illogical reasoning, correcting misunderstandings by providing accurate information, and devising more realistic alternatives to the maladaptive ways of thinking. NB More 'realistic' or 'balanced' are better terms to use than more 'positive'.

- Treatment takes the form of a *graded* series of tasks and activities. Feasibility is enhanced by patients gaining confidence in dealing with less challenging problems before attempting more challenging ones.

- Tasks and activities are presented as *experiments* in which the achievement of a goal is a success, while non-achievement is not a failure but an opportunity to learn by analysing constructively what went wrong. This helps to maintain motivation.

- *Behavioural experiments* are used to test out a patient's beliefs/predictions (invariably negative, due to active *cognitive biases*) of what will happen in a particular circumstance, and thereby to change beliefs about their vulnerability/resilience (e.g. running up and down stairs, to increase heart rate and give 'palpitations', and to thereby demonstrate a benign cause of 'palpitations'). Don't get confused: *behavioural* experiments are used to change *cognitions*.

- *Outcome monitoring* is routine. Patients are asked to rate their symptoms/problems, and to complete validated rating scales. This both helps to evaluate the success of treatment and increases collaboration with treatment.

CBT for anxiety disorder

The core techniques of CBT for anxiety include the following:

- **Using a symptom diary/dysfunctional thought record** (see Table 14.1) to assess the nature and severity of symptoms, situations in which anxiety occurs, and associated avoidance. Although standard diary templates are widely available, there is no fixed design, and the professional and patient can design one together that will work for that patient's particular circumstances.
- **Identifying and challenging maladaptive thoughts and beliefs,** which often relate to the perception of threat in particular everyday situations or from particular physical symptoms. Palpitations, chest pain, and lightheadedness, for example, are typically due to normal 'fight or flight' anxiety response or hyperventilation, rather than to serious illnesses such as heart attack or stroke.
- **Increasing understanding of the vicious circle of anxiety,** including the importance of fearful concerns about the symptoms ('fear of fear')
- **Increasing understanding of the maintaining effects of avoidance,** both overt and covert (safety behaviours).
- **Relaxation** (see p. 161).
- **Graded exposure** (see p. 161).
- **Distraction** (see p. 160), to reduce the anxiogenic effect of remaining maladaptive thoughts.

In panic disorder, for example, cognitions are key to the aetiology of the disorder. Patients are convinced that some of their physical symptoms are not caused by anxiety but are the first indications of a serious physical illness (e.g. that palpitations signal an imminent heart attack). This conviction causes further anxiety, which worsens physical symptoms such as palpitations, so that a '*vicious cycle*' of mounting anxiety is set up. Treatment includes the therapist working with the patient to demonstrate that there is a viable alternative understanding of this reality, in which physical symptoms are part of the normal response to stress, and fear of these symptoms sets up a vicious circle of anxiety.

CBT for depressive disorder

In CBT, *cognitive* and *behavioural* theories and techniques are used alongside each other, in a synergistic way.

Cognitive abnormalities in depressive disorder include the following:

1 **Intrusive thoughts,** usually of a self-deprecating kind (e.g. 'I am a failure'). When they are weak, such thoughts can be counteracted by *distraction*, but when they are strong, they are difficult to control.

2 **Logical errors** distort the way in which experiences are interpreted, and maintain the intrusive thoughts (Box 14.5). The therapist helps the patient recognize these irrational ways of thinking and change/challenge them into more *realistic/balanced* thoughts.

3 **Maladaptive assumptions** are often about social acceptability; for example, the assumption that only good-looking or successful people are liked by

Box 14.5 Logical errors/cognitive distortions in depressive disorders

- **Exaggeration:** magnifying small mistakes or problems and thinking of them as major failures/issues, that is, 'making a mountain out of a molehill'. At its worst, this is termed catastrophizing.
- **Catastrophizing:** expecting serious consequences of minor problems (e.g. thinking that a relative who is late home has been involved in an accident).
- **Minimization:** minimizing or ignoring successes or personal positive qualities.
- **Overgeneralizing:** thinking that the bad outcome of one event will be repeated in every similar event in the future (e.g. that having lost one partner, the person will never find a lasting relationship).
- **Mental filter:** dwelling on personal shortcomings or on the unfavourable aspects of a situation while overlooking favourable aspects.

others. The patient is helped to examine how ideas of this kind influence the ways in which they think about themselves and other people.

Behavioural abnormalities in depressive disorder include underactivity, due to withdrawal from or avoidance of their usual social and occupational activities, which may be precipitated and maintained by cognitive factors such as concerns about the attitude or responses of others. The therapist uses a *behavioural* intervention, *activity scheduling* (sometimes called *behavioural activation*), to help the patient to steadily increase their activity levels, by building more activities into their lives that are either satisfying or enjoyable.

CBT in a stepped-care model

Even though CBT is a time-limited, focused intervention, when it is delivered one-to-one it demands a significant amount of a healthcare professional's time. Therefore, CBT is usually delivered in a '*stepped-care model*':

- The first step or level, applicable to most patients, is *bibliotherapy*: written self-help materials, based on CBT principles, are recommended or provided, and actively endorsed by a healthcare practitioner. Some examples are given at the end of this chapter.

- The second step, applicable to some patients, might be group CBT for anxiety.

- The final step, for only the few patients who have not been helped by steps one and/or two, is individual CBT for anxiety.

In this way, the most intensive and expensive intervention is restricted to those patients who need it most. This stepped-care approach is the key guiding principle to the UK NHS IAPT programme (see, e.g. http://www. england.nhs.uk/mental-health/adults/iapt). Powerful arguments are being made for further resources to extend the reach of evidence-based psychological treatments such as CBT, delivered by a stepped-care approach (see Layard and Clark (2014) in 'Further reading').

Formal CBT is a complex and time-consuming procedure that requires special training and resource. However, simple cognitive-behavioural techniques can and should be used every day, in psychiatric and general hospitals, and indeed in the brief consultations in general practice (see David (2013) in 'Further reading').

Dynamic psychotherapy

In this treatment, patients are helped to obtain a greater understanding of aspects of their problems and of themselves, with the expectation that this will help them to overcome these problems. The focus of treatment is on aspects of the problems and of the self of which the person was previously unaware (unconscious aspects). The treatment may be brief and focused on a small number of specific problems (**brief focal dynamic psychotherapy**) or long term and dealing with a broader range of problems (**long-term dynamic psychotherapy**). Dynamic psychotherapy is a specialist treatment requiring training.

Brief focal dynamic psychotherapy

The main *indications* for brief dynamic therapy are low self-esteem and difficulties in making relationships, either of which may be accompanied by emotional disorders, eating disorders, or sexual disorders. Patients referred for dynamic psychotherapy need to be insightful and willing to consider links between their present difficulties and events in their earlier life. Because treatment is focused on self-concept and relationships, involving judgements about the kind of change that is desirable, it highlights ethical problems concerned with values (Box 14.6).

The principal steps are as follows:

1 Patient and therapist *agree on the problems* that are the focus of treatment.

2 Patients *discuss recent and past experiences* of the problem. To encourage the necessary self-revelation, the therapist speaks infrequently and responds more to the emotional than the factual content of what is said. For example, instead of asking for more factual detail, he or she may say 'You seemed angry when you spoke about that'.

Box 14.6 Ethical issues of imposing values in dynamic psychotherapy

Therapists should always respect their patients' values and never impose their own. This rule applies to all therapeutic situations, for example, when counselling about a possible termination of pregnancy. It is especially important in dynamic psychotherapy in which value judgements are often involved, for example, in deciding what relationship changes would be desirable. Therapists risk imposing their own values:

- *directly*, by expressing their values or challenging those of the patient;
- *indirectly*, for example, by giving more attention to arguments against a course of action than to arguments for it.

3 Patients *review their own part in problems* that they ascribe to other people.

4 Patients *identify common themes* in what they are describing; for example, fear of being rejected by other people.

5 Patients *recall similar problems* at an earlier stage of life. They are encouraged to consider whether the present maladaptive behaviour may have originated as a way of coping that was adaptive at that time but is now self-defeating. For example, failure to trust others following the experience of sexual abuse in childhood.

6 The *therapist makes interpretations* to help patients discover connections between past and present behaviour, or between different aspects of their present behaviour. Interpretations are presented as hypotheses to be considered, rather than truths to be accepted.

7 The patient is encouraged to consider *alternative ways of thinking and relating*, to try these out first with the therapist and then in everyday life.

Long-term dynamic psychotherapy

This treatment, originating from Freud's psycho-analysis, aims to change longstanding patterns of thinking and behaviour that contribute to personal, relationship and psychiatric problems. Patients are seen three or more times a week, for at least a year. The problems of dependency are significant with long-term therapy, and the end of treatment ('termination') should be anticipated and discussed very early. The evidence base for long-term dynamic psychotherapy is rather thin, although a small number of RCTs provide some evidence of benefit in some disorders. This relative lack of evidence compared to the copious evidence for CBT has contributed to a dwindling in NHS long-term dynamic psychotherapy in the UK, alongside a simultaneous burgeoning of NHS CBT.

Alongside basic psychotherapy procedures, these special techniques are used:

1 **Free association.** The patient is encouraged to allow their thoughts to wander freely, and potentially illogically, from a starting point of relevance to the problem. This technique and the next are used to encourage the recall of previously repressed memories.

2 **Recall of dreams** and discussion of their meaning.

3 **Interpretation of transference.** Transference (see Box 14.7) is used as a tool of treatment on the assumption that it reflects patients' relationships

Box 14.7 Transference and countertransference

In psychotherapy, an intense relationship between the patient and doctor is called a *transference*. This originates from Freud's theory that the patient transfers to the 'therapist' feelings and thoughts that originated in a close relationship during childhood, usually with a parent. When the feelings are positive, it is a *positive transference*, and, when negative, a *negative transference*.

Therapists may also transfer to their patients feelings that properly belong elsewhere, developing strong positive or negative feelings because a particular patient reminds them, consciously or unconsciously, of a parent or another close figure in their lives. This is called *countertransference*. Countertransference may impair the doctor's ability to maintain an appropriate relationship and provide impartial advice.

with their parents in earlier life. The therapist comments on the significance of the transference reactions, and helps the patient to practise controlling these strong emotion, which are likely to be similar to emotions experienced outside the therapy sessions.

4 **Control of countertransference.** The factors that encourage transference in the patient also provoke *countertransference* on the part of the therapist. For this reason, therapists are required to understand their emotional reactions better by undergoing dynamic psychotherapy themselves before using these methods with patients.

Treatment in groups

Rationale

Some psychological treatment takes place in groups. There are two main reasons for this:

1 **Cost-effectiveness and availability.** Psychological treatment staff may be expensive and scarce. Providing individual, one-to-one, treatment may therefore lead to expensive and delayed services. It is often possible to provide initial psychological treatment in a group. Any disadvantage of the reduction in personalized care may be balanced out by additional treatment processes that may arise in groups.

2 **Additional treatment processes in groups.** These processes are useful both in psychiatric treatment and in the more general practice of medicine where groups can be used to support patients or their relatives. They include:

- *understanding you are not alone*, this is sometimes called 'normalization'—meeting other people with similar problems to your own can be reassuring;
- *support from others* both in the group and outside the group (e.g. meeting for coffee afterwards);
- *learning from others*, for example, how others have overcome problems similar to the patient's own;

- *pressure from others in the group to modify behaviour within the group*, for example, disruptive outbursts, dominating the group, or excessively criticizing others may trigger feedback from group members;
- *practising social behaviour*, especially by those who are socially anxious or awkward.

Specific issues

In individual psychological treatment, patients have a confidential relationship with the therapist. Members of a psychological treatment group reveal their personal problems not only to the therapist but also to each other. Patients therefore need to agree some 'group rules', which usually include (1) that they *will* speak about personal matters *in* the group, so that they can play an active role; and (2) that they *will not* speak about matters discussed in the group *outside* the group.

Small group treatment

A small group usually has about eight patients. Group therapy can be used for any of the purposes for which individual therapy is used, that is, for *support, problem-solving, behavioural treatment, CBT*, and *dynamic psychotherapy*. The length of treatment, its intensity, and the techniques vary according to the purpose, as they do with individual therapy.

Large group treatment

Large groups are used in two ways:

- In some **psychiatric wards**, patients meet regularly in a group of 20 or more people. This enables patients to talk about the problems of living together in the ward, and thereby reduce these problems whenever possible.
- In a **therapeutic community**, group methods are used to treat personality disorder, especially emotionally unstable personality disorder. Patients reside in the community for months, living and working together, and attending small and large groups in which they

discuss relationship problems and help each other to recognize and resolve problems. The approach is available in only a few special centres. In some centres, this approach has been modified to be suitable for delivery to outpatients.

Self-help groups

These groups are organized by people who have a problem in common, for example, obesity, alcoholism, postnatal depression, or the rearing of a child with a congenital disorder. The group is often led by a person who has coped successfully with the problem. The members usually meet without a professional therapist although the leader may have a professional adviser. *Alcoholics Anonymous*, *Bipolar UK* groups, *Mind* self-help groups, and the *Alzheimer's Association* caregiver support groups are prominent examples of such groups. They are important sources of support and advice, and many can and should be recommended to patients/carers.

Treatment for couples and families

Couple therapy

Couple therapy (or **marital therapy**) is used to help couples who have problems in their relationships. In medical practice, this is used when relationship problems are maintaining a psychiatric disorder (e.g. a depressive disorder). Treatment focuses on the ways in which the couple interact. The aim is to promote concern by each partner for the welfare of the other, tolerance of differences, and an agreed balance of decision-making and dominance. The couple first identify the difficulties that they wish to put right. The therapist does not take sides but helps the couple understand each other's point of view. Communication problems are pointed out, for example, failure to express wishes directly, failure to listen to the other's point of view, 'mind reading' (A knows better than B what is in B's mind), and

following positive comments with criticism (the 'sting in the tail'). Behavioural approaches may help, by focusing on the ways that each person reinforces, or fails to reinforce, the behaviour of the other.

Family therapy

Family therapy is usually employed when a child or adolescent has an emotional or conduct disorder. In addition to the young person, the parents are involved together with any other family members (such as siblings or grandparents) who are involved closely with the young person. The aim of treatment is to reduce the problem(s) rather than to produce some ideal (and unrealistic) state of family life. Specific forms of family therapy have been devised to deal with factors thought to lead to relapse in eating disorders and schizophrenia.

Further reading

Butler G, Grey N, Hope T. *Manage Your Mind: The Mental Fitness Guide.* 3rd ed. Oxford: Oxford University Press; 2018. [This comprehensive self-help text makes extensive use of cognitive and behavioural techniques and insights. It includes chapters on, e.g. anxiety, panic, depression, alcohol, smoking, sleep, and relationships. It is relevant for all healthcare professionals—to help them educate patients, and for their own emotional well-being.]

David L. *Using CBT in General Practice: The 10 minute CBT handbook.* 2nd ed. Bloxham: Scion; 2013. [A practical text, on how to use cognitive and behavioural techniques in the inevitably time-constrained setting of primary care consultations.]

Layard R, Clark DM. *Thrive: The Power of Evidence-Based Psychological Therapies.* London: Penguin; 2014. [A highly readable and persuasive text arguing for widespread availability and use of CBT to improve well-being and other important societal outcomes, such as employment.]

Resources suitable for patients

The Oxford Cognitive Therapy Centre publishes various booklets and books based on cognitive behavioural approaches. These are ideal for patients wanting to know about their illness and how to manage it. See http://www. octc.co.uk/online-shop. Examples include:

Kennerley H. *Managing Anxiety: A User's Manual*. [An eight-part self-help programme for managing anxiety, including a relaxation CD/tape.]

Rouf K, Close H, Rosen K. *Managing Psychosis: a guide for relatives, carers and friends*. [Carers are an invaluable resource, but they need support, knowledge, and skills.]

Sanders D. *Overcoming Phobias*. [Dealing with specific phobias such as insects, animals, blood and needles, loud noises or enclosed spaces.]

Westbrook D. *Managing Depression*. [Information and self-help advice for people who are depressed.]

Whitehead L. *Overcoming Eating Disorders*. [A CBT approach to overcoming eating disorders, focusing on getting ready to change, providing suggestions for how to manage key eating disorder features, and how family and friends can help.]

15 Social treatments

The most common approach to providing comprehensive treatment for patients with mental health problems is the biopsychosocial model. This chapter will focus on social interventions.

Rehabilitation

The majority of patients with a mental disorder will have some social difficulties. This might include needing time off work temporarily while unwell, or finding more appropriate accommodation or employment. These patients can usually be helped by giving general support and advice, perhaps with minimal input from a social worker or the voluntary sector. Patients with severe, enduring mental illnesses often have much more complex social challenges. These typically involve multiple areas and have usually come about due to the individual's illness reducing the skills they can draw upon to live independently. The process by which medicine helps patients to regain their independence after illness is called **rehabilitation**. The aim of rehabilitation is to reintegrate the individual back into their community and ensure their ongoing well-being. Ideally, rehabilitation aims to change the natural course of a psychiatric disorder, but more frequently it just assists the patient in making life changes that allow them to manage more satisfactorily in their environment. The patients who most commonly benefit from rehabilitation are those with features including:

- persistent psychopathology (e.g. ongoing hallucinations in schizophrenia);
- frequent relapses (e.g. mania or depression in bipolar disorder);
- social maladaption (e.g. isolation, chaotic anti-social behaviour).

The key benefits of rehabilitation include:

- that the patient moves away from the 'sick role' and starts to see him- or herself as a well individual again;
- improvement in quality of life;
- reduction in relapses of bipolar disorder and psychotic illnesses;
- reduction in social stigma surrounding mental health disorders.

In the UK and many other countries, social workers are key players in arranging social interventions for patients. However, in order for a rehabilitative process to be successful, it is essential that the multidisciplinary team (psychiatrist, GP, CPN, and social worker) all work together. The usual areas that a social worker can help with include the following:

- Finances: help with claiming and managing benefits, managing money.
- Accommodation: applying for funding for social or supported accommodation, liaising with social housing associations or landlords.
- Meaningful activities: helping find daytime activities, for example, groups, courses, exercise, voluntary or paid work, home-based hobbies or activities.
- Employment: assisting with finding and keeping suitable employment. This could be in the voluntary or supported-employment sectors as well as standard paid employment.
- Safeguarding: assisting with child protection or vulnerability issues.
- MHA: social workers trained as AMPHs play a role in MHA proceedings (see Chapter 12), for example, attending MHA assessments or helping patients to stay within the limits of their community treatment order.

A rehabilitation programme will usually include help with housing, employment/education, finances, daily activities, medication management, social skills training, and family interventions. There is often some overlap between psychological and social treatments. For example, a patient who appears to have a problem with lack of employment may actually have two problems: (1) anxiety leading to problems getting to the job centre/benefits office and therefore (2) unemployment and lack of money. Treatment of the anxiety may well sort out the apparent social difficulties too. Many social interventions are also very specific to the particular country or region a patient is living in; as a clinician you should find out what your local options are.

The voluntary sector plays a huge role in the provision of social treatments. In other chapters in this book, specific voluntary organizations have been mentioned—for example, Mind and Alcoholics Anonymous—but there are thousands of local charities providing invaluable support in their community.

Housing

Since the Second World War, there has been huge change in the way people with mental health problems are housed. Previously, many lived in long-term institutions whereas now the emphasis is on providing appropriate accommodation in the community. The majority of people who have a mental health disorder will live independently, but those with more severe debilitating illnesses may need extra support. There is good evidence that patients living in the community in a supported environment are much less likely to be rehospitalized than those who go straight from inpatient care to independent living. In most countries there is a hierarchy of accommodation available, depending on the individual's needs:

- **Twenty-four-hour staffed sheltered accommodation.** These houses or 'group homes' have staff available at all times to provide meals, manage medications, and sort out problems. The staff are usually trained in mental health and provide basic behavioural therapy to help patients adapt to living more independently over time. Some group homes are diagnosis specific—for example, specializing in schizophrenia or learning disabilities—and others only provide accommodation for young people or the elderly. Usually people will live there for a long period, but sometimes just as a step-down between hospital and more independent living.

- **Sheltered accommodation staffed in the daytime.** This is the most commonly available type of supported accommodation in the UK, and provides less intensive assistance to residents. Sometimes help with medication management is available, and the staff frequently encourage and help the inhabitants to organize cooking meals, cleaning, and finding daytime activities.

- **Supported accommodation.** Here the person has their own apartment and manages life almost independently, but a support worker (sometimes called a warden) is available to help with problems and check up on them. There are some larger organizations which provide staffed sheltered accommodation, but with the option for patients to move into apartments once they are able to manage.

- **Independent living.** Patients living in rented or owned accommodation can live completely independently, but occasionally a little support is required. A social worker or community support worker can be invaluable in helping them to remember to pay the rent, sort out utility bills, or keep the house clean.

In the UK, some supported accommodation is funded through the social housing budget but much needs to be privately funded. The voluntary sector also provides some accommodation, but usually with very specific referral criteria.

Employment and education

In most societies, education and/or employment take up the majority of our time and play a large part in defining us 'as a person'. Mental health problems frequently disrupt education in the adolescent and early adult years, and often people with severe psychiatric conditions are not able to continue with their chosen career. It is extremely important to provide individuals with help to re-establish themselves in the world of work. Return to employment has been shown to have many benefits. It:

- provides a daily routine and structure;
- improves social contact;
- increases quality of life;
- improves self-esteem: people develop a sense of 'mastery';
- reduces the likelihood of living in poverty.

Employment (or education) should be carefully chosen to minimize stress and the risk of relapses. The best approach uses graded steps to return to work:

1 Patients frequently have not been in employment for prolonged periods and usually need help in learning the process of looking for, applying for, and maintaining employment. In the UK, some trusts have specific mental health employment advisers who meet with patients to help them with this, but often this is provided by the job centre or voluntary sector. Practical assistance includes, for example, putting together a curriculum vitae or writing covering letters to potential employers.

2 Learning new skills—sheltered workshops or college classes are invaluable in helping people with few transferable skills to improve their chances of finding work. A common example is learning how to use a computer, but specific skills relating to a trade (e.g. welding, decorating, etc.) are widely taught.

3 Temporary, part-time, sheltered employment that helps patients get used to the work environment greatly increases the chance that, in the long term, mainstream employment will work out. These jobs might include volunteering in a charity shop, serving lunch at a local mental health day centre, or working with a supportive employment. This is another opportunity for learning new skills.

4 Supported employment—there are a surprising number of employers who are sympathetic to those with mental health problems and will support them in maintaining employment. Social workers, CPNs, and community support workers provide assistance to help the patient get used to going to work and to managing their wages sensibly.

5 Mainstream independent employment.

For young people who have been out of education due to illness, finding an appropriate educational environment can be a challenge. Many adolescents can return to their previous school (e.g. after an acute episode of depression or anorexia nervosa) but some may need more specialist environments. There are schools that cater for specific conditions (e.g. autism, schizophrenia, or learning disabilities) but the trickiest situations concern those with substance misuse problems, conduct disorder, or other ongoing risky behaviours.

In the UK, a scheme called 'Building Bridges' has become used widely within mental health services. The course runs as a series of group sessions over 6–9 weeks, and may take place in a hospital, day centre, or the community. The aim is to help patients think about making a new start in their life, and point them in the right direction for achieving this. The focus is on learning social and communication skills and improving confidence and self-belief. Patients can also learn about what opportunities are available for education, employment, and housing, and start to investigate them. Building Bridges is extremely popular among patients and carers.

Benefits and finances

Unfortunately, many patients with mental health problems find themselves reliant on state benefits and may be living on very restricted incomes. This may well be due to an objective low income, but frequently habits such as smoking, alcohol, and substance abuse eat into what little there is. Sometimes patients with mania or disorganized behaviour find managing their money very difficult, and will go out on spending sprees for unnecessary items. While patients are in hospital, it is common for limits to be put on the money they can withdraw daily/weekly to help with budgeting. Where possible, this should be continued in the community—often sheltered accommodation staff or family can assist with this. Social workers or community support workers can help with setting up direct debits for utilities, or working out a budget.

Most countries have state benefits available for those with long-term illnesses. As an example, some UK benefits which those with mental health problems may be eligible for are listed here:

- **Employment and support allowance (ESA).** If a person is unable to work (and is under state retirement age) due to illness or disability then ESA is available to help them with general living costs. Depending on their illness, and as an incentive to help get them back into the workplace, some people can work up to a certain number of hours per week and still receive ESA.

- **Disability living allowance.** This benefit is specifically aimed at people who need assistance with activities of daily living (cooking, dressing, washing) due to illness. The money is supposed to be used to pay/assist the person who cares for them.

- **Carer's allowance.** This a benefit to help people who look after someone who is disabled.

- **Income support.** This is extra money to help those who are working but are on a low income.

- **Housing benefit.** This is a monthly payment to help with rent payments for those on low incomes.

- **Council tax benefits.** Those on a low income—whether they are working or not—can be eligible for a reduction in their council tax payments.

- **Job seeker's allowance.** This is the 'dole' payment that those currently unemployed but actively looking for work are entitled to.

- **Help with health costs.** Those in receipt of certain benefits are entitled to various help with various health-related costs, for example, reimbursement of travel expenses or free prescriptions.

A social worker is the best person to advise on appropriate benefits and to help patients fill out the application forms, although this is often done by family or carers.

Social interaction and activities

An integral part of many mental health disorders is the tendency for isolation. Many patients cut themselves off from friends or family, and if they are unable to work then they become very isolated and sometimes housebound. A very important aspect of rehabilitation is encouraging the patient to engage with activity scheduling—to build a structure back into their days and to interact with other people. This may be as simple as visiting the local swimming pool twice a week or meeting a friend regularly for coffee. CPNs are particularly well placed to help develop an activity schedule and encourage the patient to stick to it.

There are many options available in the community, including the following:

- **Specialist community or day centres.** These are open on most weekdays for at least half a day and often provide lunch. Some will provide transport to and from the day centre free of charge. During the day, there may be scheduled activities—for example, art or creative writing, help with daily problems, an opportunity to mingle with others, or a therapeutic group.

- **Voluntary sector organizations.** Many charities provide a range of services, including day centres as just mentioned. In the UK, the largest charity is Mind, who provide daily drop-in sessions for socialization, a rota of activities, and specialist advice (on legal problems, medication, benefits, housing) free of charge. Mind also has supported housing in the community and runs therapeutic groups covering areas such as anxiety management and problem-solving.
- **Classes and courses.** These may be evening classes, run at a local college, or be part of mental health services. Not only can patients learn new skills but they can also engage in exercise (e.g. dance classes) or other hobbies (e.g. fishing club or painting).

- **Structured projects.** One example is the Root and Branch project in the UK. This provides therapeutic gardening and training in rural crafts for people experiencing mental health difficulties. The benefits of this scheme include meeting new people, learning new skills, and becoming more physically active. Some patients go on to gain employment with their new skills (see Box 15.1).

Social skills training

Social skills training is a behavioural therapy-based programme which helps patients improve their interpersonal skills and coping skills, learn workplace essentials, and improve their self-care. It is delivered as a structured course and in the UK is available from the NHS, voluntary organizations, or the private sector. There are various adaptations for specific diagnoses or age groups. Social skills training

Box 15.1 Oxfordshire Mental Health Partnership

Oxfordshire Mental Health Partnership is an example of how organizations from the NHS and voluntary sector have come together to provide rehabilitation services to patients with mental health problems in a coordinated way. The idea is that when a patient presents for assessment (the NHS services provide a single point of multidisciplinary assessment), they can be easily referred onto or signposted to any service within the partnership. This should make it easier for patients to receive comprehensive, joined-up rehabilitation. The partnership consists of six organizations:

- Connections Floating Support: a charitable organization that aims to help people with severe, enduring mental illness to achieve recovery and live in the community. They provide support workers to help with finding work/education/training, help with finding and keeping accommodation, and money management services.
- Elmore Community Services: this charity helps people in the community who have complex needs. These might be related to mental health, physical health, homelessness, substance misuse, offending behaviour,

or learning difficulties. They work on an assertive outreach-based model and try to help difficult-to-engage patients with accommodation, activities, and accessing other services.
- Oxford Health NHS Foundation Trust: provides comprehensive NHS mental health services.
- Oxfordshire Mind: local branch of a national charity who provide peer support, psychoeducational courses, benefits advice, and supported housing to anyone with a mental health disorder.
- Response: a charity providing a range of supported housing options to those with mental health difficulties. They specialize in helping those with complex co-morbid problems.
- Restore: a charity supporting those with mental illness to get back into employment. As well as providing general advice and support with finding work, Restore helps people gain new skills. For example, it has a garden and attached cafe, through which people can learn horticultural skills, then learn to cook and sell their own produce to the public.

has been shown to be particularly useful for groups such as:

- adults and adolescents with schizophrenia (especially with predominantly negative symptoms and/or chaotic, disorganized behaviour);
- adults and adolescents with severe bipolar disorder;
- adults with personality disorders;
- adolescents with autism spectrum disorders, ADHD, or conduct disorders;
- children with ADHD.

Family interventions

Formal family therapy is an essential part of the management of many major psychiatric conditions—for example, most childhood disorders, eating disorders, schizophrenia, bipolar disorder, severe depression, and personality disorders. It addresses problems within the family—for example, interpersonal communication difficulties and unrealistic expectations—and provides education. Skilled family therapists or clinical psychologists usually facilitate the sessions.

There is also a role for less formal psychoeducation and involvement of the family, especially if the patient is continuing to live with them. Frequently, a CPN is in a good position to deliver this, but it may also be done by allied health professionals. The prognosis of a patient can be highly dependent upon the environment in which they are living and the support within it. There is good evidence that a reduction in highly expressed emotions in the home reduces the chance of relapse in schizophrenia and bipolar disorder. CPNs use basic CBT techniques to educate and change the behaviours of the family to reduce the emotional load within the household. Working with the family can have a range of other benefits, including:

- they can be taught to encourage the patient to stick to their activity schedule and to help them to engage in work or hobbies;
- helping with managing medications, belongings, and money;

- learning to be more tolerant of abnormal behaviours;
- monitoring for signs of relapse and taking responsibility for informing the patient's care team immediately;
- encouraging the family to talk to their friends and advocate a reduction in social stigma surrounding mental illness.

Medication

Compliance with medications is one of the greatest challenges in psychiatry. Studies estimate that only about 40–60 per cent of patients take medications regularly, and only about 30 per cent take them according to the doctor's instructions. Teaching patients and their carers the importance of taking medications and helping them to do so is therefore essential. While medications may be initially given in hospital, most patients are treated entirely in the community. Psychiatrists and GPs provide prescriptions and encourage patients to take their medications, but it falls to family, carers, community support workers, CPNs, and other health professionals to try and enforce this. It can be a difficult situation if the patient has limited insight into their condition but is not subject to a community treatment order. There are a variety of simple ways of helping patients with medication compliance:

1 Doctors should use the best available evidence to choose effective drugs with positive side effect profiles. They should enquire about side effects regularly and treat them aggressively or change the medication.

2 Avoid prescribing complex regimens (e.g. take four times daily vs take once daily). This may mean using slow-release formulations or choosing a different medication.

3 Offer a depot injection.

4 Arrange for prescriptions to be produced in advance and sent to the pharmacy automatically. Many pharmacies offer a free home delivery service if it would be helpful for the patient.

5 Use medication aids such as prefilled trays for each day of the week.

6 CPNs can remind patients about the importance of taking their medication, and help to educate their family/carers to support the patient with this.

7 In limited areas, SMS text messaging is being used to deliver automatic reminders to patients when their medication is due. Special applications for smartphones are now available that sound an alarm at a set time and remind the patient exactly which tablets to take.

Allied health professionals

While the provision of specific services for psychiatric disorders lies with the mental health services, there are various allied professions based in the community which patients can benefit from. Frequently the physical health of patients is poor and they may be overweight, lacking in regular exercise, and living in poverty. Maximizing overall health—including mobility and pain reduction—is an essential part of a rehabilitation programme. Some helpful professionals include the following:

- **Occupational therapists (OTs).** Within the UK, OTs provide a limited community service within the NHS and are also available through voluntary organizations and privately. They are experts in providing equipment to increase safety at home and to assist with activities of daily living. Specifically targeting mental health, OTs can reinforce behavioural modifications to daily activities at home and in the community (e.g. shopping, swimming) and help patients to develop coping skills. Some OTs work within mental health teams to provide specialist support.

- **Physiotherapists.** Physiotherapists work to maintain maximum function and mobility of the body. Patients may have co-morbid musculoskeletal disorders, have been bed-bound due to severe psychiatric disturbance, or had a restricted environment in which to exercise while in hospital. Most people benefit from the individual input the physiotherapist can give in strengthening the body and preventing further injury.

- **Podiatrists.** Many individuals with self-neglect secondary to their mental disorder can benefit from some treatments on their feet.

- **Dietitians.** There is a strong association between severe mental health problems and obesity, partly related to medications. A community-based dietitian can give practical advice on weight loss or avoiding further weight gain, especially while on a restricted budget. For patients with eating disorders, advice on a healthy balanced diet should be given alongside psychological therapy.

- **Sports/personal fitness instructors.** Exercise promotes both a healthy body and a healthy mind. For patients with anxious or depressive disorders, a structured exercise programme (three × 45 minutes per week) has been shown to reduce symptoms and the risk of relapse. Sports are also a good way to meet people and engage in a structured activity. Some gyms and sports centres offer discounted rates for patients referred in from health services, and local clubs (e.g. badminton in a school hall) are usually very cheap.

Legal support

While the majority of individuals who experience mental health disorders will never have the need for any legal support, a minority may find themselves having committed an offence or needing advice on treatment under the MHA. Each country has individual structures for providing this support, but it is widely available.

In the UK, voluntary organizations provide the majority of legal support to those with limited resources or a disability. The mental health charity Mind (http://www.mind.org.uk) has a legal unit which offers general advice regarding the MHA, mental capacity, community care, human rights, and discrimination/equality related to mental health. Community Legal Advice is a charity that provides free, confidential, and independent legal advice to any member of the public (http://www.communitylegaladvice.org.uk). This includes advice on family issues, finances, employment, benefits, crimes, and healthcare. They also have specific advisors trained in dealing with criminal acts undertaken during an acute psychiatric illness.

There is more information about the safeguarding and rights of patients being treated under the MHA in Chapter 12.

Cultural considerations

When designing a rehabilitation programme for a patient, it is important to take into consideration the cultural background from which they come. This may mean having to ask for assistance from colleagues or specialists who know more about a specific religion, culture, or community than you do. Appropriate interpreters should always be provided for patients if the interviewer does not speak the same language as them; these should be independent interpreters rather than family members wherever possible. It is not acceptable to leave the patient out of discussions regarding their care because of a language barrier. There are various specific points to consider:

- Cultural beliefs may be very different from those of the clinician's culture. Certain events or experiences may be interpreted differently and these need to be handled sensitively; for example, a woman who has been raped may find it hard to find a husband from her community now that she is no longer 'clean' or a virgin.

- Roles within the family and community may differ. It may be difficult for some women to leave the home and attend medical services; more of their care should therefore be provided in the home. Activity scheduling and engaging with others can be a particular problem in this situation. It may not be possible for a patient to live in supported housing if this would ostracize them from their community.

- Patients may present with very different symptoms to those usual for a specific diagnosis; for example, 'total body pain' is a common manifestation of depression in Afro-Caribbean people. Early warning signs, and relapse plans must take this into account.

- Expectations and acceptance of treatments may be different. Some cultures do not believe in mental health problems and it may be very difficult to persuade a patient or carer of the need for treatment. Medication compliance can be challenging. One key factor is to make sure the patient is able to leave the house and visit the pharmacy and there are no ingredients in the tablets that are forbidden in their religion.

Further reading

Gelder MG, Andreasen NC, López-Ibor JJ, Geddes JR, eds. Section 7: Social psychiatry and service provision. In: *New Oxford Textbook of Psychiatry*. 2nd ed. Oxford: Oxford University Press; 2012:1425–1504.

Mind. http://www.mind.org.uk/. [A UK national charity providing support and rehabilitation services to people with mental health disorders.]

Oxfordshire Mental Health Partnership. http://omhp.org.uk/.

16 Managing acute behavioural disturbance

Acute behavioural disturbance is a common phenomenon in mental health and acute general hospital settings and refers to agitation, aggression, and/or violent behaviour towards property, self, or others. Behavioural disturbances may be due to mental or physical causes. In psychotic patients, agitation may be due directly to psychosis (e.g. paranoia or grandiose delusions, or hallucinations) or accompanying non-psychotic symptoms (e.g. high levels of arousal or anxiety).

In the UK, NICE published detailed guidance on the management of acute behavioural disturbance in 2015, but most hospitals and emergency rooms will also have local guidelines.

A useful framework for thinking about managing behavioural disturbance is as follows:

1 **Predicting** the risk of behavioural disturbance.

2 **Preventing** behaviour escalating once a patient starts to become disturbed.

3 **Intervening** to prioritize safety of staff and patients.

4 **Reviewing** of events and planning for future risk reduction.

Many mental health trusts now have psychiatric intensive care units (PICUs), which specialize in providing a safer and more secure environment for patients at high risk of acute behavioural disturbance. These wards are locked, have a higher ratio of staff to patients, and have facilities for physical restraint and seclusion. As a rule, patients are transferred to the PICU for the shortest time possible, before being 'stepped down' on to the open wards as soon as it is safe to do so.

Prediction

Predicting the likelihood of behavioural disturbance should be part of the overall risk assessment done when a patient is first seen and/or admitted to hospital. This is frequently undertaken in mental health services, but rarely done in the general hospital. It is helpful to think of both the common causes of disturbed behaviour and the personal or situational variables relating to the individual patient (Boxes 16.1 and 16.2). Simple measures such as searching the patient's belongings and person for potential weapons and making sure that basic needs (e.g. warmth, hunger) are considered can reduce risks considerably.

Box 16.1 Causes of acute behavioural disturbance

Organic disorders

- Acute confusional state (delirium) (see p. 362)
- Dementia
- Intracranial pathology (e.g. tumours, chronic degenerative conditions, epilepsy)
- Endocrine conditions (e.g. thyroid disorders)
- Infections (e.g. sepsis, HIV, syphilis)
- Autoimmune disorders (e.g. systemic lupus erythematosus)

Psychiatric disorders

Any disorder may be associated with behavioural disturbance but it is most common in the following:

- Schizophrenia and other psychoses
- Bipolar disorder
- Personality disorders
- Learning disabilities

The following clinical features carry an increased risk:

- Acute psychosis
- Delusions or hallucinations focused on one individual
- Command hallucinations
- Delusions of control
- Preoccupation with violent fantasy
- Paranoia and overt hostility
- Antisocial or impulsive personality traits
- Co-morbid organic disorders

Substances

- Intoxication or withdrawal from alcohol
- Intoxication or withdrawal from illicit substances
- Difficult drug adverse effects (e.g. extrapyramidal side effects)

Prevention

In some cases (e.g. acute confusional state secondary to sepsis), it may be very difficult to predict or prevent behavioural disturbance, but within mental health services it is much easier. All staff should undergo mandatory training covering risk assessment, warning signs of violence, de-escalation techniques, and breakaway. If a patient does start to

Box 16.2 Personal and social risk factors for acute behavioural disturbance

Personal history

- Previous violent behaviour
- Previous use of substances
- Use of weapons
- History of impulsivity
- Lack of insight
- Known personal triggers for violence
- Verbal threats
- Recent severe stress or loss
- As a child: cruelty to animals, bed wetting, fire setting
- Reckless driving

Social circumstances

- Lack of social support
- Availability of weapons
- Relationship difficulties
- Access to potential victims
- Difficulty complying with rules and limit setting

become aggressive, the first stage is to recognize this and to take steps to de-escalate the situation immediately. All mental health facilities should have an inbuilt alarm system within the building, and many staff carry individual alarms which they can activate to summon immediate support. Some common warning signs of impending aggression are shown in Box 16.3.

Box 16.3 Warning signs of violent behaviour

- Angry facial expression
- Restlessness or pacing
- Shouting
- Prolonged, direct eye contact
- Refusal to communicate or cooperate
- Evidence of delusions or hallucinations with violent content
- Verbal threats or reporting thoughts of violence
- Blocking escape routes
- Evidence of arousal (sympathetic nervous system activation)

De-escalation techniques

The aim is to anticipate possible violence and to *de-escalate* the situation as quickly as possible. Many situations will respond to such measures, and medication, physical restraint, or seclusion should only be used when appropriate psychological and behavioural approaches have failed or are inappropriate. One member of staff should be in charge of the situation and should carry out the following steps:

1 Encourage the patient to go into a room or area designated for reducing agitation, away from other patients and visitors.

2 Speak confidently, using clear, slow speech and avoiding changes in volume or tone.

3 Adopt a non-threatening body posture—reduce direct eye contact, keep both hands visible, and make slow movements (or pre-warn 'I am going to get up now').

4 Use non-threatening verbal and non-verbal communication.

5 Explain clearly to the patient what is happening, why, and what will happen next.

6 Ask the patient to explain any problems, how they are feeling, and why the situation has arisen. Try and develop a rapport with the patient, show empathy and concern, and offer realistic solutions to any problems.

7 If weapons are involved, make sure the minimum number of people are in the room and ask the patient to put the weapon down in a neutral position.

Intervention

While non-pharmacological de-escalation techniques are the first line of management, pharmacological treatments ('rapid tranquillization'), physical restraint, or seclusion may need to be used if the risk is not reduced. The aim of drug treatment in such circumstances is to calm the person and reduce the risk of violence and harm, rather than treat the underlying psychiatric condition. One disadvantage of using sedation is that the patient is then unable to participate in further assessment and treatment at that time.

Rapid tranquillization should only be carried out by teams with appropriate training and who can manage the risks of using medications. This is especially vital in patients about whom they have limited information. The equipment and expertise to do cardiopulmonary resuscitation should be available, as should antidotes to commonly used sedatives (e.g. flumazenil, a benzodiazepine antagonist).

Ideally, a drug would be used that has a rapid onset, short half-life, minimal side effects, and is easily reversible. However, the realistic situation is that all medications have disadvantages and there are a number of risks of rapid tranquillization whatever treatment option you choose (Box 16.4). It is important that after administration of a medication, the appropriate observation and care is carried out.

Fig. 16.1 gives a frequently used rapid tranquillization algorithm and some safety considerations that go along with it. Even if the rapid tranquillization medications are prescribed on the 'as needed' part of a medication chart and given at nursing discretion, a doctor should be called to examine the patient as soon as possible. In the UK, the maximum daily doses specified in the *BNF* should not be exceeded.

Box 16.4 Risks of rapid tranquillization

- Oversedation and loss of consciousness
- Loss of airway
- Cardiovascular or respiratory collapse
- Interactions with other medications
- Arrhythmias (check admission ECG for pre-existing abnormalities)
- Hypo- or hyperthermia
- Neuroleptic malignant syndrome (antipsychotics)
- Seizures (antipsychotics, benzodiazepines)
- Involuntary movements (antipsychotics)
- Damage to the therapeutic relationship

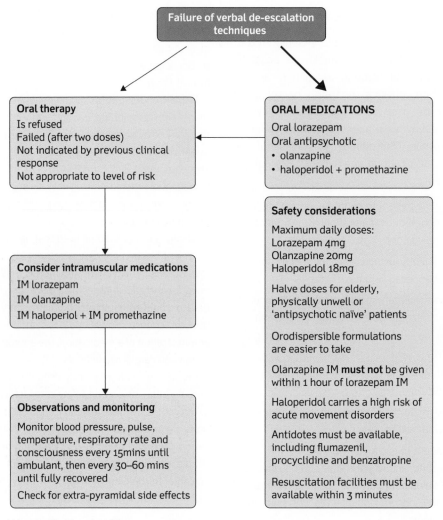

Fig. 16.1 Rapid tranquillization algorithm.

Physical interventions and seclusion

Physical restraint of a patient should be avoided wherever possible, and only used for the shortest amount of time possible. It should only be carried out by trained members of staff according to a specific protocol. Some examples of when it may be appropriate to use physical restraint include:

- to administer essential intramuscular medications;

- to allow a doctor to perform an essential physical examination or conduct investigations (e.g. a blood test or vital signs monitoring);

- in order to move a patient to a place of safety so as to reduce the risk to others;

- to prevent continued serious self-harm.

Throughout the restraint, you should continue to use de-escalation techniques and to keep the patient as calm as possible. It is essential that the patient's head and neck are supported and vital signs are monitored.

After the event, it is important to explain to the patient why restraint was needed and help them to understand how to avoid it happening again.

Seclusion is the last resort in managing behavioural disturbance with high risk to others, and should only be carried out on specialized units with a designated seclusion room and highly trained staff.

The seclusion room must:

- have clear facilities for staff observation (within eyesight);
- have a comfortable area for the patient to lie down and sleep (e.g. a mattress);
- be well insulated and ventilated;
- have a private toilet and washing facilities;
- be able to withstand attacks/damage.

Patients should only be put into seclusion if verbal de-escalation has failed and rapid tranquillization is not possible or has not had the desired effect. UK law states that patients in seclusion must be reviewed by staff every 2 hours, and by a doctor every 4 hours. They must be offered adequate food and drink. It is not appropriate to use seclusion if this may increase the risk of suicide. If rapid tranquillization starts to take effect while the patient is in seclusion, they should be moved back into their usual environment.

Review

If a patient has required rapid tranquillization, physical restraint, or seclusion, a post-incident review should take place within 24–72 hours. This will usually be done by the nursing staff on the ward with the involvement of the patient's usual medical team. It is important to review what happened, the triggers, what was successful/unsuccessful in management, and the ongoing impact upon the patient and staff. This helps to provide a more realistic risk management plan for the patient in the future.

Further reading

Allison L, Moncrieff, J. 'Rapid tranquillisation': an historical perspective on its emergence in the context of the development of antip

sychotic medications. *History of Psychiatry* 2014;25:57–69.

National Institute for Health and Care Excellence. Violence and aggression: short-term management in mental health, health and management in mental health, health and community settings community settings. NICE guideline 10. Published May 2015. **https://nice.org.uk/guidance/ng10.**

Taylor DM, Barnes TRE, Young AH. Acutely disturbed or violent behaviour. In: *Maudsley Prescribing Guidelines in Psychiatry*. 12th ed. Chichester: Wiley-Blackwell; 2015:611–617.

Part 4 Management of specific groups

Child and adolescent psychiatry: general aspects of care

CHAPTER CONTENTS

Introduction

Child and adolescent psychiatry is a broad discipline relevant to any health professional who has regular contact with young people. Childhood emotional, behavioural, and developmental problems are common, especially in children with other medical or social difficulties. This chapter aims to provide an approach to child mental health difficulties, while Chapter 32 deals with common and/or important psychiatric disorders that are specific to childhood. You may find it helpful to revise some basic child development—this can be found in any general paediatrics text (see 'Further reading'). An overview of the differences between child and adult psychiatry is shown in Box 17.1.

Classification

As in adult psychiatry, diagnosis of psychiatric disorders often relies on the clinician being able to recognize variants of and the limits of normal behaviour and emotions. In children, problems should be classified as either a delay in, or a deviation from, the usual pattern of development. Sometimes problems are due to an excess of what is an inherently normal characteristic in young people (e.g. anger in oppositional defiance disorder), rather than a new phenomenon (e.g. hallucinations or self-harm) as is frequently seen in adults.

There are four types of symptoms that typically present to child and adolescent psychiatry services:

1 **Emotional symptoms:** anxiety, fears, obsessions, mood, sleep, appetite, somatization.

Box 17.1 Child and adolescent psychiatry versus adult psychiatry

- Development is a dynamic process; children's behaviour and emotions change with age.
- A child is not an isolated individual; the family unit must be assessed and treated as a whole.
- It is usually the parents who present with a concern about their child, rather than the child themselves identifying a difficulty.
- Medication prescribing must be tailored to paediatric requirements.
- Children are dependent on others for all of their needs.

- Young people tend to have less choice about their home and social environment.
- Children are highly receptive to changes in their environment. Therefore, many forms of treatment (behaviour, art, play therapy) that use this have much greater importance.
- There are some conditions (e.g. enuresis) that the majority of children will 'grow out of'.
- Those less than 18 years of age are legal minors, and therefore others can make decisions for them.

Table 17.1 ICD classification of childhood psychiatric disorders

Category of disorder	ICD-10	Beta draft ICD-11, 2016
Pervasive developmental disorders	• Childhood autism • Atypical autism	• Autism spectrum disorders • Developmental learning disorder (reading, writing, mathematics)
Attention deficit disorders	• Attention deficit disorder with hyperactivity • Hyperkinetic disorder, unspecified	• Attention deficit hyperactivity disorder • Attention deficit disorder, without hyperactivity
Disruptive behaviour disorders	• Conduct disorder • Mixed disorder of conduct and emotions	• Oppositional defiance disorder • Conduct-dissocial disorder
Feeding and eating disorders *(Anorexia and bulimia nervosa are categorized as in adults)*	• Pica • Rumination disorder • Feeding disorder of infancy or childhood	• Pica • Rumination-regurgitation disorder • Avoidant-restrictive food intake disorder
Tic disorders	• Tourette's disorder • Chronic motor or vocal tic disorder • Transient tic disorder • Tic disorder NOS	• Tourette's disorder • Chronic motor or vocal tic disorder • Primary tic disorder, unspecified
Elimination disorders	• Non-organic encopresis • Non-organic enuresis	• Encopresis • Enuresis (nocturnal or diurnal)
Other disorders	• Separation anxiety disorder • Selective mutism • Reactive attachment disorder	• Separation anxiety disorder • Selective mutism • Reactive attachment disorder

NOS, not otherwise specified.
Source data from *International Classification of Diseases*, 10th Revision (ICD-10), World Health Organization 2016, and *International Classification of Diseases*, 11th revision (ICD-11), World Health Organization Beta draft 2016.

Box 17.2 Psychiatric disorders found in all ages, including children and adolescents

- Schizophrenia and other psychotic disorders
- Bipolar disorder
- Depression
- Suicide and deliberate self-harm
- Anxiety disorders and obsessive–compulsive disorder
- Post-traumatic stress disorder
- Eating disorders
- Substance abuse
- Somatoform disorders
- Sleep disorders

2 **Behavioural disorders:** defiant behaviour, aggression, antisocial behaviour, eating disorders.

3 **Developmental delays:** motor, speech, play, attention, bladder/bowels, reading, writing and maths.

4 **Relationship difficulties** with other children or adults.

There will also be other presenting complaints which fit the usual presentation of an adult disorder (e.g. mania, psychosis), and these are classified as they would be in an adult. Occasionally, there will also be a situation where the child is healthy, but the problem is either a parental illness, or abuse of the child by an adult. Learning disorders are covered in Chapter 19. Table 17.1 outlines specific psychiatric conditions diagnosed at less than 18 years, and Box 17.2 lists general psychiatric conditions that are also commonly found in children.

Epidemiology

Epidemiological studies carried out in the UK and the USA consistently report that the prevalence of any psychiatric disorder in children and adolescents is approximately 10 per cent (Table 17.2). While one in five children may have a mental health problem, only one in ten need specialist treatment by psychiatrists. Boys are more likely than girls to receive a psychiatric

Table 17.2 Prevalence of psychiatric conditions in children and adolescents

Diagnosis	Prevalence (%)	Male: female
Any mental disorder	10	
Anxiety disorder	3	1:>1
Depression	1	1:2
ADHD	1.5	4:1
Conduct disorder or oppositional defiance disorder	5	3:1
Anorexia nervosa	0.4	1:1 prepubertal 1:9 postpubertal
Autistic spectrum disorders	0.9	>1:1
Tic disorder	0.4	>1:1
Self-harm	1.2% overall 10–15% of children with emotional disorders	1:>1

Adapted from *Annual Report of the Chief Medical Officer 2012, Our Children Deserve Better: Prevention Pays*. Contains public sector information licensed under the Open Government Licence v3.0. https://www.nationalarchives.gov.uk/doc/open-government-licence/version/3/.

diagnosis, and those aged 10–15 years have a higher prevalence (12 per cent) than children under 11 years (8 per cent). Girls are more likely to have an emotional disorder while boys tend to have behavioural disorders. It is important to remember that research in adults has shown two-thirds of all patients' psychiatric disorders started in childhood. By 24 years, 75 per cent of individuals who are going to develop a psychiatric disorder at some point will have been diagnosed.

Aetiology

As in adult psychiatry, aetiological factors are typically heterogeneous and fall into four interacting groups: **genetics**, **physical disease**, **family**, and **sociocultural factors** (Box 17.3). Of these, family factors are particularly important.

The structure of child and adolescent mental health services (CAMHS)

In the UK, and many other countries, CAMHS work via a tiered system. The idea is the child receives the lowest intensity treatment (with the least disruption to normal life) that is appropriate for their current problems, and can move up or down the tiers as their requirements change.

- **Tier 1:** non-specialists who work with children (e.g. primary care, social work, education, and the voluntary sector).
- **Tier 2:** CAMHS specialists working in the community and primary care.
- **Tier 3:** multidisciplinary service working in specialist child psychiatry outpatient clinics. It is for children with more severe, persistent, or complex disorders. The team will include psychiatrists, psychologists, occupational therapy, social workers, family therapists, dieticians, and play therapists.
- **Tier 4:** comprehensive services such as day-patient and inpatient units, and highly specialized outpatient teams.

Box 17.3 Causes of childhood psychiatric disorder

Genetics
- Polygenic conditions, currently poorly elucidated
- Heritability 50–80% for common conditions, for example, ADHD, 70–80% heritability, 5-fold risk increase in first-degree relatives

Physical disease
- Any serious physical illness, especially if requiring hospital admissions or time away from school

Family factors
Anything preventing a stable and secure family environment in which children are loved, accepted, and provided with consistent discipline:
- Care provided by social services
- Child abuse and neglect
- Parental discord, separation, or divorce
- Poor parenting skills
- Losses and bereavements
- Illness of a parent or sibling (physical or mental, including personality disorders)
- Large family size

Social and cultural factors
These become increasingly important in the teenage years:
- Large changes in lifestyle (new school, new house, new baby)
- Influences at school
- Bullying
- Peer group behaviours
- Racism or discrimination
- Break-up of peer relationships (teenagers)
- Substances and alcohol

Assessment of a psychiatric problem in childhood

The aims of assessing a child are not fundamentally different to those within adult psychiatry (Chapter 5), but need to include the elements of developmental level and family context:

1 To obtain a clear account of the presenting problems and detect psychopathology; this

includes understanding parental attitudes and family problems.

2 To relate the problems to the child's temperament, development, and physical condition.

3 To produce a treatment plan.

4 To identify factors inherent to the child, home, or school that may influence the effectiveness of treatment, and work out how to manage these.

Differences between the assessment of children and adults

Although the psychiatric assessment of children resembles that of adults, there are three important differences:

1 When the child is young, the *parents supply most of the verbal information*. Despite this, the child should usually be seen without the parents at some stage.

2 When interviewing a child, it is often difficult to follow a set routine, and *a flexible approach is required*.

3 The child should be assessed by *at least two members of the multidisciplinary team*, including a psychiatrist.

An assessment may be done in an outpatient clinic, at school, or at the child's home.

Interviewing the parents

The parents are usually seen together, with siblings and any other relevant family members. They should feel that they are part of the solution to the child's difficulties rather than part of the problem. While interviewing the family, it is important to note the patterns of interaction between family members (alliances, scapegoating, avoidance), and how easily they communicate with one another. The important areas to cover in the interview are shown in Box 17.4.

Box 17.4 History taking in child psychiatry

The presenting problem

- Who initiated the referral and why
- Nature, severity, and frequency of symptoms
- Factors that make it better or worse
- Where the symptoms occur (home, school, elsewhere)
- Stresses at home, school, or elsewhere that might be important

Other current problems

- Mood and energy level, including thoughts of self-harm or suicide
- Anxiety level and specific fears
- Activity level, attention, concentration
- Eating, sleeping, elimination
- Relationship with parents and siblings
- Relationships with other children, special friends
- Antisocial behaviour
- School performance and attendance
- Sexual interest and behaviours
- Physical symptoms, hearing and vision

Previous psychiatric history

- Previous problems, treatments (and efficacy)

Family history

- Family structure—draw a family tree
- Current emotional state of parents, children, and wider family
- Separations from and illness of parents
- Siblings: age, temperament, health problems
- Home circumstances, sleeping arrangements
- Psychiatric problems in the wider family

Personal and developmental history

- Problems in pregnancy, type of delivery, birth weight, and gestation
- Early life—need for special care, early feeding and sleeping patterns, maternal postpartum depression, mother–child relationship
- Developmental history, age key milestones reached
- Current level of development (language, motor skills)
- Past illness and injury, hospital stays
- Schooling history: difficulties, abilities, and attainments
- Interests, hobbies, talents, and strengths of the child

Interviewing and observing the child

Starting the interview. It is important to establish a friendly atmosphere and win the child's confidence before asking about the problems, and explain how the team may be able to help. With younger children, an indirect and gradual approach is needed, starting with general topics that may engage the child's interest such as toys or birthdays, before asking about the problems. With older children and adolescents it may be possible to follow an approach similar to that for adults.

Continuing the interview. Older children can usually talk about their problems directly but young children need to be helped, for example, by asking what they would ask for if given three wishes. Children who have difficulty in expressing their problems and feelings in words may be able to show them in other ways, for example, in imaginative play or writing.

Observing behaviour. While trying to engage a child, the interviewer should observe how the child interacts with clinicians and with the parents when they are present. Specific items of the child's behaviour and mental state should be recorded (Box 17.5).

Box 17.5 Principal observations of a child's behaviour and emotional state

- Rapport with the interviewers, eye contact, spontaneous talk, disinhibition
- Relationship with parents
- Appearance (dysmorphism, nutrition state, cleanliness, evidence of neglect or abuse)
- Involuntary movements, habits, and mannerisms
- Mood (sadness, irritability, anxiety, tension)
- Presence of delusions, hallucinations, thought disorder
- Activity level and concentration
- Developmental stage, intellectual abilities, memory
- Judgement and insight into problems

Interviewing other informants

The most important additional informants, other than members of the family, are the child's *teachers*. They can describe classroom behaviour, educational achievements, and relationships with other children. They may also have useful information about the family and their circumstances. In some situations, it may be necessary to arrange a school visit to observe classroom behaviour. Useful information may also come from other clinicians, childcare providers, wider family, or social workers.

Psychological tests

Sometimes questionnaires or other psychological tests can provide information to supplement the clinical assessment, or be used as a quantitative measure of symptoms over time. Some examples are listed here:

- Assessment of IQ can help compare academic performance with potential. The Wechsler Intelligence Scale for Children is a commonly used tool.
- Conner's Rating Scales are a screening tool used in the diagnosis and monitoring of ADHD.
- The Eating Disorders Examination (child version) and Eating Disorders Inventory for Children are commonly used to screen for and assess children with suspected eating disorders.
- The Beck Youth Depression Scale or the Mood and Feelings Questionnaire are used in assessment of depression.

Physical examination

A full general examination of the child should be undertaken, especially in those presenting with eating disorders (see p. 379). Emphasis should be on a thorough neurological screening, to exclude organic pathology in the central nervous system. The examination should include:

- height, weight, body mass index (BMI), head circumference plotted on standard charts;

- standard paediatric cardiovascular, respiratory, ear, nose, and throat, and abdominal examinations;
- detailed neurological examination;
- any evidence of congenital disorders, dysmorphism features, neglect, or abuse.

Investigations

The majority of children presenting with mental health problems will need no investigations. Be guided by the presenting problems and examination results. Some examples include computed tomography (CT)/ magnetic resonance imaging (MRI) for neurological deficits, genetic testing for dysmorphic features, and thyroid function tests in mood disorders. A full list of the investigations that should be undertaken in eating disorders can be found on p. 390.

General aspects of treatment

Although treatment differs in important ways according to the type of disorder, there are many common features (Box 17.6). There is more detailed information about psychological treatments in Chapter 14, relevant to all age groups.

Choosing an appropriate setting of care

The vast majority of children will be treated as outpatients, in primary care or specialist clinics, with day- or inpatient care used only in the following situations:

1 *To treat a severe behaviour disorder* that cannot be managed in another way (e.g. unstable emaciated patients with anorexia nervosa).

Box 17.6 Treatment of child and adolescent mental health problems

Assessment

- Diagnosis of psychiatric disorders, co-morbidities, and complications
- Risk assessment (mental, physical, social, educational)
- Decide upon appropriate level of care:
  - Primary care team (Tier 1)
  - Specialist mental health workers based in primary care (Tier 2)
  - Multidisciplinary specialist CAMHS team (Tier 3)
  - Specialist outpatient team (Tier 4)
  - Day-patient or inpatient programme (Tier 4)
  - Admission to general hospital for medical stabilization

General measures for all patients

- Agree a clear treatment plan and assign a care coordinator
- Psychoeducation for parents and for the child (see p. 155)
- Self-help resources (books, websites—for parents and child)
- Reduce any stressors: problem-solving and relaxation techniques
- Recommendation of appropriate generic or specific parenting programmes
- Regular monitoring of physical and mental state

Psychological treatments

- Behavioural therapy or CBT
- Interpersonal therapy
- Group therapy
- Family therapy
- Play and art therapy

Pharmacological treatments

- As discussed in Chapter 32, for example, stimulants, antidepressants, mood stabilizers, antipsychotics

Social interventions

- Assistance with school placements (or work if over 16 years)
- Placements with social services for child protection or other issues

2 If the child is deemed to be at *high risk of suicide or deliberate self-harm*.

3 *For observation* when the diagnosis is uncertain.

4 *To separate the child* temporarily from home to assess behaviour in a different environment.

Inpatient admissions are kept as short as possible and used only as a last resort.

Parenting programmes

Parenting programmes are now commonly used in child psychiatry, and aim to teach parents techniques to appropriately reward and encourage good behaviour, while ignoring and discouraging bad behaviours. Parenting programmes are very good at reducing oppositional behaviour in young children, but are less effective for adolescents. Some commonly used programmes are the Incredible Years Programme and Triple P, but there are also specialized programmes for some specific disorders—for example, the Early Bird Programme for autism run by the National Autistic Society.

Psychological treatments

Behaviour therapy. Behavioural principles are used in the management of most kinds of childhood psychiatric problem and are usually very effective. Behavioural therapy is based on the principles of conditioning theory, and can be used either to increase desirable behaviours or decrease undesirable behaviours. It may be used alone or as part of CBT. It is frequently used in ADHD, oppositional defiance disorder (ODD), and autistic spectrum disorders (ASD). Activity scheduling is valuable in those with low mood.

Cognitive behavioural therapy. CBT in children uses the same principles as in adults (p. 163). As CBT requires the child to be able to identify and label thoughts and feelings and consider the impacts of their behaviour, it is only suitable for children at least 7–8 years old, with behavioural therapy more suitable for those younger than 7 years. Cognitive therapy is best in disorders where there is some cognitive distortion as part of the psychopathology (e.g. eating disorders, depression, or anxiety). Homework is an important part of CBT, and parents can often be involved with this. Occasionally, adolescents will be unwilling to engage as they are not yet ready to change their behaviours—in this case, it is often helpful to use motivational interviewing as a step prior to starting CBT.

Family therapy. Families are always involved in some way in the treatment of children. Family therapy refers to a specific psychological treatment in which the child's symptoms are considered as an expression of difficulties in the functioning of the family. Members of the family meet to discuss their difficulties, while the therapist helps them to find ways of overcoming the problems. It is commonly used in mood disorders, eating disorders, somatization, and psychosis.

Group therapy. Group therapies are used extensively in child and adult day-patient and inpatient programmes for almost every psychiatric condition, and are usually based on CBT principles. They are a cost-effective way of providing therapy, but also help to make the child feel less isolated, learn social skills, and have the chance to explore common issues with peers.

Play and art therapies. For young children, often the best method of making them feel at ease and expressing their true emotions and behaviour is to engage them in an activity they enjoy. It allows the child to communicate with a therapist without speech. Play can be used to show how the child is feeling at that moment, and to recreate past experiences and try to make sense of them. Play therapy is particularly useful for issues surrounding neglect, abuse, loss, bereavement, or separation.

Pharmacological treatments

Medication is considered last because it has only a limited place in the treatment of childhood psychiatric disorders. Medication is first-line treatment for very few conditions, and should only be prescribed in a more severe disorder when psychological and social interventions have failed. Table 17.3 gives an overview of which drugs are used in children, and for which conditions. Benzodiazepines are not recommended for use in those less than 18 years of age.

Table 17.3 Use of medications in child and adolescent psychiatry

Class of medication	Indications
Stimulants	ADHD
	ADHD with co-morbid ODD or conduct disorder
	ASD
Antidepressants (SSRIs unless otherwise stated)	Depression
	Anxiety disorders and OCD
	Enuresis (tricyclics)
	Tics with co-morbid anxiety
	Bulimia nervosa
Antipsychotics	Schizophrenia
	Other psychoses
	ASD
	Tics and Tourette's syndrome
	Bipolar disorder
Mood stabilizers	Bipolar disorder
	ASD
Alpha-agonists (e.g. clonidine)	Tics and Tourette's syndrome

ADHD, attention deficit hyperactivity disorder; ASD, autism spectrum disorders; OCD, obsessive–compulsive disorder; ODD, oppositional defiance disorder.

Ethical and legal issues

Consent for treatment

In most legal systems, including the UK, a 'child' is anyone under the age of 18 years. Children develop psychologically at different speeds, but the law has to decide on set age-related guidelines for obtaining consent, below which the parents typically provide proxy consent. The only caveat is that adolescents may have the right to consent to or refuse treatment if deemed to have capacity to make the specific decision (Gillick competence). Even below the age of consent, the child's agreement should be obtained whenever possible since without it treatment will be more difficult. Parents may refuse treatment for a child, though only when this does not conflict with their duty to protect the child. If the parents' refusal seems not to be in the interests of the child, most countries provide for a decision by a court of law. The MHA may be used at any age and can be very useful in older children who are disengaging with essential treatment.

Consent for psychiatric research follows the rules just discussed. Parents may find it difficult to balance the risks to their child against the benefits for others in the future; adequate explanation and discussion are therefore essential.

Conflicts of interest

Usually, the interests of the child are the same as those of the parents. When they are not, those of the child generally take precedence—for example, in suspected abuse. Occasionally, the decision is less obvious—for example, when a depressed mother is neglecting her child but is likely to become more depressed if substitute care is arranged. If the problems are anticipated, they can usually be resolved by discussion with the parents and between the professionals caring for the mother and child.

Confidentiality

Patients of any age have the right to expect that information about them will be held in confidence by their doctor. Careful thought should be given to information that it is deemed essential to share (especially with non-medical agencies) and the need should be discussed with the parents and, if they are old enough, with the children concerned.

Child protection issues and child abuse

Breakdown of the normal caring relationship between adults in the parental role and children can lead to abuse (see Box 17.7).

Box 17.7 Forms of child abuse

- Child abuse
  - Physical abuse
  - Sexual abuse
  - Emotional abuse
  - Neglect
- Fetal abuse: behaviour detrimental to the fetus (e.g. physical assault on the mother, taking of substances toxic to the fetus by the mother)
- Munchausen syndrome by proxy

Both the United Nations *Convention on the Rights of the Child* and the WHO have produced a basic set of rights and standards relating to a child's health and living circumstances. Child abuse or neglect may not necessarily occur in the home; it includes child labour, sexual exploitation, and children involved in conflict. Abuse, neglect, or exploitation of a child affects their development in every domain, and is never acceptable.

In the UK, unlike many other countries, there is no legal obligation for anyone except social workers and the police to report suspicions of child abuse. However, the GMC recommends to all doctors that they report to authorities whenever they have reasonable concern about a child's safety. Investigation of a child protection case usually involves social workers, the police, paediatricians (physical investigations), and child psychiatrists. Each hospital trust will have a designated team to deal with these situations, and all doctors should be aware of how to contact them.

Prevalence

It is extremely difficult to obtain accurate figures regarding the epidemiology of child abuse, because most cases never come to the attention of health services. Official incidence statistics report maltreatment of 2–12 per 1000 children in the UK, the USA, and Australia. Of these, neglect is the most common (30–50 per cent of cases), followed by physical abuse (15–30 per cent), sexual abuse (10–20 per cent), and then emotional abuse. The sex ratio is equal, except for sexual abuse, which is more commonly against girls. Physically disabled children are three times more likely to be abused. The most vulnerable age group is 0–3 years.

Physical abuse (non-accidental injury)

These terms refer to deliberate infliction of injury on a child by any person having custody, care, or charge of that child. Each year, about 1 per 1000 children receive injuries of such severity as to cause a fracture or cerebral haemorrhage. Less severe injury is more frequent, but rarely comes to professional attention. Failure to prevent injury is considered neglect rather than abuse. Discipline through smacking or hitting is common in some countries; there is a blurred line between acceptable and non-acceptable acts.

Detecting abuse

Physical abuse is usually detected when a child presents with injuries for which no other explanation can be found. The problem may become apparent when the parents bring a child to the doctor with an injury said to have been caused accidentally. Alternatively, relatives, neighbours, or teachers may become concerned and report the problem to the police, social workers, or voluntary agencies. Rarely a child or witness may come forward directly. Suspicion of physical abuse should be aroused by:

- the nature of the injuries (Box 17.8);
- previous suspicious injury;

Box 17.8 Injuries caused by physical abuse

- Multiple bruising
- Abrasions
- Bites
- Burns
- Torn lips
- Fractures
- Retinal haemorrhage
- Subdural haemorrhage

- unconvincing explanations of the way in which the injury was sustained;
- delay in seeking help;
- incongruous reactions to the injury by the carers;
- fearful responses of the child to the carers ('frozen watchfulness');
- evidence of distress, such as social withdrawal, regression, low self-esteem, or aggressive behaviour.

Aetiology

There are three sets of aetiological factors relating to the parents, the child, and the social circumstances (Table 17.4). The common factor is a failure of the normal emotional bonding between the parent or other carer and the infant. Knowledge of these risk factors assists in the detection of child abuse.

Table 17.4 Risk factors for physical abuse

In the parents	Young age
	Single parent
	Poverty and/or unemployment
	Social isolation
	Mental health or personality disorder
	Personal experience of abuse
	Criminal record
In the child	Premature and/or needing special neonatal care
	Age 0–12 months
	Congenital malformations or disability
	Difficult temperament
In the environment	Poor housing
	Family violence
	Lack of community support

Management

Assessment of the injuries. When abuse is suspected, a specialist assessment should be arranged, giving a full account of the reasons for suspicion. Usually, the child will be admitted to a paediatric ward for assessment, which includes taking photographs of the injuries and a radiological examination, which may show evidence of previous fractures. Occasionally, an organic cause of the injuries will be found—for example, osteogenesis imperfecta. All findings should be clearly and fully documented since evidence may be needed at subsequent legal proceedings.

Subsequent action. Each area has a child protection team who will take over the case and follow the local protocols. If it appears that non-accidental injury is probable, an experienced senior doctor and social worker should *talk to the parents* and arrange to examine other children in their care.

Returning the child. Sometimes the abused child can return home if support and close supervision are provided for the parents. Others need temporary foster care or a permanent alternative home. These very difficult decisions are usually made by a paediatrician or child psychiatrist and a social worker, both specialists in such situations.

Prognosis

Children who have been subjected to physical abuse are at high risk of delayed development, learning difficulties, and emotional and behavioural disorders extending into adult life. As adults, former victims of abuse may have difficulties in rearing their own children, and some abuse them. Abuse in childhood is a risk factor for almost every psychiatric condition, and there is a strong association with suicide and deliberate self-harm.

Sexual abuse

The term sexual abuse refers to the involvement of children in sexual activities to which they cannot give legally informed consent, or which violate generally accepted cultural rules, and which they may not fully comprehend. The term covers penetrative sexual contact, touching of genitalia, exhibitionism, pornographic photography, and inciting children to engage in sexual practices together. The abuser is usually known to the child and is often a member of the family (see Science box 17.1).

Prevalence

The prevalence of sexual abuse is difficult to determine; UK figures currently suggest approximately 6 per cent of children experience sexual abuse. Half of these cases involved penetration or orogenital contact.

SCIENCE BOX 17.1

Are retinal haemorrhages a good indicator of non-accidental injury in young children?

Head injuries caused by child abuse are the most common cause of traumatic death in children less than 1 year old. Being able to spot which children presenting with injuries are likely to have been victims of non-accidental injury (NAI) is a frequent diagnostic dilemma, and one which can have grave consequences if missed. In 1974, a radiologist named John Caffey first described the association between retinal haemorrhages (RHs) and 'shaken baby syndrome'.[1] The presence of RH is highly suggestive of intracranial bleeding, and carries a high risk of long-term brain damage. Subsequently, RHs have been widely taught to be a good indicator of NAI, and much research on the topic has been conducted. So, with the hindsight of 40 years' experience and an extensive evidence base, is it still the case that RHs are a sensitive and specific marker of NAI?

As of early 2016, Maguire and colleagues had carried out the largest systematic review on this topic.[2] They included studies primarily comparing the clinical characteristics of children up to 18 years presenting with accidental injury (AI) versus NAI. Unfortunately, this did exclude papers only describing characteristics of children with either NAI or AI. In total, 1655 children were included, 779 with NAI and the rest with AI. They report that in a child with an intracranial injury, apnoea and RH were the features most predictive of NAI, with odds ratios of 17.0 (positive predictive value (PPV) 93 per cent) and 3.5 (PPV 71 per cent), respectively.

A large proportion of severe head injuries caused by abuse occur in less mobile infants and toddlers, primarily those under 2 years. In 2015, Kelly et al. retrospectively described the characteristics of 345 cases of suspected abusive head trauma.[3] Sixty per cent of these were proved as NAI, with this group significantly more likely to have RH than those diagnosed as AI. This is similar to earlier findings by Keenan et al.[4] Bechtel and colleagues published a smaller prospective study of

infants presenting with head injuries.[5] They also report RH to be significantly more frequent in children with NAIs ($P < 0.01$).

There is a good evidence base backing the association between RH and NAI. One important point made in many publications is unless NAI is strongly suspected on first contact with medical services, fundoscopy is often not performed. With the added knowledge that non-ophthalmologists conducting fundoscopy miss up to 15 per cent of RHs, it is imperative that all children should be thoroughly assessed when attending the emergency room with head injuries, including slit-lamp examination by an ophthalmologist.[6]

1   Caffey J. The whiplash shaken infant syndrome: manual shaking by the extremities with whiplash-induced intracranial and intraocular bleedings, linked with residual permanent brain damage and mental retardation. *Pediatrics* 2974;54:396–403.

2   Maguire S, Pickerd N, Farewell D, et al. Which clinical features distinguish inflicted from non-inflicted brain injury? A systematic review. *Archives of Diseases of Childhood* 2009;94:860–7.

3   Kelly P, John S, Vincent AL, Reed P. Abusive head trauma and accidental head injury: a 20-year comparative study of referrals to a hospital child protection team. *Archives of Disease in Childhood* 2015;100:1123–1130.

4   Keenan HT, Runyan DK, Marshall SW, et al. A population-based comparison of clinical and outcome characteristics of young children with serious inflicted and noninflicted traumatic brain injury. *Pediatrics* 2004;114:633–639.

5   Bechtel K, Stoessel K, Leventhal JM, et al. Characteristics that distinguish accidental from abusive injury in hospitalized young children with head trauma. *Pediatrics* 2004;114:165–168.

6   Morad Y, Kim YM, Mian M, et al. Nonophthalmologist accuracy in diagnosing retinal hemorrhages in the shaken baby syndrome. *Journal of Pediatrics* 2003;142:431–434.

Clinical features

The children are more often female and the offenders usually male. Sexual abuse may be reported directly by the child or by a relative or other person. Children are more likely to report abuse when the offender is a stranger than when he is a family member. Sometimes, sexual abuse is discovered during the investigation of other conditions; for example, symptoms in the urogenital or anal area, behavioural or emotional disturbance, inappropriate sexual behaviour, or pregnancy.

The *immediate consequences* of sexual abuse include anxiety, depression, anger, inappropriate sexual behaviour, and unwanted pregnancy. *Long-term effects* include low self-esteem, mood disorder, self-harm, difficulties in relationships, and sexual maladjustment.

Assessment

It is important to be alert to the possibility of sexual abuse, and to give serious attention to any complaint made by a child of being abused in this way. It is also important not to make the diagnosis without adequate evidence from a thorough social investigation of the family, and from physical and psychological examinations of the child.

It is essential that information from children is obtained carefully. The child should be encouraged sympathetically to describe what has happened. Drawings or toys may help younger children to give a description, but great care should be taken not to suggest answers to the child. When the circumstances make it appropriate, a physical examination is carried out by a paediatrician, including inspection of the genitalia and anal region. If intercourse may have taken place in the past 72 hours, specimens should be collected from the genital and any other relevant regions.

Management

The initial management and the measures to protect the child are similar to those for physical abuse. In families where sexual abuse has occurred, the members may deny the seriousness of the abuse and the existence of other family problems. The discovery of abuse may lead to family conflict that adds to the child's distress. Decisions about treatment and removal from home are taken only after the most careful consideration of all the implications. The sexual development of the abused child is often abnormal, requiring help long after the event. A variety of forms of therapeutic work are used with victims of sexual abuse—the exact type of therapy depends largely upon the needs of the individual child. There is some evidence that group and individual CBT-based programmes reduce the longer-term effects of sexual abuse.

Emotional abuse

The term emotional abuse usually refers to severe and persistent emotional neglect, verbal abuse, or rejection sufficient to impair a child's physical or psychological development. Emotional abuse often accompanies other forms of child abuse but may occur alone. Management resembles that for cases of physical abuse. The parents require help for their own emotional problems, and the child needs counselling, and, in severe cases, a period of separation from the parents.

Neglect

Child neglect includes neglect of the child's physical or emotional needs, upbringing, safety, or medical care, all of which may lead to physical or psychological harm. It may occur within the family home, or within institutions such as children's homes or schools. Neglect may begin prenatally (e.g. maternal substance abuse) and continue through to 18 years old. There are four types of neglect:

1 **Physical neglect:** inadequate provision of food, shelter, and clothing.

2 **Supervisory neglect:** inadequate parental supervision or interest in the child—this includes failing to provide an education, healthcare needs, and using unsafe care situations.

3 **Emotional neglect:** insufficient parental attention to the child's need for affection.

4 **Cognitive neglect:** insufficient attention to the child's intellectual, speech, and neurological development, including the provision of adequate schooling.

Neglect of a child's emotional needs and nutrition may lead to **failure to thrive** physically in the absence of a detectable organic cause; height and weight are reduced and development is delayed. The aetiological factors associated with neglect are shown in Table 17.5.

Neglected children soon recover their physical health when provided with adequate nutrition and healthcare. However, they often show significant developmental delays, especially in speech, language, attention, and school achievements. Many children remain attention-seeking, passive, and helpless.

Munchausen syndrome by proxy

This rare disorder is where a parent or carer repeatedly fabricates an illness or disability in a child they are looking after, for the benefit of themselves. The adult involved is most frequently the child's mother, but not always. There are several important aspects to this condition, including:

- the physical harm caused to the child through falsification of illness;
- the impact upon the child's physical and emotional development;
- the psychological status of the adult involved.

The clinical presentation may be with any symptom or sign. Fabrication may be at the level of the history of presenting complaint given, an inaccurate past medical history, interference with hospital notes/blood specimens/equipment readings, or induction of an illness (e.g. by poisoning or hurting the child). The diagnosis is usually made by an alert paediatrician, for whom the story does not quite add up. The majority of children involved are under 5 years, and over 80 per cent of fabricators are females. Half of these fit diagnostic criteria for a personality disorder. Once the diagnosis is made, the child usually recovers quickly from any physical consequences, but remains at high risk of developing genuine psychiatric conditions in later years. Treatment of the fabricator is paramount.

Table 17.5 Risk factors for child neglect

Parental characteristics	Living in poverty
	Personality difficulties: immaturity, impulsivity, chaotic lifestyle
	Low self-esteem
	Unrealistic expectations of the child
	Psychiatric illness (mood disorders, schizophrenia, substance misuse)
Family characteristics	Lack of affection between family members
	Household disorganization
	Lack of cognitive stimulation
	Poor intrafamilial relationships

Further reading

BMJ Learning. Child abuse: a guide to recognition and management. Published June 2009, updated 2012. **https://learning.bmj.com/learning/module-intro/child-abuse-recognition-management.html?locale=en_GB&moduleId=10012420**. [A useful online learning module covering recognition of child abuse.]

Gelder MG, Andreasen NC, López-Ibor JJ, Geddes JR, eds. Section 9: Child and adolescent psychiatry. In: *New Oxford Textbook of Psychiatry*. 2nd ed. Oxford: Oxford University Press; 2012:1587–1816.

Lissauer T, Carroll W. Normal child development, hearing and vision. In: *Illustrated Textbook of Paediatrics*. 5th ed. London: Mosby Elsevier; 2017:27–43. [A useful guide to normal child development.]

Murphy M, Fonagy P. Mental health problems in children and young people. In: Lemer C, ed. *Our Children Deserve Better: Prevention Pays*. Annual Report of the Chief

Medical Officer 2012. Published October 2013. https://www.gov.uk/government/uploads/system/uploads/attachment_data/file/252660/33571_2901304_CMO_Chapter_10.pdf.

National Institute for Health and Care Excellence. Child maltreatment: when to suspect maltreatment in under 18s. Published July 2009, updated October 2017. http://guidance.nice.org.uk/CG89.

Sapera J, Lakhanpaul M, Kemp A, et al. When to suspect child maltreatment: summary of NICE guidance. *BMJ* 2009;339:b2689. [Useful summary of the NICE guidance.]

18 Psychiatry of older adults

Epidemiology and principles of management

The provision of mental health services for older adults faces two main challenges:

1 The world population is ageing, leading to increased numbers of elderly patients (Fig. 18.1).

2 These patients are more likely to present with multiple, complex co-morbidities which must be managed alongside acute or chronic psychiatric problems.

To provide effective care, services must combine treatment for mental, physical, and social needs of older people. The multidisciplinary team is key to delivering this, often in specialized environments such as a day centre programme.

Normal ageing

A huge number of physical, psychological, and social changes occur within the normal process of ageing. A basic understanding of these is necessary in order to identify those individuals in whom there is pathology. Covering theories behind the ageing process is outside the scope of this text, but some references are given on p. 220.

Physical changes

The following changes are seen in the brain during normal ageing:

- The weight of the brain decreases by 5–20 per cent between 70 and 90 years, with a compensatory increase in ventricular size.
- There is neuronal loss, especially in the hippocampus, cortex, substantia nigra, and cerebellum.
- Senile plaques are found in the neocortex, amygdala, and hippocampus.
- Tau proteins form neurofibrillary tangles, found normally only in the hippocampus.
- Lewy bodies are seen in the substantia nigra.
- Ischaemic lesions (reduced blood flow, lacunar infarcts) are seen in 50 per cent of normal people over 65 years.

Psychological changes

From mid life there is a decline in intellectual functions, as measured with standard intelligence tests,

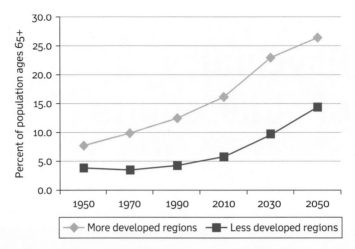

Fig. 18.1 The percentage of the population aged 65 and over for more developed and less developed countries. Source data from *World population prospects*, the 2015 revision, United Nations.

together with deterioration of short-term memory and slowness. IQ peaks at about 25 years, remains stable until 60–70 years, and then declines. Problem-solving reduces after about age 60. There may be alterations in personality and attitudes, such as increasing cautiousness, rigidity, and 'disengagement' from the outside world.

Social changes

Later life presents a series of major changes. Many individuals retire, lose partners, lose their physical health, and are forced to live on much lower incomes and in poorer-quality housing than younger people. These are difficult transitions which may predispose to mental illness. The majority of older people remain living at home: half with a partner, and 10 per cent with other family members. Those who live alone may become isolated and lonely.

Use of medical services

Older people consult their family doctors more often than younger people and they occupy two-thirds of all general hospital beds. These demands are particularly great in those aged over 75. Treatment is often made difficult by the presence of more than one disorder and by increased sensitivity to drug side effects.

Epidemiology

The United Nations estimated in 2015 that by 2030, there will be 1 billion people aged over 65 years, of whom 70 per cent are found in developed countries. Psychiatric disorders, like physical illness, are especially prevalent in older adults (Fig. 18.2). Although psychiatric disorders in old age have some special features, they do not differ greatly from the psychiatric disorders of younger adults. Table 18.1 compares the prevalence of some common psychiatric conditions in the older and general adult populations. The greatest burden of disease is in two areas: mood and anxiety disorders, and cognitive impairment. Dementia makes up a large proportion of an old age psychiatrist's caseload, and its prevalence is highly correlated to increasing age (Fig. 18.3) (see 'Further reading').

What types of mental disorder are seen in older patients?

Many of the same disorders affect older people as affect younger people. They can be subdivided into three types:

1 Pre-existing problems that continue into older age.

2 New diagnoses after the age of 65.

3 Mental health disorders associated with ageing.

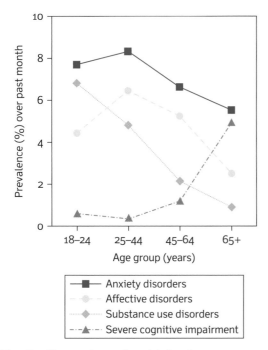

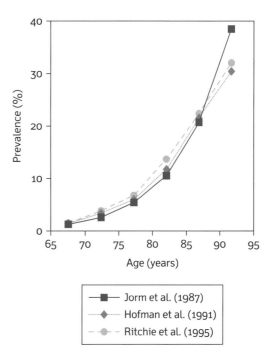

Fig. 18.2 The prevalence of mental disorders across age groups.

Source data from 1-month prevalence rates from the Epidemiologic Catchment Area Study using DSM-III criteria; from Jorm, A. F. (2000). Fratiglioni, L. & Henderson, S. (2009). The ageing population and epidemiology of mental disorders among the elderly. In *New Oxford Textbook of Psychiatry*, 2nd edn. Eds Gelder, M., Andreasen, N., Lopez-Ibor, J, & Geddes, J. Oxford University Press, Oxford.

Fig. 18.3 Prevalence rates for dementia across age groups: data from three meta-analyses.

Source data from: Jorm, A. F. (2000). Fratiglioni, L. & Henderson, S. (2009). The ageing population and epidemiology of mental disorders among the elderly. In *New Oxford Textbook of Psychiatry*, 2nd edn. Eds Gelder, M., Andreasen, N., Lopez-Ibor, J, & Geddes, J. Oxford University Press, Oxford.

Table 18.1 Prevalence of common psychiatric conditions in older adults

Diagnosis	Prevalence in adults aged 18–64	Prevalence in adults over 65
Depression	6%	10%
Psychosis	0.5%	<1%
Bipolar disorder	1.5%	1%
Generalized anxiety disorder	5–6%	10%
Alzheimer's disease	<1% before 65 years	1% aged 60
		5% aged 70
		40% aged 85
Completed suicides per year	11.9/100,000	14.5/100,000

Management and prognosis may depend on which of these subgroups are relevant, information which is usually gained from a comprehensive history. Common diagnoses include:

- dementia;
- delirium;
- mood disorders:
- anxiety disorders;
- psychoses: schizophrenia and delusional disorder;
- suicide and deliberate self-harm (DSH);
- alcohol and substance misuse.

Assessment of mental health disorders in older patients

The assessment of older people presenting with a psychiatric problem is fundamentally the same as in the younger population, but extra consideration must be given to the following:

1 Is this an episode of a recurrent problem, or a completely new diagnosis?

2 Are the symptoms being caused by mental illness, or could it be an organic pathology (e.g. brain tumour, dementia)?

3 What physical illnesses does the patient have, and how do these complicate the situation?

4 What is the patient's social situation, and what is their level of function in activities of daily living?

Referrals into psychiatric services may be from a GP, geriatrician, social worker, residential home staff, or family member. The referral should clearly state the problem and its context. In the UK, specialist old age psychiatry teams will assess the patient, either at home (to get a realistic view of the pathology) or in clinic.

The assessment should be undertaken by a multidisciplinary team including a psychiatrist, psychologist, occupational therapist, physiotherapist, and social worker. A full assessment will include:

- full history from the patient, family, and involved professionals;
- full physical and neurological examination;
- full cognitive assessment, including a Mini Mental State Examination (MMSE);
- functional assessment (activities of daily living and mobilization);
- social assessment (housing, finances, activities);
- assessment of carers' needs.

History

Most older adults are able to give a full, accurate account of their symptoms and situation themselves, but if they are unable to do so, the information can be gathered from other sources. The general history in terms of presenting symptoms is no different to that in younger patients (Box 18.1).

Box 18.1 Taking a psychiatric history in an older adult

The following specific information should be obtained during the assessment:

- Timing of onset of symptoms and their subsequent course
- Previous similar episodes
- A description of behaviour over a typical 24 hours
- Previous medical and psychiatric history (including previous intellectual ability and personality characteristics)
- Accurate drug history
- Family history of psychiatric problems
- Living conditions
- Ability for self-care, shopping, cooking, and laundry
- Ability to manage finances and deal with hazards such as fire
- Any behaviour that may cause difficulties for carers or neighbours
- The ability of family and friends to help
- Other services already involved in the patient's care

The mental state examination

This is fundamentally the same as in other age groups. One important point is to try to distinguish between depression and dementia.

Appearance and behaviour. Observation of the patient's clothing, personal cleanliness, and home environment often provides valuable information. Look for signs that suggest these are chronic problems rather than caused by an acute illness. Agitation or psychomotor retardation may be obvious. Wandering, incontinence, and disorientation may point to dementia.

Speech. Dysphasia is frequently seen in moderate to advanced dementia, or after a stroke. In delirium, dementia, or alcohol excess, speech may be inappropriate. Lack of speech may suggest depression, and excessive quantities of rapid speech may suggest mania.

Mood. Older people may not admit to low mood, sadness, or depression. Anhedonia, fatigue, weight loss, anorexia, and insomnia are common. Suicidal ideation and passive death wish are more common in older than in younger adults. Florid mania is rare, but presents as in younger patients.

Thoughts. There are no specific differences in older people. Anxiety is very common. Delusions are seen in depression, delusional disorder, delirium, and dementia.

Perceptual disturbances. Hallucinations are common in dementia and delirium, but also in pre-existing or late-onset psychoses. Visual hallucinations are particularly associated with delirium and alcohol withdrawal.

Cognition. The MMSE (see following section) is the best tool to assess cognition. A 10-point abbreviated mini mental test score may also be helpful.

Insight. This is frequently poor. Good insight into low mood suggests depression rather than dementia.

Examination and investigation

Physical examination. A detailed physical examination should be carried out on all patients, as there are likely to be physical co-morbidities. This should include a neurological examination, and an assessment of vision and hearing.

Physical investigations. These should aim to exclude an organic cause for the symptoms. Those in *italics* are needed for patients presenting with relatively acute symptoms, primarily to exclude delirium:

- blood for full blood count, urea and electrolytes, liver function tests, thyroid function tests (calcium, phosphate, magnesium, glucose, lactate, troponin, albumin, haematinics, syphilis serology);
- chest X-ray;
- imaging (e.g. CT head);
- *blood and urine cultures;*
- *arterial blood gas;*
- *ECG;*
- *urinalysis.*

Psychological and cognitive assessment

Tests should be used within the wider context of obtaining information from the history and clinical examination. They should be regularly repeated, especially after any acute illness or stressor. The Geriatric Depression Scale or Beck Depression Index may be used to screen for depression. Complex cognitive investigations are usually not needed, but the following are useful simple tests to quantify the level of impairment.

- **Abbreviated Mental Test Score (AMTS)** out of 10 points, score of 6 or less taken as delirium (http://en.wikipedia.org/wiki/Abbreviated_mental_test_score).
- **MMSE** out of 30 points, with more than or equal to 25 taken as normal, mild dementia 21–24, moderate 10–20 and severe less than 10 points. It tests the domains of orientation, attention, calculation, memory, and language.

The AMTS is often used sequentially to monitor for improvement or decline in functioning. The MMSE is primarily used for dementia, but may be helpful in delirium. In severe depression, the phenomenon of 'pseudodementia' may occur, in which the patient complains of poor memory. However, on formal memory testing they show no deficit.

Provision of psychiatric services for older adults

The WHO's CARITAS consensus is a set of values agreed by many countries as to which mental health services should be available for older people. As in the rest of psychiatry, there is a basic separation of services into outpatient, day-patient, and inpatient facilities, with some additional settings of care (Table 18.2). The voluntary sector also provides services in some countries, mostly in the form of day centres or home visiting schemes, which are accessible free of charge. These are helpful in providing help or advice on social and financial aspects, and are complementary to traditional medical services. Admission to an inpatient facility should only occur when less intensive treatment options have not been successful, or when life is at risk.

Table 18.2 Types of psychiatric services available for the older patient

Type of service	Setting	Characteristics and treatments provided
Psychiatric inpatient units	Hospital	• 24-hour specialist care • MDT assessment • Treatment with drugs, ECT, specialist nursing, talking therapies • Rehabilitation • Usually short admissions • Can accept patients under section
Acute medical wards	Hospital	• Treatment of acute physical illness • Basic assessment of mental state • Usually as a temporary or emergency measure
Consultation and liaison services	Hospital	• Psychiatrist visits patients in the general hospital • Support for acute medical services • Direct referrals to appropriate follow-up on discharge
Day hospitals	Hospital	• Often cater for specialist groups (e.g. advanced dementia) • Hospital-level treatment while remaining at home • Respite for carers
Community outpatient services	Community	• MDT assessment at home • Case management • Drug treatments and talking therapies
Specialist residential care	Community	• May be private, state funded, or run by a voluntary agency • For those unable to live independently • 24-hour personal and nursing care • Often specialize in particular diagnoses • Psychiatrists may visit the home to see patients
Respite care	Hospital or community	• Brief admissions to a residential home or hospital • Gives carers some time off • Financially difficult to support
Primary care	Community	• Consistent support and treatment • Basic assessment • Treatments • Integrating treatment for mental and physical health problems

MDT, multidisciplinary team.

Principles of treatment

In most situations, the treatment of psychiatric disorders in older adults resembles that of the same conditions in younger adults, although there are some differences in emphasis, such as:

• it is more often necessary to treat concurrent physical disorders;

• maintaining function and independence is paramount;

• special caution is needed in drug dosages;

• social measures must be considered;

• families need to be involved and supported, even more than with younger patients;

• capacity and other ethical issues are important (Box 18.2).

Box 18.2 Ethical and legal issues in the elderly

- Confidentiality in relation to information from carers
- Confidentiality of information about financial circumstances
- Consent to treatment:
  - Capacity to consent to physical and psychological treatment
  - Advance directives
  - Decisions 'not to treat'
- Management of financial affairs:
  - Nominating another to take responsibility (power of attorney)
  - Procedures to enable others to take responsibility
- Entitlement to drive a car

Specific treatments for particular conditions are covered in the latter half of this chapter, or in Chapter 26 for cognitive disorders. Patients may be treated involuntarily or voluntarily in the usual way. One specific consideration is safety at home—they may be unable to provide adequately for their own physical needs (such as warmth, food, and personal hygiene), or lack a physically safe environment (trip-free floors, risk-free heating, and cooking facilities). Boxes 18.3 and 18.4 outline the major considerations for treatment in old age psychiatry.

Box 18.3 Social considerations in treating older adults

- Psychosocial treatments
- Encourage self-care
- Social contacts
- Legal and financial advice
- Financial
- Driving
- Determining mental capacity
- Social services
- Domiciliary
- Day care
- Residential and nursing care
- Voluntary services

Ethical issues

Ethical issues are similar to those in younger people but problems relating to impaired capacity are much more common (Box 18.2). It may be necessary to consider practical matters as well as the ability to consent to treatment. In the UK, the Mental Capacity Act 2005 sets out to protect those individuals who do not have the capacity to make decisions for themselves, and provides the principles by which decisions of capacity may be made (see Chapter 12).

Specific psychiatric disorders

Cognitive impairment: delirium and dementia

These common disorders are covered in Chapter 26 (p. 361).

Depressive disorders

Depression in older adults is associated with poorer outcomes, higher co-morbid physical illness, and increased mortality compared to younger patients. Historically, it has been poorly diagnosed and treated, but this is now starting to improve.

Clinical features

There are no fundamental differences in depressive disorders in older and younger people, but some symptoms are more common. Anxiety, somatic, and hypochondriacal symptoms are frequent. Psychomotor agitation or retardation occurs in 30 per cent of depressed older patients. Depressive delusions of poverty, nihilism, and physical illness are more common among severely depressed patients, as are hallucinations of an accusing or obscene kind. DSH is rare, and should be taken seriously. Occasionally, behavioural changes can be an indicator of depression; for instance, new-onset incontinence, poor oral intake, or alcohol misuse.

Some depressed patients have conspicuous difficulty in concentrating and remembering but there is no corresponding defect in clinical tests of memory function (**pseudodementia**). The differences between

Box 18.4 Treatment options in old age psychiatry

Assessment

- Physical, psychological, cognitive, and social

Decide on an appropriate level of care

- Can the patient be treated at home or do they need admission to hospital or a supported residential environment?
- Where do I need to make a referral?
  - Primary care team
  - Specialist mental health workers based in primary care
  - Specialist outpatient, day patient, or inpatient care
  - Admission to general hospital for acute medical treatment

General measures

- Appoint a care coordinator and make a written care plan
- Detect and treat any physical disorders (e.g. electrolyte abnormalities in delirium or hypothyroidism in depression)
- Psychoeducation of patient, family, and carers
- Make decisions regarding capacity and end-of-life care
- Offer physiotherapy, occupational therapy, and a nutritional assessment
- Provide training courses, support groups, legal advice, and respite care for carers

Pharmacological

Principles to consider:

1 Use non-pharmacological treatments where possible to minimize side effects

2 Start at low dose, titrate slowly, and monitor carefully, especially for extrapyramidal and anticholinergic symptoms

3 Drugs that commonly cause psychiatric side effects include those which treat cardiovascular disorders (antihypertensives, diuretics, and digoxin), act on the central nervous system (antidepressants, hypnotics, anxiolytics, antipsychotics, antiparkinsonian drugs), or the endocrine system (steroids, thyroxine, hormones)

4 Avoid hypnotics—high risk of daytime drowsiness, confusion, falls, incontinence, and hypothermia

5 Consider use of memory aid medicine dispensers or supervised dosing

Psychological

- There is good evidence talking treatments are as effective in the elderly as in younger adults and are of benefit in those with mild cognitive impairments

Consider:

- Problem-solving and relaxation techniques
- CBT (group or individual)
- Group supportive psychotherapy
- Psychological support for carers

Social

(See Box 18.3.)

- Arrange suitable living environment and personal care if required
- Financial advice and assistance
- Arrange appropriate social activities

dementia and pseudodementia are shown in Table 18.3. The possibility of a depressive disorder should be considered whenever a patient develops apparent cognitive impairment, anxiety, or hypochondriacal symptoms.

The diagnostic criteria are the same as for younger adults, and are described on p. 261.

Prevalence

The prevalence of clinically significant depressive disorders in older people living at home is 10–15 per cent. In residential care or general medical wards, the prevalence is higher, at 20–40 per cent. Many of these disorders are found in people who have had a depressive disorder at an earlier age; first depressive illnesses decline in incidence after the age of 60, and are rare after the age of 80. Unlike in younger adults, the sex ratio is more equal, with a slight female excess. The incidence of **suicide** increases steadily with age and is usually associated with depressive disorder.

Table 18.3 Distinguishing the pseudodementia of depression from dementia

Dementia	Depression ('pseudodementia')
Insidious onset over months	Quicker onset, days to weeks
Mood and behaviour fluctuate	Mood and behaviour consistent
Biological symptoms absent	Biological symptoms present
Denies (or attempts to hide) poor memory	Admits to poor memory
Impaired orientation	Normal orientation
Reduced MMSE on testing	Normal MMSE on testing
Less often a personal history of depression	Often a personal history of depression
No response to antidepressants	Responds to antidepressants

MMSE, Mini Mental State Examination.

Differential diagnosis

- **Dementia.** The distinction depends on a detailed history from other informants, and careful observation of the mental state and behaviour of the patient (Table 18.3). The diagnostic problem is made more difficult as 30 per cent of patients with dementia have comorbid depression.
- **Paranoid disorder.** In a depressive disorder, paranoid delusions are usually egosyntonic and follow a decline in mood; in a paranoid disorder, the persecution is perceived as unjustified and mood may be euthymic.
- **Anxiety disorder.** Look for low mood, anhedonia, and fatigue in a patient presenting with agitation.
- **Stroke.** It may be difficult to distinguish between mood symptoms caused by cerebral damage (especially of left frontal lobe) and depression secondary to an adverse situation caused by the stroke. Practically, treatment should be as for any depressive episode.
- **Parkinson's disease.** Mood symptoms may be an intrinsic part of Parkinson's disease itself, or be side effects of antiparkinsonian medications.
- **Organic mood disorders.** The most common are hypothyroidism, cancer, chronic infection, and medication side effects.

Aetiology

In general, the aetiology of depressive disorders in late life resembles that of similar disorders occurring in earlier life (see Chapter 21), except that genetic factors may be less important. As in other groups, a depressive episode tends to present when a precipitating event occurs in a vulnerable individual. The most important risk factors are neurological or other chronic physical illnesses, and loss of a partner. Common stressors include the following:

1 Physical illness, such as:
   - any chronic physical illness, especially cardiovascular disease, cancer, endocrine or metabolic conditions;
   - neurological disease;
   - chronic pain or disability.
2 Social factors, such as:
   - bereavement and loss;
   - retirement and change in role;
   - loss of mobility leading to social isolation;
   - change in financial circumstances;
   - caring responsibilities;
   - lack of support from family or friends;
   - moving from own home into a residential or nursing home;
   - hospital admission.
3 Personal history of depression or other mental health disorders.

Course

Unfortunately, depression in older adults can be challenging to treat. Untreated episodes may last for years, but with treatment 85 per cent will recover within months. Long-term follow-up of recovered patients shows that relapse is frequent. Suicide is more likely than in younger people.

The factors predicting a better prognosis are:

- onset before the age of 70;
- short duration of illness;
- good previous adjustment;
- no concurrent disabling physical illness;
- good recovery from previous episodes.

There is some evidence that depression is a risk factor for later developing dementia. This is not yet well characterized and is probably multifactorial, but may be due to hippocampal atrophy, hypercortisolaemia, vascular disease, or that the depressive episode is prodromal to dementia.

Assessment

A full assessment should be carried out as outlined in the previous section. A good clinical screening tool is the **Geriatric Depression Score**: a score of greater than 5/15 indicates depression. A full set of blood tests is usually all that is needed in terms of investigations.

Management

In the UK, management of depressive disorders is as outlined in the NICE guidelines, last updated in April 2018. Full details can be found in Chapter 21, so what follows are specific points relating to treatment in older adults. Box 18.5 contains a summary of the various options.

Antidepressant drugs are effective, but should be used at low dose, titrated slowly, and with close monitoring of side effects and response. A Cochrane systematic review of patients over 55 years has found no difference in the efficacy of SSRIs compared with tricyclic antidepressants. However, NICE recommends the use of SSRIs as the first-line treatment, as they have fewer anticholinergic side effects and are safer in overdose. Tricyclic antidepressants should be avoided in those at risk of cardiac arrhythmias or postural hypotension. After recovery, antidepressant medication

Box 18.5 Treatment of depression in older people

General measures

- Optimize treatment of physical conditions
- Psychoeducation of patient and carers
- Offer advice about social and financial support
- Offer advice about sleep hygiene

Mild depression

- Antidepressants are not recommended
- Choices include activity scheduling, supervised exercise programmes, guided self-help, or computerized CBT

Moderate depression

- SSRI antidepressant

Or

- Individual CBT or IPT
- Continue with social activities and exercise

Severe depression

Antidepressants *and* individual CBT/IPT:

- Antidepressants: SSRIs (or tricyclic antidepressant, or plus mirtazapine, venlafaxine if needed)
- Consider lithium augmentation
- Consider augmentation with antipsychotics for psychosis
- Consider ECT
- Continue social activities and exercise as above in list

should be reduced slowly and then continued for at least 2 years.

Electroconvulsive therapy (ECT) is useful for the small minority of patients with severe and distressing psychosis or agitation, life-threatening stupor, or failure to respond to drugs. Special care is needed with the anaesthesia. It may be necessary to space out treatments at longer intervals or give unilateral treatment to reduce post-treatment memory impairment.

Psychological treatments. CBT and interpersonal therapy (IPT) are proven to be efficacious, in either individual or group format. As anxiety is often a large part of mood disorders, specific anxiety-reduction and relaxation techniques may be helpful.

Bipolar disorder

The natural course of bipolar disorder is such that most patients who are diagnosed as young adults will continue to have episodes throughout life. The diagnostic criteria are outlined in Chapter 21. For those patients who develop bipolar disorder after the age of 50, the prognosis is significantly worse. Depressive episodes in the context of bipolar disorder present and are treated as in younger adults.

Clinical features

The symptoms of mania are predominantly the same at all ages (p. 277). However, confusion, disorientation, paranoia and new focal neurology (which resolves with treatment) are more common in the elderly. Euphoria and grandiosity are less frequently seen. There is a greater propensity for sudden switching between mania and depression. Mixed episodes are also common, and may lead to misdiagnosis as delirium or dementia.

Prevalence

The prevalence of bipolar disorder in the general population is 1.5 per cent, reducing to 1 per cent in the over 65s. Only about 10 per cent of new diagnoses of bipolar disorder occur in patients over 50 years, and in retrospect it is usually possible to see that the patient has had episodes earlier in their life. Males and females are equally represented.

Differential diagnosis

The differential diagnosis depends upon whether the presenting episode is mania or depression. For the latter, the list in the earlier section is relevant. The main differentials of a manic episode are as follows:

- **Schizophrenia or schizoaffective disorder.** As manic episodes frequently include psychotic elements, search carefully for the characteristic features of schizophrenia. Delusions are typically mood congruent in a mood disorder, and not in schizophrenia. In mania, the content of delusions or hallucinations often changes rapidly, and

usually ceases with a reduction in the overactive state.
- **Delirium.** A sudden-onset, acute confusional state with disorientation in a patient with no history of a mood disorder is highly suggestive of delirium. Look for a precipitating cause (infection, electrolyte abnormality, etc.).
- **Dementia.** It is rare for dementia to present suddenly; symptoms have usually taken months to develop, whereas a mood disorder is relatively quick in onset.
- **Organic causes.** Endocrine disorders (hyperthyroidism, Cushing's) may present exactly as a manic episode. Neurological conditions such as space-occupying lesions, epilepsy, stroke, head injuries, multiple sclerosis, HIV, or systemic lupus erythematosus may also present with mood symptoms. Extreme social disinhibition is characteristic of frontal lobe lesions.
- **Abuse of stimulant drugs.** Amphetamines, hallucinogens, and opiates can all cause a mania-like state.
- **Medications.** Virtually any drug affecting the central nervous system can cause mania. Other culprits include antituberculosis drugs, antihypertensives, respiratory drugs, steroids, analgesics, and antacid preparations (see Science box 18.1).

Aetiology

For late-onset bipolar disorder, heritability is somewhat reduced, but is still important. Many of these patients have mild cognitive impairment, and MRI scans have shown an increased number of white matter lesions, especially in those with soft neurological signs.

Course and prognosis

In those presenting with a first episode of mania in late life, 80–90 per cent recover fully with treatment. About half of these will go on to have recurrent episodes. In patients with a long history of bipolar disorder, there is a reduced rate of full response, and the chance of further (and often more severe) episodes is higher.

SCIENCE BOX 18.1

Cognitive behavioural therapy for depression in older adults

There is good evidence that CBT is an effective treatment for moderate to severe depression and it is now included in most treatment guidelines.[1] Depression in older people is often resistant to treatment, but only 5–10 per cent of patients currently receive psychological therapies. There appears to be a general belief that therapies such as CBT are less effective with increasing age, but this has not been evidence based.[2] So is CBT as effective in the older population as in younger patients?

In 2008, Cochrane published a meta-analysis of RCTs comparing various psychotherapies with 'waiting list' or active control interventions.[3] The latter included advice and a non-therapeutic bibliography. The mean duration of the trials was 12 weeks, delivering 16–20 sessions of individual therapy. The patients who received CBT showed a significantly greater reduction in symptoms compared with waiting list controls. As of December 2018 Cochrane has not updated this review.

It was widely recognized that the Cochrane study (and several similar reviews) involved relatively small groups of patients with heterogeneous 'control' groups. In 2009, Sertafy et al. conducted a larger primary care-based trial of 204 patients, mean age 74 years, who were randomized to treatment as usual (TAU), TAU plus a talking control, or TAU plus CBT.[4] The CBT arm improved significantly when compared with either of the other groups, based on response to standard mood disorder questionnaires.

As it stands, the evidence does confirm that CBT is an effective treatment for older people with depression. It should be routinely available to patients presenting with mood disorders, irrespective of their age.

1 National Institute for Health and Care Excellence. Depression in adults: recognition and management. Clinical guidance [CG90]. Published October 2009, updated April 2018. http://www.nice.org.uk/CG90.

2 Pinquart M, Duberstein PR, Lyness JM. Treatments for later-life depressive conditions: a meta-analytic comparison of pharmacotherapy and psychotherapy. *American Journal of Psychiatry* 2006;163: 1493–1501.

3 Wilson KCM, Mottram PG, Vassilas CA. Psychotherapeutic treatments for older depressed people. *Cochrane Database of Systematic Reviews* 2008;1:CD004853.

4 Serfaty MA, Haworth D, Blanchard M, et al. Clinical effectiveness of individual cognitive behavioral therapy for depressed older people in primary care. *Archives of General Psychiatry* 2009;66:1332–1340.

Management

Treatment of bipolar disorder is discussed in detail in Chapter 21: a summary of its guidance is shown in Box 18.6.

Drug treatments

As in a manic episode at any age, the basic treatment is with an antipsychotic (usually an atypical) and a mood stabilizer. The usual choices for the latter are lithium or sodium valproate. Older people tend to metabolize drugs more slowly than younger patients, and may need lower doses. The advised therapeutic level of lithium in adults is 0.5–1.0 mmol/litre for maintenance, which can be raised slightly in an acute episode. Older patients may become toxic at these levels, and many old age psychiatrists work to a lower range. There is an increased risk of falls on sedating medications, which needs to be carefully monitored.

Schizophrenia and paranoid disorders

Patients with psychosis in later life can be divided into three groups:

1 Those with pre-existing schizophrenia.

2 New diagnoses of schizophrenia ('late-life schizophrenia', or 'late paraphrenia').

3 Other conditions producing hallucinations or delusions (dementia, delirium, mood disorders, delusional disorder, paranoid personality disorders).

Box 18.6 Management of bipolar disorder in older adults

General measures
- Optimize treatment of physical conditions
- Psychoeducation
- Organize calming activities, structured supported routine
- Offer psychological and social support

Manic episodes (not already on antimanic drugs)
- Stop antidepressants
- Atypical antipsychotic
- Mood stabilizer: lithium or valproate
- Short-term use of benzodiazepines
- Consider ECT for resistant cases

Manic episodes (already on antimanic drugs)
- Stop antidepressants
- Check doses and compliance with antipsychotic medications
- Increase dose of antipsychotic
- Add (or increase dose of) mood stabilizer: lithium or valproate
- Check blood levels of lithium regularly

Depressive episode
- Antidepressant: SSRI
- Add 'antimanic cover': lithium, valproate, or an antipsychotic
- Consider ECT for severe resistant cases
- Consider CBT or IPT
- Psychological and social measures as usual

As the population ages and treatments improve, the first group is getting significantly larger and making up a greater proportion of mental illness.

Clinical features

The classical clinical features and diagnostic criteria of schizophrenia are described in Chapter 22. Generally, older patients have less florid positive symptoms than younger adults, and not all develop negative symptoms. Persecutory delusions are the most common symptom (>90 per cent of late-life schizophrenic patients), followed by auditory hallucinations. Hallucinations in other senses (visual, tactile, olfactory) are more frequent. Some degree of cognitive impairment is typical, and may precede the onset of positive symptoms, making the diagnosis more difficult.

Prevalence

The prevalence of all psychotic disorders over 65 years of age is 4–6 per cent, rising to 10 per cent over 85 years. However, a large proportion of these cases are related to dementia. True schizophrenia or delusional disorder in the over 65s has a prevalence of 0.5–1.0 per cent. There is a female preponderance, with a ratio of female to males of 5:1, which is partly because the onset of schizophrenia tends to be later in females. Sixty per cent of cases are paranoid schizophrenia, 30 per cent delusional disorder, and only 10 per cent all other forms of psychosis.

Differential diagnosis

- **Dementia.** Memory testing is paramount; those with schizophrenia usually have a good memory. Persecutory delusions are common in dementia, but other forms of delusion are not. The timescale of symptom development will also be useful, as dementia usually has an insidious onset.
- **Delirium.** An acute confusional state with disorientation and florid visual hallucinations is typical of delirium.
- **Bipolar disorder with psychosis.**
- **Severe depression with psychosis.**
- **Paranoid personality disorder.** In paranoid personality disorder there is *lifelong* suspiciousness and distrust, with sensitive ideas but no delusions.
- **Organic cerebral disease.** Stroke, tumours, temporal lobe epilepsy, variant Creutzfeldt–Jakob disease, HIV, syphilis, multiple sclerosis, and any other diffuse brain disease should all be excluded.
- **Drug-induced states.** Amphetamines, cannabis, cocaine, and ecstasy all cause psychosis. Prescribed medications—especially steroids, antiparkinsonian

drugs, and psychoactive drugs—may be the primary cause, or exacerbate symptoms.

- **Hallucinations of sensory deprivation (Charles–Bonnet syndrome).** Complex visual hallucinations may occur in older people with low vision, especially in the context of significant hearing loss. Usually, there are no other psychotic symptoms, and the patient has more insight than in schizophrenia.

Aetiology

See Chapter 22. The significant social changes of old age may well trigger the onset of the condition, or precipitate another episode.

Course and prognosis

There is little evidence currently on the prognosis of late-life schizophrenia.

Treatment

In general, the treatment of these disorders in older people is similar to that for younger people (see Chapter 22 and Box 18.7). Outpatient treatment may be possible, but admission to hospital is often required, and is essential if there is risk of suicide or violence, severe psychosis or catatonia, lack of capacity or willingness to comply with treatments, no social supports, or complex co-morbidities. Day hospitals are often very useful in this patient group, helping to reduce time in hospital,

avoid social isolation, ensure adequate supervision, and prevent relapse. Any sensory deficit, such as deafness or cataract, should be assessed and, if possible, treated.

Most patients require antipsychotic medication but the dosage is usually less than that needed for younger adults. There is a higher risk of extrapyramidal symptoms and tardive dyskinesia than in younger people, so the older typical antipsychotics should be avoided. Medications should be introduced at the lowest dose and the patient carefully monitored for physical side effects. The most common side effects are postural hypotension (and therefore falls), urinary retention, and constipation. As with younger patients, a depot preparation should be considered. It is recommended that medications be continued for at least 2 years after full recovery (see Case study box 18.1).

Stress-related and anxiety disorders

These 'minor' psychiatric disorders are the mostly common mental health problems of old age, and are encountered throughout medicine. Ten per cent of the elderly fit diagnostic criteria for an anxiety disorder with another ten per cent having subclinical symptoms. Anxiety is highly associated with physical illness, and is very costly to health services in time and money. The main features of all of the separate conditions are described in detail in the relevant chapters; what follows is a summary of the differences seen in older patients.

Clinical features

In an older population, there is much less distinction between different types of stress-related and anxiety disorder. Generalized anxiety disorder is by far the most common condition. Symptoms frequently encountered are shown in Table 18.4.

Differential diagnosis

Patients usually present to the GP or general hospital with physical symptoms; it is therefore important (but sometimes impossible) to distinguish them from symptoms caused by organic pathology. It is frequently the case that symptoms may be an exaggeration of those caused by an underlying pathology—for example, shortness of breath in

---

Box 18.7 Treatment of late-life schizophrenia

- Refer urgently to mental health services
- Choose appropriate setting of care
- Allocate a CPN and a social worker
- Offer an antipsychotic to all patients (first-line, atypical antipsychotic)
- Consider clozapine after trials of two other antipsychotics
- Short-term low-dose benzodiazepines for agitation or poor sleep
- Offer a course of 16–20 sessions of individual CBT
- Consider group therapeutic sessions
- Social interventions: appropriate housing, activities, financial assistance

CASE STUDY BOX 18.1

Paranoid symptoms

The son of an 82-year-old widow visits your surgery to say that he is concerned about his mother. She is complaining of her neighbours shouting abuse from within their house and persecuting her. She believes that they have stolen objects and that there is a complex conspiracy that involves a number of her neighbours and which is intended to drive her out of her own home. The son has realized that the allegations are a fantasy, but his mother maintains that she is perfectly well and that the problem lies with her neighbours' behaviour. There is no past history of mental disorder. You organize a home visit; on arrival, the patient is highly suspicious but tells you about her beliefs that she is being persecuted. When you express some doubt, it is clear that she will not be dissuaded from these beliefs but her mood is euthymic, she looks physically well and does not appear cognitively impaired. You conclude that she is probably suffering from primary paranoid psychosis.

You confer with an age old psychiatrist and discuss the option of starting olanzapine 2.5 mg once daily by mouth. The patient is suspicious but agrees if it will 'help sort out the neighbours'. A CPN is allocated and her son helps to supervise the medication initially. Screening bloods and a CT head are normal. Unfortunately, the following week the patient gets distressed by hearing the neighbours plotting against her. You increase the olanzapine to 5 mg daily which starts to be effective within a week and organize a CPN and day centre to monitor progress.

chronic obstructive pulmonary disorder—which are extremely difficult to treat. It is helpful to distinguish between the following:

- **Depression.** Anxiety and stress-related disorders often coexist with depression. In depression the physical symptoms are more stereotyped—sleep disturbance, anorexia, weight loss, fatigue—and are usually in the context of low mood.

- **Dementia.** Early dementia often presents with anxiety or obsessions. It may not be possible to

Table 18.4 Symptoms of stress-related and anxiety disorders in older adults

Psychological	Physical (somatic)	Behavioural
Fearful anticipation	Abdominal pain	Phobic avoidance
Irritability	Diarrhoea	Fear of mobilizing
Hyperacusis	Dry mouth	Social isolation
Restlessness	Dysphagia	Use of alcohol or drugs
Poor concentration	Tight chest	Frequent attendance at the GP or hospital admissions
Worrying thoughts	Shortness of breath	
Fear of losing control	Palpitations	
Depersonalization	Chest pain	
Panic attacks	Sweating	
	Urinary symptoms	
	Tremor	
	Headache	
	Fatigue	
	Pain	
	Insomnia	
	Nightmares	

make a definite diagnosis until more characteristic symptoms of dementia develop.

- **Delirium.** This is characterized by a relatively sudden onset of disorientation and other features of confusion, and is usually associated with common physical problems in the elderly such as chest infection, urinary tract infection, constipation, or electrolyte disturbance.

- **Paranoid delusional disorder or schizophrenia.** The presence of hallucinations or delusions is usually relatively obvious.

- **Physical illness.** There is a high correlation between the diagnosis of a physical illness and the onset of anxiety symptoms. Frequently, it is best to treat both concurrently, if only to try and maximize symptom relief.

Aetiology

The likelihood of developing an anxiety disorder in later life is primarily related to prior vulnerability, personality, and life experiences. It is rare for a clinically significant disorder (especially if unrelated to physical illness) to develop *de novo* in a patient with no previous history of any anxiety or mental health disturbance. The genetic predisposition to anxiety continues into later life. Psychosocial factors that may predispose to or precipitate an episode are similar to those for depression (p. 261).

Course and prognosis

Anxiety disorders tend to become chronic and are very difficult to treat. Those illnesses that develop without an obvious precipitating factor have a poorer prognosis.

Treatment

There is a little evidence on the treatment of anxiety and stress disorders in older people. Most patients are treated in primary care and do not need to be referred to a psychiatrist: treatment should follow the recommendations for younger people (see Chapters 23 and 24). There is some evidence that CBT is effective in this group of patients. Frequently, the techniques need to be altered for those with sensory losses, physical disability, or cognitive impairment. Individual treatment is usually more appropriate than group therapy, but there is a role for group social activities. Antidepressants are the first-line choice for generalized anxiety, and an SSRI is the safest option. Benzodiazepines carry a high risk of sedation, falls, tolerance, and dependence and therefore should be avoided wherever possible.

Suicide and deliberate self-harm

Suicide and DSH are relatively common in older adults, with the highest rates of suicide being amongst men over 75. In the UK, the overall population rate of completed suicide in 2013 was 11.9/100,000, but in older adults was 14.5/100,000. The male-to-female ratio is 3:1, similar to younger people. With an increasing proportion of society reaching old age, suicide in this group is likely to become a more prominent problem. In younger people there is a spectrum of self-harm, from suicidal thoughts to acts of DSH to suicide attempts and completed suicide. Older people are more likely to go straight to completed suicide. They are also prone to passive methods of self-harm: refusing to eat and drink, non-compliance with medical treatments, or complete withdrawal from the world.

Deliberate self-harm

There are many fewer cases of active DSH in the old compared with the young. It is therefore important to consider every act as a failed suicide, and treat accordingly. Unlike completed suicide, DSH is more common in females, although there is less preponderance than seen in young adults. Deliberate overdose of prescribed medications (typically benzodiazepines, analgesics, or antidepressants) is the most common presentation, with few cases of over-the-counter paracetamol or aspirin-based attempts. Self-cutting is seen, but only occasionally. A psychiatric disorder is present in at least 90 per cent of patients, most of whom will be depressed. Two-thirds have severe physical illness of some type, and most have a psychiatric history. Risk factors for DSH (and suicide) are shown in Box 18.8.

Box 18.8 Risk factors for deliberate self-harm and suicide in the elderly

- Age
- Physical illness
- Widowed, divorced, or separated
- Social isolation
- Loneliness
- Grief
- Threat of moving to a residential home
- Alcohol abuse
- Depression, past or present
- Recent contact with a psychiatrist

Completed suicide

Completed suicide is a natural progression from DSH, but in many patients it is the first and final act. Only one-third have had a previous attempt at DSH or suicide. The method of suicide is highly dependent on geographical location; for instance, in the UK 'hanging, strangling, and suffocation' account for approximately 50 per cent of completed suicides, whereas in the USA (with looser firearms legislation) they account for only 15–20 per cent. More so than in younger patients, older people plan their suicide carefully, leaving an explanatory note and their affairs in order. Surprisingly, fewer patients who kill themselves appear to have been suffering from a psychiatric illness prior to their death than those who commit DSH. The figure is thought to be around 70 per cent, with almost all of these having depression.

Risk assessment

As mentioned previously, all acts of DSH should be taken seriously. Clinicians also need to be alert to the chance of depressed patients having suicidal thoughts, even with no previous history. Careful prescriptions—for instance, only prescribed 1–2 weeks' medication at a time—and/or monitoring the taking of medications may be necessary. In some cases, it may be appropriate to move a patient temporarily into accommodation where they are not alone for long periods, and involve family and friends in the care plan.

Abuse of alcohol

Alcohol use disorders are common in older adults, and are under-recognized and undertreated. One-third of those who develop a problem with alcohol only do so after the age of 65, and most have no prior psychiatric history. As liver metabolism slows and reduces in efficiency with increasing age, lower levels of alcohol are needed to provoke the characteristic symptoms and alcohol dependence syndrome. In the UK, the national recommendations for alcohol are not more than 14 units per week for all adults. There are no separate guidelines for the over 65s, for whom this is probably too much. Community-based prevalence studies have reported alcohol dependence to be around 2–4 per cent of older patients, but for those in institutional care or hospitals the figure is 15–20 per cent. It is not known how accurate these figures are. The clinical features are similar to those in younger patients, described in Chapter 29. Alcohol can cause a range of neuropsychiatric symptoms including cognitive impairment, depression, Wernicke–Korsakoff syndrome, cerebellar atrophy, psychosis, or a withdrawal syndrome.

The aetiology of alcohol use disorders in older patients is as complex as in younger ones. There remains a genetic risk, but social factors are probably more important. Retirement, bereavement or divorce, reduced socioeconomic status, and physical ill health are common precipitating events. Those patients who exhibited antisocial personality traits, hyperactivity, or impulsivity in former years are at higher risk.

Patients should be assessed as usual, with an emphasis on determining the type, amount, and pattern of drinking. Extensive physical investigations should be carried out to determine the secondary effects of alcohol excess (Box 18.9).

Treatment is similar to that in younger adults. Any underlying psychiatric or physical illness should be treated along normal guidelines. If a reducing benzodiazepine regimen is used, the doses should be significantly lower than in standard guidelines as there is a high risk of sedation and falls. Chlordiazepoxide or lorazepam are the safest choices. Concurrently, either oral or parenteral thiamine should be given to avoid Wernicke–Korsakoff syndrome. Evidence suggests

Box 18.9 Physical investigations into harmful use of alcohol

Physical examination

Look for signs of hepatic damage, malnutrition, focal neurological deficits, and cognitive decline.

Blood tests

- Full blood count: mean cell volume is raised in 60% of people with drinking problems; anaemia may occur in cases of malnutrition
- Liver function tests
- Gamma-glutamyltranspeptidase (GGT) is raised in 80 per cent of people with chronic drinking problems
- Renal function: always worth checking in older people, especially before starting any new medications
- Clotting: alcohol disturbs platelet function

Imaging

- Abdominal ultrasound/CT may be useful to identify hepatomegaly ± cirrhosis
- Chest X-ray: if patients present acutely unwell, excluding a chest infection is important

that oral thiamine is as effective as intravenous thiamine complexes (Pabrinex®). Newer therapies for alcohol abuse, such as disulfiram, acamprosate, and naltrexone, are licensed for use in all ages, but there remains only minimal evidence on safety or efficacy in those over 65 years.

Abuse of older adults

The mistreatment of older people is often known as elder abuse, and is much more commonplace than the general public realize. Abuse may occur in any setting, not just in institutions or residential care. Epidemiological studies report a prevalence of 5 per cent in the community, rising to 10 per cent in residential care. As in children and other vulnerable groups, there are a variety of different forms that abuse may take, including:

- **neglect:** refusal or failure to provide basic rights, or other obligations;

- **physical abuse:** the infliction of pain or injury, physical or drug-induced restraint;
- **emotional abuse:** the infliction of mental anguish;
- **sexual abuse:** any non-consensual sexual contact;
- **financial or material exploitation:** illegal or improper use of financial or other resources belonging to the elderly person.

Risk factors for elder abuse tend to depend strongly upon the context, but the most vulnerable people are those with cognitive and/or physical impairments, or those who are socially isolated. The consequences of abuse may be great, as older people are weaker physically, and bones or other wounds may not heal in the same way as in younger victims. They often live in financially tighter circumstances, where the loss of relatively small amounts of money may push them into poverty. One devastating result of abuse is the loss of confidence—this sets up a spiral of social isolation and increasing vulnerability to further abuse.

Clinicians need to be aware of the possibility of abuse and be prepared to intervene in whatever way will prevent continuing abuse and to deal with underlying problems. If there is any concern, a social worker and senior clinicians with experience in such cases should be contacted, and a thorough history, physical examination, and investigations undertaken. A similar process should be gone through as for child abuse, which is discussed in Chapter 17. Alternative accommodation and care may need to be found for the patient, if only in the short term. Many developed countries now have mechanisms in place to prevent elder abuse, but there is still a lack of education among the general population.

Further reading

Dening T, Thomas A. *Oxford Textbook of Old Age Psychiatry*. 2nd ed. Oxford: Oxford University Press; 2013.

Ferri CP, Prince M, Brayne C, et al. Global prevalence of dementia: a Delphi consensus study. *Lancet* 2005;366:2112–2117.

Gelder M, Andreasen N, López-Ibor JJ, Geddes J, eds. Section 8: The psychiatry of old age. In: *New Oxford*

Textbook of Psychiatry. 2nd ed. Oxford: Oxford University Press; 2012:1505–1586.

Goldsmith TC. Solving the programmed/non-programmed aging conundrum. *Current Aging Science* 2015;8:34–40.

Jin KL. Modern biological theories of aging. *Aging and Disease* 2010;1:72–74.

Kirmizioglu Y, Doğan O, Kuğu N, et al. Prevalence of anxiety disorders amongst elderly people. *International Journal of Geriatric Psychiatry* 2009;14:1026–1033.

Mojtabai R. Diagnosing depression in older adults in primary care. *New England Journal of Medicine* 2014;370:1180–1182.

National Institute for Health and Care Excellence. Dementia: assessment, management and support for people living with dementia and their carers. Published June 2018. https://www.nice.org.uk/guidance/ng97.

Rodda J, Walker Z, Carter J. Depression in older adults. *BMJ* 2011;343:d5219.

19 Learning disability

Disorders of intellectual development—or learning disability (LD)—denote a permanent impairment of intelligence associated with limitations of social functioning. A distinction is to be made between LD and dementia, the former originating early in life and the latter after 18 years of age. Although not reversible, much can be done to enable people with LDs to live as normally as possible. It is helpful for doctors to have basic knowledge of LD so they have an approach when the patient presents with physical or mental health problems and know when to refer to psychiatry.

Overview of aetiology and clinical features

Classification and terminology

Several interchangeable terms are used to describe people with intellectual impairment originating early in life, including:

- LD (common term used in Europe)
- Intellectual disability
- Disorder of intellectual impairment
- Mental retardation (*this term is being phased out for ICD-11 and has been removed from the DSM-5*).

The term LD implies more than intellectual impairment. It aims to separate those who cannot lead a near-normal life from people of the same IQ level who can. Patients with LD can be subdivided into categories which tend to be prognostically very useful (Table 19.1 and Box 19.1). A LD is not a clinical diagnosis in its own right, just a way of describing a particular clinical syndrome of impairments with disability and handicaps. The underlying diagnosis is the cause(s) of these impairments, which may or may not have been identified. The terms impairment, disability, and handicap are not interchangeable. The value of their use is in describing an individual's specific needs, irrespective of their aetiological diagnosis.

- **Impairment** is any loss or abnormality of psychological, physical, or anatomical structure or function. It is not dependent upon aetiology.
- **Disability** is any restriction in the ability to perform an activity within the range considered normal for a human at a corresponding level of development.
- **A handicap** is a disadvantage for a person, due to their impairment or disability, that prevents them from fulfilling a role that is normal for that individual.

Table 19.1 Classification and epidemiology of learning disability

Learning disability	IQ level	Proportion of patients (%)	Prevalence in general population (%)
Mild	50–69	80	2.5
Moderate	35–49	12	0.4
Severe	20–34	7	0.1
Profound	<20	1	

Epidemiology

The definition of LD as an IQ less than 70 (in combination with an impairment of function) is based upon the assumption that IQ is normally distributed with a mean of 100 and standard deviation of 15. Two standard deviations below the mean is 70, representing 2.5 per

Box 19.1 Diagnostic classification for learning disability

ICD 10 Criteria: F70-79 Mental Retardation

A condition of arrested or incomplete development of the mind, which is especially characterized by impairment of skills manifested during the developmental period, skills which contribute to the overall level of intelligence, that is, cognitive, language, motor, and social abilities. Retardation can occur with or without any other mental or physical condition. Subcategories of mild, moderate, severe, and profound (Table 19.1).

Proposed changes for ICD-11

(From Beta-draft, January 2017.)

- Change in terminology to 'Disorders of Intellectual Development'—subcategorized as mild, moderate, severe, or profound.
- Disorders of intellectual development are a group of conditions originating during the developmental period characterized by significantly below-average intellectual functioning and adaptive behaviour that is approximately two or more standard deviations below the mean.

cent of the population—a typical UK GP will have six to eight patients with at least moderate LD. However, reported rates of LD are actually slightly higher at 2–3 per cent. This is because average IQ varies with a number of factors:

- **Country.** LDs are more common in developing than developed countries. This is primarily due to preventable causes (e.g. iodine deficiency).
- **Genetics.** Different ethnic groups show variable intellectual abilities.
- **Age.** Prevalence of LD is higher in child than adult cohorts, with a peak at 10 years. This is partly due to the reduced life expectancy of some individuals with LD, but also due to diagnostic bias.
- **Method of data collection.** Ascertaining the true level of LD is difficult. Data collected from education registers of special needs or specialist health services underestimate the general population figures.

The **prevalence** of LD has changed little since the 1930s even though the **incidence** of severe LD has fallen by one-third to one-half in the same period, partly as a result of improved antenatal and neonatal care. The reason that the prevalence has not changed despite the lower incidence is that people with LD are living longer.

Causes of learning disability

There are a myriad of different causes of LD, representing a heterogeneous group of individuals. A specific cause can be identified in 80 per cent of severe cases, but only in 50 per cent overall. The heritability of IQ is estimated to 70 per cent, but we do not currently know which (combination of) genes are responsible for this. There are three main reasons for making an aetiological diagnosis for a given patient:

1 A diagnosis may guide treatment options.

2 It allows prediction of likely disabilities and prognosis, allowing for planning of services, education, finances, and family life.

3 It may provide information relating to the likely risk of recurrence in future pregnancies.

Mild LD is usually due to a combination of genetic and adverse environmental factors, such as extreme prematurity or damage to the brain during birth. **Severe and profound LD** is usually due to specific pathological conditions, most of which can be diagnosed in life and about two-thirds of which can be diagnosed before birth. The causes of **moderate LD** are varied. An overview is shown in Table 19.2.

Prevention and early detection

Primary prevention depends mainly on genetic screening and counselling, together with good antenatal and obstetric care (Box 19.2). In some developing countries, correction of iodine deficiency and malnutrition is important.

Secondary prevention aims to reduce the effect of the primary disorder; for example, by providing 'enriching' education.

Genetic screening and counselling. Most parents seek advice only after the birth of a first child with LD. Those asking for advice before or during the first pregnancy usually do so because there is a person with LD in the extended family. Specialist advice is usually needed to assess the risk that an abnormal child will be born, and to explain this risk to the parents so that

Table 19.2 Aetiology of learning disability

Aetiology	Subgroup	Examples
Genetics	Dominant genes	Neurofibromatosis, tuberose sclerosis, myotonic dystrophy
	Recessive genes (mostly errors of metabolism)	Phenylketonuria, homocystinuria, urea cycle abnormalities
		Tay–Sachs disease, Gaucher's disease
	Chromosomal abnormalities	Down's syndrome (trisomy 21), Klinefelter syndrome (XXY), Turner's syndrome (XO)
	X-linked disorders	Lesch–Nyhan syndrome, fragile X syndrome
	Genomic imprinting	Prader–Willi syndrome (paternal 15q11–13), Angelman's syndrome (maternal 15q11–13)
Antenatal	Intrauterine infections	Rubella, cytomegalovirus, syphilis
	Intoxication (via maternal ingestion)	Alcohol, cocaine, lead
	Physical damage	Injury, radiation, hypoxia
	Endocrine disorders	Hypothyroidism, hypoparathyroidism, diabetes
Perinatal	Late pregnancy maternal conditions	Pre-eclampsia, placental insufficiency, bleeding
	Birth and newborn complications	Birth injuries, hypoxia, hypoglycaemia, intraventricular haemorrhage, kernicterus, neonatal infections
Postnatal	Injury	Accidental or non-accidental
	Infections	Meningoencephalitis
	Intoxication	Lead, drugs
	Early physical disorders	Brain tumours, vascular events
Malnutrition		Protein–energy malnutrition, Iodine deficiency

Box 19.2 Prevention and early detection of learning disability

Prevention

- Before pregnancy:
  - Test for rubella immunity, syphilis, HIV, and hepatitis B and C
  - Folic acid supplementation (5 mg daily from conception to 12 weeks)
  - Genetic counselling and preimplantation diagnosis
  - Reduce smoking and alcohol
- During pregnancy:
  - Avoid excess alcohol, drugs, and toxic substances
  - Protection against sexually transmitted diseases
  - Promote good maternal health including nutrition and exercise
- During and after delivery:
  - Care of premature infants

Early detection

- During pregnancy:
  - Ultrasound screening, amniocentesis, and fetoscopy
- After delivery:
  - Screening for phenylketonuria, hypothyroidism, and galactosaemia (heel-prick)
  - Aggressive treatment of neonatal complications in special care
  - Good nutrition

Table 19.3 Levels of learning disability

Mild (IQ 50–70)	• Specific causes uncommon • Many need practical help and special education • Few need special psychiatric or social services
Moderate (IQ 35–49)	• Most can manage some independent activities • Require special education, sheltered occupation, and supervision
Severe (IQ 20–34)	• Specific causes usual • Many physical impairments • Social skills and communication severely limited • Require close supervision and much practical help
Profound (IQ below 20)	• Specific causes usual • Little or no language and communication skills • Multiple complex physical problems • Require help with basic self-care

problem-solving. Sometimes, one specific function is impaired more than the rest, such as the use of language. The clinical features are described best by reference to the subgroups of mild, moderate, severe, and profound disability (Table 19.3).

Mild learning disability (IQ 50–70)

About 80 per cent of people with LD fall into this group. Their appearance is usually normal and any sensory or motor deficits are slight. Most develop more or less normal language abilities and social behaviour during the preschool years so that in the least severe cases, the LD may not be identified until the child starts school. In adult life, most can live independently, although some need help with housing and employment, and support when they are experiencing stress.

they can make their own decision whether to start or continue the pregnancy.

Clinical features

The clinical features of each specific diagnosis are obviously different, but some general points that may assist with management can be made. People with LD perform badly on all kinds of intellectual task including learning, short-term memory, the use of concepts, and

Moderate learning disability (IQ 35–49)

Individuals in this group account for about 12 per cent of those with LD. Most have enough language development to communicate, and most can learn to care for themselves, albeit with supervision. As adults, most continue to do this and are able to undertake simple routine work.

Severe learning disability (IQ 20–34)

About 7 per cent of the people with LD are in this group. In the preschool years their development is greatly slowed, and so is their learning when they go to school. With special training, many can eventually look after themselves under supervision and they can communicate, albeit in simple ways. As adults, most are able to undertake simple tasks and limited social activities. Many have associated physical disorders. A small number of these people have a single, highly developed cognitive ability of a kind normally associated with superior intelligence, such as the ability to carry out feats of mental arithmetic or memory. Such people were historically called **idiots savants**.

Profound learning disability (IQ below 20)

Less than 1 per cent of those with LD are in this group. Few learn to care for themselves completely. A few achieve some simple speech and social behaviour. Physical disorders are very frequent.

General problems in people with learning disability

From a medical perspective, the problems that patients with an LD (and/or their families) present with can be divided into four categories: emotional and behavioural problems, physical disorders, effects of the LD upon the family, and psychiatric disorders.

Emotional and behavioural problems

Behavioural disorders, at any given age, are more common in individuals with LDs than in the general population. As well as the direct effects of intellectual impairment, children with LD may show any of the common behavioural problems of childhood (see Chapter 32). These problems tend to occur at a later age than in a child of normal intelligence, and to last longer, although they usually improve slowly with time. A minority show severely disordered behaviour that threatens the well-being of the patient or the carers. Such behaviour is referred to as **challenging behaviour**. There are a variety of common behaviours which can be difficult to manage:

- Aggression and/or antisocial behaviour: this may be shouting and screaming, faecal smearing, and self-induced vomiting in youngsters. Aggressive outbursts towards people or property are common in adolescence, but dangerous physical violence is not. These behaviours usually reduce in early adulthood.

- Self-injury: biting, cutting, burning, and head banging. These are inversely proportionate to IQ in frequency. Overall, 40 per cent of children and 20 per cent of adults with LD self-injure.

- Stereotyped behaviours such as rocking, mannerisms, and flapping. The presence of these does not necessarily mean the child is autistic.

- Hyperactivity.

- Anxiety.

- Social withdrawal.

Behavioural problems are usually multifactorial in origin, combining genetics, characteristics inherent to the specific cause of the LD, and environmental factors (Table 19.4). It is important to recognize the cause of the problem if possible, for this may aid management.

Sexual problems. Some people with LD show a child-like curiosity about other people's bodies, which can be misunderstood as sexual. Many need sympathetic help in understanding sexual feelings at and after puberty. Concern is sometimes expressed that people with LD may give birth to children with LD. However, many of the causes of LD are not inherited, and most of those that are inherited are associated with infertility. A more important concern is that people with severe LD may struggle to be able to function well as parents. If termination of pregnancy or sterilization is considered,

Table 19.4 Causes of behavioural problems in learning disability

Causal factor	Description and examples
Stressful events	Distress is often displayed through behaviour rather than words; for example, in agitation, fearfulness, irritability, and dramatic behaviours
Over- or understimulation	An overstimulating environment may cause problems such as agitation or aggression, while an understimulating environment may lead to withdrawal, self-stimulation, or self-injury
Undiagnosed physical illness	Gastrointestinal disorders, epilepsy, otitis media, migraine, and pain are common examples
Psychiatric illness	For example, schizophrenia, depression, anxiety disorders
Brain damage	The underlying damage causing the LD may also cause behavioural problems
Epilepsy	The first sign of epilepsy may be the onset of challenging behaviour
Behavioural phenotypes	Some genetic causes of LD also cause a specific pattern of behaviour problems, e.g. individuals with: <ul><li>Prader–Willi syndrome have voracious appetite, pick and scratch their skin, and show outbursts of unprovoked rage</li><li>Lesch–Nyhan syndrome injure themselves seriously by biting their lips and fingers</li><li>Fragile X are shy, anxious, and avoidant</li></ul>
Frustration	With lack of communication, sensory deprivation, etc.
Iatrogenic	Medication side effects are commonplace

difficult ethical and legal problems can arise relating to consent, and specialist advice is necessary.

Physical disorders among people with learning disability

Physical disorders are most frequent among those with severe and profound LD, many of whom have motor disabilities (20–30 per cent) or epilepsy (40 per cent). Impaired hearing or vision may add an important additional obstacle to normal cognitive development, and is found in 10–20 per cent of those with an IQ less than 35. Motor disabilities, which are frequent, include spasticity, ataxia, and athetosis, and are often due to cerebral palsy. Only a third of such people are continent and ambulant, and a quarter are highly dependent on other people. The majority of genetic phenotypes (e.g. Down's syndrome, fragile X) produce physical and cognitive impairments. It is important to recognize these, but also to look for non-associated conditions in every individual.

Epilepsy is frequent in LD—found in 40 per cent of those with severe/profound LD and 10 per cent of those with mild LD—and may present at any age. It needs to be carefully distinguished from stereotypies or mannerisms (e.g. rolling eyes) and from episodes of complete social withdrawal. All forms of epilepsy may occur, and the seizure pattern may change over time. Increased frequency of seizures may indicate physical illness, stress, or non-epileptic seizures. Severe epilepsy can cause permanent loss of intellectual ability in anyone, and this is more frequent in those with LD to begin with. Epilepsy can usually be controlled effectively with antiepileptic drugs.

Effects of learning disability on the family

The effects of a child with LD upon their family should not be underestimated. Common challenges include the following:

- Making difficult prenatal decisions about an unborn child, especially when the diagnosis is unclear or prognosis variable.

- Distress around the time of diagnosis. This often includes a period of bereavement, depression, guilt, shame, or anger as parents have to abandon preconceived hopes and expectations for the child.

- Emotional and practical challenges of having a special needs child, especially if they have a physical disability as well. This may involve career changes and financial pressures.

- Depression is very common among parents, and siblings may be affected by family stress or reduced parental attention.

Psychiatric disorder in people with learning disability

Psychiatric disorders are more common in individuals with LD than in those within the normal range of intelligence and add an additional burden to the patient, their carers, and the community. All types of mental disorder may occur at any degree of LD, but at the severe level the most frequent are autism, hyperkinetic syndrome, stereotyped movements, pica, and self-mutilation. Those patients with epilepsy have a higher risk of serious psychiatric disorders. The assessment and management of all psychiatric diagnoses are generally as for any patient presenting with the corresponding symptoms.

Diagnosis

There are several reasons why psychiatric diagnosis is difficult in people with LD:

1 Patients may have *insufficient verbal ability* to describe abnormal experiences accurately (the level of ability corresponds to an IQ level of about 50).

2 Some people with LD are *suggestible* and may answer positively to a question about a symptom when they have not in fact experienced it.

3 *Some causes of LD also cause abnormal behaviour.* Behaviour problems due to psychiatric disorder may be wrongly ascribed to this other cause, or vice versa.

4 LD is *associated with autism*, and some of the symptoms of autism can be mistaken for those of another psychiatric disorder, for example, obsessive–compulsive disorder (OCD). Psychiatric disorder should be diagnosed only after deciding whether a pervasive developmental disorder is present (see p. 476).

5 *Physical illness* or *stressful events* can cause changes in behaviour, and both should be considered before the diagnosis of mental disorder is made.

It is always best to gather third-party information about symptoms and changes in the patient's behaviour. Normal diagnostic criteria can be used for those with LD; however, the reliability and validity of these criteria in LD are poorly characterized, especially for children. The criteria that include judgements based on whether or not a symptom is consistent with developmental level are particularly difficult.

Specific psychiatric disorders

Attention deficit hyperactivity disorder (ADHD). ADHD is seen in up to 20 per cent of children with LD. It should be diagnosed using the usual criteria and observation of the patient. Attention and concentration should be judged against those of a child of a comparable developmental, not chronological, age. Hyperactivity is typically the most prominent symptom, and usually responds well to stimulants.

Autistic spectrum disorders (ASD). ASD are more common in people with LD than in the rest of the population, with an estimated prevalence of 20–30 per cent. Looked at in another way, about two-thirds of children with ASD also have some degree of LD. There is a particular association with tuberous sclerosis, congenital rubella, severe epilepsy, and phenylketonuria. It can be quite difficult to tell between those children with LD who have stereotypies and a limited range of interest, and those with autism. Most children with LD will try to communicate, use gestures/facial expressions, and display emotions, whilst these are reduced or absent in ASD.

Mood disorder. When people with LD develop a **depressive disorder** they are less likely than people of normal intelligence to complain of low mood or to express depressive ideas. Look for observable features such as an appearance of sadness, reduction of appetite, disturbance of sleep, retardation, or agitation. Atypical features such as a regression to child-like behaviours, incontinence, and loss of social skills are more common. A severely depressed patient with adequate verbal abilities may describe depressive ideas, delusions, or hallucinations. Any change in behaviour in someone with a LD should lead to the exclusion of a mood disorder as the cause. Rarely, these patients may make attempts at suicide, although these are usually poorly planned. Classic bipolar disorder I is occasionally seen in LD, with rapid cycling being a prominent feature. Mania has to be diagnosed mainly on overactivity and behavioural signs indicating excitement and irritability.

Anxiety disorders. The most commonly reported anxiety disorders are simple phobia, social phobia, and generalized anxiety disorder (GAD). Behaviour problems, irritability, withdrawal, insomnia, and somatic complaints are the usual symptoms seen. In GAD, conversion and dissociative symptoms are more conspicuous than in the corresponding disorders of people of normal intelligence. Anxiety disorders may improve with stress reduction strategies, but tend to be hard to treat. SSRIs are frequently used, but there is less good evidence of their efficacy. Similarly, stress-related and adjustment disorders occur commonly among people with mild and moderate LD, especially when they are facing changes in the routine of their lives.

Psychosis. In individuals with mild LD, the classic symptoms of schizophrenia (or other psychoses) are present, and diagnosis is relatively simple. However, delusions are often less elaborate than they are among schizophrenics of normal intelligence, and hallucinations may have a simple and repetitive content. Delusions frequently contain ideas gathered from the person's immediate environment (e.g. television shows). 'First-rank' symptoms of schizophrenia are uncommon, and often the main features are a further impoverishment of a person's already limited thinking, and an increased disturbance of behaviour and social functioning. Catatonic symptoms are much more common. The negative symptoms of schizophrenia appear early, and are relatively treatment resistant. When the IQ is below 45, it is difficult to make a definite diagnosis of schizophrenia. Sometimes a trial of antipsychotics is sensible even if the diagnosis remains 'probable' rather than definite.

Delirium and dementia. As at the extremes of age, the threshold for delirium is lower in those with LD. Disturbed behaviour resulting from delirium may be the first indication of physical illness. Dementia causes a progressive global decline in intellectual and social functioning from the previous level. It presents at a younger age, and may progress more quickly in those with severe or profound LD. The typical symptoms are present, but may be difficult to identify. Nocturnal confusion ('sun downing'), forgetting a usual routine, and late-onset epilepsy are sensitive markers of dementia. All forms of dementia may occur, but Alzheimer's disease is especially common in Down's syndrome.

Personality disorder. There is debate as to whether or not personality disorders are a valid concept in those with moderate to profound LD. Epidemiological data suggest that personality disorders are common among people with mild LD and sometimes lead to greater problems in management than the learning problems. Because psychological development is delayed, the diagnosis is not generally made until the age of 20 years. There is no specific treatment, and management has to be directed at finding an environment as suitable as possible for the patient's temperament.

An approach to assessment and management

Assessment

Severe LD is usually diagnosed in infancy, as it is often associated with physical abnormalities or with delayed motor development. It is more difficult to diagnose less severe LD, which may present at any age. A distinction should be made between assessing the level and type of the intellectual impairment and related psychiatric or behavioural difficulties. The assessment aims to:

- to make a diagnosis of LD and consider its aetiology;
- to diagnose co-morbid physical and psychiatric disorders;
- to identify the specific needs of the patient and their family;
- to put together a coherent, long-term management plan.

A multidisciplinary team should be involved and usually includes the family GP, psychiatrist, developmental paediatrician, psychologist, social workers, community psychiatric nurse, occupational therapist, physiotherapist, speech and language therapist, audiologist, and play specialist.

History taking

The aim of the history is to understand why the patient is presenting at that specific time and to gather relevant information about symptoms and their context. The parents and other relevant adults (e.g. teachers, paediatrician) should be interviewed in every case; patients who have reasonable language ability should be interviewed as well. Particular points which should be covered (see also Box 17.4 in Chapter 17) include:

- presenting symptoms (e.g. aggressive behaviour, social withdrawal, failure to learn at school);
- previous medical and psychiatric history; current medications;
- the pregnancy, maternal infections/complications (e.g. pre-eclampsia); use of alcohol or drugs in pregnancy; labour and birth; neonatal complications, early feeding and weight gain;
- developmental history, including dates of passing key developmental milestones, review of growth charts;

- behaviour and physical disorders in the early years; head injuries;
- school/nursery attendance, attainment, and behaviour; for older patients, exam performance;
- family history; age of parents, consanguinity, family history of LD/congenital abnormalities/psychiatric disorders; current family structure and set-up.

Interviewing and suggestibility

When interviewing people with LD, the interviewer should remember that some are unusually suggestible. There are several reasons for this increased suggestibility including:

- a strong wish to please others, especially people in authority;
- reliance on cues from the interviewer when deciding what answer to give, rather than reliance on factual information;
- a tendency to reply 'yes' rather than 'no' to yes/no questions, regardless of the appropriateness of this response.

When interviewing patients, try to follow these pointers:

1 **Ask simple questions,** avoiding complexities of grammar.

2 **Allow adequate time** for the patient to respond, and do not appear impatient.

3 **Check answers to closed questions** (e.g. 'Do you feel sad?'), which may have to be used because the patient cannot volunteer information. A positive answer can be checked by asking the opposite (e.g. 'Do you feel happy?').

4 **Avoid leading questions and check responses.** Some people with LD repeat the interviewer's last words—e.g. interviewer: 'Do you feel sad?'; patient: 'Sad'.

5 **Check information received with an informant.**

In younger children or those with limited communication, interviewing is not possible. A behavioural assessment will therefore need to be based on the account from others and on observations of (1) the child's *ability to communicate*, (2) *sensorimotor skills*, (3) any *unusual behaviour*, and (4) ability to *self-care*. The child may need to be visited at home or school to build a full picture of the behavioural problems. In older patients, a mental state examination should be carried out in the usual way, making adaptations as necessary.

Developmental and psychological testing

This is a complex procedure, which is performed usually in a specialist unit. IQ testing is important, usually using the Wechsler Intelligence Scales. Developmental delay and adaptive skills can be measured using the Griffiths or Bailey Developmental Scales, and the Vineland Adaptive Behaviour Scales. These quantify the problems the patient has, and can be useful aids when planning appropriate interventions and applying for social benefits. Conners scales for ADHD can be used as for any child, if necessary.

Physical examination

The physical examination is best carried out by a paediatrician with knowledge of developmental and neurological disorders. It should include the recording of *head circumference, height*, and *weight*. Look carefully for dysmorphic features and congenital abnormalities. It may be helpful to examine close relatives to determine if any abnormalities are present in them too. A full neurological examination is essential, including speech and language, hearing, and vision assessments.

Investigations

In some cases, the clinical phenotype will clearly point to a cause for the LD (e.g. Down's syndrome) and little further investigation will be necessary. However, in cases of moderate to profound LD without obvious causation, a series of investigations should be carried out. Some examples of these include:

- blood tests for full blood count, urea and electrolytes, liver function, renal function, clotting, thyroid function, glucose, and lipids;

- infection screening or serology (blood, urine, occasionally cerebrospinal fluid (CSF)) for rubella, toxoplasmosis, HIV, cytomegalovirus, Epstein–Barr virus, herpes simplex virus, and syphilis;

- metabolic screening of blood for inborn errors of metabolism;

- genetics: karyotyping, single-gene disorder testing (e.g. fragile X DNA testing);

- imaging of dysmorphia or abnormalities seen on physical examination, e.g. X-rays, CT/MRI (especially cranial);

- ECG, echocardiography;

- electroencephalogram (EEG), visual evoked potentials, and muscle biopsy.

Overall assessment

At the end of the assessment, the clinician should have an idea of the cause of the LD and a clear view of the current behavioural, psychiatric, and social problems the patient has. These should be carefully documented, with specific individuals assigned to managing particular problems (e.g. ADHD—psychiatrist; schooling—social worker and educational psychologist).

Management approaches

The management of a patient with LD should be as for any other complex patient, with special attention to the psychological and social needs of the family (Box 19.3).

Box 19.3 Goals of service provision for a person with learning disability

- 'Normalize' the person's life
- Recognize individual needs
- Develop abilities
- Offer choice and involve the patient in management decisions
- Provide the best possible care for physical and psychiatric problems
- Support the family or carers

Few people with mild LD need specialist services. Most live with their families, cared for when necessary by the family doctor. When specialist treatment is needed, it is usually for an associated physical disability or illness, emotional disorder, or psychiatric illness. When placement away from home is needed, it is usually because of complex physical or behavioural needs. In these cases, group homes or boarding school placement for children or residential care for adults is arranged. Adults with mild LD may need extra support when they are facing problems with housing and employment or with the problems of growing old (Box 19.4).

As people with LD live longer, provision is needed increasingly for the later years of their lives. At this stage, parents may not be around to provide care and physical illness or dementia may add to the person's disability. It is important to recognize these problems when planning services (see Case study box 19.1).

Box 19.4 Components of a service for people with learning disability

Social and psychological

- Support for family at home; respite admissions
- Education, training, and occupation
- Social activities
- Accommodation
- Help with financial and other problems

Medical

- Treatment of physical disorders
- Management of challenging behaviour
- Behavioural therapy
- CBT

Treatment of psychiatric disorders

- Psychological treatments
- Pharmacological treatments

CASE STUDY BOX 19.1

The value of collateral information in learning disability

Philip, a 43-year-old forklift truck driver, presented to the emergency room with abdominal pain. He was unable to give much history, just saying that he was ill. On examination, he was distended, diffusely tender, had tinkling bowel sounds, and had had a right orchidectomy. Philip seemed surprised to hear he was missing a testicle, and couldn't remember why it had been removed. He was admitted under the suspicion of bowel obstruction. During the night, Philip kept running about and was aggressive towards staff. A doctor was called, who gave him intramuscular sedation. In the morning, the surgeons called the on-call psychiatrist for help with his management. A psychiatrist came, who immediately called Philip's mother and his GP. This revealed that Philip had moderate LD, and had had testicular cancer for which he had received a radical right orchidectomy and radiotherapy 25 years earlier. He also tended to become anxious at night without his mother, and usually took stimulants (for hyperactivity) and low-dose zopiclone to help him sleep. That night, Philip's mother was invited to stay in hospital with him, and his usual medications were given. There were no behavioural problems. Philip underwent a laparoscopy, revealing small bowel obstruction secondary to adhesions, probably related to radiotherapy. He did well postoperatively, and was discharged on day 3. His community psychiatric nurse was contacted, and she arranged for the district nurses to help his mother with dressing the wounds, and also visited more regularly for the next 3 weeks.

Learning points

- Always gather as much collateral history and information as possible; this may not be possible from the patient.

- Remember, changes in routine can upset those with LD, who may show distress as challenging behaviour.

- Consider carefully if the patient has capacity, and, if not, how to make a medical decision ethically.

Social interventions

Help for families. Parents need help as soon as the diagnosis of LD is made. It is seldom enough to explain the problem once; most parents need to hear the information several times before they can recognize its implications. Adequate time is needed to explain the prognosis, indicate what help can be provided, and discuss the part the parents can play in helping their child achieve their full potential. As explained previously, parents need continuing psychological support and help with practical matters. These provisions are needed in particular at times of change for the patient, especially leaving school, and at times when there are additional problems in the family such as the illness of another child. The rise of self-help and support groups for parents has been useful, and volunteers can play a valuable part in the arrangements. The Internet is now providing a huge support base for parents with children suffering from rare conditions.

Education. Education and training should begin early. Extra education and training from preschool age helps children with LD to realize their potential. When the normal school age is reached, the least disabled children can be educated in a mainstream school with extra help. More disabled children benefit more from attendance at a school for children with LDs. For intermediate levels of disability, a choice has to be made between education in an ordinary school or a special school. The former offers the advantages of more normal social surroundings and greater expectations of progress; it has the disadvantages of lack of special teaching skills and the risk that the child may not be accepted by more able children. Since learning is slow, education may need to extend into adult life.

The period after leaving school is difficult for people with LD and they need a lot of help from those around them. It is important to review the prospects for employment, suitability for further training, and requirements for day care. At this stage of life, it may be difficult for the parents to look after a young person with severe LD and residential care may be required. Wherever the person is living, there is a need for sheltered work or other occupation after leaving school.

Training and work. Most people with mild LD are capable of work and benefit from appropriate training. Most school-leavers with moderately severe LD need sheltered work or further training when they leave school. Most need these special provisions throughout their lives, although some do progress to normal employment.

Accommodation. Most people with LD live with their families. For the rest, a variety of accommodation is required ranging from ordinary housing to 24-hour nursing-type homes. A useful intermediate level of supervision is provided in a 'core and cluster' system in which several group homes are sited near to a central staffed unit. When parents grow old and can no longer care for their disabled son or daughter, special accommodation is required. In most places, the supply of such accommodation has not kept pace with the increasing life expectancy of people with LD.

Help with financial and other practical problems. People with LD may need help in managing their money, dealing with forms, regulations, and other problems of daily life. In most developed countries there are various social benefits available for people with special needs; patients and their families may need help and advice in order to access these. Special equipment for the home is also available and occupational and physiotherapists can be very helpful in arranging this.

Medical and psychological interventions

General medical services. People with LD sometimes receive substandard medical care because doctors do not detect their needs or do not provide the extra support needed to enable these patients to cooperate with treatment. It is good practice to keep a register of these patients and arrange regular health checks. Basic physical problems (e.g. toothache, hay fever) are a great source of behavioural disturbance, and should be actively sought and aggressively managed.

Treatment of challenging behaviour. The most important step in treating challenging behaviour is to identify the cause; if possible, this is then removed/treated. If the behaviour persists, behavioural treatment may be tried, directed to changing any factors that appear to be reinforcing the behaviour.

- **Behavioural therapy.** Behavioural techniques are very helpful in teaching basic self-care skills and establishing normal patterns of behaviour. Eating, sleep, and disobedience problems respond well to simple parenting skills such as ignoring poor and rewarding good behaviour. Phobias and anxiety disorders can be treated in the standard way. It can be used in people without verbal skills, which is a benefit over most other treatments.

- **Cognitive behavioural therapy.** CBT can be successfully used in people with mild to moderate LD. Anger management, aggression, interpersonal skills, low self-esteem, and problem-solving skills can all be treated with CBT in LD. There has been particular success in the treatment of sex offenders. It has been found that CBT for LD actually works best when delivered in a group format.

Family members and carers may also benefit from counselling, or a CBT course for mood disorders.

Treatment of psychiatric disorder. Treatment of mental disorder among people with LD is similar to that of the same disorder in a patient of normal intelligence. There is typically a lower threshold for admission to hospital, which is usually related to the family/carer's ability to cope at home, rather than the patient being a risk to themselves or society.

Psychopharmacological treatments are widely used in LD, partly because the patients frequently have physical disorders (e.g. epilepsy) which are independent indications for them. While medications do have a role to play in relieving specific symptoms and behaviours, they should not be used without a good indication. Because patients are less likely to report the side effects of drugs, particular care is needed in adjusting dosage. They are also more prone to atypical or idiosyncratic reactions.

- **Antipsychotics.** Antipsychotic drugs are used for psychosis, challenging behaviour (especially in autism, self-injury, and social withdrawal), tic disorders, and in severe mood disorders. Patients with LD are more prone to the metabolic side effects of atypical antipsychotics (weight gain, metabolic syndrome) and should be carefully monitored. There is good randomized controlled evidence for the use of risperidone in challenging behaviour, especially in the context of autism (see Science box 19.1).

- **Antidepressants.** SSRIs are helpful for depression, OCD, anxiety disorders, and self-injury. Lithium is also licensed for use in self-injury and aggression.

- **Mood stabilizers** are used in the treatment of bipolar disorder and severe depression, and are a particularly good choice in patients with co-morbid epilepsy.

- **Stimulants** are now widely used to tackle hyperactivity and ADHD, and there is some evidence that they can improve behaviour more globally (improving eating, sleep, and mood).

- **Opiate antagonists.** There is a hypothesis that opioid excess may underlie autism and self-injury, and naltrexone has been used to treat both these conditions. There is little evidence that it improves symptoms in autism, but it does reduce the frequency and severity of self-injury.

Ethical problems in the care of people with learning disability

Most of the ethical problems encountered in the care of people with LD are similar in type to those in the care of other patients. Two problems will be mentioned further.

Normalization, autonomy, and conflicts of interest

If people with LD are to live as normally as possible, they require support. Often this support comes from their family and arrangements that were entered into willingly at one time may become unduly burdensome if the needs of the disabled person increase, other children have additional needs, or the carers grow older. The problem can usually be resolved by discussion between all the various people involved. Comparable conflicts of interest may arise also when deciding whether a disabled child should be educated in an ordinary school or a special school for disabled children.

SCIENCE BOX 19.1

What is the evidence for the use of antipsychotic drugs in the treatment of challenging behaviour in patients with learning disability?

Challenging behaviour is exhibited by 5–20 per cent of individuals with a LD, dependent upon the severity of LD and setting in which studies are conducted. It is difficult for patients, carers, and clinicians to manage and behavioural strategies may not be entirely effective. So, is there any evidence to support antipsychotic usage in this patient group?

One of the first studies to describe the use of antipsychotics in the LD population was published by Bair and Herold in 1955.[1] They concluded that chlorpromazine (in high dosage) was an effective method of treatment: this led to an upsurge in antipsychotic prescriptions.

A recent, UK-based cohort study found the prevalence of antipsychotic prescribing in 33,016 adults registered as having a LD as 49 per cent.[2] Only 21 per cent of these individuals were recorded as having a mental illness, with an additional 25 per cent coded for challenging behaviour. This suggests that modern prescribing is still favouring the use of antipsychotics for this indication.

Large systematic reviews are now possible in this area—for example, McQuire et al. combined 14 RCTs (*N*=912) examining risperidone vs placebo in children with LD and challenging behaviour.[3] They reported a small, statistically significant reduction in challenging behaviour in the short term, but considerable levels of hyperprolactinaemia and weight gain. Other systematic reviews, including those in adults, have found similar weakly positive results, although the evidence is more robust for those with co-morbid aggression and mental illness. The best evidence is for use of risperidone.

There is now UK national guidance in this area, covering all age groups, which recommends the use of antipsychotics **if** other methods of behaviour modification have failed **and** it is combined with psychological input.[4] Efficacy should be monitored with the Aberrant Behaviour Checklist (or similar scale) and frequent reviews undertaken.

Given the current evidence, the NICE[4] recommendation seems a reasonable strategy, but clinicians should ensure they treat any underlying mental or physical health issues first, then balance the risks and benefits for the patient before giving a trial of antipsychotic.

1 Bair HV, Herold W. Efficacy of chlorpromazine in hyperactive mentally retarded children. *Archives of Neurology and Psychiatry* 1955;74:363–364.

2 Sheehan R, Hassiotis A, Walters K, et al. Mental illness, challenging behaviour, and psychotropic drug prescribing in people with intellectual disability: UK population based cohort study. *BMJ* 2015;351:h4326.

3 McQuire C, Hassiotis A, Harrison B, Pilling S. Pharmacological interventions for challenging behaviour in children with intellectual disabilities: a systematic review and meta-analysis. *BMC Psychiatry* 2015;15:303.

4 National Institute for Health and Care Excellence. Challenging behaviour and learning disabilities: prevention and interventions for people with learning disabilities whose behaviour challenges. Published May 2015. https://www.nice.org.uk/guidance/ng11.

Consent to treatment and research

Most learning disabled people can give informed consent provided that explanations are in clear and simple language, and adequate time is set aside for discussion. In the UK, when an adult with (usually severe) LD cannot give informed consent, no one can consent for them and the doctor has to decide what is in that person's best interests. The new Mental Capacity Act (see Box 18.2, p. 209) has made the process of making these decisions clearer. It is sensible for a parent/carer to apply for power of attorney in these cases.

Specific clinical syndromes

While the majority of people with mild LD do not have a unifying diagnosis for their problems, one can be identified in the majority of those with moderate to profound LD. In many cases, the diagnosis is of a 'clinical syndrome': **a syndrome is a characteristic pattern** of clinical features, including both signs and symptoms. It may include physical, genetic, cognitive, and emotional features. A syndrome may not necessarily have only one aetiological basis. While some diagnoses will inevitably produce certain characteristics (e.g. LD in Angelman's syndrome), others are more variable in their phenotype (e.g. cardiac abnormalities in Down's syndrome). In these latter cases, the syndrome is said to be associated with the abnormality, or it is said that the patients will have vulnerability towards it. One of the advantages of recognizing a syndrome is that it allows clinicians to look for associated anomalies and treat them early; it also helps parents to plan for the future and families to access specialist support and services.

There are a large number of clinical syndromes that include or are associated with LD, but by far the most common are Down's, fragile X, and Klinefelter syndromes. These three examples will be explored in some detail, and Table 19.5 outlines the features of some rare conditions.

Down's syndrome

Down's syndrome was described by John Langdon Down in 1887, but it was not until 1959 that it was discovered to be (in the majority of cases) caused by the chromosomal abnormality trisomy 21. Down's syndrome is the most common autosomal trisomy, and the most prevalent cause of moderate to profound LD. The natural prevalence of Down's syndrome is 1 in 600 live births, but this has been significantly reduced by prenatal screening, and in the UK is now 1 in 1000 live births. The rate of Down's syndrome increases with increasing maternal age, such that the risk is 1 in 37 births once the mother is aged 44.

There are three different ways in which trisomy 21 may come about:

1 **Non-disjunction (94 per cent of cases).** One pair of chromosome 21 fail to separate at meiosis, such that one gamete has two chromosome 21s, rising to three after fertilization.

2 **Translocation (5 per cent).** An extra chromosome 21 is joined on to another chromosome (usually

14, 15, or 22), so that while the child has 46 chromosomes, there are three copies of the chromosome 21 material.

3 **Mosaicism (1 per cent).** This is due to non-disjunction at mitosis. Some of the cells in the body have three chromosome 21s and others have two. The clinical phenotype is often less severe.

Clinical features

The characteristic clinical features are shown in Box 19.5. The syndrome can usually be accurately diagnosed soon after birth, but nowadays most parents have had prenatal testing, and know in advance that their child has trisomy 21. For further information about the physical abnormalities typical of Down's syndrome, see the 'Further reading' section on p. 243.

Learning disability. In Down's syndrome, the degree of LD varies considerably from person to person; usually the IQ is between 20 and 50, but in 15 per cent it is greater than 50. Many people are able to self-care (with prompting) by adolescence, and the majority to live with their families.

Temperament. The temperament of children with Down's syndrome is usually affectionate and easy-going, and many show an interest in music. Most have some obsessional characteristics and behaviours, and may be very stubborn about their daily routine, but these are usually subclinical problems.

Behaviour problems are less frequent than in most other forms of LD; nevertheless, about a quarter of children with Down's syndrome are chaotic and difficult to engage. They relish attention and do very well with behavioural therapy approaches.

Ageing. In the past, many people with Down's syndrome died in infancy, but with improved medical care about half now live beyond the age of 50. Signs of ageing appear prematurely and **Alzheimer-like neuropathological changes** are found in the brain of most of those dying at the age of 40 years or more. However, for unknown reasons, survivors do not show signs of dementia until later, with a mean age of onset of about 50 years.

Table 19.5 Notes on some causes of learning disability

Syndrome	Aetiology	Clinical features	Comments
Chromosome abnormalities			
Down's, fragile X, and Klinefelter syndromes are described in the text			
Triple X	Trisomy X	Tall and thin Mild LD	1 in 1000 female births
Cri du chat	Deletion in chromosome 5	Microcephaly, hypertelorism, typical cat-like cry, failure to thrive Hyperactivity Language problems	1 in 35,000 births
Angelman's syndrome	Deletion of 15q11–q13 from maternal chromosome	Excessive laughter Epilepsy and ataxia Blond hair, blue eyes Severe to profound LD Fewer than 6 words by adulthood	Genomic imprinting condition
Prader–Willi syndrome	Deletion of 15q11–q13 from paternal chromosome	Hypotonia Short stature Hypogenitalism Overeating DSH Mild to moderate LD	Genomic imprinting condition; complement of Angelman's syndrome
Inborn errors of metabolism			
Phenylketonuria	Autosomal recessive causing lack of liver phenylalanine hydroxylase Commonest inborn error of metabolism (1 in 10,000)	Lack of pigment (fair hair, blue eyes) Retarded growth Epilepsy, microcephaly, eczema, hyperactivity, autism, and self-injury Untreated leads to severe LD	Detectable by postnatal screening of blood or urine Treated by exclusion of phenylalanine from the diet during early years of life
Homocystinuria	Autosomal recessive causing lack of cystathionine synthetase	Ectopia lentis, fine fair hair, joint enlargement, skeletal abnormalities similar to Marfan's syndrome Associated with thromboembolic episodes Variable severity of LD	Sometimes treatable by methionine restriction

Table 19.5 Continued

Syndrome	Aetiology	Clinical features	Comments
Galactosaemia	Autosomal recessive causing lack of galactose-1-phosphate uridyltransferase	Presents after the introduction of milk into the diet Failure to thrive, hepatosplenomegaly, cataracts	Detectable by postnatal screening for the enzymic defect Treatable by galactose-free diet Toluidine blue test on urine
Tay–Sachs disease	Autosomal recessive resulting in increased lipid storage (the earliest form of cerebromacular degeneration)	Progressive loss of vision and hearing Spastic paralysis Cherry red spot at macula of retina Epilepsy	Death at 2–4 years
Hurler's syndrome (gargoylism)	Autosomal recessive affecting mucopolysaccharide storage	Grotesque features Protuberant abdomen Hepatosplenomegaly. Associated cardiac abnormalities Severe LD	Death before adolescence
Lesch–Nyhan syndrome	X-linked recessive leading to enzyme defect affecting purine metabolism Excessive uric acid production and excretion	Normal at birth Development of choreoathetoid movements, scissoring position of legs, and self-mutilation (finger and lip biting) IQ 40–80 Death in second or third decade from renal failure	Can be diagnosed prenatally by culture of amniotic fluid and estimation of relevant enzyme Postnatal diagnosis by enzyme estimation in a single hair root Self-mutilation may be reduced by treatment with hydroxytryptophan
Other inherited disorders			
Neurofibromatosis (von Recklinghausen's syndrome)	Autosomal dominant inheritance, mutation in neurofibromin gene	Neurofibromata, café au lait spots, vitiligo Associated with symptoms determined by the site of neurofibromata Astrocytomas, meningioma LD in a minority Speech defects	1 in 3000 births High spontaneous mutation rate, 50% have no family history
Tuberous sclerosis (epiloia)	Autosomal dominant (very variable penetrance)	Epilepsy, adenoma sebaceum on face, white skin patches, shagreen skin, retinal phakoma, periungual fibromata	1 in 7000 in UK

(continued)

Table 19.5 Continued

Syndrome	Aetiology	Clinical features	Comments
	Up to 80% arise from spontaneous mutations	Associated multiple tumours in kidney, spleen, and lungs LD in about 70% High rates of autism, OCD, ADHD, and self-injury	
Lawrence–Moon–Biedl syndrome	Autosomal recessive	Retinitis pigmentosa, polydactyly, obesity, infertility, diabetes Mild to moderate LD	Common in Kuwait and Canada
De Lange syndrome	Mutation in *NIPBL* gene on chromosome 5	Growth retardation Distinct facial features Feeding problems Self-injury Autism Severe to profound LD	1 in 60,000 births
Rett's syndrome	Mutation of *MECP* gene on X chromosome, affects females only	Normal to 1 year, then loss of motor skills Scoliosis, spasticity, leg deformities Epilepsy Sleep disturbance Profound LD	Few girls survive beyond mid adolescence
Infection			
Rubella	Viral infection of mother in first trimester	Cataract, microphthalmia, deafness, microcephaly, congenital heart disease	If mother infected in first trimester, 10–15% of infants are affected (infection may be subclinical)
Toxoplasmosis	Protozoal infection of mother	Hydrocephaly, microcephaly, intracerebral calcification, retinal damage, hepatosplenomegaly, jaundice, epilepsy	Wide variation in severity
Cytomegalovirus	Virus infection of mother	Brain damage Only severe cases are apparent at birth	
Congenital syphilis	Syphilitic infection of mother	Many die at birth Variable neurological signs 'Stigmata' (Hutchinson teeth and rhagades often absent)	Uncommon since routine testing of pregnant women

Table 19.5 Continued

Syndrome	Aetiology	Clinical features	Comments
Cranial malformations			
Hydrocephalus	Sex-linked recessive Inherited developmental abnormality (e.g. atresia of aqueduct, Arnold–Chiari malformation, meningitis, spina bifida)	Rapid enlargement of head in early infancy, symptoms of raised CSF pressure Other features depend on aetiology	Mild cases may arrest spontaneously May be symptomatically treated by CSF shunt Intelligence can be normal
Microcephaly	Recessive inheritance, irradiation in pregnancy, maternal infections	Features depend on aetiology	Evident in up to 20% of institutionalized patients with LD
Miscellaneous			
Spina bifida	Aetiology multiple and complex	Failure of vertebral fusion Spina bifida cystica is associated with meningocele or, in 15–20%, myelomeningocele Latter causes spinal cord damage, with lower limb paralysis, incontinence, etc.	Hydrocephalus in 80% of those with myelomeningocele LD frequent in this group
Cerebral palsy	Perinatal brain damage Strong association with prematurity	Spastic (commonest), athetoid, and ataxic types Variable in severity	Majority are below average intelligence Athetoid are more likely to be of normal IQ
Congenital hypothyroidism	Iodine deficiency or (rarely) atrophic thyroid	Appearance normal at birth. Abnormalities appear at 6 months Growth failure, puffy skin, large tongue, lethargy, constipation Moderate LD	Now rare in the UK Responds to early replacement treatment
Hyperbilirubinaemia	Haemolysis, rhesus incompatibility, and prematurity	Kernicterus Choreoathetosis, opisthotonus, spasticity, convulsions	Prevention by antirhesus globulin Neonatal treatment by exchange transfusion
Fetal alcohol syndrome	Exposure to alcohol during development	Mild to moderate LD Hyperactivity Facial dysmorphia Stunted growth Skeletal, heart, and urological abnormalities	0.3 per 1000 live births

Box 19.5 Abnormalities found in Down's syndrome

External abnormalities at birth

- Flat occiput
- Oblique palpebral fissures
- Epicanthic folds
- Small mouth, high-arched palate
- Macroglossia
- Short, broad hands
- Single transverse palmar crease
- Curved fifth finger
- Hypotonia and extensive joints
- Brushfield spots in the iris
- Congenital heart disease (40 per cent)
- Deafness (and recurrent otitis media)
- Duodenal atresia or Hirschsprung's disease

Later physical problems

- Delayed motor milestones
- Short stature and obesity
- Immunocompromise—high risk of bronchopneumonia
- Visual problems
- Leukaemia
- Atlantoaxial instability
- Hypothyroidism (25 per cent)
- Epilepsy

Behavioural and psychiatric characteristics

- Moderate to severe LD
- Speech and language delay
- Early-onset Alzheimer's disease
- Obsessional and stubborn behaviours

Co-morbidities. The most common psychiatric co-morbidities are ADHD, depression, OCD, and schizophrenia.

Fragile X syndrome

The condition is so called because a break is seen in an X chromosome of a proportion of cells when cultured in a medium deficient in folate. Fragile X is a trinucleotide repeat expansion mutation, similar in mechanism to those seen in Huntington's or Friedrich's ataxia.

The basis of the abnormality is a region of CGG repeats in the gene *FMR1*. The repeats accumulate with successive copying, and affect the function of the gene when their number exceeds 200. Men and women with 50–200 repeats are carriers, though men are unlikely to pass on the condition as *FMR*, which is found active mainly in the brain and testis, probably modifies the activity of other genes. Testing can identify heterozygous females who are clinically normal, and males who are carriers. As the condition is inherited as an X-linked recessive disorder, all mothers of affected males are carriers, but there are some affected women, and unaffected males can pass the condition on to their grandsons via a daughter.

The disorder occurs in about 1 in 4000 males and in a milder form in 1 in 8000 females. The condition is the second most frequent cause of LD (Down's syndrome is the first), accounting for about 7 per cent of moderate and about 4 per cent of mild LD among males, and about 3 per cent of moderate and mild LD among females.

Clinical features

Affected children have *characteristic features*, none of which is diagnostic, and the clinical picture varies greatly from one affected person to another.

Physical characteristics

The most specific physical feature is that 95 per cent of postpubertal men have large testes (macroorchidism). Other typical features include a high forehead, prominent supraorbital ridges, and large everted ears. Connective tissues are often abnormal, leading to mitral valve prolapse (and other cardiac anomalies), hyperflexibility, cataracts, flat feet, and ear infections. Approximately 30 per cent of affected men have epilepsy. Since the absence of these physical characteristics does not exclude the diagnosis, it is appropriate to test for the disorder in all unexplained cases of LD.

Behavioural and psychiatric characteristics

People with fragile X almost inevitably have LD, with an IQ varying from 20 to 80. They have increased rates of abnormalities of speech and language, with speech that is rapid and disorganized with frequent repetition of words and phrases (a disorder known as **cluttering**). There are behaviours similar to those seen in autism: hand flapping, gaze avoidance, repetitive movements, and social anxiety. However, they can usually self-care and are more socially responsive than autistic children. Poor attention and concentration, and hyperactivity are almost universal.

Klinefelter syndrome (47, XXY)

Klinefelter syndrome is a trisomy of the sex chromosomes, resulting in the karyotype 47, XXY. Prevalence at birth is 1–2 per 1000 live males, although this is being reduced by prenatal diagnosis. The majority of males with Klinefelter syndrome do not present until young adulthood, when they are found to be infertile. The most common clinical features are:

- small testes (>95 per cent);
- increased height (typically >75th centile);
- gynaecomastia (60 per cent);
- decreased facial and pubic hair;
- increased gonadotrophin levels and reduced testosterone levels;
- LDs (70–80 per cent);

While LDs are very common in Klinefelter syndrome, the severity is variable, with 95 per cent of individuals having an IQ in the range 50–110. Delays in language development and verbal cognitive function are extremely common: the majority need speech and language therapy at school and underperform in literacy based tasks. Psychiatric co-morbidity is frequently seen in adults. There is a four- to fivefold increase in the risk of schizophrenia in Klinefelter syndrome, plus increased rates of schizotypal and schizoid traits, mood disorders, and ADHD. Testosterone therapy is effective at producing development of sexual characteristics and reducing physical risks, but there is no evidence at present to suggest it helps with neuropsychological complications.

Further reading

Gelder MG, Andreasen NC, López-Ibor JJ, Geddes JR, eds. Section 10: Intellectual disability (mental retardation). In: *New Oxford Textbook of Psychiatry*. 2nd ed. Oxford: Oxford University Press; 2012:1819–1887. [Chapter 10.4 has a useful guide to rarer syndromes causing LD.]

Hagerman RJ, Polussa J. Treatment of the psychiatric problems associated with fragile X syndrome. *Current Opinion in Psychiatry* 2015;28:107–112.

Jensen KM, Bulova PD. Managing the care of adults with Down's syndrome. *BMJ* 2014;349.

Lissauer T, Carroll W. Normal child development, hearing and vision. In: *Illustrated Textbook of Paediatrics*. 5th ed. London: Mosby Elsevier; 2017:27–43. [A useful paediatrics text.]

Royal College of Psychiatry. *DC-LD: Diagnostic Criteria for Psychiatric Disorders for Use with Adults with Learning Disabilities/Mental Retardation*. 1st ed. London: RCPsych Publications; 2001. [This is likely to be updated to coincide with the publication of ICD-11.]

20 People presenting with physical disorder

All healthcare professionals dealing primarily with physical disorder need a working knowledge of relevant psychological factors and psychiatric disorders. Despite the geographical and, often, cultural separation of most 'general' (i.e. physical) and psychiatric hospitals, there are close links (1) between physical and psychological disorders, and (2) between physical and psychological factors in the aetiology, presentation, and management of all illness. This chapter aims to stimulate you to think about these issues in primary care and in the general hospital, and to equip you with the knowledge required to think about them in an integrated, biopsychosocial way.

The links between physical and psychological factors are multiple. They include:

- *psychiatric and physical disorders occurring together by chance*—as they are both common;
- *psychiatric disorders causing physical symptoms*— for example, depression is associated with low physical energy (anergia), amenorrhoea, and constipation;

- *psychiatric disorder adversely affecting the outcome of physical disorder*—for example, a depressive disorder might impair self-management of diabetes mellitus, because low motivation is a common symptom of depression, and may reduce adherence to self-monitoring of glucose;

- *psychological factors increasing disability associated with physical disorder*—for example, if a patient recovering from a myocardial infarction believes that it has led to a permanent reduction in their cardiac function, they are less likely to return to work, to take regular exercise, and to have a normal sex life;

- *untreated psychological problems leading to the inappropriate use of medical resources and to poor compliance with medical advice*—for example, people with panic disorder are more likely to attend emergency departments with acute 'cardiac' symptoms;

- *physical symptoms and disorders having psychological consequences, which include psychiatric disorder*—for example, hypothyroidism and cerebrovascular disease may lead to depression;

- *physical disorder exacerbating unrelated psychiatric symptoms*—for example, a viral infection could delay recovery from a depressive disorder, by impairing the person's usual activities, at work and at home, which would otherwise provide therapeutic distraction and stimulation.

Epidemiology

In the *general population*, psychiatric disorder is two to three times more likely when physical ill health is present (Fig. 20.1). Also, disabling functional somatic (bodily) symptoms are frequent (see Chapter 25). In *primary care*, psychological issues are important in the management of many patients with serious acute or chronic physical illness. Functional somatic symptoms are among the commonest reasons for seeking treatment and are often related to psychiatric disorder. In *secondary care,* psychological problems are especially frequent in emergency departments, in gynaecological and medical outpatient clinics, and in specialist inpatient units such as stroke units. In general hospital outpatient clinics, about 15 per cent of patients with a definite medical diagnosis have an associated psychiatric disorder, and about 40 per cent of those with no medical diagnosis have a psychiatric disorder. About 25 per cent of patients in medical wards have a psychiatric disorder of some kind.

Psychological factors as causes of physical disorders

Psychological factors contribute to the aetiology, presentation, and outcome of physical illness. They may, for example:

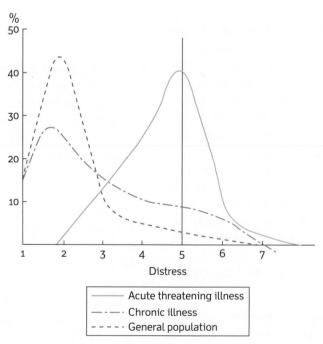

Fig. 20.1 The distribution of emotional distress in the general population and in those with physical illness. Level 5 and over indicates a diagnostic psychiatric disorder.

- lead to *unhealthy habits*—such as overeating, smoking, and excessive use of alcohol, which are risk factors for physical disease;

- result in *hormonal, immunological*, or *neuro-physiological changes*, which contribute to the onset or affect the course of the physico-pathological process. This may explain the increased mortality seen among patients depressed after myocardial infarction;

- affect *symptom perception*—such as people experiencing more physical pain when they are depressed;

- affect *medical help-seeking*—for example, a person who would not seek help for backache when in a normal mood may do so when depressed, or vice versa;

- affect *treatment adherence*—for example, a patient with diabetes, in which depression is common, may become depressed and neglect self-care of his/her diabetes.

Psychological complications of physical disorders

Most people are remarkably resilient when ill and are able to carry on without undue distress. However, **acute illness**, unless mild and brief, often leads to anxiety, which may be followed by depression. In a quarter of patients, these reactions reach the diagnostic threshold for disorder—whether anxiety, depressive, or adjustment. Other possible reactions include anger and the denial (complete or partial) of a life-threatening diagnosis, leading to poor collaboration with treatment. In **chronic illness**, anxiety and depressive disorders are twice as common as in the general population, and psychological and social variables are strongly predictive of important outcomes such as return to work.

Although adjustment disorder, anxiety, and depression are the commonest psychiatric complications of physical illness, other psychiatric disorders may also be precipitated by physical illness (Table 20.1).

Table 20.1 Common psychiatric disorders in the physically ill

More common

- Adjustment disorder
- Depressive disorder
- Anxiety disorder
- Delirium

Less common

- Somatoform disorders
- Dementia
- Post-traumatic stress disorder
- Mania
- Schizophrenia and delusional disorder

Physical disorders cause psychological complications via several important mechanisms:

- *Acute global impairment of cognitive functioning* (delirium), which is frequent in those who are severely ill, is often not diagnosed, and is caused by one or more *generalized* impairing mechanisms such as hypoxia, cardiac failure, urinary infection, electrolyte abnormalities, or constipation (see Chapter 26).

- *Direct effects of physical disorder, via specific pathophysiological mechanisms*—for example, depression caused by hypothyroidism or cerebrovascular disease; anxiety caused by hyperthyroidism or hypoglycaemia.

- *Indirect effects of physical illness*, causing disability and handicap, leading to anxiety, depression, and other symptoms such as irritability.

- Finally, some *medicines* used in the management of physical disorders have psychiatric side effects, and it is important to be aware of the possibility of iatrogenic psychiatric disorder (Table 20.2).

Determinants of the psychological consequences of physical illness

Some illnesses and treatments are particularly threatening. However, psychological reactions depend

Table 20.2 Some medications reported to cause depression

- Antihypertensives, e.g. beta-blockers, calcium channel blockers, reserpine
- Gastrointestinal drugs, including cimetidine, ranitidine
- Interferon
- NSAIDs
- Corticosteroids, e.g. dexamethasone, prednisolone (although mood elevation is much more common)
- Combined oral contraceptive pill
- Roaccutane® (isotretinoin)
- l-Dopa

as much upon a patient's *perception* of the illness as on its objective nature (Table 20.3). If patients see their illness as particularly unpleasant or if their ability to cope with stress is poor, then severe distress is more likely. The reactions of others may also affect patients' perceptions and their ability to cope.

Patients at high risk are especially likely to be encountered in emergency departments and in specialized units such as those responsible for terminal care, cancer, severe neurological problems, and pain.

Table 20.3 Factors associated with a higher risk of psychiatric problems

Physical factors

- Severe illness—unpleasant, threatening, relapsing, progressive, or terminal
- Unpleasant treatment—e.g. major surgery, chemo- or radiotherapy
- Uncertain outcome of treatment
- Very demanding self-care
- High or progressive disability
- Conspicuousness to others—e.g. deforming

Psychological factors

- Previous psychiatric disorder
- Dysfunctional beliefs about the illness, its impact, and its treatment

Social factors

- Poor social support, social isolation
- Adverse reactions of family, friends, or employer
- Other adverse social circumstances

Psychiatric assessment of a physically ill patient

Among severely ill patients, distress is often seen as understandable and inevitable and no help is offered. This is incorrect: most people cope remarkably well with even the most severe medical problems, and, by implication, marked distress is abnormal and requires assessment and treatment.

The psychiatric assessment of a physically ill patient is similar to that of a patient presenting solely with psychiatric symptoms, except that it requires knowledge of the nature and prognosis of the physical illness. Box 20.1 lists some screening questions. It is best if these questions do not come out of the

Box 20.1 Recognition of emotional disorder in the physically ill

Psychiatric symptoms

- How have you been feeling in yourself?
- How worried have you been about your health?
- How have you been sleeping?
- Are you taking any tablets for your nerves or for your sleep?

Social factors

- Have you had any other problems recently that have upset you?
- Do you have any problems at home or at work?
- How is your relationship with your husband/wife/partner/children?

Beliefs and concerns

- What do you think is the cause of your symptoms/illness?
- To what extent do you understand the causes of your symptoms/illness?
- What effects do you think your symptoms/illness will have on your life?
- To what extent can *you* make a positive difference to your symptoms/illness?
- To what extent can *treatment* make a positive difference to your symptoms/illness?
- How hopeful are you for your future?
- How do you think things will turn out?

blue, but, rather, that there is a clear introductory rationale—for example, 'It's clear that your illness has been tough on you, and we do find that some people with illnesses like yours have trouble coping. Has that been the case with you? ... I'd like to ask you about that.'

It is important to:

- speak to relatives—they can provide extra information, and may also need help themselves;
- review medical notes—they often contain useful medical history and other information;
- be aware that some symptoms (e.g. mental and physical fatigue, poor sleep) may occur in both physical and psychiatric disorders.

Management

A vital part of good psychological care in *acute illness* is effective patient education, which should comprise five key elements:

1 *What*—what their illness is called, and what it is.

2 *Frequency*—how common it is.

3 *Cause*—what might have caused it and be maintaining it (i.e. provide a coherent aetiological model, on which to base the treatment plan—the degree of 'fit' between a patient's understanding of cause and a patient's understanding of treatment predicts patient adherence with treatment).

4 *Healthcare*—what health services can do to help.

5 *Self-care*—what the patient can do to help (i.e. self-care).

In addition, three simple approaches improve the effectiveness of communication:

6 Involve the *patient's closest relative/main carer* in the discussion.

7 Give *written information* to back up verbal messages, and copy patients in to medical letters, which should be written clearly, with the patient in mind.

8 Finally, ask the patient if they have any queries or concerns.

Management of the psychological problems of *chronic illness* is best organized as a process of 'stepped' care:

In **step one**, psychosocially informed medical care is provided for everyone, and includes:

- *self-care*—information about and encouragement of self-care including symptoms management;
- *family involvement*—discussion of how the patient and their family will be involved in care;
- *who*—explanation of who will be providing treatment, and routine and emergency contact arrangements, including a named keyworker where possible;
- *practical support*—with occupational, financial, and accommodation problems, perhaps with the assistance of a social worker or benefits expert;
- *systematic monitoring*—of progress (by patient and/or healthcare professionals);
- *identification*—of those needing step two care.

In **step two**, care is provided by the patient's GP or by the team providing the patient's physical care, and comprises initial treatment of common psychiatric disorders such as depression, perhaps following telephone advice from mental health specialists. The treatment of any specific psychiatric disorder among the physically ill is similar to that of the same condition in a physically healthy person, with one important proviso: particular attention should be paid to (1) the *side effects of medicines*, and (2) *interactions between medicines*.

In **step three**, care is provided by mental health professionals, based either within the physical setting (as a liaison psychiatry service) or within community mental health teams. This step is appropriate if the problem persists despite step two care, or if there are specific concerns, such as significant suicidality.

Some specific problems

Depressive disorder

Mild depression can often be helped by illness support, advice, or problem-solving, and encouragement of re-engagement with aspects of the patient's occupational, home, and social life that they have given up following diagnosis. These are simple approaches which can be delivered by a member of the team treating the physical disorder. *Moderate or severe depression* requires antidepressant medication or formal psychological treatments such as CBT. The choice of antidepressant may be affected by side effects, cautions and contraindications, and drug interactions, so it is vital to consult the *BNF*. As an example, SSRIs increase bleeding risk, which may be relevant in the very elderly, with gastrointestinal ulceration, with NSAID use, in the third trimester of pregnancy, or when undergoing orthopaedic surgery.

Acute distress

Distress, anxiety, or anger often reflects patients' uncertainties and fears about what is happening to them. It is important to try to understand, to show empathy, and to correct misunderstandings. Remain calm and take time to understand the patient's concerns. When anxiety remains severe, small amounts of anxiolytic medication, prescribed for a short period of time within *BNF* guidelines, may be helpful.

Patients who refuse consent to medical treatment

Occasionally, patients are unwilling to accept their doctor's advice about treatment that seems essential for a serious medical condition. There are many reasons for this. Commonly, this is because the patient is frightened or angry, does not understand fully what is happening, has had aversive previous experience of medical care, or knows someone that has. Remember that your views and experiences, as a member of the healthcare team, may be very different to many members of the public, who may have good reason to hold different views to you. Frequently, taking time to explain and to discuss the patient's situation, perhaps involving a close relative, and steadily building trust over a series of meetings, will result in informed

consent. Occasionally, the cause of refusal is a mental illness that interferes with the patient's ability to make an informed decision and, if so, the illness should be treated, if appropriate under the Mental Health Act (MHA). Importantly, the MHA does *not* give the right to treat physical disorder, except in the unusual case when physical disorder is the direct cause of the mental disorder.

Inevitably, some mentally healthy patients will continue to refuse treatment even after a full and rational discussion of the rationale. *It is the absolute right of a conscious, mentally competent adult to refuse treatment.* In the UK, the Mental Capacity Act provides the statutory framework in this area, supported by comprehensive guidance (see Chapter 18).

Psychiatric emergencies in general hospital practice

However urgent the problem, the successful management of a psychiatric emergency, like any other medical emergency, depends greatly on a thorough clinical assessment. The aims are to:

- establish a satisfactory relationship with the patient;
- take a brief history, from patient and key healthcare professional;
- assess the mental state, including observing behaviour.

When the patient's behaviour is very disturbed, the history may have to be obtained from other people, such as relatives or nurses. Although in managing emergencies there may not be the time or opportunity to follow the usual systematic scheme of history taking and examination, mistakes will be avoided and time saved if the assessment is as complete as the circumstances permit. Several common problems are discussed elsewhere, including deliberate self-harm (see Chapter 9), substance intoxication (see Chapter 29), acute stress reactions to trauma (see Chapter 23), and delirium (see Chapter 26).

Psychiatric services for a general hospital

GPs are responsible for all aspects of their patients' care: physical, psychological, and social. Similarly, in a general hospital, a consultant team is responsible for psychological aspects of illness and for social aspects such as arranging appropriate discharge and social support. Step one psychological care (assessment, advice about self-care, simple cognitive behavioural strategies, first-line medication) should be within the domain of the physical healthcare team. Sometimes, specialist psychiatric advice is needed. In larger hospitals this advice may be from a **psychological medicine** (also known as liaison psychiatry) **service**. The psychological medicine service may provide:

- *assessment*—of patients admitted after deliberate self-harm;
- *emergency assessment*—of other emergency department attenders;
- *advice*—on the psychiatric management of inpatients;
- *outpatient care*—for patients referred with psychiatric complications of physical illness or functional somatic symptoms;
- *regular visits to selected medical and surgical units*—in which psychiatric problems are especially common (e.g. neurology, renal dialysis, terminal care), to develop knowledge and skills among the physical healthcare team.

Because specialist psychiatric care is provided by a multidisciplinary team, referral is usually made to that team rather than to a specific doctor. The team will decide (1) which of its members is best placed to respond (availability, skill set) and (2) how they will respond (phone call, visit, or phone call followed by visit; emergency, urgent, or routine). Referral to the psychological medicine team should provide basic information about:

- *medical problem(s)*;
- *reason(s) for the referral*;
- *specific question* to be answered, or specific nature of the help required;
- *urgency of the referral* (not all referrals can be seen immediately!).

Cancer

Cancer causes considerable distress to many patients and their families. Psychological and social problems include family worries, financial and work difficulties, and worries about appearance. Patients may be angry. Sexual difficulties are common, sometimes due to direct effects of the illness or its treatment, but often due to cancer's impact on self-esteem, self-confidence, and personal relationships. Only a minority develop a psychiatric disorder, such as adjustment disorder (on diagnosis or recurrence), anxiety, depression, or rarer psychiatric syndromes due to metastases or paraneoplastic syndromes. Cancer and its treatment vary considerably in the nature, intensity, and duration of its physical impact on an individual and, by implication, in the nature of its psychological impact. Distress is particularly likely to occur at particular points during the patient's experience of cancer, including at diagnosis, during treatment (surgery, radiotherapy, or chemotherapy), and at the point (or points) of recurrence.

Care should involve patients and families to prevent or minimize psychological and social problems. Almost all psychological care is provided in primary care or in specialist cancer services in secondary care, which are increasingly well equipped to think in an integrated, biopsychosocial way about the management of cancer. This includes information and explanation, provided in a staged manner as patients and families require it. It is accompanied by practical and social support and willingness to encourage patients to talk about their worries. Specific psychiatric treatments (pharmacological and psychological) are effective for anxiety and depression and in helping patients to cope with physical symptoms. In many cases, cancer is a chronic disease, and there are repeated opportunities to provide advice, information, and re-assurance; to screen for psychological problems; and to intervene if necessary.

Surgical treatment

Most patients are anxious before major surgery; those who are most anxious before surgery are also most likely to be distressed afterwards. Anxiety can be reduced by a clear explanation of the operation, its likely consequences, and the plan for postoperative care, including the effective treatment of pain. In addition, written information is helpful since anxious people do not remember all that they have been told. Delirium is common after major surgery, especially in the elderly. When surgery leads to changes to the body's appearance (e.g. mastectomy) or function (e.g. colostomy) there may be additional psychological problems. These patients benefit from information, advice, and support.

Pregnancy and postpartum disorder

Pregnancy and the immediate postpartum period are times of major *biological* change, but also times of major *psychosocial* change. It is therefore unsurprising that mental illness can present particular challenges, for the woman, her partner and other carers, and for healthcare professionals. For any student interested in mental health, women's health, and the health of infants and children, this is a fruitful area for further enquiry, and we have recommended 'Further reading' at the end of this chapter.

Psychiatric disorder is more common in the first and third trimesters of pregnancy than in the second. In the *first* trimester, unwanted pregnancies are associated with anxiety and depression, and the news of the pregnancy, even when welcomed by both partners, brings the prospect of uncertainty and significant lifestyle change. In the *third* trimester, there may be fears about coping as a parent, the impending delivery, or the normality of the fetus. Psychiatric symptoms in pregnancy are more common in women with a history of previous psychiatric disorder, although some women with chronic psychiatric disorders may improve during pregnancy. Women with chronic psychiatric problems may attend irregularly for antenatal care, and are at increased risk of obstetric problems.

Abuse of *alcohol* and *street drugs* may affect the fetus and should be strongly discouraged, especially in the first trimester when the risk to the fetus is greatest. Current advice about alcohol consumption (see 'UK Chief Medical Officers' low risk drinking guidelines' in 'Further reading') is that 'if you are pregnant or planning a pregnancy, the safest approach is not to drink alcohol at all, to keep risks to your baby to a minimum; drinking in pregnancy can lead to long-term harm to the baby, with the more you drink the greater the risk'.

Treatment of psychiatric disorder during pregnancy

Please note carefully: *during pregnancy (and during pre-pregnancy, when a woman is attempting to get pregnant)* **great care** *must be taken in the use of psychotropic drugs because of the possible risk of fetal malformations, impaired growth, and perinatal problems* (Box 20.2). The current *BNF* provides up-to-date guidance.

Loss of a fetus and stillbirth

Loss of a fetus during pregnancy ('miscarriage' or spontaneous abortion) or at delivery (stillbirth) may have substantial and immediate psychological impacts for the mother and the father. The loss leads to significant depression, which may continue for several weeks. Stillbirth is typically associated with greater distress than earlier loss of the pregnancy. The distress is likely to be greatest when the pregnancy was particularly wanted, for example, when there have been previous miscarriages or stillbirths. Termination of pregnancy for medical reasons is especially likely to cause distress, depression, and feelings of guilt, which usually improve over a period of 2–3 months. After abortion, termination, or stillbirth, mothers and fathers should be encouraged to grieve the loss as they would the death of an infant.

Box 20.2 Use of psychiatric medicines during pregnancy and breastfeeding

Pregnancy

Ensure medicines-related decisions are discussed with the patient with or without their partner. Avoid all medication *if possible*, especially during the first trimester. Use only if the expected benefit to the mother is greater than the possibility of risk to the fetus. Clearly there will be circumstances, such as perceived high risk of relapse of a challenging mental disorder, when continued prescription is considered appropriate, despite theoretical risks to the fetus. In that case, use the lowest effective drug with the greatest evidence of safety (often an older drug). Review prescriptions regularly. Pharmacokinetics (e.g. hepatic metabolism) change markedly through pregnancy.

Antidepressants. The data are complex, but there is no robust evidence that tricyclics or SSRIs cause fetal abnormality. However, use only where there are very clear indications and in minimal dosage, and avoid paroxetine (possible cardiac malformations with first-trimester exposure). Possibility of SSRI withdrawal syndrome in neonates. Current SSRI use increases (by 30–60 per cent) risk of postpartum haemorrhage. Emerging evidence suggests that second- and third-trimester SSRI use may increase risk of autism.

Valproate and carbamazepine. Avoid. These mood stabilizers are associated with a high rate of congenital malformation, which may be reduced but not eliminated by preconception use of folate.

Lithium. The risks of this mood stabilizer have historically been overestimated. There is a *small* absolute risk of cardiac malformations early in the first trimester; therefore, ideally lithium should be avoided in preconception and early pregnancy. Pharmacokinetics change during the third trimester (increased body water) and abruptly return to normal after delivery—risks are reduced by monthly monitoring of levels, and dose reduction immediately postpartum. Consider careful screening for cardiac abnormalities in exposed pregnancies.

Antipsychotics. Continue in minimal dose if there are major clinical indications—risks of exposure to high doses during relapse probably exceed risks of exposure to low maintenance doses. Most experience with common typicals, and the atypicals olanzapine and quetiapine. Occasional side effects seen in neonates, so *consider* dose reduction or withdrawal.

Breastfeeding

Take care with all medications, as data are often scanty, especially regarding long-term outcomes. This general advice is motivated by a relative absence of evidence of safety, rather than by actual evidence of harm.

Antidepressants. Although there is no convincing evidence of possible harm, most manufacturers advise avoiding during breastfeeding. Avoid if possible, but if risks to the woman's mood are considered high, carefully consider the risks and benefits with the parents. Sertraline may be preferred.

Lithium. Excreted in breast milk, with theoretical risk of toxicity. Careful assessment of risks and benefits, with the mother involved in the decision-making (helped by lithium being a medicine in which high levels of patient involvement are required, outside pregnancy and breastfeeding).

Antipsychotic drugs. The risk is probably very small, but there is a theoretical risk to nervous system development, so avoid if possible. Olanzapine may be preferred.

Postpartum mental disorders

Terminology is tricky in the 'puerperium': the period of about 6 weeks after delivery. Strictly, the '*postnatal*' period refers to the period after the child has been born, and '*postpartum*' refers to the period after the mother has given birth—but they are often used interchangeably. There are three kinds of postpartum psychiatric disorder:

- 'baby blues';
- postpartum depression;
- postpartum psychosis.

'Baby blues'

At least 50 per cent of women experience a brief episode of irritability, tearfulness, and lability of mood after delivery. Typically, this starts after 2–3 days, and lasts 1–2 days. The patient and her partner should be reassured that the condition is common, short-lived, and not the onset of 'depression'. No treatment is needed.

Postpartum depression

Postpartum depression occurs in 10–15 per cent of women within 6 months of delivery. Tiredness, irritability, and anxiety (including phobic anxiety) are often prominent alongside depressive mood. There may be concerns about the health of the baby, or about the quality of mothering. Most cases (90 per cent) are short-lived (≤1 month). These episodes are caused mainly by the psychological adjustments required after childbirth, by sleep disturbance, and by the hard work involved in baby care. Risk factors include history of psychiatric illness, psychosocial stressors, and poor support; but, notably, not obstetric complications.

Postpartum depression adversely affects the mother–infant relationship and may have a small adverse effect on cognitive and emotional development of the infant. Early identification of postpartum depression is therefore important. In the UK, the Edinburgh Postnatal Depression Scale is commonly used to screen by community midwives and health visitors, but the Patient Health Questionnaire (PHQ)-9 is also recommended. *It is vital to ask the mother (sensitively and thoughtfully) about thoughts of harming herself or harming her child.*

Management may include advice about child care, help with child care, advice on sexual relationships, and more general relationship guidance. Otherwise, management of postnatal depression is similar to that of depression in general.

Postpartum psychosis

Postpartum psychosis occurs after less than 0.2 per cent of births. It begins, typically, 2–3 days after delivery and nearly always in the first 2 postpartum weeks. This is because childbirth is a powerful precipitant of psychosis and mood disturbance. *Suicide is an important cause of maternal death, often in the context of postpartum psychosis.*

There are three common presentations, namely:

- **mood** syndromes (elation, depression, mood-congruent psychotic features) are easily the most common in high-income countries; followed by
- **schizophreniform** syndromes; and, finally,
- **delirium** (confusional syndrome, including psychotic features), which was common before antibiotics were introduced to treat puerperal sepsis, but is now rare.

Established risk factors include:

- history of bipolar disorder;
- previous postpartum psychosis;
- primiparity (for possible biological and psychosocial reasons);
- absence of a supportive partner.

Assessment. *It is essential to ascertain the mother's ideas concerning the baby.* Severely depressed patients may have delusions that the child is malformed or diseased and some patients may attempt to kill the child to end its suffering. Assessment of *suicidal intent* is also important.

Treatment is as described for mood disorder and schizophrenia occurring outside pregnancy. For moderate–severe depressive disorders, *ECT* is often the best treatment because its rapid effect enables the mother to resume the care of her baby quickly. When the disorder is not severe and the mother has no ideas of harming herself or the baby, treatment can be at home with appropriate help to ensure safety of baby and mother. When the disorder is more severe, or there are ideas of harm to self or baby, the mother should usually be admitted to hospital, if possible to a specialist mother and baby unit. If psychiatric medicines have to be prescribed, the safety of breastfeeding must be assessed.

Treatment during subsequent pregnancies. Women who have had a postpartum psychosis should be referred to a psychiatrist and monitored very closely in the hours and days after delivery. Women who have a history of bipolar disorder may require lithium prophylaxis, avoiding the first trimester and stopping for a short period at delivery.

Menstrual disorders

Premenstrual syndrome

This term denotes psychological and physical symptoms starting a few days before, and ending at or around, menstruation. Psychological symptoms include anxiety, irritability, depression, reduced concentration, and sleep disturbance; physical symptoms include fatigue, headache, breast tenderness, abdominal discomfort, and distension. Impact on daily life varies from mild to severe: this is not a trivial illness. Estimates of the frequency of premenstrual syndrome (PMS) in women of reproductive age vary from 50–80 per cent (at least mild PMS) to 5–10 per cent (severe). The cause is uncertain, but is clearly related to cyclic ovarian function, and the role of SSRIs in treatment suggests an important serotonergic role. Psychological factors may exacerbate distress and disability originating from physiological changes around menstruation.

To determine whether a particular treatment is effective in a particular patient, a daily symptom diary (main emotional and physical symptoms) should be completed for 1 or 2 months before the treatment starts; and then continued after treatment, to determine full, partial, or absent response. Retrospective recall of symptoms is unreliable, and this approach offers a scientific, objective assessment of treatment response.

Treatment options (see 'Further reading') supported by RCT evidence include the following:

- *SSRIs*—prescribed either continuously or during the luteal phase only of the menstrual cycle (the 14 days prior to expected menstruation). SSRI side effects are common, but are typically better tolerated than PMS symptoms, and may respond well to a dose reduction.

- *CBT*—which can help by improving coping with symptoms and their consequences, and enabling them to feel more in control of their PMS rather than feeling controlled by it. Availability is likely to be limited, although a variety of self-help books are available, some of which have a cognitive behavioural element.
- *The combined oral contraceptive pill.*
- *Vitamin B6.*

Menopause

Some menopausal women complain of physical symptoms of flushing, sweating, vaginal dryness, headache, and dizziness, and psychological symptoms such as depression and anxiety. Although there is a widespread belief that emotional problems are an inevitable part of the menopause, it is not certain whether psychological symptoms are more common in menopausal women than in other women of similar age. Depressive and anxiety-related symptoms around the time of the menopause could be related to hormonal changes but this has not been proved. Alternatively, or additionally, the symptoms could result from changes in the woman's role as her children leave home, her relationship with her partner alters, her own parents become ill or die, and her career develops and potentially becomes more challenging. Hormone replacement therapy should not be seen as a treatment of depressive illness in those of menopausal age. Psychiatric disorders around the menopause should be treated as at other times of life.

Further reading

Department of Health. UK Chief Medical Officers' low risk drinking guidelines. Published August 2016. https://www.gov.uk/government/uploads/system/uploads/attachment_data/file/545937/UK_CMOs__report.pdf.

Green LJ, O'Brien PMS, Panay N, Craig M, on behalf of the Royal College of Obstetricians and Gynaecologists. Management of premenstrual syndrome. *BJOG: An International Journal of Obstetrics and Gynaecology* 2017;124:e73–e105.

The Lancet published an important series on perinatal mental health, with an introductory comment:

Howard LM, Piot P, Stein A. No health without perinatal mental health. *Lancet* 2014;384:1723–1724.

Howard LM, Molyneaux E, Dennis CL, Rochat T, Stein A, Milgrom J. Non-psychotic mental disorders in the perinatal period. *Lancet* 2014;384:1775–1788.

Jones I, Chandra PS, Dazzan P, Howard LM. Bipolar disorder, affective psychosis, and schizophrenia in pregnancy and the post-partum period. *Lancet* 2014;384:1789–1799.

Stein A, Pearson RM, Goodman SH, et al. Effects of perinatal mental disorders on the fetus and child. *Lancet* 2014;384:1800–1819.

Part 5 The specific disorders

21 Mood disorders

Introduction

Variations in mood are part of normal experience; we all have our 'good' and 'bad' days and different ways of managing these. Sadness is a natural response to loss, adversity, stress, or other negative life experiences and is not necessarily abnormal. The main difference between normal sadness and a mood disorder is that normal sadness is usually a temporary state strongly relating to the person's current situation, whereas mood disorder is a more persistent pervasive change in mood which affects social and occupational functioning. Primary mood (or 'affective') disorders are very common, and are also seen in most other psychiatric disorders or co-morbid to a physical illness.

Classification of mood disorders

The distribution of mood variation in the general population is probably continuous, producing a spectrum of severity (see Fig. 21.1). As with all psychiatric disorders, classification is descriptive and based on clinical characteristics.

The most useful current approach to classification is based on the clinical course. Fundamental elements of this approach include:

- classifying an illness as a single episode, recurrent, or persistent;
- distinguishing between people who have only low mood (unipolar depression) and those who also have elated mood (bipolar disorder);
- classifying episodes of illness according to severity: depressive episodes are mild, moderate, or severe; elated mood is hypomanic or manic (Table 21.1).

The classification includes two categories for less severe and more chronic illnesses:

- **Dysthymia:** chronic mildly low mood which lasts at least several years but does not meet criteria for a recurrent depressive disorder.
- **Cyclothymia:** chronic instability of mood with periods of mild depressive and elation, none of which are severe enough to meet criteria for bipolar disorder or recurrent depressive disorder. It is often seen in relatives of those who have bipolar disorder, and some patients may eventually meet criteria for bipolar disorder themselves.

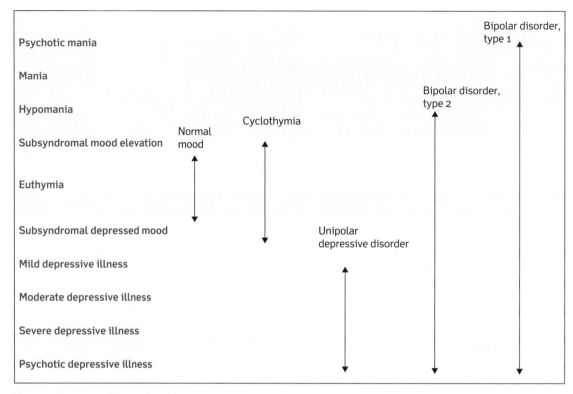

Fig. 21.1 Spectrum of mood disorders.

Table 21.1 The classification of mood disorders in ICD-10

Hypomania	
Manic episode	
Bipolar affective disorder	
Depressive episode	• Mild • Moderate • Severe
Recurrent depressive disorder	
Persistent mood (affective) states	• Cyclothymia • Dysthymia

The ICD-11 will change 'bipolar affective disorder' to 'bipolar disorder' to bring it in line with the DSM. The diagnostic criteria will remain the same

Adapted from *International Classification of Diseases*, 10th Revision (ICD-10). Copyright (2016) World Health Organization.

Epidemiology of mood disorders

The prevalence of mood disorders is hard to accurately ascertain, as many patients with low mood do not seek professional help. This is especially common in men. However, data from research studies (which tend to use structured diagnostic criteria) and large national surveys (self-report) give very similar results, outlined in Table 21.2. Bipolar disorder epidemiology is well captured, as patients tend to seek help and the diagnostic criteria are well defined. Overall, unipolar depressive disorders are twice as common in women as in men, a finding only partly explained by selective reporting. The aetiology of this gender difference is poorly understood.

Unipolar depressive episodes are common in patients attending primary care (up to 40 per cent of attenders) and general hospital. It is one of the most important causes of disability and an important cause of mortality, through suicide. Depressive disorders are more common in urban than rural populations and, in general, the prevalence is higher in groups

Table 21.2 Epidemiology of mood disorders

Diagnosis	12-month prevalence (%)	Lifetime risk (%)	Male:female	Average age of onset
Depressive episode	4–6	15–20	1:2	27 years Second peak age 60–70 years
Dysthymia	2–3	4	1:2	25 years
Bipolar disorder	1–1.5	1–2	1:1	17 years (IQR 15–25)

IQR, interquartile range.

with adverse socioeconomic factors (e.g. in homeless people) and in patients with physical disorder. There is a genetic element, such that the risk is increased in first-degree relatives. Bipolar disorder has a particularly high heritability: first-degree relatives have a 5–10 per cent lifetime risk of bipolar disorder, a 12 per cent lifetime risk of recurrent depressive disorder, and a 12 per cent risk of dysthymic or other mood disorders.

The high prevalence means that depressive disorders are one of the most important causes of disability in all countries. Depressive disorders cause both direct costs to health services, but much greater indirect costs due to inability to work. As mood disorders tend to start during the second and third decades of life, they can significantly impact education, employment, and family life.

Unipolar depressive disorder

Unipolar depressive disorder (typically known as 'depression') is a syndrome in which mood is consistently low, energy levels are reduced, and there is a lack of enjoyment of life. It is important to detect depression, as unrecognized depressive disorder may slow recovery and worsen prognosis in physical illness. It is important, therefore, that all clinicians should be able to recognize the condition, treat the less severe cases, and identify those requiring specialist care because of suicidal risk or for other reasons.

General clinical features

Pathological low mood is the central symptom of depressive disorder and needs to be distinguished from normal sadness commonly experienced by healthy people in response to misfortunes, especially loss events such as the loss of a partner. Low mood can be viewed as a spectrum from normal mood variability through to profound and severe depressive disorder (see Fig. 21.1). In depressive disorder, the low mood is **persistent**; causes **impairment of functioning** in normal daily activities such as in employment or childcare; and is **accompanied by other symptoms**, including loss of pleasure (*anhedonia*), lack of energy, poor concentration, anxiety, and poor sleep. Low mood, reduced energy, and anhedonia are the core symptoms of depression. Low mood may be hidden because the patient smiles and denies feeling miserable. Some patients may present with physical symptoms rather than complaining of low mood, or appear primarily anxious. Diagnosing depressive disorder therefore requires a careful search for the whole range of symptoms and the psychosocial context in which the patient presents. Diagnostic criteria for a depressive episode are shown in Box 21.1 and a fuller explanation of symptoms in Table 21.3.

A depressed patient's appearance may be characteristic. They may fail to smile or laugh, or do so less than they would usually. In more severe conditions, there may be evidence of self-neglect or a reduction in interest in appearance. Psychomotor retardation, which is a slowing of mental and motor activity, is frequent. There may be agitation, and a feeling of restlessness, which may manifest itself as an inability to relax accompanied by restless activity. When agitation is severe, the patient cannot sit for long and may pace up and down.

It is usual in a mild depressive episode for the patient to be able to continue with their usual activities (e.g. work, domestic responsibilities, and hobbies). They may reduce the intensity of these or not be able

Box 21.1 ICD-10 F32 Depressive Episode

Main features

- Low mood
- Reduced energy levels (or fatigue)
- Anhedonia

Associated features

- Reduced activity
- Changes in appetite
- Changes in sleep pattern
- Loss of libido
- Poor concentration and attention
- Reduced self esteem
- Feelings of guilt or worthlessness

Duration

- Symptoms for most of the day, on almost all days for at least 2 weeks

Disability

- Reduced occupational and social functioning

Exclusions (which should be considered in the differential diagnosis)

- Symptoms in context of major life event (adjustment disorder)
- Symptoms part of a recurrent depressive disorder
- Previous episodes of hypomania or mania (bipolar disorder)
- Depressive syndrome caused by physical disorder (e.g. hypothyroidism)

Mild depressive episode: at least two main features present but patient able to continue with most of their usual daily activities.

Moderate depressive episode: all main features present plus several other symptoms; patient is distressed and has great difficulty continuing with usual activities.

Severe depressive episode: patient has all main features and typically has significant deficits in self-esteem and feelings of worthlessness and/or suicide. Very severe deficits in functioning are present.

Severe depressive episode with psychotic symptoms: above-mentioned features plus presence of hallucinations, delusions, psychomotor retardation, or catatonic symptoms.

ICD-11 beta-draft does not contain any changes to these criteria.

Adapted from *International Classification of Diseases*, 10th Revision (ICD-10). Copyright (2016) World Health Organization.

to do them to their usual standard, but there is only a mild impairment. In moderate to severe depression, the degree of functional impairment is more significant, and the patient might find it very difficult to work or look after the family.

Depressive thinking ('depressive cognitions') are a core part of the illness, and play a key role as a maintaining factor. Typically, there is a 'triad' of unrealistically negative thoughts about the past, present, and future:

- **Thoughts about the past.** These thoughts often take the form of unreasonable **guilt** and **self-blame** about objectively minor matters: for example, patients may feel guilty about some trivial act of dishonesty in the past or about letting someone down. Usually, the patient has not thought about these events for

years, but as the depression develops, they flood back into memory accompanied by intense feelings of guilt. Other memories are focused on unhappy times: patients remember occasions when they were sad, when they failed, or when their fortunes were at a low ebb.

- **Thoughts about the present.** Patients see the unhappy side of every new event; think that they are failing in everything they do, that other people see them as a failure, and develop low self-esteem; and they lose confidence and discount any success as a chance happening for which they should take no credit.

- **Thoughts about the future.** Patients expect the worst: they foresee failure in their work, the ruin of their finances, misfortune for their families, and

Table 21.3 Symptoms of depressive disorders

Symptom of depression	Typical characteristics
Core symptoms	
Low mood	• Mood is usually low, sad, or flat but may be more irritable than usual • Family/friends may describe the patient as having changed or being different • Mood has diurnal variation; frequently worse in mornings
Reduced energy levels	• Majority of patients complain of tiredness or fatigue. • Reduced motivation *(Note: reduced energy may be present even when the patient appears restless, so specifically enquire for this)*
Anhedonia	• Lack of enjoyment in life or activities they previously liked • Social withdrawal is common
Biological (somatic) symptoms	
Changes in appetite	• Loss of appetite and weight • (Less common: overeating)
Changes in sleep pattern	Typical patterns include: • early morning waking (often 4–6 am): patient wakes early, unrefreshed, and has pessimistic thoughts about the day ahead • insomnia • repeated awakenings overnight • frequent daytime napping • oversleeping (often in those who have increased appetite)
Loss of libido	• Decreased interest in sex
Psychomotor retardation or agitation	• Patient is slower than usual in thoughts and movements. They appear 'slowed up'. Seen in more severe depression • Occasionally patients may appear agitated, restless, and pacing
Psychological symptoms	
Poor concentration and attention	• Ability to sustain attention on tasks is reduced. Patient is unable to do activities such as reading, studying, etc. • Subjective poor memory may be reported; on testing, this deficit is not demonstrated. More common in the elderly, where it may present as a 'depressive pseudodementia'
Low self-esteem	• Feelings of worthlessness • Feelings of guilt • Loss of self-confidence
Depressive thinking	• Hopelessness and helplessness • Pessimism about the future • Feelings of suicide

(continued)

Table 21.3 Continued

Symptom of depression	Typical characteristics
Anxiety	• May be about any topic • Health anxiety/hypochondriasis is common
Physical symptoms commonly reported in depression	
	• Headaches • Abdominal pain (especially in some cultures) • Gastrointestinal symptoms: constipation, nausea • Pain • Chest pains
Other symptoms which may occur as part of the depressive syndrome	
	• Depersonalization • Obsessions • Phobias • Conversion symptoms
Psychotic symptoms	
Delusions	Delusions may be of any content, but nihilistic (or negative) delusions are common, e.g. of poverty, disease, guilt, or worthlessness. Patient may be paranoid
Hallucinations	Usually mood congruent, often second-person auditory hallucinations (e.g. 'you are a bad person')

an inevitable deterioration in their physical health. These ideas of hopelessness are often accompanied by the thought that life is no longer worth living and that death would come as a welcome release. These gloomy preoccupations may progress to thoughts of, and plans for, suicide. It is important to ask about suicide in every case of depressive disorder.

In more severe depression, some patients may have psychotic symptoms. These are usually delusions and hallucinations, the content of which are mood congruent, that is, they fit with the depressive mood.

Typical depressive delusions include:

• **delusion of guilt** in which a person believes that some dishonest act, such as a minor concealment in making a tax return, will be discovered, that he will be punished severely, and that he deserves this punishment;

• **delusion of hypochondriasis** in which a person believes that he has cancer, serious heart disease, or a sexually transmitted disease;

• **delusion of poverty** in which a patient believes that he has lost all his money in a business venture;

• **nihilistic delusion,** in which a patient believes that he has no future, or that some part of him has ceased to exist or function (e.g. that his bowels are wholly blocked);

• **delusion of persecution** in which a patient believes, for example, that other people are about to take revenge on him, and that such persecution is deserved/reasonable.

If mood-**incongruent** delusions are present, then the patient may lie somewhere along the spectrum between mood disorder and schizophrenia.

Typical depressive hallucinations are auditory, in the form of voices, speaking to the patient (i.e. in the second person), and may address repetitive words and phrases to the patient. These voices confirm the patient's beliefs about their guilt or worthlessness (e.g. 'you are evil; you should die'), that is, they are mood congruent. More worryingly, they may urge suicide, and such hallucinations need to be noted and considered carefully in the risk assessment. Occasionally, visual hallucinations occur, such as scenes of death and destruction.

Suicidal ideas should be enquired about carefully in any patient with a moderate or severe depressive disorder. Rarely, there are homicidal ideas and, when these occur, they may concern family members including children. This possibility must be considered when assessing women with symptoms of postnatal depression.

Variants of depressive disorder

The clinical picture of severe depressive disorders is varied and several terms are sometimes used to describe common patterns:

- **Agitated depression** is a condition in which agitation is particularly severe. Agitated depression occurs more commonly among older patients.
- **Retarded depression** is marked by prominent psychomotor retardation.
- **Depressive stupor** is a rare variant of severe depressive disorder in which retardation is so extreme that the patient is motionless, mute, and refuses to eat and drink. On recovering, patients can recall the events taking place at the time they were in stupor.
- **Atypical depression** is characterized by *reversed biological symptoms* such as *increased* sleep, *increased* appetite and severe anxiety, fatigue, and interpersonal sensitivity.

Seasonal affective disorder

Some people repeatedly develop a depressive disorder at the same time of year. In some cases, this timing reflects extra demands on the person at a particular time of year; in other cases, there is no such extra demand, and it has been suggested that the cause is related to changes in the season, for example, in the length of daylight. Although these mood disorders are characterized mainly by the season in which they occur, they are also said to be characterized by some symptoms that are less common in other mood disorders, for example, hypersomnia and increased appetite with cravings for carbohydrates. The most common pattern is onset in the autumn or winter, and recovery in the spring or summer. This pattern has led to the suggestion that shortening of daylight is important. Some patients improve after exposure to artificial light given usually in the early morning (see p. 153). It is uncertain for which patients the treatment is effective, or how lasting are its effects.

Differential diagnosis

In a patient with a depressive syndrome, this may be a 'standalone' depressive episode or part of recurrent depressive disorder or bipolar disorder:

- **Depressive episode** (i.e. the only mood episode in the person's life to date).
- **Recurrent depressive disorder, currently depressive episode** (i.e. the person is currently depressed, and there has been at least one other episode of depression).
- **Bipolar disorder, currently depressive episode** (i.e. the person is currently depressed, and there has been at least one previous episode of mania/ hypomania). For this reason, it is important to ask the patient about a history of elevated mood.

Other possibilities to consider include the following:

- **Normal sadness.** The distinction depends upon severity, persistence, and the presence of other symptoms.
- **Grief.** Depressive disorder resembles uncomplicated grief in many ways, but severe pessimism, suicidal thoughts, profound guilt, and psychotic symptoms are all rare in grief. Severe symptoms persisting more than 6 months after bereavement suggest a depressive disorder.

- **Anxiety disorder.** Mild depressive disorders are sometimes difficult to distinguish from anxiety disorders. Accurate diagnosis depends on assessment of the relative severity of anxiety and depressive symptoms, and of their order of appearance. Similar problems arise when there are prominent phobic or obsessional symptoms.

- **Unexplained physical symptoms** (see p. 349). It is not uncommon for depressive disorder to present with concern about non-specific and medically unexplained physical symptoms, without a direct complaint of the psychological symptoms. Careful enquiry will elicit these additional symptoms.

- **Schizophrenia or schizoaffective disorder.** The differential diagnosis of depressive disorder from schizophrenia depends on a careful search for the characteristic features of schizophrenia (see Chapter 22). Diagnosis may be difficult when a patient has both depressive symptoms and persecutory delusions, but the distinction can usually be made by examining the mental state carefully and by establishing whether the delusions followed, and are consistent with, the depressive symptoms (mood congruent—depressive disorder) or the delusions came first or are not congruent with the mood disorder (schizophrenia). For example, in depressive disorder, persecution is usually accepted as the deserved consequence of the patient's own failings; in schizophrenia it is strongly rejected. Some patients have symptoms of both depressive disorder and of schizophrenia; these schizoaffective disorders are discussed in Chapter 22. A depressive syndrome may also occur following treatment of the psychotic symptoms of schizophrenia, when it is called post-psychotic depression.

- **Dementia.** In middle and late life, depressive disorders may be difficult to distinguish from dementia because some patients with depressive disorder complain of considerable difficulty in remembering and some demented patients are depressed. In depressive disorders, difficulty in remembering occurs because poor concentration leads to inadequate registration. The distinction between the two conditions can often be made by careful cognitive testing; standard psychological tests are required in doubtful cases, but even these may not decide the issue. If memory disorder does not improve with recovery of normal mood, dementia is probable (see also p. 361).

- **Substance abuse.** Depressive symptoms are common in substance abuse and some patients with depressive disorder abuse alcohol or non-prescribed drugs to relieve their distress. The sequence of the depressive symptoms and substance abuse should be determined, as well as the presence of the features of depressive disorder other than low mood.

Aetiology of depressive disorders

In broad terms, mood disorders are caused by an interaction between (1) stressful events and (2) constitutional factors resulting from genetics and childhood experience. These aetiological factors act through biochemical and psychological processes, which have been partly identified by research. An overview is shown in Table 21.4. It is also important to remember that as well as predisposing factors, precipitating factors (typically stressful life events) and maintaining factors play important roles.

Genetics

Genetic factors have been studied mainly in moderate to severe cases of mood disorder, rather than in milder cases. First-degree relatives of depressed patients have a higher lifetime risk for mood disorder than the general population. Twin studies indicate that these high rates among families are due to genetic factors. Monozygotic twin studies have reported 35–40 per cent concordance for a moderate depressive episode, compared to approximately 20 per cent in dizygotic twins. Studies of adopted children confirm the importance of genetic causes of depressive disorder. In children raised by adoptive parents without a history of depressive disorder, the risk of developing depression in adult life is higher in those children born to a parent with a history of serious depressive disorder than in those children born to parents with no such history.

Table 21.4 Aetiology of depressive disorders

Biological	Psychological	Social
Genetics: • Twofold increased risk in first-degree relatives • Heritability estimated at 37% • Inconsistent evidence from research linking depression to the serotonin transporter gene, tryptophan hydroxylase, and brain-derived neurotrophic factor	Personality traits: • Lifelong tendency towards anxiety • Need for approval • Tendency towards negative outlook • Low self esteem	• Acute stressful life events (typically within the past 12 months) • Chronic stressors (e.g. long-term marital discord, problems with children, financial difficulties)
Low birth weight (weak association) General medical conditions: Strong associations have been demonstrated with: • stroke • ischaemic heart disease • endocrine disorders • influenza • Parkinson's • pregnancy and the puerperium	Adverse early life experiences: • Childhood abuse (especially emotional neglect) • Lack of positive parental attachments • Parental separation/divorce • Family discord or difficulties during childhood	• Lack of social support or criticism by main supporters • Deprivation or poverty • Main carer for 3 or more children under 5 years • Lower levels of education • Association with substance misuse
Medications (e.g. antihypertensives, steroids, Parkinson's treatments, interferons)	Severe maternal postnatal depression (or other cause of lack of response to the child's emotional needs) Emotional enmeshment with close family members	

There is no single gene for depression, it appears to be a combination of multiple background genetic effects and altered gene expression as a response to stress. It is proving very difficult to identify the genes associated with a risk of depression, which suggests it is a complex polygenetic risk. Genome-wide association studies have identified several hundred candidate genes—but results from different studies are not consistent and there appears to be considerable variety between racial groups. For example, a polymorphism in a serotonin transporter gene has been linked to a higher risk of depression in multiple studies. However, a recent meta-analysis of more than 14,000 patients did not find any greater risk of depression in those with the polymorphism compared to controls.

Mediating processes of depression

Two kinds of complementary mediating processes have been studied: psychological and biochemical.

Psychological mediating processes

Depressed patients may process information in a way that causes and then prolongs the initial change of mood (**cognitive biases**). Several abnormalities have been proposed:

1 Abnormalities of emotional processing—for example, people who are susceptible to depression may be more likely to interpret facial expression as negative.

2 Tendency to remember unhappy events more easily than happy ones.

3 Unrealistic beliefs, for example, 'I cannot be happy unless I am liked by everyone I know'.

4 Cognitive distortions in drawing a general conclusion from a single event; for example, 'I have failed in this relationship, so I will never be loved by anyone'. These illogical ways of thinking allow the intrusive gloomy thoughts and the unrealistic expectations to persist despite evidence to the contrary.

Biochemical mediating processes

There is clear evidence of biochemical abnormalities, at least in the more severe depressive disorders, but their nature is uncertain. Also, it is not known whether there is a single abnormality present in every patient with depressive disorder, or different abnormalities leading to the same clinical picture. The strongest evidence is for an abnormality of serotonin (5-HT) function. There are several strands of evidence:

- The main serotonin metabolite (5-HIAA) is reduced in the CSF of patients with severe depressive disorders.

- Serotonin is reduced in the brains of depressed patients who have died by suicide.

- Neuroendocrine functions that involve serotonin transmission are reduced in depressed patients. Tryptophan (an amino acid precursor of serotonin) depletion via diet can lead to increased depressive mood in people who have recovered.

- Finally, if low serotonin function is important in causing depressive disorder, then increasing this function should be therapeutic, and this is a common effect of most antidepressants.

Noradrenergic function also seems to be reduced in depressive disorders and antidepressant agents that effect both serotonin and noradrenaline may be moderately more effective that agents that work on one neurotransmitter (e.g. SSRIs vs mirtazapine).

Endocrine abnormalities

A causal role for endocrine abnormalities is suggested by the association of mood disorder with Cushing's syndrome, Addison's disease, and hyperparathyroidism (Cushing's syndrome is sometimes associated with elation rather than depression of mood). It has also been suggested that depressive disorders occurring after childbirth or at the menopause are related to endocrine changes but there is no strong evidence for this.

Plasma cortisol is increased in about half of patients with depressive disorder. However, this increase in cortisol is not specific to depressive disorder; it occurs also in mania and schizophrenia. The change does not seem to be just a reaction to the stress of being ill, for it involves a change in the diurnal pattern of secretion of cortisol (being high in the afternoon and early evening after which time it normally decreases), a change not seen after exposure to stressors. It has been suggested that the elevation of cortisol may arise after a prolonged life stress and may predispose to depression by interfering with brain 5-HT function.

Prognosis of depressive disorders

There are three important aspects to the prognosis of depressive disorders:

- **The prognosis of individual episodes.** Untreated episodes last 6 months or more with a significant minority lasting for years. With treatment, an episode typically lasts 2–3 months. Most patients eventually recover from the episode. Some patients will continue to have subsyndromal persistent symptoms beyond the main recovery period.

- **The risk of recurrence.** Recurrence is common: 80 per cent of those who have a single episode followed by recovery will eventually have another episode.

- **The risk of suicide.** This is much higher among patients with depressive disorder than among the general population. The lifetime risk of suicide is about 10 per cent in severe depressive disorder—about 15 times higher than in people without depression.

Management of depressive disorders

Most patients with depressive disorders are treated in primary care. Those managed in secondary care tend to have moderate to severe depression, or co-morbid diagnoses, or significant risks.

Detection of depressive disorders

It is important that all doctors remain aware of the high prevalence of depression in all settings. This includes patients presenting primarily with physical complaints. The detection of depression can be improved if the doctor always remembers to ask two simple screening questions (which are very similar to the PHQ-2):

1 During the last month, have you often been bothered by feeling down, depressed, or hopeless?

2 During the last month, have you often been bothered by little interest or pleasure in doing things?

Doctors with good interviewing skills are more likely to detect depression when it exists, and also to lead to better outcomes. This may be because good interviewing provides non-specific benefits as well as leading to improved diagnosis and treatment.

Assessment

A patient who is suspected of having a depressive disorder needs a comprehensive assessment that includes a consideration of medical, psychological, and social needs and an assessment of the risk (Table 21.5).

Diagnosis depends on careful, focused assessment that is appropriate to the setting: clearly assessment in primary care will be much briefer than in secondary care. History taking, mental state examination, and physical examination are required. Particular care should be taken:

- to consider the possibility of depressive disorder in a patient who complains of physical symptoms of depression (e.g. fatigue/poor sleep/abdominal discomfort) rather than depressed mood ('**masked depression**');

- to consider whether the patient has suffered from a previous episode of mania/hypomania, that is, the diagnosis is **bipolar depression** (see p. 278);

- to consider the possibility of an **organic psychiatric syndrome** (caused by, e.g. cerebral neoplasm, hypothyroidism);

- to remember that **certain medicines** can cause depression;

- to remember that **alcohol and certain street drugs** can cause depression.

The severity of the disorder is judged from the symptoms, behaviour, and the level of functional impairment. Whenever possible, an informant should be

Table 21.5 Assessment of depressive disorder

Diagnosis	• History (including medications) • Mental state • Relevant physical examination and investigation • Informants' accounts
Severity	• Number of depressive symptoms • Extent of functional impact (on work, domestic, and other responsibilities) • Risk of suicide or self-harm • Other risks: occupational risks, care of dependents, driving, engagement with treatment, self-neglect
Aetiology	• An exploration of the biological, psychological, and social factors predisposing to the patient's illness. • Identify precipitating and maintaining factors • Co-morbid physical illness? • Drug history and use of substances and alcohol
Social situation	• Community support from friends/family • Housing • Work • Finances

interviewed as well as the patient. The risk of suicide must be assessed in every case (the methods of assessment are described in Chapter 9). It is also important to assess how far the depressive disorder has reduced the patient's capacity to work or to engage in family life and social activities. In this assessment, the duration and course of the condition should be taken into account as well as the severity of the present symptoms and disability. The length of history not only affects prognosis, it also gives an indication of the patient's capacity to tolerate further distress. A long continued disorder, even if not severe, can bring the patient to the point of desperation.

The impact on the patient's everyday life should be considered by asking about ability to work, ability to carry out caring responsibilities, effects on leisure interests, and relationships with other people. The effect of the disorder on other people should be considered. It is important to consider whether the patient could endanger other people by remaining at work (e.g. as a bus driver). Effects on the family are important, especially on young children. A severely depressed mother may, for example, accidentally neglect her children. Danger may also arise when there are depressive delusions that could lead to action. Very rarely, severely depressed mothers may sometimes kill their children because of the belief that they are doomed to suffer if they remain alive. Severely depressed patients occasionally kill their spouses. In the longer term, depressive disorder in either parent is associated with the development of emotional disorder in the children.

Treatment of the acute phase of depression

Treatment of depressive disorder can be divided into three main phases:

- An **acute** phase to relieve symptoms of depression and achieve recovery.
- A **continuation** phase to preserve the improvement while the illness fully resolves.
- A **maintenance** phase to protect the vulnerable patients from further episodes (see also Fig. 21.2).

There are several effective treatments for depressive disorders. The choice of treatment for each individual patient depends largely on four factors, namely:

- the **severity** of the disorder;
- **previous treatment response** (if any);
- the **patient's preference**;
- the **availability** of specific treatments.

An overview of currently recommended treatment options is shown in Table 21.6.

General aspects of the treatment of the acute phase

As well as specific treatments, non-specific and supportive measures are very important. The patient may have an unclear view of the nature of depressive disorder and its treatment. The doctor should therefore provide a clear outline of the nature of the disorder and the available treatments (including likely benefits and possible adverse effects), should discuss the patient's preferences, and agree a treatment plan with them.

Active follow-up with early identification of any problems leads to better adherence to the prescribed therapy and improved outcomes. During the initial weeks of treatment, patients should be seen and supported; those with severe disorders may need to be seen every 2 or 3 days; others usually weekly. The possibility of the emergence of a manic episode should be kept in mind when depression is being treated because the first manic episode follows treatment for a depressive disorder in some patients with bipolar disorder.

It is important to discuss with the patient ways in which they can help themselves to recover from depression. If possible, involve their closest relative in the conversation. Key self-help interventions include the following:

- **Increased activity ('behavioural activation').** Depressed patients give up activities and withdraw socially. They therefore become deprived of social stimulation and rewarding experiences, and their depression increases. For most patients, a graded

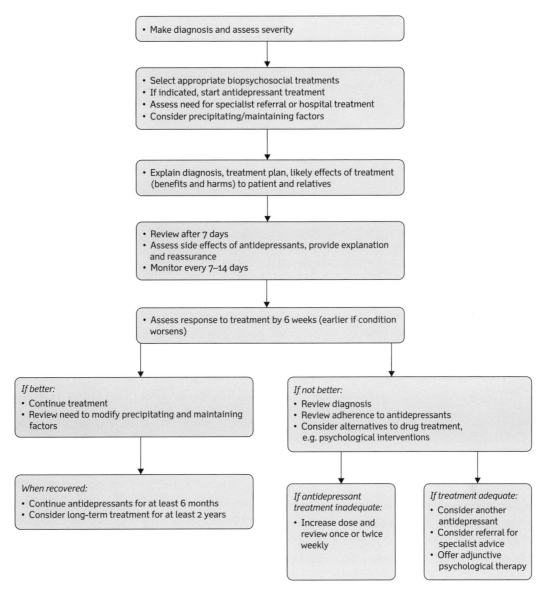

Fig. 21.2 Treatment of depressive disorders.

increase in activity is likely to lead to and consolidate improvement. Activities should include both those that aim to provide enjoyment and those that aim to provide satisfaction. Equally, it is important that patients with more severe depression are not pushed into activities in which they almost inevitably fail because of slowness or poor concentration: it is important to get the balance right.

- **Diet.** Appetite may be diminished, and the patient should be encouraged to eat regularly and healthily. Alcohol should be avoided.

- **Sleep.** Simple advice should be given on how to deal with insomnia, if present (see p. 403). Depressed patients may well be spending an excessive amount of time in bed, and returning to bed in the afternoon to 'catnap'. Time in bed should be restricted to

Table 21.6 Treatment options for depression

All patients presenting with depression	• Full assessment • Psychoeducation • Advice about sleep hygiene (use hypnotics for short periods only) • Active monitoring with early follow-up
Mild depression	• Note: antidepressants are *not* recommended. • Low-intensity psychosocial interventions, e.g. sleep hygiene, regular exercise, befriending services • Low-intensity psychological interventions, e.g. computerized CBT or guided self-help, group CBT • Encourage patient to continue usual activities, including work
Moderate depression	• Antidepressants • High-intensity psychological interventions (CBT, IPT, behavioural activation) • May need referral to secondary care
Severe depression	• Antidepressants • High-intensity psychological interventions • Referral to specialist services • May require: crisis interventions or hospital admission
Severe depression with psychosis, severe self-neglect or risk to life	All of the above, plus: • immediate liaison with specialist care • hospital admission • use of mental health act may be needed • consideration of ECT

appropriate levels, and catnapping discouraged. Specific guidance may be needed.

• **Regular exercise.** There is considerable evidence that physical activity can improve both mood and self-esteem. It is unclear what type of exercise is best, or if it should be undertaken individually, in a group, or with a qualified instructor. Current guidelines suggest at least three sessions of 45 minutes should be undertaken per week, but again the evidence base for these specifics is limited. The potential benefits of exercise to a patient's physical health are an important way in which the mortality gap between people with and without mental illness may be reduced.

Psychological help

Even when not being treated with a specific psychological treatment, all depressed patients require support, encouragement, and repeated explanation that they are suffering from illness not moral failure. When the depressive disorder appears to have been precipitated by life problems, discussion and problem-solving counselling may be required. However, when the depressive disorder is severe, consideration of problems may increase hopelessness, or the patient's poor concentration may prevent meaningful discussion. In that situation, problems should be reconsidered when the mood improves.

Is psychiatric referral appropriate?

Moderately severe depression is usually treated by non-specialists, for example, GPs. However, it is essential to consider in every case whether psychiatric referral is required (Box 21.2) and, if so, whether the referral should be for outpatient treatment, or hospital admission.

Box 21.2 Referral for specialist advice

- In all severe and some moderately severe cases, especially when there is a substantial risk of suicide or harm to the welfare or life of another person (particularly dependent children)
- When the diagnosis is in doubt
- When a patient has failed to respond to antidepressant treatment
- When day- or inpatient care is required
- When intensive CBT may be required

Is hospital care needed?

In deciding the need for hospitalization, consideration is given to:

- the severity and risk to the self and to others, especially to any dependent children;
- the patient's ability to look after themselves;
- the availability of social support (a patient living alone may need hospital care for a disorder that could be treated at home if there was a supportive family member who could be present day and night.)

Should the patient remain at work?

When the disorder is more severe, retardation, poor concentration, and lack of drive are likely to impair performance, and this failure may add to feelings of hopelessness. Sometimes, poor performance at work may endanger other people, and when the potential for such danger is great (as in the case of driving a heavy goods vehicle), the patient should not work even if the risk of failure is small. In larger employers, an occupational health department may support a patient to remain in work by making adjustments, and facilitate their return to work as they recover.

Specific treatments for depressive disorder

Antidepressant drug treatment

Antidepressant drugs are effective for most patients with a depressive disorder of at least moderate severity, and particularly those with 'biological' symptoms. Their potential for adverse effects, and relative lack of evidence of effectiveness in mild depression, justify their use only in moderate and severe (rather than mild) depressive episodes, and also in long-term preventative 'maintenance' treatment. A history of previous response to medication and severe symptoms both suggest a good response to treatment. No single antidepressant is clearly more effective than another. The choice for a particular patient depends on:

- response to any previous antidepressant medication;
- specific illness features;
- adverse effects;
- concurrent medical illnesses;
- concurrent medication;
- toxicity in overdose;
- cost.

There are five main groups of antidepressant drugs (see Table 13.4 in Chapter 13):

- **SSRIs** including fluoxetine, paroxetine, sertraline, citalopram (both enantiomers), escitalopram (active enantiomer only). They have specific serotonin uptake-blocking effects. SSRIs are generally well tolerated, being a little better tolerated overall than tricyclic antidepressants. Common side effects include nausea, agitation, insomnia, and sexual dysfunction. They are relatively safe in overdose. Network meta-analyses have suggested that while only minor differences in efficacy exist between the SSRIs, overall sertraline and citalopram have the best profiles of efficacy and safety. SSRIs are the first-line choice of antidepressant.

- **SNRIs** including venlafaxine and duloxetine. They block both 5-HT and noradrenaline reuptake. There is evidence that venlafaxine is more effective than some SSRIs, but is more likely to cause adverse effects. SNRIs are particularly associated with hypertension. They are not recommended for first-line use due to poorer tolerance and higher toxicity in overdose.

- **Tricyclic antidepressants** (imipramine, amitriptyline, dosulepin) were standard first-line therapy until about 1990 when the SSRIs were introduced. They are now much less frequently prescribed, largely due to their high toxicity in overdose. These drugs are slightly more effective in severe depressive disorders than SSRIs, but less well tolerated. They have a range of adverse effects, and anticholinergic symptoms are frequently the reason why patients stop taking these drugs. The main hazards are in patients who have heart disease, glaucoma, prostatic hypertrophy, or epilepsy.

- **Mirtazapine** is an atypical antidepressant which is commonly prescribed due to its unique combination of properties. It is an effective antidepressant, is relatively safe in overdose, is relatively non-cardiotoxic, and has other properties which may be of use in specific settings, including being sedating, antipruritic, and antiemetic. The main adverse effects are appetite stimulation (leading to weight gain) and oversedation.

- **MAOIs** (e.g. phenelzine, tranylcypromine, and moclobemide) **and reversible inhibitors of monoamine oxidase (RIMAs)** (moclobemide) are generally less effective than tricyclics for severe depressive disorders, but some patients with less severe disorders with atypical features (see p. 261) respond better to MAOIs than other drugs. MAOIs potentiate the effects of naturally occurring pressor amines including tyramine, found in some common foods (see p. 145), and of synthetic amines used as decongestants and vasoconstrictors. These interactions can cause dangerous increases in blood pressure. Although these reactions can be avoided by careful choice of diet and by avoiding prescription of synthetic amines, prescription is generally only by specialists and for patients with treatment resistance or atypical depression. The reversible MAOI, moclobemide, is less likely to cause a tyramine reaction than the conventional MAOI drugs.

Treatment with more than one drug may be useful when patients have not responded to monotherapy, although there is limited evidence. In many cases, trying another drug (e.g. another SSRI or a different tricyclic) is the best first option. Combinations of drugs are more likely to lead to interactions and adverse effects and

should generally be initiated by a specialist, used cautiously and monitored carefully. The current UK recommended combination treatments are:

- an SSRI, SNRI, or tricyclic plus mirtazapine (these can usually be initiated in primary care);
- any antidepressant plus lithium (see Chapter 13, p. 147);
- any antidepressant plus a low dose of an atypical antipsychotic.

Electroconvulsive therapy

ECT is described more comprehensively on p. 151. The antidepressant action of ECT is quicker than that of antidepressant drugs, but it causes more adverse effects, especially impairment of short-term memory. For these reasons, ECT is mainly used to treat severe depressive illness when:

- depressive disorder has **not responded** to several adequate trials of different antidepressant drugs (by adequate is meant at adequate dose, for at least 6 weeks, and with high levels of compliance);
- **rapid response is necessary** because of high suicidal risk, untreatable severe distress, or severe psychomotor retardation with failure to eat and drink.

Psychological treatment

CBT (see p. 163) is effective in the treatment of mild and moderate depressive illness, and may also prevent relapse. In moderate depressive episodes, it is as effective as antidepressants, and patients should therefore be offered a choice of physical (antidepressant) or psychological (CBT) treatment. CBT is increasingly available in England due to the IAPT programme, in which CBT is 'scaled' via self-help, computer-assisted, or group interventions. CBT for depression has two core elements: **behavioural activation**, in which patients are encouraged to plan and engage in more activities that are enjoyable or satisfying; and **cognitive retraining**, in which patients identify and challenge negative automatic thoughts, and practise replacing them with more realistic thoughts.

Supportive and problem-solving treatments. All depressed patients and their families need supportive care to sustain them until improvement takes place. Persistent interpersonal problems maintain depression and problem-solving can resolve the difficulties.

Interpersonal psychotherapy (IPT) (see p. 159) is a standardized form of brief psychotherapy that focuses on improving the patient's interpersonal functioning and identifying the problems associated with the onset and maintenance of depression.

Dynamic psychotherapy. Although depressed patients often express guilt and regrets about experiences in their recent or remote past, these feelings generally resolve as mood improves and there is no good evidence that dynamic psychotherapy speeds this process. Indeed, it is generally better not to dwell on past events in the early stages of treatment for this may only increase the patient's guilty introspection.

Failure to respond to treatment

Around 30 per cent of patients with a depressive disorder do not respond within 6 weeks to a combination of antidepressant drugs, graded activity, and psychological treatment. In these cases, the treatment plan should be reviewed at 6 weeks and earlier in severe cases (Box 21.3). It is important to reassure the patient that they will almost invariably eventually recover.

Box 21.3 Lack of response to antidepressant treatment

- Review diagnosis (are you missing alcohol/substances/physical disorder/personality factors/other psychiatric disorder?)
- Check compliance with treatment
- Review psychosocial stressors
- Increase antidepressant dose to maximum
- Consider change of antidepressant
- Obtain specialist opinion concerning need for hospital admission and further treatment[a]
- Combined drug treatment[a]
- Consider ECT[a]

[a] These steps usually require a specialist opinion (see text).

Continuation therapy

The continuation phase of treatment focuses on maintaining the improvement during the first 6 months or so following the successful treatment of the acute phase. After recovery from a depressive disorder, the patient should be followed up for several months either by the family doctor or by a psychiatrist. At this stage, it is often valuable to discuss possible precipitants of the illness with the patient and also in joint interviews with close relatives. This discussion is particularly important when there have been repeated depressive disorders provoked by life events.

Some residual symptoms may take several months to disappear and many patients are particularly vulnerable to relapse during this period. With antidepressant medicines, the same dose of the successful treatment should be continued during the continuation phase. Patients will need encouragement to continue with treatment, deal with any adverse effects, and advice about the appropriate level of activity and about returning to work.

Prevention of relapse

Maintenance medication. Patients who have responded to acute-phase treatment, remained well during the continuation phase, and are at moderate or high risk of relapse (e.g. those with a history of relapse relatively soon after successful treatment of depression, or on the ending of continuation therapy) will benefit from long-term therapy for at least 2 years with antidepressants at the same dose that was effective in the acute phase. Long-term drug treatment will halve the risk of relapse.

Cognitive therapy (see p. 163) may also reduce the relapse rate after a moderately severe depressive disorder but there is less evidence than for drug maintenance. Cognitive therapy is sometimes tried for patients who have repeated episodes of depression despite maintenance medication, and apparently related to depressive forms of thinking.

Life changes. If the depressive disorder was clearly related to stressors such as overwork or complicated social relationships, the patient should be helped to address these factors.

Recognizing early signs of relapse. It can also be helpful to have a written, agreed care plan should depressive symptoms recur. The patient should be fully involved in this process by being helped to understand the risk of relapse, taught to recognize warning signs, and agreeing an appropriate action plan. When appropriate, the patient's relatives should be involved.

Bipolar disorder

Bipolar disorder (bipolar affective disorder, manic depressive disorder) is characterized by unusually high variability of mood, with periods of **both** elation and depression which significantly impair function. Bipolar disorder comprises a wide spectrum of illnesses, and can be thought of as part of a continuum of mood abnormalities (Fig. 21.1). It is, in essence, an intensification of the mood variability that we all experience, due to a relative lack of the homeostatic mechanisms that keep mood stable. It is a relatively common condition (see p. 260), and the 12-month prevalence and lifetime risks are very similar; this relates to the chronicity of the disorder.

The diagnostic criteria for bipolar disorder are potentially confusing, as the ICD-10 does not subcategorize (although this will change in the ICD-11), whereas the DSM-5 includes subcategories of bipolar 1 and bipolar 2 under the broad term of bipolar disorders. The current ICD-10 definition of bipolar disorder is:

- two or more episodes of mood disorder, at least one of which must have been of low mood (depression) and the other of elevated mood (hypomania, mania, or mixed).

It is expected that the ICD-11 will come into line with the DSM-5; the online beta-draft currently has the following definitions (accessed September 2017):

- Bipolar type 1 disorder: an episodic mood disorder in which at least one manic or mixed episode has occurred, with or without episodes of depression.

- Bipolar type 2 disorder: an episodic mood disorder in which one or more hypomanic episodes AND at least one depressive episode have occurred.

Mania

The central features of the syndrome of mania are elation or irritability, increased activity, self-important ideas, poor judgement, and disinhibition (Table 21.7). It is important that abnormal mood elevation is recognized in its early stages because in the later stages the patient becomes increasingly unwilling to accept treatment. Most manic patients can exert some control over their symptoms for a short time. Many do so when the interviewer is assessing the need for treatment, with the result that the severity of the disorder may be underestimated. For this reason it is important, whenever possible, to interview an informant as well as the patient.

Clinical patterns

- **Hypomania.** This term refers to a state in which manic symptoms are present and noticeable, but they do not cause a serious degree of functional impairment.

- **Mild mania.** Physical activity and speech are increased; mood is labile, mainly euphoric but at times irritable; ideas are expansive, the patient often spends more than he can afford. By definition, there is significant social impairment in this and the other patterns of mania.

- **Moderate mania.** There is marked overactivity with pressure and disorganization of speech; the euphoric mood is increasingly interrupted by periods of irritability, hostility, and depression; and grandiose and other preoccupations may become delusional.

- **Severe mania.** There is frenzied overactivity; thinking is incoherent and delusions become increasingly bizarre; hallucinations are experienced. Very rarely, however, the patient becomes immobile and mute instead of overactive and talkative (manic stupor).

Table 21.7 Clinical features of mania

Appearance and behaviour	• May be inappropriately dressed or wear bright clothing and make-up. Can become dishevelled as mood deteriorates • Overactivity—*sometimes to the point of exhaustion* • Socially inappropriate behaviour (e.g. overfamiliarity) • Increased appetite—*although overactive patients may be too busy to eat regularly* • Increased libido • Risky behaviours: overspending, dangerous driving, risky business decisions, use of substances, sexual promiscuity, neglect of self or dependents
Speech	• Fast (pressurized), copious, and loud
Mood	• Elation or euphoria • Irritability
Thoughts	• Racing thoughts • Loosening of associations and flight of ideas • Grandiose or expansive ideas—*patients have ideas which they believe are original or important. They may attempt to embark on outrageous or impractical schemes* • Delusions: paranoid, religious, or grandiose
Perceptions	• Hallucinations—*usually mood congruent, e.g. a voice telling the patient how special they are or confirming their paranoid beliefs*
Cognition and insight	• Poor concentration, distractibility—*patients tend to start activities and fail to complete them* • Impaired insight

Mixed, alternating, and rapid cycling states

In a **mixed** mood state, manic and depressive symptoms occur together, at the same time. For example, an overactive and overtalkative patient may have profound depressive thoughts including suicidal ideas. Mixed states are associated with the highest risk of suicide, as the combination of depressive cognitions and manic energy levels can lead to impulsivity.

In an **alternating** mood state, mania and depression follow one another in a sequence of rapid changes. Thus, a manic patient may be intensely depressed for a few hours and then quickly become manic.

In **rapid cycling** disorder, states of mania and depression follow one another regularly with intervals of a few weeks between them. There need to be four or more mood episodes (depressive, manic, or mixed) in a 12-month period.

Differential diagnosis of manic disorders

Manic disorders have to be distinguished from the following:

• **Schizophrenia.** The diagnosis from schizophrenia can be challenging. In manic disorders, auditory hallucinations and delusions can occur, including some delusions that are characteristic of schizophrenia such as delusions of reference. However, in mania, these symptoms usually change quickly in content, are mood congruent, and seldom outlast the overactivity. In schizophrenia, the delusions are typically more static and may be bizarre and mood incongruent. When there is a more or less equal mixture of features of the two syndromes, the term 'schizoaffective' is used. These conditions are discussed further in Chapter 22.

- **Dementia** should always be considered, especially in middle-aged or older patients with expansive behaviour and no past history of affective disorder. In the absence of gross mood disorder, extreme social disinhibition (e.g. urinating in public) strongly suggests frontal lobe pathology. In such cases, appropriate neurological investigation is essential.

- **Endocrine disorders.** Hyperthyroid states may cause symptoms suggestive of mania. Physical signs of elevated thyroid should be sought and blood levels of thyroid hormones estimated.

- **Abuse of stimulant drugs.** The distinction between mania and excited behaviour due to abuse of amphetamines depends on the history together with examination of the urine for drugs before treatment with psychotropic drugs is started. Drug-induced states usually subside quickly once the patient is in hospital and free from the drugs (see Chapter 29).

Bipolar depression

The features of bipolar depression are fundamentally the same as a unipolar depressive episode. It is important to examine the mental state fully to look for features of mania that would suggest a mixed state. Bipolar depression can be severe and difficult to treat, and carries a higher risk of suicide than a standalone unipolar depressive episode.

Course and prognosis of bipolar disorders

Bipolar disorders usually begin in the first half of life, 90 per cent starting before the age of 50 years. They run a recurring course with recovery between episodes of illness. Each episode generally lasts several months—on average about 3 months. Most patients experience depressive as well as manic episodes, but a few have only manic episodes. Untreated, epidemiology suggests that bipolar patients will experience approximately ten major mood episodes in their lifetime. Some patients will return to their usual mood and their previous level of functioning between episodes, while others will not. Recent research suggests it is very common for patients to have considerable mood instability (subclinical mood variation over short time periods) over the long term.

Suicide is substantially more frequent among patients with bipolar disorder than among the general population. Fifty per cent of patients with bipolar disorder will attempt suicide during their lifetime, with rates of completed suicide at approximately 10 per cent. The highest risk for suicide is during a mixed episode or a severe depressive episode, but patients coming to terms with their lifelong illness during a period of normal mood are also at risk.

Aetiology of bipolar disorder

As with all psychiatric disorders, the aetiology of bipolar disorder is a complex interaction between biological, psychological, and social factors. However, bipolar disorder is among the most heritable conditions (estimated at 70 per cent), with genetic load making up the greatest part of an individual's risk. Many of the psychosocial risk factors are the same as for unipolar depression (Table 21.4). Biological factors in the aetiology of bipolar disorder include the following:

1 Genetics:
   - Heritability estimated to be approximately 70 per cent.
   - Lifetime risk of bipolar disorder in first-degree relative is 5–10 per cent.
   - Monozygotic concordance for bipolar disorder is 60–70 per cent, versus 5–10 per cent in dizygotic twins.

2 Paternal age: sixfold greater risk of bipolar in offspring of fathers over 45 years.

3 Neuroimaging:
   - Neuroimaging has consistently shown smaller grey matter total volumes in bipolar disorder.
   - Inconsistent reports of abnormalities in prefrontal cortex and limbic system.

4 Inflammation: markers of inflammation are increased in bipolar disorder, although the significance of this is unknown.

5 Medications: prescribed medications (e.g. corticosteroids, antiretrovirals, thyroxine, l-dopa) or illicit substances (stimulants, anabolic steroids) may all trigger mania. The pathogenesis of this is not understood. In some patients with undiagnosed bipolar disorder, antidepressants prescribed for low mood may trigger a mood elevation.

Management of bipolar disorder

Assessment

The assessment of a depressive episode in a patient with bipolar disorder is essentially the same as the assessment of a unipolar depressive episode (described earlier), although the treatment is different as described here.

The assessment of a manic patient may need the help of a specialist. In the assessment of mania, the steps are those already outlined for depressive disorders. They are (1) decide the diagnosis, (2) assess the severity of the disorder, (3) form an opinion about the causes, (4) assess the patient's social resources, and (5) judge the effect on other people.

Diagnosis depends on a careful history and examination. Whenever possible, the history should be taken from relatives as well as from the patient because the patient seldom recognizes the full extent of the abnormal behaviour. Differential diagnosis has been discussed earlier in this chapter; it is important to remember that mildly disinhibited behaviour can result from intoxication with drugs or alcohol or, rarely, from frontal lobe lesion causes (e.g. by a cerebral neoplasm).

The severity and the degree of psychosocial dysfunction should be carefully considered because this has important implications for diagnosis (e.g. for discriminating between hypomania and mania, see p. 276) and management. For this purpose, it is essential to interview an informant. Manic patients are able to exert a degree of self-control during an interview with a doctor, and then behave in a more disinhibited and grandiose way immediately afterwards (see p. 276). At an early stage of the disorder, it is easy to be misled by patients in this way and to miss the opportunity to persuade them to enter hospital before causing difficulties for themselves, for example, through ill-judged decisions at work or unaffordable extravagance.

A full risk assessment should be undertaken, taking into consideration:

● deliberate risk to self: suicide;

● accidental risk to self: self-neglect, accidents (e.g. while driving), use of substances, unfortunate incidents in the workplace;

● risks to others: getting into arguments, neglect of dependents, risks while driving, occupational risks (teachers, care workers, assembly line workers);

● undesirable results of risky behaviours: sexually transmitted diseases, pregnancy, overspending;

● risks from others: vulnerability, potential to irritate others accidentally leading to assaults.

The general treatment of bipolar disorder can be divided into two phases:

1 Treatment of an acute mood episode (depression or mania).

2 Maintenance treatment to promote mood stability.

Acute treatment of mania

General aspects of the treatment of mania

Treatment for mania must be started quickly, without delay, due to the likelihood of serious personal and social consequences following errors of judgement that are characteristic of the disorder. Milder manic episodes (hypomania) may be treated as an outpatient, but more severe disorders with associated loss of judgement will almost always need initial treatment as an inpatient. When the disorder is more severe, compulsory admission is likely to be needed.

During treatment, a careful watch should be kept for the appearance of depressive symptoms because transient but profound depressive mood change and depressive ideas are common among manic patients. Also, the clinical picture may change rapidly from mania to a sustained depressive disorder. In either case, suicidal ideas may appear. A sustained change to a depressive syndrome may require treatment, including with antidepressant drugs which should be used cautiously to avoid precipitation of a manic relapse. Following recovery, regular follow-up is necessary to detect relapse into mania or the onset of depression. Patients should be helped to deal with or to come to terms with any precipitating causes of the episode, and with the consequences of any ill-judged actions during the acute illness.

Specific treatments for mania

The pharmacological treatment of mania is outlined in Fig. 21.3. In the vast majority of patients, antidepressants should be stopped as they may aggravate a manic episode.

Antipsychotic drugs

An atypical antipsychotic such as olanzapine, quetiapine, or risperidone is the first-choice treatment. First-generation antipsychotics such as haloperidol

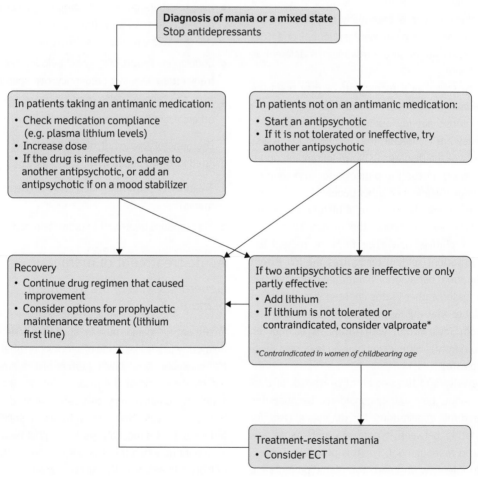

Fig. 21.3 Treatment of mania.

are effective but may be less well tolerated. Doses may need to be titrated to achieve a full therapeutic effect. In the early stages, a regular dose of a short-acting benzodiazepine (e.g. lorazepam) may be needed to help promote sleep and control behaviour.

Lithium

Lithium is effective in mania, but less so than anti-psychotic drugs and it can be very difficult to use safely in severely disturbed patients. The effect in mania may take several days to begin. Lithium is therefore used mainly in patients with milder manic episodes, or those who are already taking it for prophylaxis. The advantage is that lithium can then be continued long term for maintenance. The plasma range to aim for in mania is 0.8–1.0 mmol/litre, higher than prophylaxis. This needs careful monitoring. Lithium is also a useful adjunct to an antipsychotic.

Antiepileptic drugs

Valproate is effective in acute mania, but similarly to lithium takes a few days to begin working. It is slightly less effective than antipsychotics, but causes fewer adverse effects. Thus, it may be particularly useful in patients who are not currently taking a long-term mood stabilizer, and who have a mild manic illness without psychotic features. However, it is contraindicated in women of childbearing age.

Electroconvulsive therapy

Although there is no evidence from randomized trials, clinical experience indicates that ECT has a powerful therapeutic effect in mania. Nevertheless, ECT is not a first-line treatment; its use is mainly in the uncommon cases when antipsychotic drugs are ineffective and the patient is so seriously disturbed that to spend time trying further medication or awaiting natural recovery is not justified (see p. 151).

Treatment of acute bipolar depression

Depressive episodes cause more disability then manic episodes in most people with bipolar disorder. The general aspects of treatment are the same as those described previously for unipolar depression, but there are important differences in both the effectiveness of treatments and the risks associated with treatment. The aim is to return mood to euthymia without accidentally tipping the patient into hypomania or mania. In many patients, mood stabilizers or an antipsychotic with some mood-stabilizing properties can be used to achieve this, without the need for antidepressants. However, while a risk of a 'manic switch' is present when using an antidepressant alone in bipolar disorder, if it is combined with antimanic medication this risk is considerably reduced. Psychological treatments are helpful for promoting long-term recovery and prevention of relapse. In the UK, the current suggested options for treating bipolar depression are shown in Table 21.8.

Treatment of mixed episodes

Manic symptoms usually predominate over depressive symptoms in mixed states and treatment of mixed states is therefore usually the treatment of a manic episode, with antipsychotics alone or in combination with a mood stabilizer. Mood stabilizers may also be used alone. Antidepressants should not be used when manic symptoms predominate, although may be used when depressive symptoms are prominent.

Maintenance therapy

Bipolar disorder has a strong tendency to relapse. Following the first severe episode of mania, the risk of a serious manic relapse occurring in any year is about 10–20 per cent. The risk is greater when patients have suffered multiple previous episodes—for example, after three previous episodes, the annual risk of relapse is about 20–30 per cent. For this reason, long-term prophylactic treatment is strongly recommended. Long-term active management substantially reduces the risk of relapse. Such management includes both pharmacological management and non-pharmacological management (Table 21.9).

Table 21.8 Management of bipolar depression

Pharmacological treatments	
Patients not already on long-term treatment	• Quetiapine • Olanzapine (± fluoxetine) • Lamotrigine • Lithium • Valproate[a] • Antidepressant + mood stabilizer or antipsychotic
Patients already taking long-term treatment	• Check compliance • Increase dose of medication • Add lithium or an antipsychotic if not already taking.
Refractory depression	• Antipsychotic plus lithium and valproate[a] • ECT
Rapid cycling bipolar disorder	• Lithium plus valproate[a]
Psychological treatments	• Psychoeducation • CBT or IPT

[a] Valproate is contraindicated in women of childbearing age.

Pharmacological management

There are several available drug treatments and the choice will depend on patient preference, adverse effects (including risks in women of childbearing age), and previous response to treatment (Table 21.9). Antidepressants should be avoided long term in bipolar disorder.

Lithium

Lithium is the first-line choice. It has the strongest evidence base for both preventing recurrence of manic or depressive episodes, and reduces the risk of suicide. The benefits outweigh the risks of adverse events for most patients who are at least at moderate risk of relapse (those with three or more previous episodes, very severe previous episodes, or a strong family history of recurrent bipolar disorder). As the therapeutic index of lithium is low, it needs careful monitoring (see p. 147). If lithium is only partly effective, then the addition of valproate (especially in rapid-cycling illnesses) or an antipsychotic may be helpful. If lithium is not tolerated or contraindicated,

then the other options outlined in Table 21.9 should be considered.

Non-pharmacological management

Non-drug approaches are not an optional addition to pharmacological management; they should be at the core of every patient's management plan.

Lifestyle management

Everyone's mood responds to environmental/lifestyle factors. People with bipolar disorder are especially sensitive to such factors, and so they need careful consideration in the management plan.

Relevant factors:

• **Sleep.** Standard recommendations include a regular sleep–wake pattern, going to bed at a similar time, and getting up at a similar time, even at weekends. Shift work should be avoided if possible (this may mean involving occupational health), as a week of 'nights' may trigger a manic episode. Remember that, in people with mood disorder,

Table 21.9 Long-term maintenance treatment of bipolar disorder

Pharmacological interventions	
First line	Lithium
Second line (if lithium is not tolerated or ineffective)	Valproate[a]
	Lithium and valproate (if lithium only partly effective)
	Olanzapine or quetiapine
Third line	Lithium/valproate plus antipsychotic
	Lamotrigine
	Carbamazepine
Psychological interventions	• Psychoeducation of patient and carers about bipolar disorder, risk of relapse, and identification of early warning signs
	• Individual mood monitoring
	• Family therapy if appropriate
	• Individual CBT for bipolar disorder
Social interventions	• Housing, appropriate daytime activities, finances

[a] Contraindicated in women of childbearing age.

sleep may function as a depressant, and so consider limiting time in bed for people with depression, and increasing time in bed for people with emergent elation/hypomania.

- **Work.** Employment with regular hours provides important benefits, due to the structure of daily work, and the sense of purpose and social contact associated with it.

- **Socialization.** Regular contact with other people, at work, at home or in leisure activities. If the person's mood is low, socialization should be increased; if the person's mood is high, socialization may need to be managed or reduced.

- **Compliance.** Keep taking prescribed drugs, and especially mood stabilizers, even when mood is in the normal range. Possible changes should be discussed with and agreed by a healthcare professional who knows the patient well, before being implemented.

- **Exercise.** Regularly, independent of mood.

- **Street drugs.** To be avoided, due to their unpredictable effect on mood.

- **Alcohol.** To be used either not at all, or within accepted limits.

Mood monitoring

This is an important, and core, part of the long-term management of mood disorders and, especially, bipolar disorder. The patient records their mood, each day or each week, either on paper or, increasingly, in an electronic format. Mood monitoring has several benefits, including (1) improved communication with clinicians about the person's mood, over a period of weeks, months or years (the patient has a contemporaneous record, rather than relying on their memory); (2) regular prompts to the patient to assess their mood, leading to improved recognition of early signs of relapse; and (3) helping the patient to understand how environmental/lifestyle factors influence their mood. If an electronic system is used, symptom data can be shared effortlessly with a key clinician and a key relative, so that mood management is a genuinely shared endeavour.

True Colours® is an effective electronic system. The patient is prompted, usually each week but more frequently if necessary, to record their mood. They receive an email message or a text message, with reminder messages if required. If they have bipolar disorder, they complete both a depression measure (the 16-item QIDS-SR scale) and a mania measure (the five-item Altman SRM scale). The patient's responses are automatically saved in a secure database. Over time, copious data become available to help the patient, their carer(s) and their family to understand both the nature of their mood variability and the factors that influence it. These data are available online in an easy-to-use graphical format, which allows those viewing to look at a graph of mood fluctuations over long periods of time (e.g. 2–3 years) or shorter periods (e.g. 2–3 months). Further information on how patients use True Colours® is available at https://truecolours. nhs.uk/demo/documents/PatientGuide.pdf.

Education to recognize early signs of relapse

Many patients develop characteristic prodromal symptoms before a relapse (see Box 21.4). These patients can be helped to recognize these symptoms and given an agreed plan of action to use when the prodromal signs occur. This approach can help patients avoid manic episodes but it is less certain that it helps avoid depressive episodes.

Psychological treatments

Family therapy can help prevent relapse. The evidence that cognitive therapy prevents relapse in bipolar

Box 21.4 Common early warning signs of manic relapse

- Reduced need for sleep
- Increased physical activity
- Racing thoughts
- Elated mood
- Irritability or rage if plans or wishes are not satisfied
- Unrealistic plans
- Overspending
- Increased drinking or street drug use
- Reduced compliance with medication

disorder is equivocal. The most important psychological treatment is psychoeducation, delivered in a group or individually, which addresses medication issues, lifestyle factors, mood monitoring, and the identification of and response to early warning signs of relapse.

Mood disorders in pregnancy and following childbirth

Mood disorders are common during pregnancy and the first postnatal year. While postnatal depression is routinely screened for in many countries, antenatal (prenatal) depression is less well appreciated. Psychotic symptoms in pregnancy are usually due to a pre-existing illness, but new symptoms or a postnatal psychosis are strongly linked to bipolar disorder. Any mood disorder carries significant risks to mother and baby, so prompt diagnosis and the starting of appropriate treatment is essential. The majority of women will need referral into specialist services for advice on the use of medications during pregnancy and breastfeeding. Suicidal thoughts, or thoughts to harm the baby, should be discussed with every patient each time they are seen.

Antenatal depression

Research consistently reports the prevalence of a depressive episode to be 6–8 per cent of expectant mothers. The symptoms are typical of any depressive episode, but more frequently include ideas of being undeserving of the baby, or the notion that she will be a 'bad mother'. The main risk factors for depression in pregnancy are:

- previous episodes of depression or anxiety;
- unplanned pregnancy;
- multiple life stressors (especially relationship difficulties or financial strain);
- domestic abuse;
- poor social support.

It is unclear exactly what effect depression in the mother may have on the developing fetus. Antenatal depression has been linked to **small** increases in the risk of:

- spontaneous miscarriage;
- bleeding during pregnancy;
- an instrumental delivery or caesarean section;
- premature birth

Mothers who have been depressed during pregnancy (even if they have recovered fully by delivery) are at high risk of developing postnatal depression and should be closely monitored. In mothers with bipolar disorder, there is an increased risk of a bipolar depressive episode or of mania. This is particularly high if the mother decides to stop her maintenance treatment during pregnancy (see later).

Postnatal mood disorders

The postnatal period is generally considered to be the first 12 months after delivery. During this period, 10–20 per cent of mothers will experience a mental disorder, the majority of which are depression or anxiety disorders. As it is a formative time in development of the infant, especially in developing a secure mother–baby attachment, it is very important to detect and treat these mood disorders.

Baby blues

The 'baby blues' is a normal phenomenon occurring in about 70 per cent of mothers. It is self-limiting, usually disappearing within a few days. The main symptoms are irritability, lability of mood, and tearfulness. They peak on the third or fourth postpartum day. Both the frequency of the emotional changes and their timing suggest that maternity 'blues' may be related to re-adjustment in hormones after delivery. No treatment except reassurance and general support is required.

Postnatal depression

Postnatal depression occurs in about 10 per cent of mothers. Two-thirds of cases develop within 12 weeks of delivery and, for some women, their symptoms are a continuation of an episode which began in pregnancy.

As with antenatal depression, the risk factors for postnatal depression are as for any depressive episode, but with some additional factors such as:

- previous depressive episodes or anxiety disorders;
- stressful life events during late pregnancy or after delivery (especially relationship difficulties);
- maternal age less than 25;
- single mothers;
- domestic violence;
- unwanted pregnancy;
- perinatal complications;
- difficulties in establishing breastfeeding;
- difficult infant temperament.

The symptoms are similar to depressive disorder occurring at any other time although tiredness, irritability, and anxiety may be more prominent than depressive mood and there may be prominent phobic symptoms. Symptoms are undoubtedly exacerbated by loss of sleep, and by the hard work involved in looking after the baby. Screening tests such as the Edinburgh Postnatal Depression Scale are helpful at distinguishing depression from transient low mood. Potential adverse consequences of postnatal depression are shown in Table 21.10.

Postnatal psychosis (also known as postpartum psychosis or puerperal psychosis)

Postnatal psychosis is rare, only occurring in about 0.1–0.2 per cent of mothers. It is highly associated with bipolar disorder. The risk of postnatal psychosis in a mother who already has a diagnosis of bipolar disorder is 30–40 per cent, while 50 per cent of those without prior psychiatric history later acquire a diagnosis of bipolar disorder, schizophrenia, or schizoaffective disorder. Risk factors include previous serious major psychiatric disorder, a family history of bipolar/psychosis, and primiparity.

Postnatal psychosis usually begins in the first or second week after delivery. The usual clinical picture is of a severe psychotic mood disorder although

Table 21.10 Potential consequences of postnatal depression

Impact upon baby	Impacts upon mother
• Impaired bonding with mother	• Impaired bonding with infant
• Lower rates of breastfeeding	• Increased rates of relationship discord
• Poorer infant nutrition	• Self-neglect (e.g. poor nutrition)
• Lower rates of childhood vaccinations	• Suicide (rare—1/100,000 live births)
• Higher risk of delayed development	
• Harm to baby/infanticide (very rare)	

confusion and disorientation can lend an organic 'flavour' to the clinical picture. About one-third of patients have delusions about their baby, although it is rare that these pose a threat to the baby. More common is paranoia about the baby's safety, which can lead to the mother preventing other people (e.g. health professionals) from getting adequate access to the infant.

A careful risk assessment should be undertaken, considering mother, baby, and any other dependents. The greatest risks are of self-neglect and/or accidental neglect of the infant or other children. Risks of suicide and infanticide are considerably increased, but remain objectively low. Recurrence of psychosis after subsequent deliveries is high, and family/professionals should monitor the mother closely in the postnatal period.

Management of mood disorders in pregnancy and following childbirth

The general principles of management are the same as for any other patient, but the following should be taken into account:

- Low threshold for referral into specialist services.
- Assessment should exclude an antenatal/postnatal complication leading to an organic cause or exacerbating factor for the symptoms (e.g. anaemia, pain, etc.).
- Careful consideration of risks to the fetus/child.
- Close cooperation between primary care, midwives, health visitors, and psychiatric services. Social services may need to be involved if there is a risk to mother or child.
- The family may need additional support with childcare, especially for older siblings.
- If admission to hospital is necessary (e.g. for psychosis, self-neglect, severe depression, thoughts of harm to baby) then a referral to a mother and baby unit should be made if possible, where mother and baby can be nursed together.
- Use of medications is often needed, but advice should be taken about the best choice to limit risks to the fetus/infant.

Medications

While it would be preferable to not expose the fetus or infant to medications, in many cases the risks posed by the mother's mood disorder outweigh the potential risks to the baby. These need to be carefully weighed up for each individual. No drug has been shown to be completely safe in pregnancy or during breastfeeding.

- **Antidepressants.** Sertraline is the first-line choice during pregnancy and breastfeeding, but the other SSRIs also have a good safety and tolerance record. Tricyclics (imipramine or amitriptyline) were used historically, but are less well tolerated.
- **Sedatives.** Use non-pharmacological approaches where possible. Benzodiazepines should be avoided (risk of dependence, risk of cleft lip/palate), but Z-drugs may be used in low doses short term.

- **Antipsychotics.** Atypicals (olanzapine, quetiapine, risperidone) are the first-line choice. Olanzapine has the largest evidence base for safety during pregnancy and breastfeeding.
- **Mood stabilizers.** Sodium valproate is contraindicated during preconception and pregnancy due to a risk of congenital malformations. Lithium may be used in pregnancy, but there is probably a small risk (<1/1000) of heart defects in the fetus. If the risk of major mood episodes in the mother is high if lithium is discontinued, it may be best for mother and baby to continue it, with close monitoring of plasma levels throughout pregnancy. Breastfeeding is not advised when taking lithium.

Further reading

Cleare A, Pariante CM, Young AH, et al. Evidence-based guidelines for treating depressive disorders with antidepressants: a revision of the 2008 British Association for Psychopharmacology guidelines. *Journal of Psychopharmacology* 2015;29:459–525.

Goodwin GM, Haddad PM, Ferrier IN, et al. Evidence-based guidelines for treating bipolar disorder: revised third edition recommendations from the British Association for Psychopharmacology. *Journal of Psychopharmacology* 2016;30:495–553.

McAllister-Williams RH, Baldwin DS, Cantwell R, et al. British Association for Psychopharmacology consensus guidance on the use of psychotropic medication preconception, in pregnancy and postpartum. *Journal of Psychopharmacology* 2017;31:519–552.

National Institute for Health and Care Excellence. Bipolar disorder: assessment and management. Clinical guideline [CG185]. Published September 2014, updated April 2018. https://www.nice.org.uk/guidance/cg185.

National Institute for Health and Care Excellence. Depression: in adults: recognition and management. Clinical guideline [CG90]. Published October 2009, updated April 2018. https://www.nice.org.uk/guidance/cg90.

Risch N, Herrell R, Lehner T, et al. Interaction between the serotonin transporter gene (5-HTTLPR), stressful life events, and risk of depression: a meta-analysis. *JAMA* 2009;301:2462–2471.

22 Schizophrenia and related psychotic disorders

Schizophrenia and related disorders are a group of conditions characterized by psychotic symptoms which lead to impairments in thinking, feelings, behaviour, and social interactions. There is a spectrum of severity. In **schizophrenia**, the patient suffers from both psychotic symptoms and functional impairment. In **delusional disorders**, the patient experiences delusions, but there is no evidence of hallucinations and their functional level may remain normal.

Schizophrenia can be a particularly disabling illness because its course, although variable, is frequently chronic and relapsing. The care of patients with schizophrenia places a considerable burden on all carers, from the patient's family through to the health and social services. GPs may have only a few patients with chronic schizophrenia on their lists but the severity of their problems and the needs of their families will make these patients important.

This chapter aims to provide sufficient information for the reader to be able to recognize the basic symptoms of schizophrenia and related disorders and to be aware of the main approaches to treatment.

Diagnosis and clinical features

As the clinical presentation and outcome of the disorder vary, schizophrenia can be a confusing illness to understand. It is best to start by considering simplified descriptions of two common presentations: (1) the acute syndrome, and (2) the chronic syndrome. It is then easier to understand the core features as well as the diversity of schizophrenia. In the acute syndrome, the patient **gains** symptoms; they start to have unusual experiences or thoughts they did not previously, and act in bizarre or atypical ways. This is in contrast to the contrast to the chronic syndrome, in which there is a loss of function—the **negative symptoms**.

CASE STUDY BOX 22.1

Acute schizophrenia

A previously healthy 20-year-old male student had been behaving in an increasingly odd way. At times he appeared angry and told his friends that he was being followed by the police and secret services; at other times he was seen to be laughing to himself for no apparent reason. For several months he had spent more time on his own, apparently preoccupied with his own thoughts, and his academic work had deteriorated. When seen by the family doctor he was restless and appeared frightened. He said that he had heard voices commenting on his actions and abusing him. He also said that the police had conspired with his university teachers to harm his brain with poisonous gases and take away his thoughts, and that the police had arranged for items referring to him to be inserted into television programmes.

The acute syndrome (positive symptoms)

The positive symptoms of schizophrenia may appear within a few days, or more insidiously over a period of weeks. A typical presentation is described in Case study box 22.1, and symptoms outlined in Table 22.1. It is not necessary for the patient to have all of these symptoms; they usually have a selection which may change over time.

Appearance and behaviour

Many patients with acute schizophrenia appear entirely normal. Some appear awkward in their social behaviour, preoccupied and withdrawn, or otherwise odd. Others smile or laugh without obvious reason, or appear perplexed by what is happening to them. Some are restless and noisy, and a few show sudden and unexpected changes in behaviour. Others retire from company, spending much of their time alone.

Speech

Speech may be difficult to follow. In the early stages, a patient's talk may be vague so that it is difficult to grasp the meaning. Later, there may be more definite abnormalities (formal thought disorder). These abnormalities are of several kinds. Some patients have difficulty in dealing with abstract ideas (a phenomenon called concrete thinking) while others become preoccupied with vague pseudoscientific or mystical ideas. There may be a lack of connection between the ideas expressed by the patient (loosening of associations). The links between ideas may be illogical, or they may wander from the original theme. In its most extreme form, loosening of association leads to totally incoherent thought and speech (word salad).

Table 22.1 The acute syndrome (positive symptoms)

Appearance and behaviour	Preoccupied, withdrawn, inactive
	Restless, noisy, inconsistent
Mood	Mood change
	Blunting
	Incongruity
Disorders of thinking	Vagueness
	Formal thought disorder
	Disorders of the stream of thought
Hallucinations	Auditory
	Visual
	Tactile, olfactory, gustatory
Delusions	Primary
	Secondary (especially persecutory)
Orientation	Normal
Attention	Impaired
Memory	Normal
Insight	Impaired

Mood

Abnormalities of mood are common. There are three main kinds:

1 Mood change such as depression, anxiety, irritability, or euphoria. Patients are often suspicious or guarded. Depressive symptoms in the acute syndrome may develop in one or more of three ways:

   (a) As an integral part of the disorder—caused by the same processes that cause the other symptoms such as the delusions and hallucinations.

   (b) As a response to insight into the nature of the illness and the problems to be faced.

   (c) As side effects of antipsychotic medication.

2 A reduction in the normal variations of mood, which is called blunting (or flattening) of affect. A patient with this disorder may seem indifferent to others because of unchanging mood.

3 Emotion not in keeping with the situation, a condition known as incongruity of affect. A patient may, for example, laugh when told about the death of his mother.

Abnormalities of the form and content of thought

There may be disorders of the stream of thought, such as pressure of thought, poverty of thought, and thought blocking (all of which are described on p. 37).

Delusions occur commonly in schizophrenia. Primary delusions (see p. 39) occur occasionally and when present are important because they occur seldom in other disorders and are therefore of value in diagnosis. Most delusions are secondary, that is, they arise from a previous mental change. Delusions may be preceded by so-called delusional mood (see p. 40), which is seldom found in conditions other than schizophrenia, or by hallucinations. Several kinds of delusion occur. Persecutory delusions are common, but not specific to schizophrenia. Less common but of greater diagnostic value are delusions of reference (false beliefs that objects, events, or people have a special personal significance, see p. 41), delusions of control (the feeling of being controlled by an outside agency, see p. 41), and delusions about the possession of thought (the idea that thoughts are being inserted into or withdrawn from the person's mind, or 'broadcast' to other people, see p. 42).

Perception

Patients with schizophrenia may have any type of perceptual abnormality (p. 44). **Auditory hallucinations** are among the most frequent symptoms of schizophrenia. They may be experienced as simple noises or complex sounds of voices or music. Voices may utter single words, brief phrases, or whole conversations. The voices may seem to give commands to the patient. A voice may speak the patient's thoughts aloud, either as he thinks them or immediately afterwards. Sometimes, two or more voices may seem to discuss the patient in the third person. Other voices may comment on his actions. As explained later, these last three symptoms have particular diagnostic value (see p. 294).

In schizophrenia, **visual hallucinations** are less frequent than auditory ones, and seldom occur without other kinds of hallucination. A few patients experience **tactile**, **olfactory**, **gustatory**, and **somatic** hallucinations, which are often interpreted in a delusional way; for example, hallucinatory sensations in the lower abdomen may be attributed to unwanted sexual interference by a persecutor.

Cognition

In the acute phase, cognition is usually relatively normal, although attention may be impaired. Patients are often preoccupied or distracted by their hallucinations and delusions.

Insight

Insight is usually impaired. Most patients do not accept that their experiences result from illness, often ascribing them instead to the malevolent actions of other people. This lack of insight is often accompanied

---

CASE STUDY BOX 22.2

The chronic syndrome

A middle-aged man lives in a group home for psychiatric patients and attends a sheltered workshop. In both places, he withdraws from company. He is usually dishevelled and unshaven, and cares for himself only when encouraged to do so by others. His social behaviour is odd and awkward. His speech is slow, and its content vague and incoherent. When questioned, he says that he is the victim of persecution by extraterrestrial beings who beam rays at him. He seldom mentions these ideas spontaneously and he shows few signs of emotion about them or about any other aspects of his life. For several years, this clinical picture has changed little except for brief periods of acute symptoms, which are usually related to upsets in the ordered life of the group home.

---

by unwillingness to accept treatment. In many cases, this lack of insight leads to the patient to lack capacity to consent to treatment, and they may need to be treated under the MHA (see p. 118).

The chronic syndrome (negative symptoms)

The syndrome can be illustrated by a brief case study of a typical patient (see Case study box 22.2). This description illustrates several of the features of what is sometimes called a 'schizophrenic defect state'. See also Table 22.2.

Impairment of volition

The most striking feature is diminished **volition**, that is, a lack of drive and initiative. Left to himself, the patient may be inactive for long periods, or may engage in aimless and repeated activity.

Impairment of daily living skills

Social behaviour often deteriorates. Patients neglect personal hygiene and their appearance. They may withdraw from social encounters. Some behave in ways that break social conventions, for example, talking intimately to strangers, shouting obscenities in public, or behaving in a sexually uninhibited manner. Some patients hoard objects, so that their surroundings become cluttered and dirty.

Table 22.2 The chronic syndrome (negative symptoms)

Lack of drive and activity	Underactivity or disorganized behaviour
Social withdrawal	
Abnormalities of behaviour	
Abnormalities of movement	Stupor and excitement
	Abnormal movements
	Abnormal tonus
Speech	Reduced in amount
	Evidence of thought disorder
Mood disorder	Blunting
	Incongruity
	Depression
Hallucinations	Especially auditory
Delusions	Systematized
	Encapsulated
Orientation	Age disorientation
Attention	Normal
Memory	Deficits in working and semantic memory
Insight	Variable

Movement disorders

A variety of disturbances of movement occur which are often called **catatonic**. They will be described only briefly here (they are detailed in the *New Oxford Textbook of Psychiatry*). Catatonic symptoms have become much less common with the introduction of atypical antipsychotics and trend away from using high doses of medication over long periods of time. **Stupor** and **excitement** are the most striking catatonic symptoms. A patient in stupor is immobile, mute, and unresponsive, although fully conscious. Stupor may change (sometimes quickly) to a state of uncontrolled motor activity and excitement.

Patients with chronic schizophrenia sometimes make repeated, odd, and awkward movements. Repeated movements that do not appear to be goal directed are called **stereotypies**; repeated movements of this kind that do appear to be goal directed are called **mannerisms**. Occasionally, patients have a disorder of muscle tone, which can be detected by placing the patient in an awkward posture; when the sign is present, the patient maintains this posture without apparent distress for much longer than a healthy person could without severe discomfort (waxy flexibility). When catatonic symptoms are prominent, the illness is referred to as catatonic schizophrenia.

Speech and form of thought

Speech is often abnormal, reflecting **thought disorder** of the same kinds as those found in the acute syndrome (described earlier).

Affect and perception

Affect is generally blunted, and when emotion is shown, it may be incongruous. **Hallucinations** are common, and any of the forms occurring in the acute syndrome may occur in the chronic syndrome.

Thought content

In chronic schizophrenia, **delusions** are common and often systematized. They may be held with little emotion. For example, patients may be convinced that they are being persecuted but show neither fear nor anger. Delusions may also be 'encapsulated' from the rest of the patient's beliefs. Thus, a patient may be convinced that his private sexual fantasies and practices are widely discussed by strangers, but his remaining beliefs are not influenced by this conviction, nor is his work or social life affected.

Cognitive function

It is now recognized that people with schizophrenia frequently suffer from a variety of cognitive impairments and that these impairments are associated with important aspects of functional outcome, such as the acquisition of social skill and the chances of successful employment. Many areas of cognitive functioning appear to be affected; the best established are deficits in working and semantic memory, attention, and executive functioning. Verbal fluency and motor functioning also appear to be affected, although to a lesser extent.

Insight

Insight is often impaired; the patient does not recognize that his symptoms are due to illness and is seldom fully convinced of the need for treatment.

Factors modifying the clinical features

In schizophrenia, several factors can interact with the disease process to modify the clinical picture.

Age of onset

The symptoms of adolescents and young adults often include thought disorder, mood disturbance, and disrupted behaviour. With increasing age, paranoid symptoms are more common, and disrupted behaviour is less frequent.

Gender

The course of the illness is generally more severe in males.

Sociocultural background

Sociocultural factors may affect the content of delusions and hallucinations. For example, delusions with a religious content are more common among patients from a religious background. Recent technological innovations are often used to explain symptoms. For example, a patient thought that his auditory hallucinations were due to nanotechnology.

The amount of social stimulation has a considerable effect on the type of symptoms. *Understimulation* increases 'negative' symptoms such as poverty of speech, social withdrawal, apathy, and lack of drive, and also catatonic symptoms. *Overstimulation* induces 'positive' symptoms such as hallucinations, delusions, and restlessness. Modern treatment is designed to avoid understimulation; as a result, 'negative' features including catatonia are less frequent than in the past. This policy can, however, result in a degree of overstimulation, leading to more positive symptoms.

High emotional expression by people with whom the patient is living is one form of social stimulation that increases symptoms. Overt expressions of criticism seem to be particularly important. The more time the patient spends in the company of highly critical people, the more likely he is to relapse. This is a reason why some patients are less disturbed when living in supported accommodation than with their family.

Diagnosis

The diagnosis of schizophrenia is based entirely on the clinical presentation (history and examination). The only diagnostic tests used are those needed to exclude other disorders when there is clinical suspicion. Because the diagnosis is based on clinical findings, it is made more reliable when **diagnostic criteria** are used to specify patterns of symptoms which must be present to make the diagnosis.

The currently most widely used diagnostic criteria are those in the ICD-10 and the DSM-5 (see Box 22.1). Both these systems include the following:

1   Individual symptoms that have been found to be highly specific for schizophrenia and therefore

Box 22.1 ICD-10 diagnostic criteria for schizophrenia

Individuals with schizophrenia show multiple abnormalities of their mental state:

- Thoughts—delusions, thought interference, delusional perception
- Perceptions—hallucinations (typically auditory), passivity phenomena
- Affect—blunted
- Normal conscious level and normal cognition, although the latter may deteriorate with chronic illness
- Negative symptoms

Schizophrenia may be a continuous condition, or episodic with partial or complete remission between episodes. Symptoms must be present for at least 1 month.

Subtypes: paranoid, hebephrenic, catatonic, simple, residual, undifferentiated

Duration: at least 1 month of continuous symptoms.

Exclusions: diagnosis should not be made in context of significant mood symptoms, organic brain pathology or intoxication/withdrawal from substances.

Major changes in ICD-11 beta-draft: the subtypes of schizophrenia have been withdrawn.

have a high **positive predictive value**. These are called **Schneider's 'first-rank' symptoms** after the clinician who first described them (Box 22.2 and described more fully in Chapter 5). They occur

Box 22.2 Schneider's 'first-rank' symptoms of schizophrenia

- Hearing thoughts spoken aloud
- 'Third-person' hallucinations
- Hallucinations in the form of a commentary
- Somatic hallucinations
- Thought withdrawal or insertion
- Thought broadcasting
- Delusional perception
- Feelings or actions experienced as made or influenced by external agents

Note: the terms used in this list are explained in Chapter 5.

in about 70 per cent of patients who meet the full diagnostic criteria for schizophrenia.

2 Symptoms that are more frequent but less discriminating than first-rank symptoms (e.g. prominent hallucinations, loosening of association, and flat or inappropriate affect).

3 Impaired social and occupational functioning.

4 A minimum duration of 1 month of active symptoms. The DSM-5 also specifies this should be within a 6-month period of behavioural change.

5 The exclusion of (a) organic mental disorder, (b) major depression, (c) mania, or (d) the prolongation of autistic spectrum disorder (which is a mental disorder of childhood, see p. 476).

Classification of psychotic disorders which do not meet the diagnostic criteria for schizophrenia

Both the ICD-10 and the DSM-5 provide categories for disorders that resemble schizophrenia but fail to meet the diagnostic criteria for schizophrenia in one of the following three ways:

1 Duration is too short. Cases lasting for less than 1 month are called acute psychotic disorders in both classifications. The DSM-5 has an extra category for cases lasting less than the 6 months required in this classification for the diagnosis of schizophrenia. These cases are called schizophreniform. (Since the ICD-10 requires a duration of only 1 month, it does not require this extra category.)

2 Prominent affective symptoms. These cases are called schizoaffective in both classifications.

3 Delusions without other symptoms of schizophrenia. These are called delusional disorders.

Differential diagnosis

Schizophrenia needs to be distinguished from four other types of disorder (see Science box 22.1):

1 **Organic syndromes.** In younger patients, the most relevant organic diagnoses are:

(a) **Drug-induced states.**

Drugs of abuse, especially that induced by amphetamines (see p. 426), but also ketamine, methedrone, phencyclidine, cocaine, ecstasy, and LSD. Cannabis intoxication may cause perceptual distortions but rarely frank psychosis. Cannabis may, however, precipitate relapse in patients with established schizophrenia.

Prescribed drugs: many prescribed drugs can rarely cause psychotic reactions, but steroids and the dopamine agonists used in the treatment of Parkinson's disease are probably the most commonly implicated drugs.

(b) **Temporal lobe epilepsy** should be considered when the condition is brief and there is evidence of clouding of consciousness. (In a few patients, chronic temporal lobe epilepsy gives rise to a persistent state resembling schizophrenia more closely.)

In older patients, the organic brain diseases which should be excluded include the following:

(a) **Delirium** can be mistaken for an acute episode of schizophrenia, especially when there are prominent hallucinations and delusions; the cardinal feature of this disorder is clouding of consciousness (see p. 362).

(b) **Dementia** can resemble schizophrenia, particularly when there are prominent persecutory delusions; the finding of memory disorder suggests dementia.

(c) Some other **diffuse brain diseases** can present a schizophrenia-like picture without any neurological signs or gross memory impairment; for example, **general paralysis of the insane**, a form of neurosyphilis.

To exclude organic disorders, history taking and mental state examination should focus on cognitive impairment (including disorientation and memory deficit) which tends to be more severe in organic disorder but not in schizophrenia, and a thorough

SCIENCE BOX 22.1

What is schizophrenia?

When Eugen Bleuler coined the term 'schizophrenia' in 1911, he was trying to describe the splitting of psychological functions—particularly the loosening of associations—that he observed in his patients at the Burghölzli Clinic in Zurich. Bleuler felt that schizophrenia was a better description of the serious mental disorder characterized by psychotic symptoms in the absence of coarse brain pathology that had been called **dementia praecox** by his German contemporary, Emil Kraepelin. Gradually, the term schizophrenia prevailed and achieved worldwide use in clinical psychiatry. It was always seen as being somewhat unsatisfactory, however, as it referred to an uncertain psychological process and led to popular misunderstanding that the illness was 'split-mind' or even multiple personalities. Gradually, the adjective 'schizophrenic' became a commonly used description of unpredictable or inconsistent thinking. Moreover, the clinical boundaries and fundamental symptoms of schizophrenia remain uncertain, which has led some to suggest that it does not exist and/or that it is simply a catch-all for labelling people who do not fit into society.

Until recently, attempts to replace the term have been resisted in the absence of reliable knowledge about aetiology, which would allow a classification rationally based on causes. Instead, the reliability of the diagnosis has been improved by the introduction of operational diagnostic criteria—exemplified by the DSM-IV. This has fulfilled the need for a clinically valid and reliable diagnosis and has allowed the gradual development of a scientific basis for effective treatment.

Nonetheless, there has remained widespread dissatisfaction about the term schizophrenia because of the rather imprecise and arbitrary nature of the diagnostic boundaries (between both normality and other disorders), the failure of the term to provide a good description of either the neurobiology or the clinical features of the disorder, and the stigma which has gradually attached itself to the label.

The problem is what to replace it with. One proposal is **salience dysregulation syndrome**, admittedly a bit of a mouthful, but this describes the difficulty in deciding which stimuli are important, that is, characteristic of the disorder.[1,2] We shall see—but we predict that schizophrenia's days as a diagnosis are numbered!

1 Kapur S. Psychosis as a state of aberrant salience: a framework linking biology, phenomenology, and pharmacology in schizophrenia. *American Journal of Psychiatry* 2003;160:13–23.

2 van Os JA. Salience dysregulation syndrome. *British Journal of Psychiatry* 2009;194:101–103.

---

physical examination should be done, including a neurological examination.

2 **Psychotic mood disorder.** The distinction between mood disorder and schizophrenia depends on:

  (a) the degree and persistence of mood disorder;

  (b) the congruence of any hallucinations or delusions with the prevailing mood;

  (c) the nature of the symptoms in any previous episodes (if previously predominantly mood, then current mood disorder is more likely).

Sometimes, mood and schizophrenic symptoms are so equally balanced that it is not possible to decide whether the primary disorder is affective or schizophrenic. As explained earlier, these cases are diagnosed as schizoaffective disorder:

3 **Personality disorders.** Differential diagnosis from personality disorder may be difficult, especially when there have been insidious changes of behaviour in a young person who does not describe hallucinations or delusions. As well as interviewing relatives it may be necessary to make prolonged observations for first-rank and other features of schizophrenia before a definite diagnosis can be reached.

4 **Schizoaffective disorder.** Some patients have, at the same time, definite schizophrenic symptoms and definitive affective (depressive or manic)

symptoms of equal prominence. These disorders are classified separately because it is uncertain whether they are a subtype of schizophrenia, or of affective disorder. Schizoaffective disorders usually require both antipsychotic and antidepressant drug treatment. When they recover, affective and schizophrenic symptoms improve together, and most patients lose all their symptoms, although many have further episodes. Some of these subsequent episodes are schizoaffective, but others have a more typical schizophrenic or more typical affective form.

Epidemiology

Incidence

The annual incidence of schizophrenia is between 10 and 20 per 100,000 of the population. In men, schizophrenia usually begins between the ages of 15 and 35. In women, the mean age of onset of the disorder is later (Fig. 22.1). Although the incidence of schizophrenia is similar worldwide, it may be higher in certain ethnic groups (e.g. Afro-Caribbean immigrants in the UK).

Prevalence

The point prevalence of schizophrenia is about 4 per 1000 (much higher than the incidence because the disorder is chronic). The lifetime risk of developing schizophrenia is about 10 per 1000. The prevalence of schizophrenia is higher in socioeconomically deprived areas: in people who are homeless, the prevalence is 100 per 1000.

The GP with an average list of 2000 may expect to have about eight patients with schizophrenia. An inner-city doctor, with a large homeless population, may have considerably more cases (50–100). Although the numbers are usually small, the needs of these patients for medical care are great.

Aetiology

The aetiology of schizophrenia is uncertain, although there is evidence for several risk factors (Table 22.3). There is strong evidence for genetic causes, and good reason to believe that stressful life events may provoke the disorder. Structural changes have been found in the brains of some schizophrenic patients, particularly

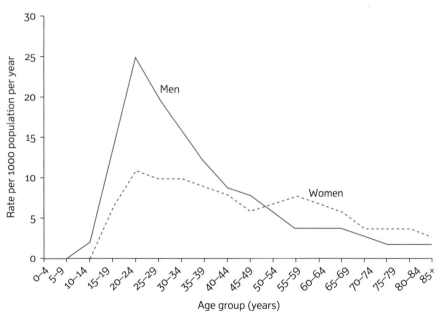

Fig. 22.1 Age- and sex-specific incidence rates for schizophrenia in men and women.

Source data from Information and Statistics Division, NHS Scotland, 1993.

Table 22.3 Risk factors for schizophrenia

	Risk factors	Relative risk of developing schizophrenia
Predisposing		
Genetic	Monozygotic twin of a schizophrenic patient	40
	Dizygotic twin of a schizophrenic patient	15
	Child of a schizophrenic patient	10–15
	Sibling of a schizophrenic patient	10–15
Environmental	Abnormalities of pregnancy and delivery	2
	Maternal influenza (second trimester)	2
	Fetal malnutrition	2
	Urban birth	2–3
	Migration	2
	Winter birth	1.1
Precipitating	Early cannabis consumption	2–3

in the temporal lobes, but it is not yet certain how they are caused.

Genetic factors

There is strong evidence for the heritability of schizophrenia from three sources.

1 **Family studies** have shown that schizophrenia is more common in the relatives of schizophrenic patients than in the general population (where the lifetime risk is approximately 1 per cent). The risk is 10–15 per cent in the siblings of schizophrenics, among the children of one schizophrenic parent 10–15 per cent, and among the children of two schizophrenic parents about 40 per cent.

2 **Twin studies** indicate that a major part of this familial loading is likely to be due to genetic rather than to environmental factors. Among monozygotic twins, the concordance rate (the frequency of schizophrenia in the sibling of the affected twin) is consistently higher (about 40 per cent) than among dizygotic twins (about

10–15 per cent). The heritability of schizophrenia is about 80 per cent.

3 **Adoption studies** confirm the importance of genetic factors. Among children who have been separated from a schizophrenic parent at birth and brought up by non-schizophrenic adoptive parents, the likelihood of developing schizophrenia is no less than that among children brought up by their own schizophrenic parent.

Specific genes and the mode of inheritance

Several susceptibility genes for schizophrenia have now been identified, which may have an effect on neurodevelopment and synaptic functioning (see Box 22.3). Genome-wide association studies (GWAS) have identified more than 100 areas within the genome which are associated with schizophrenia. Some of these are genes, others single nucleotide polymorphisms. This strongly supports a polygenic model of inheritance, in which multiple genes contribute additive small effects to the risk an individual

Box 22.3 Susceptibility genes for schizophrenia

- *DISC1*
- Dysbindin
- Neuregulin-1
- MHC locus
- *ZNF804A*
- *G72*

carries. There is probably an interaction between these genes and environmental factors. Many of the areas of the genome identified have also been linked to other psychiatric disorders (e.g. bipolar disorder).

Environmental factors

Environmental factors can predispose to the development of schizophrenia, precipitate the onset, provoke relapse after initial recovery, and maintain the disorder in persisting cases:

- **Predisposing factors.** Some factors putatively implicated in the development of schizophrenia are summarized in Table 22.3. The role of most of the environmental factors remains uncertain. Abnormalities of pregnancy and fetal development are risk factors, although the size of the association is small. The mechanism of action remains obscure, although it may involve fetal hypoxia. There is also an association with low **social class** and this is probably both cause and effect: social deprivation increases exposure to several risk factors, and it is likely that people who develop schizophrenia tend to become increasingly socially deprived. There is some evidence that heavy cannabis consumption is associated with the development of schizophrenia.

- **Precipitating factors** of schizophrenia include stressful life events occurring shortly before the onset of the disorder. Migration is a common precipitant of schizophrenia. Use of cannabis, especially in the early teenage years, is strongly associated with a two- to threefold increased risk of developing schizophrenia.

- **Maintaining factors** include strongly expressed feelings, especially in the form of critical comments, among family members ('high emotional expression'). Continued use of cannabis is frequently a factor in continuing symptoms, especially paranoid ideas. Finally, it has been suggested that inconsistent forms of **child rearing** predispose to schizophrenia, but such ideas are not supported by evidence. Such speculations have caused unjustified guilt in some parents.

Pathophysiology

The response of some schizophrenic symptoms to antipsychotic drugs suggests that they may have a biochemical basis. A disorder of dopaminergic function is implied by the efficacy of dopamine D_2-blocking antipsychotic drugs. Nonetheless, until recently, it has proved difficult to find direct evidence that there is abnormal dopaminergic transmission in schizophrenia. With the availability of more powerful brain imaging techniques, it is now clear that there is evidence of increased dopaminergic transmission in the basal ganglia and mesolimbic system in acute schizophrenia and diminished dopaminergic transmission in the prefrontal cortex. The latter may relate to the cognitive decline in chronic schizophrenia. However, dopaminergic abnormalities are probably not the primary problem—or antipsychotics would be more effective, and clozapine (a weak D_2 antagonist) less effective—a more complex dysregulation of neurotransmission is more likely. There is now evidence of significant hypofunction of NMDA receptors across the cortex, suggesting a key role for the glutaminergic system.

Schizophrenia as a disorder of brain development

It is currently thought that schizophrenia is a **neurodevelopmental disorder**; this idea is based on several pieces of evidence:

1. Evidence of brain abnormalities has been consistently found in studies performing computed

tomography (CT) and magnetic resonance imaging (MRI) scans of patients with schizophrenia. The most frequently observed abnormalities are reductions in the volumes of parahippocampus, temporal lobes, and amygdala/hippocampus, and increased lateral ventricular volumes. These abnormalities can be present before the illness and it remains uncertain to what extent they progress during the course of the disorder.

2 Patients with schizophrenia are more likely than controls to have dermatoglyphic abnormalities (sometimes associated with central nervous system developmental disorder) and separate 'soft' neurological signs.

3 Postmortem studies have not found gliosis in the brains of schizophrenic patients. This means that it is likely that the brain abnormalities occurred early in life.

4 Subjects who subsequently develop schizophrenia are more likely than controls to have developmental problems during childhood.

Taken together, this evidence suggests a pathological process, which takes place early in life and results in abnormal neurodevelopment that is sometimes observable during childhood. The current neurodevelopmental model proposes a polygenetic susceptibility interacting with early environment and leading to abnormal brain maturation (in particular, synaptic pruning, myelination, and apoptosis). This process leads to the frequently observable childhood abnormalities and, in the presence of later environmental risk factors (psychoactive drugs, stress), leads to the onset of schizophrenia.

This model needs much more validation and testing but would integrate what is currently known and would also explain why there appears to be a spectrum of severity.

Autoantibodies and psychosis

It is now known that a few cases of first-episode psychosis (~8%) have a different aetiology to that described earlier; they are autoimmune disorders. Before this was discovered, it was known that some forms of encephalitis were caused by autoantibodies directed against neuronal cell surface receptors. Patients with these encephalitides frequently present with psychiatric symptoms alongside neurological deficits, clouding of consciousness, autonomic instability, abnormal movements, and seizures. They have been treated with steroids, intravenous immunoglobulins, or monoclonal antibodies with excellent results. Recent research has shown that, in some cases, these autoantibodies are associated with psychosis in the absence of encephalitis. These include autoantibodies directed towards the NMDA receptor, VGKC complex, CASPR2, and LGI1. The clinical presentation in those with positive autoantibody status appears no different to those without it, but small-scale studies have demonstrated that immunotherapy is an effective treatment. It is now recommended in the UK that all patients presenting with a first episode of psychosis are screened for these autoantibodies, so that they can be quickly identified and appropriately treated.

Course and prognosis

The *course* of schizophrenia is variable:

- Acute illness with complete recovery: 20 per cent.
- Recurrent course with some persistent deficits: 50 per cent.
- Chronic illness with persistent functional disability: 20 per cent.
- Suicide: 10 per cent.

In contrast to traditional views of a poor long-term prognosis in the majority of patients, it is now recognized that at least 30 per cent (and possibly as many as 50 per cent) of patients either recover completely or suffer minimal symptoms in the long term. This change to a more optimistic view of the prognosis is probably due to a combination of the increased recognition of milder illnesses and better treatment. Early recognition and swift treatment ensures the best outcome for patients with schizophrenia.

Patients with recurrent acute episodes often do not recover to the previous level after each relapse and so gradually deteriorate. The risk of *suicide* is high among young patients in the early stage of the disorder when insight is still present into the likely effect of the illness on the patient's hopes and plans.

The best *outcome* is in disorders of acute onset following stress. Other predictors of outcome, some related to the illness, others to the ill person, are listed in Table 22.4. Although of some value, these predictors cannot be used to make a definite prediction for an individual patient. For this reason, advice to patients and relatives should be given cautiously, especially in the first episode of illness. The factors listed in Table 22.4 are those operating before or at the onset of schizophrenia. Factors acting after the onset are discussed next.

Life events

As noted earlier, stressful life events can precipitate relapses, and patients exposed to many life events generally have a less favourable course. In general, as

Table 22.4 Factors predicting poor outcome in schizophrenia

Features of the illness	Insidious onset
	Long first episode
	Previous psychiatric history
	Negative symptoms
	Younger age at onset
Features of the patient	Male
	Single, separated, widowed, or divorced
	Poor psychosexual adjustment
	Abnormal previous personality
	Poor employment record
	Social isolation
	Poor compliance

already explained, an overstimulating environment increases positive symptoms, while an understimulating one increases negative symptoms. Prognosis depends, in part, on how far a balance can be achieved between these extremes.

Family environment

The risk of relapse is increased when relatives make many critical comments, express hostility, and show signs of emotional over-involvement. In such families, the risk of relapse is greater if patients spend much time in contact with their close relatives (35 hours a week has been suggested as a cut-off point). Reducing this contact by arranging day care appears to improve prognosis, as may family therapy.

Cultural background

The outcome of schizophrenia may be better in less developed countries, perhaps because fewer demands are made on patients and there is greater family support, as part of a traditional rural way of life.

Assessment and management

The majority of people with schizophrenia will be treated by specialist mental health services, although the first evidence of schizophrenia is usually detected by GPs. Delay in starting treatment is associated with poorer outcome, and the importance of *early intervention* is increasingly recognized. GPs need to be familiar with the basic assessment and make a rapid referral for full assessment and management. The importance of early intervention has recently led to the development of specific services that aim to engage the patient with services and effective interventions as quickly as possible after the onset of symptoms.

Assessment in primary care

Sometimes the patient asks for help with the symptoms of schizophrenia, but more often relatives or other people draw attention to problem behaviours that could be caused by schizophrenia. For example, a GP may be asked to help a young person who is becoming increasingly withdrawn and showing odd behaviour, or an elderly woman who is reclusive and suspicious. In these situations, family doctors are in a good position to make an initial assessment because they will often know the family and the patient's background. The doctor should try to:

- obtain a good description of the patient's symptoms and behaviour. When possible this should be supplemented by information from an informant;

- assess the patient's level of functional impairment. For example, is the patient still working? Is the patient having difficulties in his or her relationships?

- make an assessment of the degree of risk the patient poses to himself and others (see Chapter 9);

- clearly inform the patient of the results of the assessment and try to persuade the patient to accept referral to the specialist mental health services;

- when the patient will not accept referral, discuss the presentation with a psychiatrist. Treatment can then sometimes be commenced, although it is advisable to maintain contact with a psychiatrist in case the situation deteriorates.

Assessment in specialist services

When psychiatric services receive a referral for a patient presenting with psychosis, the next steps depend on the urgency of the situation. Assessment may be in the outpatient setting or at home if the patient is not acutely disturbed and has capacity to consent, but in many cases it will occur after admission to hospital. Assessment should, where possible, include:

- an interview with a psychiatrist to try and establish the diagnosis, or at least begin the diagnostic process;

- gathering of psychosocial and developmental history;

- full physical examination (including detailed neurology, vital signs, weight/BMI/waist circumference);

- urine sample for drug testing and exclusion of infection/renal disease;

- routine blood tests to exclude organic causes of psychosis and provide baseline levels (e.g. lipids, prolactin);

- autoantibody screening: NMDA receptors antibodies, VGKC complex, NMDA receptor antibodies;

- baseline ECG—to establish safety to start antipsychotics;

- brain imaging (CT or MRI).

Some patients presenting with psychosis will require admission to hospital. The decision will depend on:

- the severity of the psychotic, mood, cognitive, or behavioural symptoms;

- the nature of the psychotic symptoms (e.g. command auditory hallucinations telling the patient to harm himself or others);

- the level of social support;

- the insight into illness and acceptance of need for treatment.

If the patient refuses admission to hospital when this is considered essential for his (or other people's) health or safety, compulsory powers for admission to hospital may be required (see Box 22.4 and p. 303). Increasingly, alternatives to hospital admission such as intensive community treatment or day hospital attendance can be organized.

Management of an acute episode of schizophrenia

An overview of management is shown in Table 22.5. If the diagnosis is uncertain, and if safe to do so, it may be desirable to withhold drug treatment for several days to allow the diagnosis to be clarified and to perform baseline investigations prior to treatment. When the diagnosis is sufficiently clear, antipsychotic medication is started. The antipsychotic effect may not occur immediately, but antipsychotics also have a calming effect which may reduce the need for a sedative agent.

Box 22.4 Ethics issues of compulsory treatment

Usually considered ethical when:

1 the patient is suffering from a severe mental disorder and does not consider himself ill and/or will not consent to treatment;
2 treatment is necessary for health or safety of the patient or to protect others.

Ethical issues:

1 Nature of psychiatric diagnosis; for example, in the former USSR and China, political dissidents were considered mentally ill and compulsorily detained and treated.
2 Balance between individual freedom and protection of others.
3 What is 'effective' treatment? Treatment may be defined vaguely as supportive care provided in hospital to prevent deterioration, or more specifically as a defined therapeutic intervention for which beneficial and adverse effects are known.

Table 22.5 Management of schizophrenia

Assessment	Psychiatric interviews
	Physical examination
	Investigations: bloods, ECG, imaging
Biological treatments	Antipsychotics (oral or depot)
	Short-term benzodiazepines
	Treatment of co-morbid mood symptoms
Psychological treatments	CBT
	Family therapy
	(These may need to be postponed until the acute symptoms have resolved)
Social aspects	Reduction of high expressed emotion at home
	Appropriate daytime activities or work adjustments
	Support with accommodation and finances
Long-term monitoring	Mental state
	Physical health: weight, blood pressure, lipid profile, prolactin
	ECG if on long-term antipsychotics
	Evidence of movement disorders

For treatment when a patient is very excited or abnormally aggressive, see Chapter 16 on managing behavioural disturbance. Drug treatment may be needed for immediate behavioural control, in which case a sedative benzodiazepine such as diazepam or lorazepam (see p. 179) is usually used, often in combination with an antipsychotic. These should be used for short periods at the lowest possible effective dose.

Antipsychotic drug therapy

The most effective treatment for acute psychotic symptoms is antipsychotic drug therapy (see p. 137). Most antipsychotic drugs have an immediate sedative effect, followed by an effect on psychotic symptoms (especially hallucinations and delusions), which may take up to 3 weeks to develop fully.

There are many antipsychotic drugs, which differ more in side effect profiles than in effectiveness. Antipsychotic drugs should be started at a low dose and increased gradually. Equivalent doses of some commonly used antipsychotics are shown in Table 22.6. These equivalents should only be used as a rough guide, and the manufacturer's instructions should be followed. Second-generation 'atypical' agents are often used because of the lower risk of extrapyramidal side effects. However, the decision on which drug to be used should be tailored for the individual patient and take into account the patient's preference.

Choice of antipsychotic drug

(See also p. 136.) Antipsychotic drugs are divided into two groups: the **conventional** (sometimes termed first-generation) and **atypical** (second-generation) antipsychotics (Table 22.7). With the exception of clozapine, there is no good evidence that there are real differences in efficacy between antipsychotics. It was initially thought atypicals might be more effective at

Table 22.6 Commonly used antipsychotic drugs with normal daily dose range

Conventional		Atypical	
Haloperidol	(2–30 mg)	Risperidone	(4–16 mg)
Chlorpromazine	(100–600 mg)	Olanzapine	(5–20 mg)
Trifluoperazine	(5–30 mg)	Quetiapine	(150–800 mg)
Sulpiride	(400–800 mg)	Clozapine	(100–900 mg)[a]

[a] Sometimes effective in schizophrenia resistant to conventional antipsychotics.

reducing negative symptoms, but recent evidence has not replicated these findings. The side effect profile of the various drugs is therefore important to consider (Table 22.8). In choosing an antipsychotic, consideration of the following may be helpful:

- Which antipsychotics, if any, have been effective previously?
- Is there a need for sedation?
- What is the patient's baseline metabolic and cardiac risk?
- Are there concurrent mood symptoms?
- Is a depot formulation likely to be needed?

A trial of an antipsychotic is considered to be adequate if it has been given at therapeutic dose for 6 weeks. If a patient does not respond to adequate courses of at least two other antipsychotics, this is termed 'treatment resistance'. Clozapine is currently the only drug that has been shown to be effective in treatment resistance. Unfortunately, clozapine requires a slow titration and has an array of side effects,

Table 22.7 Comparison of first- and second-generation antipsychotics

	First-generation 'typical' antipsychotics	Second-generation 'atypical' antipsychotics
Examples	Haloperidol, chlorpromazine, sulpiride, zuclopenthixol, trifluoperazine, fluphenazine	Olanzapine, clozapine, risperidone, quetiapine, aripiprazole, lurasidone, paliperidone
Action	D_2-receptor antagonists	D_2, D_4, and 5-HT antagonists (variable potency between drugs)
Extrapyramidal symptoms and hyperprolactinaemia	High risk	Low risk (NB risperidone has higher risk for hyperprolactinaemia)
Sedation	High risk	Variable: spectrum of neutral (aripiprazole) to highly sedating (clozapine)
Metabolic side effects	High risk of weight gain Relatively lower risk of diabetes and dyslipidaemia	High risk of weight gain (especially olanzapine and clozapine) High risk of diabetes and dyslipidaemia
Effects on mood	No strong evidence	Evidence emerging that quetiapine and olanzapine may have mood-stabilizing properties

Table 22.8 Side effects of antipsychotic drugs

Typical antipsychotics	• Sedation, 70–80%
	• Anticholinergic and antiadrenergic effects (including dry mouth, constipation, blurred vision, urinary retention, tachycardia)
	• Extrapyramidal side effects (parkinsonism, dystonia, akathisia, neuroleptic malignant syndrome)
	• Tardive dyskinesia: 4% per year of antipsychotic medication
	• Endocrine effects: hyperprolactinaemia leading to galactorrhoea and oligomenorrhoea
	• Weight gain
	• Sexual dysfunction
	• Prolonged QTc interval
Atypical antipsychotics	• Sedation (variable)
	• Weight gain (variable)
	• Orthostatic hypotension
	• Prolonged QTc interval (variable)
	• Dyslipidaemia
	• Increased risk of type 2 diabetes
	• Sexual dysfunction
Clozapine	• Sedation
	• Weight gain
	• Constipation
	• Hypersalivation
	• Tachycardia
	• Myocarditis
	• Orthostatic hypotension
	• Seizures, 3%
	• Agranulocytosis, <1% (neutropenia 2–3%)

including agranulocytosis, which makes it an unsuitable first-line antipsychotic.

Anticholinergic **medication** can be used to prevent or relieve extrapyramidal symptoms, including acute dystonic reactions, akathisia, or parkinsonism. However, the goal of all drug treatment should be to avoid the side effects by adjusting the dose of the chosen antipsychotic.

The effects of antipsychotics

Following commencement of an antipsychotic, symptoms of excitement, irritability, and insomnia usually improve within a few days. Hallucinations and delusions may take longer to improve, often changing gradually over several weeks. If there is no improvement, a check should be made that the patient is taking the prescribed drugs. If not, the reason should be determined and an attempt made to ensure compliance. If the patient is taking the prescribed dose, this should be increased cautiously unless it is already at the top of the recommended range. If there is concern about compliance, or the patient prefers, a depot preparation of the antipsychotic can be used.

Electroconvulsive therapy (ECT)

ECT is not used regularly in the treatment of schizophrenia but there are two important indications:

1 When there are severe depressive symptoms accompanying schizophrenia.

2 In the rare cases of catatonic stupor.

ECT is often rapidly effective in both these conditions. ECT may be effective also in acute episodes of schizophrenia, even without severe depression or stupor, but it is seldom used because drug treatment is simpler and equally beneficial. The main exception is a postpartum psychosis, when a rapid response is particularly important (see p. 151).

Drug-resistant symptoms

In about 70 per cent of acute episodes, symptoms respond to antipsychotic drug treatment. Drug-resistant symptoms can be treated in two ways:

Alternative drug therapy. Clozapine is the only agent that has clearly been shown to be effective in patients where symptoms are resistant to treatment with conventional antipsychotics (see p. 136). In practice, if a patient does not respond to two or more courses of different first-line agents, than clozapine should be considered.

Psychological treatments. There is some evidence suggesting that cognitive therapy may reduce preoccupation with drug-resistant hallucinations and delusions.

Prevention of relapse

Preventing relapse in patients who recover fully from an acute episode

If the symptoms are well controlled on discharge from hospital, the dual aims of management are to continue to control symptoms with antipsychotic drugs, while making arrangements for daily living that protect the patient from too many stressors, and enable him to return as far as possible to his previous life. Even if the patient is free from symptoms, antipsychotic medication should be continued for **at least** 6 months.

Patients should be informed there is a high risk of relapse if they stop medication within the first 2 years. For patients living with their families, family therapy aimed at reducing the number of critical comments, and improving the family's knowledge of the disorder, can reduce the relapse rate.

Long-term treatment of patients who do not fully recover from an acute episode

The general aims of treatment are similar to those for patients who return to their premorbid state, but more attention has to be given to the social aspects of care.

The main approach to management is based on a systematic assessment of the patient's medical and social needs. Patients with schizophrenia who do not fully recover may have multiple social needs (e.g. housing and occupation), which are best met by a multidisciplinary team (see p. 103). A **care plan** should be developed in which the problems are listed with the interventions proposed.

In caring for patients with chronic schizophrenia, an experienced community psychiatric nurse is often one of the key professionals. The roles of the community nurse include:

- acting as a key worker responsible for coordinating the care plan;
- monitoring the mental state;
- administering depot neuroleptic medication;
- monitoring compliance with medication and the presence of side effects;
- arranging or carrying out specific behavioural and psychological interventions;
- education and support of the patient and relatives;
- liaison with other care workers.

Where possible, primary and secondary care services should work closely to ensure the patient receives high-quality monitoring and physical healthcare as well as mental health input.

Drug therapy

Continuation therapy reduces the risk of relapse. Since adherence to medication is often poor, intramuscular depot injections are often used instead of oral medication. There are two main problems. First, 20 per cent of patients remain well without drugs and second, long-term conventional antipsychotic medication leads to persistent tardive dyskinesia in 15 per cent of subjects after 4 years of treatment. Therefore, if all patients receive continuation treatment, some will be exposed unnecessarily to the risk of developing side effects. Unfortunately, it is not possible to predict which patients will benefit from continuing drug treatment. The clinician and patient therefore need to work together to judge the benefit of continuation treatment by reducing the drugs cautiously when the patient has been free from symptoms for several months. Patients taking long-term continuation therapy should be assessed every 6 months for signs of tardive dyskinesia, weight gain, and hyperglycaemia (see p. 137).

Although anticholinergic drugs reduce parkinsonian side effects, they may increase the likelihood of dyskinesia. They should not be prescribed routinely but only if there are extrapyramidal side effects that cannot be avoided by adjusting the dose of antipsychotic drug.

Family therapy

Family psychoeducation aimed at reducing emotional involvement and criticism has been shown to reduce the rate of relapse in schizophrenic patients living with their families.

Treatment of associated depressive symptoms

Depressive symptoms in schizophrenia are common and may need specific treatment.

Antidepressants

When depressive symptoms are severe, antidepressant medication may be used although there is uncertainty about how efficacious antidepressants are in schizophrenia. Antidepressants are also indicated in schizoaffective disorder.

Lithium

Lithium may be beneficial for schizoaffective disorders, especially when there is a mixture of schizophrenic and manic symptoms (see p. 147).

Psychosocial care and rehabilitation

The main aim of psychosocial care and rehabilitation is to reduce the long-term disability experienced by many patients with schizophrenia. In practice, psychosocial care is usually tailored to the individual patient's needs. Skill is required to arrange a care plan which is optimally stimulating but not too stressful. The approach is a general one including supportive care from community nurses and others. There is only limited evidence for the effectiveness of specific methods that include the following:

- **Social skills training.** Social skills training uses a behavioural approach to help patients to improve interpersonal, self-care, and coping skills needed in normal life.
- **Employment training.** This includes a range of activities from help in developing the skills necessary to obtain and hold down a job, to the provision of sheltered employment or other occupational activities.
- **Cognitive remediation.** Cognitive remediation therapy aims to help the neuropsychological impairments that are often associated with schizophrenia and, hence, improve psychosocial functioning.

Management of aggressive behaviour in patients with schizophrenia

Overactivity and disturbances of behaviour are common in schizophrenia. There is an increased risk of violence to others, although this remains uncommon, and homicide is very rare. The risk of violence to others should be assessed in all cases; it is greater when there are delusions of control, persecutory delusions, or auditory hallucinations.

Threats of violence should be taken seriously, especially if there is a history of such behaviour in the past, whether or not the patient was ill at the time. The danger usually resolves as acute symptoms are brought under control, but a few patients pose a continuing threat and require regular, close supervision.

Treatment for a potentially violent patient is the same as for any other schizophrenic patient, although a compulsory order is more likely to be needed. While medication is often needed to bring disturbed behaviour under immediate control, much can be done by providing a calm, reassuring, and consistent environment in which provocation is avoided. A hospital with a special area with an adequate number of experienced staff is usually able to rely less on the use of large doses of medication.

Delusional disorders

A delusional disorder is a condition in which a person has one or more persistent delusions in the absence of other persistent psychotic symptoms and outside of an episode of mood disorder. Patients often have complex encapsulated delusional systems, which are usually along a specific theme. Under the diagnostic

Table 22.9 Common delusional disorders

Disorder	Clinical features
Pathological jealousy (Othello syndrome)	The patient believes that their partner is unfaithful to them. They look for evidence to support this claim, and usually find it. Sometimes the patient also thinks their partner is plotting against them in some way. The patient is typically very angry and suspicious. The beliefs of infidelity lead to significant relationship difficulties and in some cases the patient may become violent towards their partner
Persecutory	A paranoid belief system develops in which the patient believes they are being spied on, monitored, and that someone is 'out to get them'. The patient typically withdraws and acts to protect themselves. There can be a risk of violence if the patient attempts to right the wrongs directed at them or eliminate their perceived enemies
Erotomania (de Clerambault syndrome)	The patient believes that another person is secretly in love with her or him. This person is often a celebrity or of higher status that the patient. They may try to contact or see this person, which can lead to stalking. The patient may react very badly to being rejected by the individual they seek
Grandiose	The patient believes they are particularly important or have a special gift or talent. This is outside of the context of mania
Somatic	A belief develops that there is something wrong with the patient's body. This might be a specific condition (e.g. cancer or infestations with parasites), that an area of the body is misshapen or abnormal, or that they emit a foul odour. The patient typically seeks medical attention from different health professionals regularly
Mixed	A combination of delusional beliefs that do not fit one specific theme
Induced delusional disorder (folie à deux)	This is a delusional disorder shared by two or more people with close emotional links. The delusions are usually persecutory in nature. One person (typically the dominant personality) has a psychotic disorder and is the originator of the delusion; it is then induced in the second person. Usually, when the two are separated, the induced delusions quickly remit. It is more common in women

criteria, the delusions should be present for at least 3 months. Transient hallucinations or other psychotic symptoms are seen in some patients, but these should be related to the delusions and there should not be abnormalities of speech or odd behaviour. The patient's function is usually normal, except in areas where the delusional beliefs lead to changes in behaviour. Insight is typically minimal, which can make engagement with treatment very challenging. Delusional disorders may occur at any age, but are most frequent in middle age. Table 22.9 outlines the common types of delusional disorder.

Prognosis

The prognosis of delusional disorders is difficult to predict but is generally poor, and highly related to the degree of insight the person has.

Assessment

Patients should be assessed as for schizophrenia and a detailed risk assessment should be included. Some subtypes of delusional disorder are associated with violence and this should be closely monitored. If any risk of violence to others is identified, the potential victims need to be aware of this.

Treatment

The treatment of delusional disorders is often difficult, because the patient frequently lacks insight and is uncooperative. Treatment should be with an antipsychotic drug, which may need to be given as a depot if there are difficulties with compliance. If it is judged there is a risk to others from the patient, hospital admission may be necessary.

Further reading

Lennox BR, Palmer-Cooper EC, Pollak T, et al. Prevalence and clinical characteristics of serum neuronal cell surface antibodies in first-episode psychosis: a case-control study. *Lancet Psychiatry* 2017;4:42–48.

Messias E, Chen CY, Eaton WW. Epidemiology of schizophrenia: review of findings and myths. *Psychiatric Clinics of North America* 2007;30:323–338.

National Institute for Health and Care Excellence. Psychosis and schizophrenia in adults: prevention and management. Clinical guideline [CG178]. Published February 2014, updated March 2014. https://www.nice.org.uk/guidance/cg178.

Weinberger DR, Harrison PJ. *Schizophrenia.* 3rd ed. Chichester: Wiley Blackwell; 2011. [A comprehensive and definitive textbook covering aetiology, diagnosis, treatment, and prognosis.]

23 Reactions to stressful experiences

In biological terms, stress literally means *a force from the outside world acting upon an individual*, and is a phenomenon we have all experienced. The term '**stress**' was first used in the 1930s by the endocrinologist Hans Selye to describe the responses of laboratory animals to various stimuli. Originally, Selye meant 'stress' to be the response of an organism to a perceived threat or '**stressor**', but the term is now used to mean the stimulus rather than the response in some cases. When presented with a stressor of any type, everyone will produce a reaction to that stress, and this is a normal physiological event. However, if the reaction is prolonged, too intense, or atypical in some way, stress can become abnormal and cause problems.

Stressful events, even when reacted to normally, are important contributors to the causes of many kinds of psychiatric disorder. In this chapter, we consider those psychiatric disorders that are specific reactions to stressful experiences. These may occur independently or alongside other psychiatric conditions and include:

- **acute stress reactions:** short-term disorders after stressful events;

- **post-traumatic stress disorder:** a disorder following exceptionally severe stress;

- **adjustment disorders:** conditions occurring after a change in life circumstances;

- **grief reactions:** the normal and abnormal responses to bereavement;

- **reactions to special kinds of acute stress:** for example, traffic accidents, war, earthquakes, etc.

For all these conditions, an identifiable stressor is a necessary but not always sufficient factor in its aetiology.

GPs encounter the vast majority of patients with stress disorders who present to the health services, but *all* clinicians will see these patients in their clinical specialties. The reasons for this are threefold:

1. Acute physical illness and its treatment are stressful.

2. Chronic illness or disability can result in substantial changes in life circumstances.

3. Clinicians treat people involved in other kinds of stressful experiences.

What is a stressful event?

Everyone reacts to stress differently, and what constitutes a stressful event is therefore highly subjective. However, there are certain situations that are likely to be experienced as stressful by anyone. The Holmes and Rahe Stress Scale is a list of 43 life events which predispose to stress-related illnesses, weighted according to their respective probability of doing so. The list was compiled by asking a large sample of Americans which life circumstances or events they found stressful, and then giving them a ranking according to how difficult they were to adjust to. Table 23.1 shows a selection of these 43 life events.

Table 23.1 Excerpt from life events table

Life event	Stress ranking[a]
Death of a spouse	100
Divorce	73
Marital separation	65
Imprisonment	63
Death of a close family member	63
Personal injury or illness	53
Marriage	50
Dismissal from work	47
Pregnancy	40
Beginning or ending school	26
Change in residence	20
Vacation	13
Christmas	12

[a] This is a rating where 100 is the most stressful event recorded, with relatively less stressful situations having progressively lower values.
Adapted from *Journal of Psychosomatic Research*, 11, Holmes T and Rahe R, The Social Readjustment Rating Scale, pp. 213–18. Copyright © 1967 Published by Elsevier Inc.

The normal response to stressful events

The normal stress response has three components:

1 A somatic 'fight or flight' response.

2 An emotional response.

3 A psychological response that aims to reduce the potential impact of the experience and help to cope with the situation at hand.

The somatic response

Human physiology has evolved a variety of mechanisms to deal with perceived threats. The core components of the stress response are the sympathetic nervous system and hypothalamic–pituitary–adrenal (HPA) axis. When a threatening situation occurs, the sympathetic nervous system is activated, releasing epinephrine (adrenaline) from the adrenal medulla. Epinephrine then causes the fight or flight response, which activates the body ready to flee from or deal with a threat. Both stress itself and firing of the locus coeruleus (pons) activate the HPA axis, which leads to release of glucocorticoids from the adrenal cortex. These two pathways alter the body to deal with a threat, and are outlined in Fig. 23.1.

Emotional responses

Emotional responses to stressful events are of three kinds:

1 A response to danger: **fear**.

2 A response to a threat: **anxiety**.

3 A response to separation or loss: **depression**.

Table 23.2 describes coping strategies that people develop to try and reduce the impact of stressful events; these may be helpful (adaptive) or unhelpful (maladaptive).

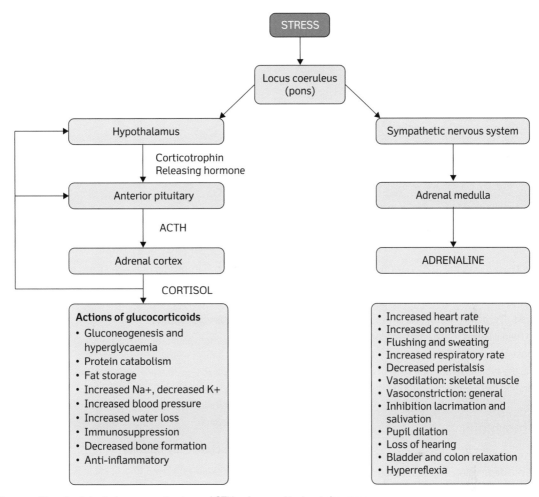

Fig. 23.1 The physiological response to stress. ACTH, adrenocorticotropic hormone.

Table 23.2 Psychological changes that reduce the impact of stressful events

Coping strategies	
Potentially adaptive	**Maladaptive** *(These may be helpful short term but soon become a secondary problem)*
Avoidance	Excessive use of alcohol or drugs
Working through problems	Histrionic or aggressive behaviour
Coming to terms with situations	Deliberate self-harm

Epidemiology

The US National Comorbidity Study has repeatedly found that 50–60 per cent of individuals experience at least one traumatic stressor in their lifetime. However, many individuals with stress-related disorders do not seek medical attention so gathering accurate epidemiology is challenging (Table 23.3).

Acute stress reaction

Acute stress reaction is *an abnormal reaction to sudden stressful events*. The basic response of the body is the same as in the normal stress reaction, but the symptoms are more severe and last for a longer period. It

Table 23.3 Epidemiology of stress-related disorders

Disorder	Prevalence *(examples where no overall figures available)*	Lifetime risk	Male:female
Acute stress reaction	13–15% after road traffic accidents 30–40% after terrorist attacks	Unknown	Unknown
Post-traumatic stress disorder	3%	1–8% overall 15% conflict zones 50% rape victims	1:>2
Adjustment disorders	5–10% hospital inpatients 20% children after moving house	Unknown	1:>1 More common in the elderly

is generally accepted that having symptoms after a stressful event is normal for up to about 48 hours, but after this point the majority of people will have recovered. By definition, acute stress reaction lasts no more than 4 weeks. Cases that last longer are described as post-traumatic stress disorder (PTSD). Box 23.1 shows the typical symptoms seen in an acute stress reaction and the diagnostic criteria are shown in Box 23.2.

Co-morbidity

The most common co-morbidities in acute stress reactions are depression and substance misuse.

Differential diagnosis

- **PTSD.** By consensus if symptoms continue beyond 4 weeks the diagnosis is PTSD.
- **Adjustment disorder.** Symptoms are more generalized and milder in response to any stressor (it does not need to be extremely threatening or horrific).
- **Brief psychotic disorder.** Watch out for hallucinations, delusions, disorganized speech, or grossly abnormal behaviour.
- **Dissociative disorders.** The presence of dissociative symptoms in the absence of a stressor.
- **Organic disorder.** A head injury or space-occupying lesion in the brain can sometimes cause similar symptoms to acute stress reaction. History of a head

Box 23.1 Symptoms of acute stress reaction and post-traumatic stress disorder

Increased arousal

- Sweating, palpitations, and tremor
- Anxiety and panic attacks
- Restlessness, impaired concentration, and purposeless activity
- Irritability, depression, anger, or despair
- Insomnia

'Dissociative' symptoms

- Emotional numbness and 'being in a daze'
- Reduced awareness of surroundings
- Difficulty in recall of the stressful events
- Depersonalization and derealization

'Re-experiencing' symptoms

- Flashbacks (*sudden and repeated re-experiencing of visual images of traumatic experiences which are often not recalled at other times*)
- Recurrent images or thoughts
- Disturbing dreams

Avoidance of reminders of the stressful events

Maladaptive coping strategies

injury, headaches, or the finding of neurological signs should raise suspicion, and appropriate imaging should be requested.

Box 23.2 ICD-10 F43.0 Acute Stress Reaction

Main features

- Acute stress reaction refers to the development of transient emotional, somatic, cognitive, or behavioural symptoms as a result of exposure to an event or situation of an extremely threatening or horrific nature
- The response to the stressor is considered to be normal given the severity of the stressor and starts within a few days

Associated features

- Symptoms are shown in Box 23.1

Duration

- Onset shortly after the event with symptoms subsiding within a few days and lasting not longer than 4 weeks

Exclusions

- Post-traumatic stress disorder

ICD-11 beta draft: key changes 7B26 Acute Stress Reaction

- None expected

Adapted from *International Classification of Diseases*, 10th Revision (ICD-10). Copyright (2016) World Health Organization.

Aetiology

Many kinds of highly stressful events can provoke an acute stress reaction, but not all those exposed will be affected. This suggests some kind of personal predisposition and is probably a combination of psychological and biological factors. Note that stress reactions can occur among bystanders as well as those directly involved, and among those involved in rescuing or caring for others.

1 **Psychological theories.** A variety of psychological mechanisms are probably at work in acute stress reaction, but dissociation is the most studied. Dissociation reduces the negative consequences of trauma by restricting awareness of the event and thereby preventing the person from being overwhelmed by the traumatic experience. Unfortunately, this prevents recovery as it does not allow the experience to be processed and integrated into existing coping mechanisms.

2 **Biological theories.** The main theory is based upon classical conditioning. When a traumatic event occurs (an unconditioned stimulus), people respond with fear (unconditioned response). As reminders of the trauma occur (conditioned stimulus), people then respond with fear reactions (conditioned response). It is thought that in some people, the stress response becomes sensitized to repeated stimuli, and a larger response is produced to each stimulus. Those people who suffer a panic attack during a traumatic event are very likely to experience increasing panic attacks in the few weeks afterwards.

Prognosis

The majority of acute stress reactions will spontaneously remit within a few days to a week. Those that do not may go on to develop PTSD, depression, and/or phobic disorders. Individuals with more severe symptoms (especially dissociation), with psychiatric co-morbidities or previous episodes of stress disorder are probably more likely to develop PTSD but this is an area of current research.

Management

Most acute stress reactions can be managed by the family doctor, with the majority only needing general reassurance and practical advice. An outline of treatment strategies is shown in Box 23.3—more severe cases may be referred to secondary care.

Debriefing. Until recently, a type of counselling known as debriefing was often made widely available after stressful events. The aim was to promote adaptation to the traumatic event, and it was usually given within 24–72 hours of the trauma. Subjects *talked* about the stressful events and were encouraged to express their

Box 23.3 Treatment of acute reactions to stressful experiences

General measures

- Explain that the majority of patients will recover within 4 weeks
- Provide emotional and practical support (latter can be essential after natural disasters, fires, assaults, etc.)
- Help with residual problems—for example, disability after a traffic accident

Psychological treatments

- Encourage recall of, and coming to terms with, the events
- Help with developing effective (rather than maladaptive) coping strategies
- CBT (best evidence for trauma-focused therapy)

Pharmacological treatments

- SSRIs:
  - Consider if: high risk of developing PTSD, evidence of depression, or if the patient is too unwell to engage with CBT
- Short-term anxiolytics

thoughts and feelings at the time and since. However, the practice lacked an evidence base. A Cochrane review of RCTs found that while the majority of people said they found the counselling useful, it did not reduce the proportion of patients developing PTSD. UK guidance is now that debriefing should not be routinely offered to patients. CBT differs from debriefing crucially in its emphasis on integrating recovered memories with existing ones, and on self-help. Evidence suggests the most effective strategy is a brief intervention, typically five sessions of individual therapy. Studies vary in their results but on average, CBT reduces the proportion of people developing PTSD by 20–50 per cent.

Post-traumatic stress disorder

PTSD is a disorder that may develop after exposure to an exceptionally threatening or horrifying event. Descriptions of psychological disturbance secondary to trauma are found frequently in literature (e.g. Shakespeare's *Henry IV*), but the first clinical descriptions of the syndrome were not published until the horrors of the World Wars and Holocaust forced the issue into mainstream practice. A variety of terms have been used to describe what we now call PTSD, including **railway spine**, **stress syndrome**, **shell shock**, **battle fatigue**, and **traumatic (war) neurosis**. Our modern understanding of PTSD began in the 1970s, when studies were undertaken in the forces that fought in the Vietnam War.

What makes a stressful event traumatic?

As discussed in the introduction, stress is a subjective experience, which makes it hard to generalize as to the severity of a given situation. It is accepted that for a stressor to be called traumatic it must be **outside the range of usual human experience** *and* **markedly distressing to almost anyone**. Experiences that are frequently associated with PTSD include rape, violence during conflicts, being held captive, genocides, and all types of abuse. However, you should always treat the patient in front of you rather than the referral letter contents: PTSD may occur in one individual after a minor car accident (perhaps within the range of usual human experience) but not in a genocide survivor.

Clinical features

The symptoms of PTSD are the same as those of acute stress reaction (Box 23.1), but they last for longer. The essential differences are that symptoms have **lasted for more than 4 weeks** and **dissociative symptoms** must be present. The change of nomenclature/diagnosis at 4 weeks may appear arbitrary, but these cases generally run a chronic course and require a different treatment strategy from those used for acute stress reaction. As explained earlier, there are a number of characteristic features. The diagnostic criteria are shown in Box 23.4; these also cover the core clinical presentation.

Box 23.4 ICD-10 F43.1 Post-Traumatic Stress Disorder

Main features

- A delayed or protracted response to an extremely threatening or horrific event or series of events
- Characterized by re-experiencing the traumatic event or events—vivid intrusive memories, flashbacks, or nightmares
- Dissociative symptoms—difficulty with recall, 'numbness', depersonalization, derealization
- Avoidance of thoughts and memories of the event or activities/people reminiscent of the event (s).
- Persistent perception of a heightened current threat—shown by hypervigilance or an enhanced startle reaction

Associated features

- Symptoms of increased arousal—anxiety, irritability, insomnia, poor concentration
- Depression

Duration

- Symptoms persist for more than 4 weeks after the stressor
- Symptoms must last for at least several weeks

Disability

- Symptoms must cause a significant impairment in functioning

Exclusions

- Acute stress reaction

ICD-11 beta draft: key changes 7B20 Post-Traumatic Stress Disorder

- None expected to PTSD but a new diagnosis added as listed below in box

ICD-11 beta draft: 7B21 Complex Post-Traumatic Stress Disorder

Main features

- A disorder that may develop following exposure to an event or series of events of an extreme and prolonged or repetitive nature that is experienced as extremely threatening and from which escape is difficult or impossible
- Examples: torture, slavery, genocide campaigns, prolonged domestic violence, repeated childhood sexual or physical abuse
- Core symptoms:
  1. Fulfils criteria for PTSD
  2. Severe and pervasive problems in affect regulation
  3. Persistent beliefs about oneself as defeated or worthless, accompanied by feelings of shame, guilt, or failure related to the stressor
  4. Persistent difficulties in sustaining relationships

Disability

- The disturbance causes significant impairment in personal, family, social, educational, occupational, or other important areas of functioning

Source data from *International Classification of Diseases*, 10th Revision (ICD-10), World Health Organization 2016, and *International Classification of Diseases*, 11th revision (ICD-11), World Health Organization Beta draft 2016.

Co-morbidity

It is often difficult to determine if co-morbidities in patients with PTSD are primary disorders or secondary reactions to the traumatic event. The most common co-morbidities are depression, anxiety disorders, somatization, and alcohol or substance misuse. In the US National Comorbidity Replication Study (see 'Further reading'), 88 per cent of patients with PTSD fitted the criteria for another psychiatric diagnosis.

Differential diagnosis

- **Acute stress reaction.** Symptoms have been present for less than 4 weeks.
- **Adjustment disorder.** The stressor is of lesser severity, with milder, more generalized symptoms.

- **Depressive disorder.** Ask about core and biological symptoms and whether the symptoms predate the stressful event.
- **Anxiety disorder.** Usually the stressful event will not fit the criteria for being traumatic, and there will be no or few dissociative symptoms.
- **Obsessive–compulsive disorder.** Intrusive repetitive thoughts, dreams, and images are also found in obsessive–compulsive disorder. The key is to identify rituals, and there should be resistance towards the obsessions and compulsions.
- **Brief psychotic disorder or schizophrenia.** The presence of hallucinations, delusions, disorganized speech, or grossly abnormal behaviour points to a psychotic disorder.
- **Dissociative disorders.** The presence of dissociative symptoms in the absence of an extreme stressor.
- **Substance-induced disorder.**

Aetiology

The necessary cause of PTSD is an *exceptionally stressful event* in which the person was involved directly or as a witness. However, only a minority of those involved in the same event develop the disorder, and the reason for this is currently unknown. PTSD is more common among those involved most directly in the stressful events, but the variation in response is not accounted for solely by the *degree of personal involvement*. The aetiology of PTSD is controversial and probably complex, a brief overview is given in Table 23.4 and common risk factors are listed in Box 23.5.

Course and prognosis

The majority of patients with PTSD will recover within 1 year of the traumatic event, but about 30 per cent will

Table 23.4 Aetiology of post-traumatic stress disorder

Predisposing factors	Precipitating factors	Maintaining factors
- **Genetics**: heritability 30–40% - **Enhanced physiological reactions to stress:** patients with PTSD show higher levels of epinephrine and corticotrophin-releasing hormone secretion to stressors than controls - **Neurotransmitter dysregulation**: reduced central serotonergic activity → therapeutic effects of SSRIs. Alpha-blockers promote flashbacks suggesting abnormal noradrenergic function - **Neuroanatomical abnormalities:** smaller hippocampi than controls in PTSD patients and heightened response to stress in limbic system and prefrontal cortex on functional MRI	- Traumatic event	- **Conditioning theory:** when a traumatic event occurs (an unconditioned stimulus), people respond with fear (unconditioned response). As reminders of the trauma occur (conditioned stimulus), people then respond with fear reactions (conditioned response). Avoidance of stimuli reinforces the conditioning, as it leads to reduced discomfort in the absence of a stimulus - **Stimuli triggering memories of the event:** frequent memories are associated with a chronic course of PTSD - **Behaviours that maintain symptoms:** Avoidance, safety behaviours (e.g. checking gas is off after being stuck in a fire), or use of alcohol/substances prevent a return to normality and cause continued symptoms - **Differing personal understanding of the event.** PTSD patients are unable to 'shake-off' an event as a one-off and may develop negative cognitions that generalize beyond it; e.g. person starts to believe they were responsible for the stressor or that they are a worthless person for becoming ill

Box 23.5 Factors associated with developing post-traumatic stress disorder

Biological

- Females
- Family or personal psychiatric disorder
- Age: children are particularly vulnerable
- Ethnic minorities
- Low intelligence and/or low educational level

Psychological

- Childhood adversity or abuse
- Exposure to previous trauma
- Low self-esteem
- Peri-traumatic dissociation

Social

- Lack of social support
- Multiple ongoing socioeconomic adversities
- Occupation with exposure to traumatic events (e.g. military personnel)

Adapted from *Evidence-Based Mental Health*, 4, Review: 14 risk factors for post-traumatic stress disorder include childhood abuse and family psychiatric history, p. 61. Copyright (2001) BMJ Publishing Group Ltd.

have chronic symptoms. There is good evidence that treatment can be effective even when symptoms have been present for a long time (see Science box 23.1).

Assessment

In the majority of cases, a diagnosis of PTSD will be relatively straightforward. However, co-morbidities are so frequent that a full psychiatric history (including third-party information where possible) should be taken. It is important to exclude depressive disorder and do a complete risk assessment (see p. 69 and p. 261, respectively). If the traumatic event included injury to the head (e.g. from an assault or a road accident), a neurological examination should be carried out to exclude an injury to the brain. Conditions related to traumatic events are particularly associated with litigation: be sure to record the assessment fully.

Treatment

Treatment of PTSD has a solid evidence base and there are clinical guidelines in most countries depending on local resources (Box 23.6). It is extremely important to reassure all patients that the symptoms they are experiencing are part of PTSD, and are not a sign that they are going crazy.

Psychological treatments for PTSD

The first-line treatment for PTSD should be psychological therapy:

1 Trauma-focused cognitive behavioural therapy (CBT); or

2 Eye movement desensitization and reprocessing (EMDR).

Meta-analysis has shown CBT and EMBR to be equally effective, but CBT is more widely available. Specialized trauma-focused CBT for PTSD includes both *exposure* and *cognitive therapy*. The exposure element involves helping the patient to remember and put together memories of the events, and to relive the stressor with an emphasis on discussing their thoughts and feelings during the process. It is thought that exposure works in two ways: getting the patient used to being in the situation again (habituation), and organizing their memories such that they can identify that intrusive re-experiences are recollections, and are not happening right now. Cognitive therapy helps the patient to identify disbeliefs that they have formed about the events and to challenge these beliefs and change their behaviours surrounding them. A completed course of CBT reduces symptoms to a clinically insignificant level in 60 per cent of patients.

EMDR is another specialized treatment that assists the patient to process memories of the traumatic event and feel more positive about it. The patient is told to track the therapist's finger as they move it rapidly back and forth, which induces saccadic eye movements. During this process the patient is supposed to focus on a trauma-related image, and then afterwards to discuss the thoughts and emotions that surround it. This is repeated many times while focusing on different

SCIENCE BOX 23.1

Is there a gene for stress?

When a group of people are exposed to the same stressor, there is a wide range of individual response. Twin studies show a heritability of PTSD between 30 and 40 per cent and recent case–control studies have found significantly higher rates of PTSD in the offspring of those with known post-traumatic stress.[1] Candidate gene studies have been used to try and identify specific 'stress-related genes'. One example is pituitary adenylate cyclase activating polypeptide (PACAP)—which modulates CRH release and therefore the HPA axis—which has various common nucleotide variants in its receptor gene that are associated with PTSD.[2] The strongest link is for females, especially those who have also suffered childhood adversity.[3] The Grady Trauma Project, looking at African Americans with high trauma exposure, has reported some evidence for PTSD being associated with variants in the C-reactive protein gene (CRP). Several polymorphisms which affect plasma CRP levels are significantly related to PTSD risk and especially the startle response.[4] Other acute-phase proteins are being similarly investigated, especially in patients whose traumatic event including physical injury. Pituitary SLC6A4, a polymorphism in the promoter region of the ST-transporter gene which reduces transcription of the transporter, was initially associated with PTSD in small trials. However, a meta-analysis has since shown no significant association.[5] Unfortunately, many candidate gene trials have been underpowered, meaning initially promising results do not provide useful answers when meta-analyses or larger trials are conducted. It is likely to be a complex genetic picture, with significant gene–environment interactions, but hopefully further investigations may help to identify those patients who may be at higher risk of developing PTSD.

1 Roth M, Neuner F, Elbert T. Transgenerational consequences of PTSD: risk factors for the mental health of children whose mothers have been exposed to the Rwandan genocide. *International Journal of Mental Health Systems* 2014;8:12.

2 Vaudry D, Falluel-Morel A, Bourgault S, et al. Pituitary adenylate cyclase-activating polypeptide and its receptors: 20 years after the discovery. *Pharmacological Reviews* 2009;61:283–357.

3 Almli LM, Srivastava A, Fani N, et al. Follow-up and extension of a prior genome-wide association study of posttraumatic stress disorder: gene x environment associations and structural magnetic resonance imaging in a highly traumatized African-American civilian population. *Biological Psychiatry* 2014;76:E3–E4.

4 Smoller JW. The genetics of stress-related disorders: PTSD, depression, and anxiety disorders. *Neuropsychopharmacology* 2016;41:297–319.

5 Gressier F, Calati R, Balestri M, et al. The 5-HTTLPR polymorphism and posttraumatic stress disorder: a meta-analysis. *Journal of Traumatic Stress* 2013;26:645–653.

Box 23.6 Treatment of post-traumatic stress disorder

General measures

- Provide support (practical, emotional, social, self-help materials)
- Information and education about PTSD
- Treatment of co-morbidities
- Short-term hypnotics if necessary

Specific interventions

- Watchful waiting: symptoms for less than 4 weeks or minimal functional deficit
- First-line interventions:
  - Trauma-focused CBT *or*
  - Eye movement desensitization and reprocessing
- Second-line interventions if therapy is unsuccessful or not possible:
  - Antidepressants: SSRIs (paroxetine), venlafaxine, and mirtazapine have the best evidence
- Combination treatments: combining therapy and antidepressants; SSRI + venlafaxine/mirtazapine; adjunctive treatment with an atypical antipsychotic (best evidence for olanzapine)

CASE STUDY BOX 23.1

Post-traumatic stress disorder

A 38-year-old man, originally from Rwanda, presented to his GP complaining of poor sleep. On questioning, he revealed that he had fled Rwanda after witnessing his entire family being massacred during the 1994 civil war. He described terrifying dreams where visions of the genocide returned to him, and he was so scared of them that it became difficult to get to sleep. He also had frequent flashbacks which sometimes led to panic attacks, and that poor concentration meant he had trouble keeping in employment. The GP explained that PTSD was the likely diagnosis, and provided a web link to self-help materials in the patient's first language. She then made a referral for CBT, which the patient initially attended for, but his English was poor and he found it very difficult to discuss what had happened. At this stage the GP referred him to a psychiatrist, who decided to prescribe fluoxetine and recommended an online CBT course. Over the next year, the patient's English improved and he felt more motivated on fluoxetine. He was then able to undertake a course of individual CBT, which improved his symptoms considerably.

images. The treatment is more effective than placebo treatment but its success has not been shown to depend on the specific eye movement component (see Case study box 23.1).

Reactions to sexual assault or abuse

Reactions to sexual assault (rape)

Sexual assault is unfortunately more common than statistics suggest, with the police estimating only one in seven incidents are reported. After a sexual assault, it is important to give the person practical, emotional, and social support. It is helpful to talk over the problems, and to put them in touch with a victim support organization. These provide practical support and information, such as help in reporting the crime and understanding the criminal justice system. In the 1970s, the term 'rape trauma syndrome' became used to describe the commonest psychological reaction to an assault. It is now recognized that this is a variant of PTSD, and it is more appropriate to use the terminology of acute stress reaction and PTSD.

Approximately one-third of people who have been sexually assaulted have long-term psychological problems relating to it: asking about sexual abuse of any type should be part of all psychiatric assessments. The symptoms are as outlined in Box 23.1. There are a number of specific psychological reactions that are common in victims of sexual assault/abuse, and should be addressed in psychological treatment including:

- feeling humiliated, ashamed, and embarrassed about what happened;
- blaming themselves for having put themselves at risk;
- loss of confidence and poor self-esteem;
- difficulty in trusting others, especially in sexual relationships;
- feeling vulnerable to further attack.

Long-term effects of sexual trauma in childhood

Sexually abused children frequently suffer psychological difficulties during the rest of their life (Box 23.7). Most adults who were sexually abused as children retain some memory of the events, though these are often incomplete. Forgotten aspects are sometimes recalled again, for example, after a chance encounter with some reminder of the events or when the person becomes sexually active as an adult. Memories may also return during the history taking and discussion involved in psychological treatment. Occasionally, an adult who is receiving counselling or psychotherapy suddenly recalls an episode of child abuse of which he or she was previously completely unaware. Sometimes such memories are confirmed by people who knew the

Box 23.7 Conditions associated with childhood sexual abuse

- Anxiety
- Depression
- PTSD
- Eating disorders
- Functional disorders (somatization)
- Chronic pain
- Substance abuse (including alcohol)
- Poor educational and work performance
- Low self-esteem and poor confidence
- Problems with sexual relationships
- Violent and destructive behaviour
- Deliberate self-harm and suicide

patient at the time, but sometimes they are vigorously denied by others, including the alleged abuser. When this happens, it has to be decided whether the reports are true memories of actual events, or false memories induced by overzealous questioning, interpretation, or suggestion (the **false memory syndrome**). It is uncertain whether memories of sexual abuse can be completely forgotten for many years and then recalled. It is, however, generally agreed that care should be taken during history taking, counselling, and psychotherapy to avoid questions or comments that could suggest childhood sexual abuse, and that any apparent recall of events of which the person had no previous recollection should be considered most carefully and supporting evidence sought, before concluding that it is a true memory.

Children who have suffered sexual abuse may present in a variety of ways, with secondary psychiatric problems, within the criminal justice system, or via social services. A full multidisciplinary assessment should be undertaken (see p. 103), and then usually family and/or individual therapy is indicated. Adults usually present for treatment with a secondary psychiatric problem (Box 23.7) and management should be aimed at the current symptoms, with consideration given to the sexual abuse being a causative factor. For example, a patient presenting with an eating disorder will require the same treatment as other patients (see Chapter 27), but in individual

therapy the issues surrounding the sexual abuse should be discussed.

Normal and abnormal adjustment reactions

Normal adjustment

Adjustment refers to the psychological reactions involved in adapting to new circumstances. Like the physiological reaction to stress, it is a normal process that is expected after major life changes such as divorce, illness, financial difficulties, or a new baby.

Symptoms of normal adjustment are mild, short-lived anxiety, depression, irritability, and poor concentration that have minimal functional impacts.

Adjustment disorder

Adjustment is judged to be abnormal if the distress involved is:

1 **greater** than that which would be expected in response to the particular stressful events (a subjective judgement); *or*

2 is accompanied by **impairment of functioning**; *and*

3 is **within a month of the stressor**; *and*

4 is **not severe enough to meet the criteria for another diagnosis**.

It is clear from the listed points that adjustment disorders are really a bridge between normal behaviour and psychiatric conditions.

Clinical features

There are no specific symptoms of an adjustment disorder, and patients usually present with mild symptoms of depression, anxiety, emotional or behavioural disturbance, or a combination of these. The diagnostic criteria are outlined in Box 23.8. A collaborative history from a relative or the GP can be helpful in making a judgement as to if the distress is abnormal for that individual in the circumstances.

Box 23.8 ICD-10 43.2 Adjustment Disorder

Main features

- A maladaptive reaction to an identifiable psychosocial stressor or multiple stressors
- Patient is preoccupied with the stressor or its consequences leading to excessive worry, recurrent and distressing thoughts about the stressor

Associated features

- Rumination

Duration

- Symptoms occur within a month of the stressor and typically resolve within 6 months

Disability

- Failure to adapt to the stressor that causes significant impairment in personal, family, social, educational, occupational, or other important areas of functioning

Exclusions

- Symptoms not severe or specific enough to meet criteria for another mental health diagnosis, for example, depressive episode or separation anxiety disorder of childhood

ICD-11 beta draft key changes: 7B23 Adjustment Disorder

- None expected

Adapted from *International Classification of Diseases*, 10th Revision (ICD-10). Copyright (2016) World Health Organization.

Co-morbidity

Alcohol and substance misuse frequently coexist with adjustment disorders.

Differential diagnosis

- **Acute stress reaction or PTSD.** Was the stressor extreme and traumatic, or a more routine change in life situation? Consider PTSD if symptoms have continued beyond 6 months.
- **Mood disorder.** Ask about core and biological symptoms and whether the symptoms predate the stressful event.
- **Anxiety disorder.**
- **Alcohol or substance misuse** (see p. 423).
- **Grief reaction.** Was the stressor a bereavement, with severe symptoms for more than 6 months?
- **Organic disorder causing psychological symptoms.** Take a full history—it is common that psychological symptoms are attributed to an adjustment disorder after diagnosis of a severe physical illness, when actually the symptoms are being caused by the physical pathology itself.

Aetiology

Adjustment disorders may be caused by any identifiable stressful event. It is thought that some people are more vulnerable to developing an adjustment disorder due to a lack of, or failure of existing, coping mechanisms. Individuals who have a broad range of flexible coping mechanisms usually adjust well to any change, whereas those who have more limited resources (especially poor problem-solving skills) fare less well.

Risk factors include:

- age—young people have fewer established coping mechanisms;
- female sex;
- past experiences of stressful events;
- past psychiatric history;
- low self-esteem.

Course and prognosis

The majority of patients with an adjustment disorder will recover without any intervention within a few months. Approximately 20 per cent of adult patients and 40 per cent of adolescents go on to develop a more serious psychiatric disorder, usually depression or substance/alcohol misuse.

Management

Many patients with an adjustment disorder do not need any formal treatment; they recover spontaneously

Box 23.9 Management of adjustment disorders

General measures

- Practical support to manage the stressor
- Information and reassurance about adjustment disorders for patient and carers

Psychological

- Self-help materials, including problem-solving techniques
- An opportunity to talk—usually a friend/relative or other sympathetic listener will suffice rather than formal therapy
- Supportive brief psychotherapy including problem-solving techniques (rarely needed)

Pharmacological

- Short-term anxiolytics (in the immediate aftermath of the stressor)
- Antidepressants: SSRI and screen carefully for depression.

with the help of friends and family. Any treatment given should aim to teach the person a wider range of coping skills to protect against future episodes (Box 23.9).

Adjustment to special situations

Adjustment to physical illness

Being diagnosed with a serious physical illness is a stressor that many people experience and, as with any stressor, they may react in a variety of different ways.

Why is being diagnosed with a physical illness stressful?

1 Unexpectedness of the diagnosis.

2 Difficulty accessing medical care.

3 Feelings of uncontrollability over what has and what might happen.

4 Poor understanding of aetiology and likely progression of the condition.

5 Treatments may be complex, unpleasant, and/or time-consuming.

6 Associated life changes—for example, giving up work or driving.

The stress associated with physical illness may lead to *anxiety* and *depression*, and sometimes to *anger*. Certain *medications* used in the treatment of physical illness may also affect mood and behaviour. Occasionally, adjustment to physical illness often involves an initial stage of denial, which protects against overwhelming distress. This is only a problem if it persists beyond the early stages and interferes with engagement with treatment. Most reactions are short-lived, subsiding as the person adjusts to the new situation. The stressful effect of physical illness cannot be judged solely in terms of its objective severity; it depends also on the *patient's appraisal* of the illness and its likely consequences. This appraisal may be unrealistic and based on false assumptions. The latter may be shared by the relatives, thus reinforcing the patient's concerns, or contradicted by them, thus leading to family conflict.

Adjustment to having a physical illness involves a set of changes known as **illness behaviour**. This behaviour includes seeking medical advice, taking medication, accepting help, and giving up activities. Some people are able to make these changes easily, but others struggle. This may lead to an adjustment disorder, another psychiatric condition, or to **abnormal illness behaviour**. Illness behaviours are at first adaptive, but if they persist too long they may become maladaptive. Occasionally, people adopt illness behaviours when they have no physical disorder. They are said to display **abnormal illness behaviour**.

The sick role

Society allows sick people to adopt a special role, which comprises two privileges and two duties:

Privileges:

- **Exemption** from some responsibilities.
- The **right** to help and care.

Duties:

- The **obligation** to seek and cooperate in treatment.
- The **expectation** of a wish to recover and efforts to achieve this.

The sick role is usually adaptive. However, some people continue to adopt a sick role long after the illness is over, avoiding responsibilities and depending on others instead of becoming independent. Others adopt the sick role without ever having experienced any physical disorder.

Treatment

When adjustment to physical illness is slow and incomplete, some support may be necessary. For serious physical conditions, there are often professionals available (e.g. a specialist nurse) who are experienced in managing patients with a particular diagnosis.

- **Psychoeducation.** A doctor should explain the nature of the physical illness, prognosis, and treatment. It is hard to remember everything said in a consultation so written material or web links are helpful.
- **Supportive talking and listening.** This may be a friend or family member, but sometimes more formal counselling is needed. The latter can address any maladaptive behaviours that may have developed and help teach problem-solving skills.
- **Managing co-morbidities.** The guidelines for co morbidities (e.g. depression) should be followed as usual. Occasionally, discussion with the patient's physical health team may be needed before initiating medications.

Adjustment to terminal illness

After terminal illness has been diagnosed, people tend to go through four stages in the journey to accepting their situation.

1 **Denial.** It may be experienced as a feeling of disbelief and a consequent initial period of calm. Denial usually reduces as the patient gradually comes to terms with the situation, but may return if there is progress of the disease which the patient is not ready to accept.

2 **Displacement.** Anger about the situation may be displaced on to professionals or relatives. It is often short lived and may reduce with psychoeducation.

3 **Dependency** is common among terminally ill people. It is adaptive at times when the patient is required to comply passively with treatment, but persisting or excessive dependency makes treatment more difficult, and increases the burden on the family.

4 **Acceptance** is the final stage of adjustment. The aim is to help the patient to reach this state before the final stage of the physical illness.

At some point during their illness, many people become anxious, depressed, guilty, angry, or adopt maladaptive ways of coping. About half of patients who die in hospital have some emotional symptoms. Understandably, these emotional reactions are more common in the young than in the old, and less common in the religious. The following symptoms are particularly common among the dying:

- **Anxiety** may be provoked by personal concerns about pain, disfigurement, or incontinence, and by concerns about others, especially the family.
- **Depression** may be provoked by the loss of valued activities and the prospect of separation from loved ones.
- **Confusion** due to delirium is frequent among dying patients, and is caused, for example, by dehydration, drug side effects, and secondary infection.
- **Guilt** may be caused by the belief that excessive demands are being placed on relatives or friends.
- **Anger** may derive from ideas about the unjustness of impending death.

Treatment

Control of physical symptoms. The first steps in treatment are to control symptoms such as pain, vomiting, or confusion.

Explaining the illness and treatment. If patients are allowed to lead the discussion, discussing the terminal nature of an illness is usually helpful rather than distressing. When patients ask about the prognosis they should be told the truth; evasive answers undermine trust. However, when patients do not at first indicate a desire to know the full extent of their problems, it is better to keep this information for a subsequent interview and time set aside for this.

Help for relatives. Relatives need information about the disease and its treatment, and opportunities to talk about their feelings and to prepare for the impending bereavement. Adjustment disorders are not uncommon in this group.

Referral to a psychiatrist is indicated when:

- there is *doubt about the psychiatric diagnosis* (e.g. between adjustment disorder and depressive disorder);
- the patient has had a *previous psychiatric disorder*;
- the patient *refuses to discuss* the illness, or to make necessary decisions;
- the patient *refuses to cooperate* with treatment, in order to determine whether this refusal is for rational reasons or has a psychiatric cause.

Grief reactions

- **Bereavement** refers to any loss event, typically the death of a loved one but it may occur after loss of one's health, home, country, or wealth.
- **Grief** is the response to bereavement, encompassing the thoughts, feelings, and emotions surrounding the event.

Normal grief

Similarly to the stress response, grief is a normal physiological process that only becomes abnormal if it is **prolonged**, **intense**, or **atypical**. The classical theory of the grief response is the Küber–Ross model, published in 1969, which was originally modelled on people suffering from terminal illness, and later adapted to those suffering from a catastrophic personal loss. The model included five stages: denial,

> **Box 23.10** The normal grief reaction
>
> **Stage 1: hours to days**
> Denial, disbelief, 'numbness'—there may be incomplete acceptance that the death has taken place.
>
> **Stage 2: weeks to 6 months**
> - Sadness, weeping, waves of grief
> - Somatic symptoms of anxiety
> - Poor sleep
> - Diminished appetite
> - Guilt, blame of others or self (*some project these feelings on to clinical staff for failing to provide optimal care for the dead person*)
> - Experience of the presence of the deceased
> - Hallucinations of the dead person's voice, illusions, vivid imagery
> - Preoccupation with memories of the deceased
> - Social withdrawal
>
> **Stage 3: weeks to months**
> - Symptoms resolve and social activities are resumed
> - Memories of good times
> - Symptoms may recur at anniversaries

anger, bargaining, depression, and acceptance, not attached to any particular timescales. More recent research suggests that this model is too restrictive, and that grief is typically more dynamic and multifactorial. However, it is relatively well accepted that there are three main stages to responding to bereavement, although these do not always occur in a restrictively linear order (Box 23.10).

Prolonged grief reaction

Grief is said to be abnormal when the symptoms are:

- **more intense** than usual;
- **prolonged** beyond 6 months;
- or **delayed** in onset.

Typically, the patient will present with symptoms of a moderately severe depressive disorder which is linked to a recent loss event (Box 23.11). There are a variety of circumstances that make it more likely that

Box 23.11 ICD-10

There is no separate diagnostic category for a grief reaction in ICD-10; it is classified as an adjustment reaction. A new diagnosis will be added to ICD-11:

ICD-11 beta draft: 7B23 Prolonged Grief Reaction

Main features

- There is a persistent and pervasive grief response following a bereavement
- Characterized by longing for the deceased or persistent preoccupation with the deceased
- Accompanied by intense emotional pain
- Clearly exceeds expected social, cultural, or religious norms for the individual's culture and context

Associated features

- Typical symptoms include sadness, guilt, anger, denial, blame, difficulty accepting the death, feeling one has lost a part of one's self, an inability to experience positive mood, emotional numbness, difficulty in engaging with activities

Duration

- Symptoms persist beyond 6 months after the death

Disability

- Significant impairment in personal, family, social, educational, occupational, or other important areas of functioning

Source data from *International Classification of Diseases*, 11th revision (ICD-11) Beta draft 2016.

an individual will have an abnormal grief reaction; these are outlined in Table 23.5.

Assessment and management

The majority of patients who suffer a loss do not require any formal intervention, but for those who do, treatment resembles that for other kinds of adjustment reaction.

Assessment should address the death and its circumstances, the relationship, and the history and course of the bereaved one's symptoms. It is important to assess available social support, and take a full psychiatric history. If there are symptoms of anxiety, depression, or another psychiatric diagnosis that are affecting functionality, it is appropriate to treat them along condition-specific guidelines.

Emotional support. The first step is to provide empathic, compassionate support by *listening* while the bereaved person talks about the loss, and to enable him or her to express feelings of sadness or anger. When the person is seen soon after the loss, it is helpful to *explain* the normal course of grieving, and to forewarn about the possibility of feeling as if the dead person were present, or experiencing illusions or hallucinations. Without this warning, these experiences may be very alarming. As time passes, the bereaved person should be encouraged to resume social contacts, to talk to other people about the loss, to remember happy and fulfilling experiences that were shared with the deceased, and to consider positive activities that the latter would have wanted survivors to undertake.

Table 23.5 Risk factors for a prolonged grief reaction

Pre-existing vulnerabilities	Nature of relationship	Circumstances of the death
• Avoidant or dependant personality traits	• Child or partner	• Death was prolonged
• Prior multiple losses	• Stillbirth, neonatal deaths, and cot deaths	• Sudden unexpected deaths
• Childhood separation anxiety		• People are missing, believed dead
• Personal psychiatric history	• Survivor dependent upon the deceased	• Homicide committed by a loved one
• Family history of psychiatric disorders		
• Co-morbid substance abuse		
• Multiple social and/or financial adversities		

Practical support. Help with death certification, funeral arrangements, and financial issues may be needed, and, following the loss of a partner, a parent may require help in caring for young children. The bereaved person may need help to move from the early stage of denial of the loss to *acceptance* of reality by viewing the body and by later putting away the dead person's belongings.

Supportive counselling. There is no evidence that one form of psychological intervention is better than another, so the choice is usually made on what is available locally. Options include:

- guided self-help programmes;
- bereavement counselling;
- specific brief CBT for traumatic grief;
- brief interpersonal psychotherapy.

Support groups and voluntary sector organizations can provide very useful peer support and specialist counselling (e.g. CRUSE).

Pharmacological treatments. If anxiety is severe or sleep disturbed in the first few days after a loss, then an anxiolytic or hypnotic drug may be appropriate. These should be prescribed in the short term only, due to the risks of tolerance and dependence, and the fact that in most cases distress can be reduced by the opportunity to talk and cry. Occasionally, grief is sufficiently intense to meet the criteria for depressive disorder—in this situation, antidepressant drug treatment may be warranted.

Further reading

Bisson J, Cosgrove S, Lewis C, Roberts N. Post-traumatic stress disorder. *BMJ* 2015;351:h6161.

CRUSE Bereavement Care. http://www.cruse.org.uk/.

Gelder MG, Andreasen NC, López-Ibor JJ, Geddes JR, eds. Chapter 4.6: Stress-related and adjustment disorders. In: *New Oxford Textbook of Psychiatry*. 2nd ed. Oxford: Oxford University Press; 2012:693–727.

National Institute for Health and Care Excellence. Post-traumatic stress disorder. NICE guideline [NG116]. Published December 2018. http://guidance.nice.org.uk/CG26.

Smoller JW. The genetics of stress-related disorders: PTSD, depression, and anxiety disorders. *Neuropsychopharmacology* 2016;41:297–319.

24 Anxiety and obsessional disorders

In the community, the term 'anxiety' is frequently associated with a stressful Western lifestyle and thought of as a modern phenomenon—but this is far from the case. Anxiety disorders were clearly described as early as the writings of Hippocrates, and have been prevalent in literary characterization to the present. Anxiety disorders are the most common type of psychiatric disorder, with one in three people experiencing them during a lifetime. They are characterized by marked, persistent mental and physical symptoms of anxiety, that are not secondary to another disorder and that impact negatively upon the sufferer's life. Anxiety disorders may be primary psychiatric conditions, or a secondary response to the stress associated with physical illness and its treatment. Many people with anxiety disorders never seek medical attention, but these are commonly seen conditions in both primary and secondary care, and they may present with either mental or physical complaints.

Obsessive–compulsive disorder is also considered in this chapter. Its relationship to anxiety disorders is uncertain—classification systems currently separate the two—but there are some important common features.

What is normal anxiety?

Normal anxiety is the response to threatening situations. Feelings of apprehension are accompanied by physiological changes that prepare for defence or escape ('**fight or flight**'), notably increases in heart rate, blood pressure, respiration, and muscle tension. Sympathetic nervous system activity is increased, causing symptoms such as tremor, sweating, polyuria, and diarrhoea. Attention and concentration are focused on the threatening situation. Anxiety is a beneficial response in dangerous situations, and should occur in everyday situations of perceived threat (e.g. examinations).

Abnormal anxiety is a response that is similar but out of proportion to the threat and/or is more prolonged, or occurs when there is no threat. With one exception, the symptoms of anxiety disorders are the

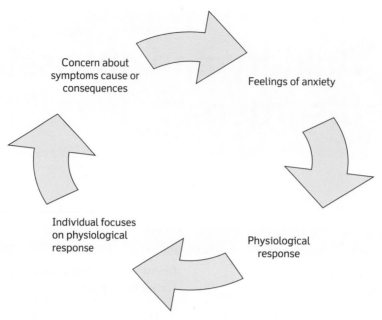

Fig. 24.1 Cycle of anxiety.

same as those of a normal anxiety response. The exception is that the focus of attention is not the external threat (as in the normal response) but the physiological response itself. Thus in abnormal anxiety, attention is focused on a symptom such as increased heart rate. This focus of attention is accompanied by concern about the cause of the symptom. For example, a common concern is that a rapid heartbeat is a sign of impending heart attack. Because these concerns are threatening, they activate a further anxiety response thus adding to the autonomic arousal, generating further concern, and setting up a vicious cycle of mounting anxiety (Fig. 24.1).

Anxiety disorders

Classification

Abnormal anxiety becomes clinically relevant when it causes distress or impairment of daily activities. Anxiety disorders are classified into those with continuous symptoms (**generalized anxiety disorder (GAD)**) and those

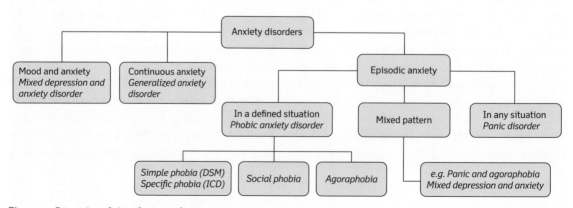

Fig. 24.2 Principles of classification of anxiety disorders.

with episodic symptoms. This is shown in Fig. 24.2. Mixed states of anxiety and depression are common; these were previously described as 'minor mood disorders' and are classified with depressive disorders, to which they are more closely related, and should be managed using the mood disorders treatment protocols (see p. 270).

Epidemiology

Anxiety disorders are common in the population, with a 1-year prevalence of about 14 per cent, or about 10 per cent if specific phobias are excluded. The approximate prevalence of the various kinds of anxiety disorder is shown in Table 24.1, along with some other useful epidemiology for all the diagnoses described in this section. Anxiety disorders frequently start early in life and often have a chronic waxing and waning course. Overall they are more common in females than males.

Generalized anxiety disorder

GAD is characterized by excessive, uncontrolled, and irrational worry about everyday things that is out of proportion to actual events. The worry typically shifts between concerns rapidly and impairs function. The diagnostic criteria for GAD are shown in Box 24.1 By convention, GAD is diagnosed only when symptoms of anxiety have been present for several months—shorter periods lead to a diagnosis of **stress** or **adjustment disorder** (see p. 312 and p. 322).

Clinical features

Patients may complain directly of anxiety, or ask for help for the many physical symptoms of anxiety. It is also important to remember physical diseases can produce the same symptoms as anxiety disorders—always take a full history and consider the differential diagnosis (see later). Symptoms are variable but the commonest are shown in Table 24.2.

Sleep is disturbed in a characteristic way. Patients lie awake worrying for long periods and then wake frequently, sometimes reporting unpleasant dreams where they feel scared upon waking for an unknown reason. Early waking is much less common among patients with a GAD than among patients with depression (see

Table 24.1 Epidemiology of anxiety disorders

Disorder	1-year prevalence (%)	Lifetime risk (%)	Age of onset	Male:female ratio
Any anxiety disorder	8.4	29.6		
Generalized anxiety disorder	0.9	2.8	Bimodal: 15–30 years then 40–60 years	1:2
Agoraphobia	0.3	0.8	Bimodal: 15–30 years then 70–80 years	1:2
Social phobia	1.2	2.4	Childhood–30 years	1:1
Specific phobia	5.4	7.7–8.3	Animals: mean 7 years Situational: teenage years	Unknown
Panic disorder	0.7	1.6	Bimodal: 15–25 years then 40–60 years	1:≥2
Obsessive–compulsive disorder	1.2	2.7	Teenage years	1:1

Box 24.1 ICD-10 F41.1 Generalized Anxiety Disorder

Main features

- Anxiety that is generalized and persistent but not restricted to, or even strongly predominating in, any particular environmental circumstances.

Associated features

- Muscular tension or motor restlessness.
- Sympathetic autonomic overactivity.
- Subjective experience of nervousness.
- Difficulty maintaining concentration.
- Irritability.
- Sleep disturbance.

Duration

- Symptoms must be present more days than not for at least several months.

Disability

- Significant distress or significant impairment in personal, family, social, educational, occupational, or other important areas of functioning.

ICD-11 beta draft: key changes 7B00 Generalized Anxiety Disorder

Change in the 'main features' definition:

Generalized anxiety disorder is characterized by marked symptoms of anxiety accompanied by either general apprehension or worry focused on multiple everyday events, most often concerning family, health, finances, and school or work.

Table 24.2 Typical symptoms of generalized anxiety disorder

Psychological	• Fearful anticipation or of losing control • Poor concentration • Irritability or low mood • Sensitivity to noise • Restlessness • Obsessive thoughts • Depersonalization or derealisation
Physical	• Difficulty in swallowing
Gastrointestinal	• Epigastric discomfort • Frequent or loose motions
Respiratory	• A 'tight' chest • Difficulty inhaling • Overbreathing
Cardiovascular	• Palpitations or awareness of missed beats • Chest pain
Genitourinary	• Frequent or urgent micturition • Failure of erection • Problems related to menstruation
Neuromuscular	• Tremor • Tinnitus • Dizziness, unsteadiness, feeling 'faint' • Headache (often tension-like) • Aching muscles (especially in the back and shoulders)
Sleep disturbance	• Insomnia and/or nightmares

p. 263). Therefore, early waking should always prompt a search for other symptoms of a depressive disorder.

Hyperventilation and panic attacks are common symptoms of GAD—see Boxes 24.2 and 24.3, and p. 333.

Co-morbidity

It is usual for patients with GAD to suffer from other mood and anxiety disorders; at least two-thirds of patients with a primary diagnosis of GAD meet criteria for another psychiatric disorder. The most common are depression, social phobia, panic disorder, and substance misuse (alcohol, benzodiazepines). Typically, substance misuse should be treated before primary anxiety-related interventions to attain a good outcome.

Box 24.2 Symptoms and signs of hyperventilation

- Rapid shallow breathing
- Dizziness
- Tinnitus
- Headache
- Chest discomfort
- Weakness
- Faintness
- Numbness and tingling in the hands and feet
- Carpopedal spasm

Differential diagnosis

GAD needs to be distinguished from other psychiatric disorders in which anxiety may be prominent, and from physical illnesses that produce similar symptoms:

- **Depressive disorder**—typically the mood symptoms are more severe than the anxiety symptoms and appeared first, and other symptoms of depressive disorder will be present.

- **Schizophrenia**—occasionally patients with schizophrenia complain of anxiety—which may be secondary to their psychotic phenomena.

- **Dementia** may first come to notice when the patient complains of anxiety. Poor memory can not necessarily be ascribed to poor concentration alone.

- **Drugs,** either prescribed or recreational, can cause anxiety-like symptoms. Alcohol, cannabis, antidepressants, antipsychotics, benzodiazepines, caffeine, and sedatives are frequent in psychiatry, but other common culprits include bronchodilators, antihypertensives, antiarrhythmics, anticonvulsants, thyroxine, chemotherapy, and antibiotics.

- **Withdrawal from drugs or alcohol**—for example, early morning anxiety in the withdrawing alcohol-dependent patient.

- **Physical illnesses**—especially if the symptoms are episodic:
  - Thyrotoxicosis leads to irritability, restlessness, tremor, and tachycardia. Check for an enlarged thyroid, atrial fibrillation, and exophthalmos, and arrange thyroid function tests.
  - Hypoparathyroidism.
  - Phaeochromocytoma.
  - Hypoglycaemia.
  - Arrhythmias.
  - Ménière's disease.
  - Temporal lobe epilepsy.
  - Respiratory disease.
  - Carcinoid tumours.

Box 24.3 Hyperventilation

Hyperventilation is overbreathing—usually in a rapid and shallow way—that results in a fall in the concentration of carbon dioxide in the blood and leads to a respiratory alkalosis. Paradoxically, overbreathing produces a feeling of breathlessness, which causes the patient to breathe even more vigorously. It is common in all anxiety disorders and should be considered when a patient has appropriate unexplained symptoms.

- **To terminate an acute episode,** the patient should rebreathe expired air from a paper bag. This increases the alveolar concentration of carbon dioxide, correcting the acid–base abnormality, and decreasing the feeling of breathlessness. Rebreathing during an episode is also an effective way of demonstrating that certain symptoms are caused by hyperventilation.
- **To prevent further episodes** of hyperventilation, patients should practise slow, controlled breathing, at first under supervision and then at home. Downloadable recordings are available free online that can help teach this skill. It is important to identify and treat the underlying anxiety disorder/diagnosis.

Aetiology

An overview of the causes of GAD is outlined in Table 24.3. **Predisposing factors** are of four kinds: genetic, neurobiological, childhood upbringing, and personality type:

1 **Genetic causes.** GAD is five times more prevalent in those with first-degree relatives with GAD than

Table 24.3 Aetiology of generalized anxiety disorder

Predisposing factors	Precipitating factors	Maintaining factors
Genetics: • Family history • Twin studies Neurobiological mechanisms Personality Childhood upbringing	Stressful events, e.g.: • Relationships • Unemployment • Financial problems • Ill health • Natural disasters	Continuing stressful life events Depressive disorder Cycle of anxiety (Fig. 24.1)

in the general population and there is a high concordance between monozygotic twins.

2 **Neurobiological mechanisms** have been implicated based on investigation of the stress response in animal models and patients. The response to stimulation of the autonomic nervous system is prolonged in patients with GAD, and negative feedback of the HPA axis by cortisol is reduced.

3 **Childhood upbringing.** Inconsistent parenting, poor attachments, a chaotic lifestyle, and traumatic events in childhood may cause anxiety which persists into later life.

4 **Personality traits.** Anxious and worry-prone personalities are linked to anxiety disorder but other personality difficulties can predispose by making people less able to cope with stressful events.

Prognosis

By convention, the diagnosis of GAD cannot be made until the symptoms have been present for several months. Without treatment, about 80 per cent of patients still have the disorder 3 years after the onset, and for many it is a lifelong problem. Unemployment and separation/divorce are higher in those with GAD than the general population. Prognosis is worse when symptoms are severe, and when there is agitation, derealization, conversion symptoms, or suicidal ideas. Brief episodes of depression are frequent among patients with a chronic GAD and it is often during one of these episodes that further treatment is sought.

Assessment and management

There are many common features in treating the various anxiety disorders: the following sections outline a general approach to all patients with anxiety disorders, plus individual guidance for GAD (Tables 24.4 and 24.5). Specific treatments for other disorders will be covered later in the chapter. The great majority of patients will not need specialist care, but if two different treatments delivered in primary care fail they should be referred into mental health services.

Phobic anxiety disorders

Phobic disorders have similar presenting features to GAD, but with three important distinguishing points:

1 **Anxiety occurs in particular circumstances only.** These are typically situations (e.g. heights, crowded rooms), living things (e.g. spiders), or natural phenomena, such as thunder.

2 **Avoidance** of circumstances that provoke anxiety.

3 **Anticipatory anxiety** when there is the prospect of encountering such circumstances.

Phobic disorders are classified in three groups: specific (or simple) phobia, social phobia, and agoraphobia. As explained earlier, some patients have both agoraphobia and non-situational panic.

Specific phobia

A person with specific phobia is inappropriately anxious in the presence of a particular object or situation,

Table 24.4 General treatment plan for anxiety disorders

Assessment	• Take a full history from the patient, referrer, old notes, and third parties
	• Ask about: current symptoms and functional impact, previous treatments, current medications (prescribed, illicit, over-the-counter, alcohol, caffeine, nicotine), premorbid personality
	• Full risk assessment
	• Make a diagnosis
	• Detect any co-morbid anxiety disorders, depression, and/or substance misuse (see Chapters 21 and 29)
	• Physical examination and investigations if suspicion of physical aetiology
General measures	• Agree a clear plan and assign one named physician to manage the patient's care (this reduces further anxiety)
	• Psychoeducation: educate to break the vicious cycle of anxiety. Provide verbal and written materials
	• Problem-solving techniques (p. 159) and relaxation help relieve stress
	• Manage hyperventilation (see Box 24.3)
Psychological treatment (see also Chapter 14)	• Self-help books, based on cognitive behavioural techniques
	• Group/computerized cognitive behavioural therapy
	• Individual cognitive behavioural therapy (minimum 16 × 1-hour sessions)
Pharmacotherapy	• Antidepressants: SSRIs (first line) or tricyclics (see Table 24.5) Try at least two SSRIs initially, if successful, continue for at least 6 months after recovery. Mental health specialists may then try venlafaxine
	• Short-term benzodiazepines—high risk of dependency
	• Buspirone: non-benzodiazepine anxiolytic with lower dependency

or when anticipating this encounter, and has the urge to avoid the object or situation. A list of common phobias is shown in Table 24.6. The urge to avoid the stimulus is strong, and in most cases there is actual avoidance. Anticipatory anxiety is often severe; for example, a person who fears storms may become extremely anxious when there are only black clouds, which might precede a storm. The diagnostic criteria for specific phobias are shown in Box 24.4.

Co-morbidity

Of individuals with a specific phobia, 83.4 per cent will meet criteria for another psychiatric diagnosis: these are most commonly other anxiety disorders or depression.

Aetiology

Most of the specific phobias of adult life begin in childhood when specific phobias are extremely common.

Why most childhood phobias disappear and a few persist into adult life is not known, except that the most severe phobias are more likely to do so. One suggestion is that phobias are due to classical conditioning, with the individual reinforcing a learned behaviour after a negative experience with an object or situation. Avoidance then maintains the fear and makes it hard to eliminate.

There is robust evidence for a genetic component to specific phobias; one in three first-degree relatives of a person with specific phobia also meet diagnostic criteria.

Prognosis

There is little reliable information about the prognosis of specific phobias. Clinical experience indicates that specific phobias that began in childhood continue for many years, while those starting after a stressful experience in adult life may improve with

Table 24.5 Psychological treatments for specific anxiety disorders

Disorder	Therapy
General treatments	
Any anxiety disorder	Psychoeducation for patient and carers
	Relaxation training
	Problem-solving skills
	Self-help: books, websites, telephone-guided treatment
	Computerized CBT
	Voluntary-sector group meetings and/or therapies
Specific therapies	
GAD	CBT
Phobias	CBT: graded-exposure therapy
Social phobias/agoraphobia	CBT: graded-exposure therapy
Panic disorder	Specialized CBT for panic disorder (usually individual sessions are required)
OCD	Mild to moderate: brief CBT, group/individual, based on 'exposure with response prevention techniques'
	Severe: full course of individual CBT

time. Often patients with specific phobias will adjust their lifestyle to avoid the object or situation, thus perpetuating the disorder. They may present for treatment only if the phobia becomes severe or if a change in circumstances leads to increased contact with the feared situation. An example of this is a new job that requires frequent air travel in a person with a fear of flying.

Treatment

The basic treatment approach is as for GAD, outlined on p. 335, including a specific type of CBT called graded exposure therapy, which is a structured programme to gradually reintroduce the patient to the phobic situation. It is worth noting that the majority of patients need no treatment beyond sensible advice unless the phobia is having a significant impact on their

Table 24.6 Common specific phobias

Objects that induce anxiety	Situations that induce anxiety
• Blood (haematophobia)	• Dentists (5% of adults; may lead to poor dentition)
• Excretion	• Darkness (scotophobia)
• Vomit or vomiting (emetopobia)	• Elevators
• Needles or injections (trypanophobia)	• Illness
• Animals (zoophobia), e.g.:	• Heights (acrophobia)
• Spiders (arachnophobia)	• Storms or thunder
• Snakes (ophidiophobia)	• Flying or aeroplanes

Box 24.4 ICD-10 F40.2 Specific Phobia

Main features

- A marked and excessive fear or anxiety that consistently occurs when exposed to one or more specific objects or situations and that is out of proportion to actual danger.
- The phobic objects or situations are avoided or else endured with intense fear or anxiety.

Duration

- Symptoms persist for at least several months.

Disability

- Symptoms result in significant distress or significant impairment in personal, family, social, educational, occupational, or other important areas of functioning.

ICD-11 beta draft: key changes 7B03 Specific Phobia

- None expected.

well-being. Prescription of benzodiazepines should be avoided wherever possible.

Social anxiety disorder

Social anxiety disorder (previously *social phobia*) is incapacitating inappropriate anxiety in social situations which leads to the desire for escape or avoidance. It typically *begins* with an acute attack of anxiety in some public place—subsequently, anxiety occurs in similar places. There are a number of principal features:

- **Specific concerns** about being observed critically by other people.
- **Situations** that provoke anxiety in public places, speaking in public, and occasions when some action is open to scrutiny, for example writing, eating, or drinking in front of another person. The theme common to all situations is the potential for being observed and negatively evaluated.
- **Anticipatory anxiety.**
- **Avoidance** of these situations. Sometimes the avoidance is partial; for example, entering a social group but failing to make conversation, or sitting in an inconspicuous place in the group.
- **Symptoms** are similar to those of other anxiety disorders, although blushing (and concern about this) is particularly frequent.
- **Use of alcohol to relieve anticipatory anxiety.**
- **Low self-esteem and perfectionism** (see Case study box 24.1).

The formal diagnostic criteria for social anxiety disorder are shown in Box 24.5.

Co-morbidity

About 80 per cent of patients with social anxiety disorder will fit diagnostic criteria for another anxiety disorder, depression, PTSD, or alcohol use disorders.

CASE STUDY BOX 24.1

Specific phobia

Louise presented to her GP asking for help to overcome a fear of vomiting as it was preventing her pursuing a career in childcare. Louise's phobia meant seeing or dealing with vomit led to panic attacks, and so she avoided ill people and small children. She was starting to feel trapped in her secretarial job and quite despondent. The GP reassured her that specific phobias are common, and that it was nothing to be ashamed of. He recommended a self-help website while awaiting a referral for CBT. Louise found the site helpful in understanding her phobia, but did not make practical progress. She attended individual CBT sessions with a therapist, who took her through a graded exposure programme. This involved talking about vomiting, seeing pictures, videos, and attending a nursery with the therapist. Finally, Louise entered training in a childcare setting where she could learn to manage unwell children gradually in a supported way.

Box 24.5 ICD-10 40.1 Social Phobias

Fear of scrutiny by other people leading to avoidance of social situations, low self-esteem, and fear of criticism. Presents as blushing, hand tremor, nausea, or urgency of micturition. Symptoms may progress to panic attacks.

ICD 11 beta draft: key changes 7B04 Social Anxiety Disorder

- *Note change in name of disorder as above, and features as below.*

Main features

- Marked and excessive fear or anxiety that consistently occurs in one or more social situations such as social interactions, being observed, or performing in front of others.
- The social situations are consistently avoided or else endured with intense fear or anxiety.

Duration

- The symptoms persist for at least several months.

Disability

- Symptoms are sufficiently severe to result in significant distress or significant impairment in personal, family, social, educational, occupational, or other important areas of functioning.

Differential diagnosis

- **GAD**—this is not situational.
- **Depressive disorder.** Screen for core symptoms of low mood.
- **Schizophrenia.** Occasionally, patients with schizophrenia are anxious in, and avoid, social situations because of paranoid delusions.
- **Anxious/avoidant personality disorder,** characterized by lifelong shyness and lack of self-confidence, may closely resemble social anxiety disorder. However, personality disorder starts at a younger age and develops more gradually than social anxiety disorder.

- **Social inadequacy** is a primary lack of social skills with secondary anxiety. People with social anxiety disorder possess these social skills but cannot use them when they are anxious.
- **Panic disorder with agoraphobia** can usually be distinguished from social anxiety disorder by the fact that panic attacks are typically unexpected, whereas the anxiety or panic that comes with social anxiety disorder occurs in anticipation of negative evaluation by others.

Aetiology

The cause of social anxiety disorder is uncertain. Symptoms usually start in late adolescence, a time when many young people are concerned about the impression they are making on other people. It is possible that social anxiety disorders begin as exaggerated normal concerns, which are then increased and prolonged by thoughts that other people will be critical of any signs of anxiety. It may be that styles of parenting and early childhood experiences influence the development of social anxiety. Patients with social anxiety often remember their mother being fearful in social situations, and frequently describe their parents as overprotective. At time of writing, there is no good evidence for a strong genetic component.

Treatment

NICE guidance in the UK recommends the following approach for social anxiety disorder:

1 General measures as described in Tables 24.4 and 24.5. Assess in primary care using a questionnaire such as the three-item Mini Social Phobia Inventory (Mini-SPIN).

2 First line: CBT for social anxiety. This should be individual treatment.

3 Second line: SSRI.

4 Third line: try combining CBT and an SSRI or considering venlafaxine.

5 Try to avoid benzodiazepines due to risk of dependence. There is no good evidence that use

of propranolol is better than placebo for treating social anxiety when used regularly.

Agoraphobia

Agoraphobia is a condition in which the patient experiences anxiety in situations that are unfamiliar, from which they cannot escape, or in which they perceive they have little control. This anxiety leads to avoidance of those situations. Agoraphobic patients are anxious when they are away from home, in crowds, in situations they cannot leave easily, in social situations, and in open spaces (this last fear explains the name—'agoraphobia' contains the Greek word for 'marketplace') (Table 24.7). Diagnostic features are shown in Box 24.6 but general anxiety symptoms and panic attacks are commonly seen. Similarly to social anxiety disorder, the *first episode* of agoraphobia often occurs while the person is away from home. Suddenly, the person develops an unexplained panic attack, and either hurries home or seeks immediate medical help. As the condition progresses, patients avoid more and more of these situations until in severe cases they may be almost confined to their homes. The anxiety experienced in these situations is reduced by the reassuring presence of a

Table 24.7 Situations feared and avoided by patients with agoraphobia

Common themes	Distance from home
	Crowding
	Confinement
	Open spaces
	Social situations
Examples	Public transport
	Crowded shops
	Empty streets
	School visits
	Cinemas, theatres

Box 24.6 ICD-10 40.0 Agoraphobias

A fairly well-defined cluster of phobias embracing fears of leaving home, entering shops, crowds, and public places, or travelling alone in trains, buses, or planes. Panic disorder is a frequent feature of both present and past episodes. Avoidance of the phobic situation is often prominent.

ICD11 beta draft: key changes 7B02 Agoraphobia

- *More structured criteria as below.*

Main features

- Agoraphobia is characterized by marked and excessive fear or anxiety that occurs in response to multiple situations where escape might be difficult or help might not be available.
- The individual is consistently anxious about these situations due to a sense of danger or fear of specific negative outcomes.
- The situations are actively avoided, or endured with intense fear or anxiety.

Duration

- The symptoms last for at least several months.

Disability

- Significant distress or significant impairment in personal, family, social, educational, occupational, or other important areas of functioning.

trusted companion, or a reassuring object such as a few anxiolytic tablets, which are carried but never taken. As the condition progresses, patients become increasingly *dependent on the partner or other relatives* for help with activities, such as shopping, that provoke anxiety. These demands on the partner sometimes lead to arguments, and serious marital problems are common.

Co-morbidity

Co-morbidity is seen in almost all patients, especially:

- panic disorder;
- social anxiety disorder (50%);

- depression;
- alcohol or anxiolytic misuse.

Differential diagnosis

- **GAD,** although this does not have the pattern of avoidance characteristic of agoraphobia.
- **Social anxiety disorder.** Is the primary fear one of negative scrutiny or of an inability to escape from danger?
- **Specific phobias** only occur in the presence of a specific situation or object.
- **Depressive disorder**—screen for low mood, anhedonia, and lack of energy.
- **Schizophrenia.** Rarely, a thorough history will discover paranoia as the true reason for avoiding social situations or going out.

Aetiology

The development of anticipatory anxiety and avoidance after the first panic attack can be understood in terms of conditioning. The cause of the first panic attack is typically uncertain. Agoraphobia is *maintained by avoidance*, which prevents deconditioning, and by *apprehensive thoughts*, such as fears of fainting or social embarrassment, which set up vicious circles of anxiety.

Prognosis

Agoraphobia that has been present continuously for a year is likely to persist for at least 5 years. Brief episodes of depressive symptoms often occur in the course of chronic agoraphobia.

Treatment

See Tables 24.4 and 24.5. There is some evidence that the most effective treatment for agoraphobia is a combination of CBT and medication.

Panic disorder

In Greek mythology, the mischievous god Pan was said to be able to inspire fear in people and animals when they were in lonely places. He could do this without warning, very suddenly, and the emotions that people experienced when he did this became known as panic. The **unprovoked, spontaneous nature of panic attacks is their defining quality**, and is essential for their recognition and diagnosis. Panic attacks are very common—9 per cent of the population experience at least one in their lifetime—and are associated with significant social and occupational disability.

A panic attack is a period of intense fear characterized by a cluster of typical symptoms that develop rapidly, last a few minutes, and during which the person fears that some kind of catastrophe will occur. Panic attacks may occur in all anxiety disorders, as well as other psychiatric and physical disorders.

Panic disorder is a condition in which a person experiences recurrent panic attacks that occur unexpectedly (i.e. not in response to a phobic stimulus), and are not associated with substance abuse, medical conditions, or another psychiatric disorder.

Clinical features

The typical symptoms of a panic attack are listed in Box 24.7, and the formal diagnostic criteria are shown in Box 24.8. The characteristic feature of a panic attack is that it occurs spontaneously and without provocation. Anxiety increases over a few minutes to a severe level, during which the patient fears some kind of catastrophic outcome such as a heart attack. The frequency and severity of panic attacks vary between patients, but one or two attacks per week is usual. Panic

Box 24.7 Symptoms of a panic attack (in order of frequency)

- Palpitations
- Tachycardia
- Sweating and flushing
- Trembling
- Dyspnoea
- Chest discomfort
- Nausea
- Dizziness or fainting
- Fears of an impending medical emergency or death
- Depersonalization

Box 24.8 ICD-10 41.0 Panic Disorder

Main features

- Recurrent unpredictable attacks of severe anxiety (panic), which are not restricted to any particular situation or set of circumstances.

Associated features

- Secondary fear of dying, losing control, or going mad.
- Behaviours intended to avoid recurrence of attacks.

Disability

- Significant impairment in personal, family, social, educational, occupational, or other important areas of functioning.

Exclusions

- Panic disorder should not be given as the main diagnosis if the patient has a depressive disorder at the time the attacks start.

ICD-11 beta draft: key changes 7B01 Panic Disorder

- None expected.

attacks are a terrifying experience, and patients often become scared of having more attacks, and of being in situations where an attack previously occurred. This can lead to agoraphobia, as discussed earlier.

Differential diagnosis

Panic attacks occur in many conditions other than panic disorder, both psychiatric and physical, so a full history and examination is important. Common examples include:

- other anxiety disorders such as GAD, phobias, social anxiety, or agoraphobia; (note: two-thirds of patients will fit criteria for more than one anxiety disorder).
- depression (did low mood precede or follow the onset of panic?);
- PTSD;

- OCD;
- drugs—intoxication or withdrawal (e.g. caffeine, cocaine, cannabis, theophylline, amphetamines, steroids);
- endocrine disorders (hyperthyroidism, hypoglycaemia, Cushing's syndrome, carcinoid tumours, phaeochromocytoma);
- cardiovascular disorders (arrhythmias, chest pain, mitral regurgitation);
- respiratory disorders (chronic obstructive pulmonary disease, asthma).

Aetiology

The causes of panic disorder are uncertain. There are three main areas of current research:

1 **Genetics.** There is good evidence that the rates of panic disorders among first-degree relatives of those with the disorder are seven to eight times higher than average. Heritability of panic disorder is estimated to be around 40 per cent.

2 **The biochemical hypothesis** suggests that panic disorder is due to an imbalance in neurotransmitter activity in the brain. Certain chemical agents can induce panic attacks more readily in panic disorder patients than in healthy people—these agents include yohimbine (an alpha-adrenergic antagonist), isoproterenol (a beta-adrenergic agonist), and inhaled carbon dioxide. It is thought that the serotonin (5-HT) and GABA systems are also involved, because SSRIs and benzodiazepines are effective at reducing panic attacks.

3 **The cognitive hypothesis** is based on the observation that, compared with other anxious patients, patients with panic disorder more often have fears concerning physical symptoms of anxiety. They fear, for example, that palpitations will be followed by a heart attack. This produces a vicious cycle, as shown in Fig. 24.1. There is experimental evidence in support of this hypothesis; for example, reducing fearful cognitions reduces panic.

Prognosis

Many individuals have occasional panic attacks across their lifespan with minimal functional impact. However, in those with panic disorder that has persisted for 6 months or more the disorder usually runs a prolonged, although often fluctuating, course which may last for many years.

Treatment

The general guidance for anxiety disorders on p. 335 and in Tables 24.4 and 24.5 all applies to panic disorder and forms the basis of treatment, but there are specific additional points listed in Box 24.9. The evidence for the efficacy of psychological, pharmacological, or self-help treatments is all robust—the patient should be involved in choosing the most appropriate approach for them.

Box 24.9 Management plan for panic disorder

Step 1

- Make a diagnosis and detect any co-morbid depressive disorder or substance misuse.
- General psychoeducation, problem-solving, and relaxation. Teach how to manage hyperventilation (Box 24.1). Recommend self-help materials.
- Avoid prescribing benzodiazepines.

Step 2

- Offer a first-line intervention: CBT or an SSRI (no evidence for any particular SSRI choice).

Step 3

- Offer the other first-line intervention, or try a different SSRI.

Step 4

- Consider use of a tricyclic (imipramine or clomipramine).
- Refer to secondary care for reassessment and consideration of more specialist therapy or pharmacotherapy.

Obsessive–compulsive disorder

OCD is a condition characterized by obsessions and/or compulsions that the person feels driven to perform according to specific rules in order to prevent an imagined dreaded event. OCD is the fourth most common psychiatric disorder and is often chronic condition—it therefore represents a high burden of morbidity within the population. Effective treatment is available, so prompt diagnosis and referral are essential.

Clinical features

OCD is characterized by obsessional thinking, compulsive behaviour, and varying degrees of other psychiatric symptomology. An overview of the symptoms that may be experienced is shown in Fig. 24.3 and described in Box 24.10, and explanations follow. Key epidemiology is shown in Table 24.1.

Obsessions are recurrent persistent thoughts, impulses, or images that enter the mind despite efforts to exclude them. The feeling of being compelled to undergo the intrusion of a thought, impulse, or image and the resistances produced against them are key characteristics of an obsession. They may come in the form of any of the following:

- **Obsessional thoughts** which intrude forcibly into the patient's mind and the patient attempts to exclude them. Obsessional thoughts may be single words, phrases, or rhymes; they are usually unpleasant or shocking to the patient, obscene, or blasphemous.
- **Obsessional images** typically appear as vividly imagined scenes, which may be violent or sexual.
- **Obsessional ruminations** are internal debates in which continuous arguments are reviewed endlessly.
- **Obsessional doubts** are thoughts about actions that may have been completed inadequately, such as failing to turn off a gas tap completely, or about actions that may have harmed other people.
- **Obsessional impulses** are urges to perform acts, usually of a violent or embarrassing kind; for example, leaping in front of a car or shouting blasphemies in church. The urges are resisted strongly, and are not

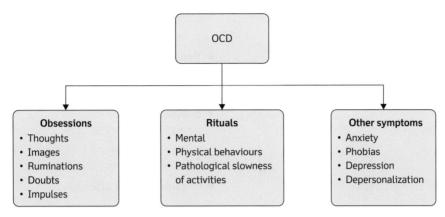

Fig. 24.3 Symptoms of obsessive–compulsive disorder.

carried out, but the internal struggle may be very distressing.

- **Obsessional rituals** or compulsions are repeated but senseless activities. They may be *mental activities*, such as counting repeatedly in a special way or repeating a certain form of words, or *behaviours*, such as excessive handwashing or lock checking. Rituals are usually followed by temporary release of distress. The ritual may be followed by doubts whether it has been completed in the right way, and the sequence may be repeated over and over again. Patients are aware that their rituals are illogical, and usually try to hide them.

Obsessional or anankastic personality is described on p. 467. Under the ICD-11 classification, individuals with functional deficits due to obsessional or anankastic traits will be described as '*mild/moderate/severe personality disorder with prominent anankastic features*'. Obsessional personality is over-represented among patients who develop OCD, but about a third of obsessional patients have other types of personality.

Box 24.10 ICD-10 F42 Obsessive–Compulsive Disorder

Main features

- Obsessive–compulsive disorder is characterized by the presence of obsessions or compulsions, or both. Patients try to ignore or suppress obsessions or neutralize them by performing compulsions.
- *Obsessions*: repetitive and persistent thoughts, images, or urges (impulses) that are intrusive, unwanted, and commonly associated with anxiety.
- *Compulsions*: repetitive behaviours or mental acts that the individual feels driven to perform in response to an obsession, according to rigid rules, or to achieve a sense of 'completeness'.

Associated features

- The patient must realize that his or her obsessions or compulsions are unreasonable or excessive.
- Often associated with anxiety or depression.

Duration

- Symptoms must be time-consuming (taking more than 1 hour daily).

Disability

- Result in significant distress or significant impairment in personal, family, social, educational, occupational, or other important areas of functioning.

Exclusions

- Obsessive–compulsive personality disorder.

ICD-11 beta draft: Obsessive–Compulsive Disorder

- None expected.

Co-morbidity

- Depression (70 per cent).
- Eating disorders.
- Other anxiety disorders.
- Body dysmorphic disorder.
- Problems with alcohol.

Differential diagnosis

- **Anxiety disorders.** Which symptom is most prominent or developed first?
- **Phobias.** The stimuli in phobias are usually specific avoidable situations (e.g. lifts, spiders, and crowds) whereas phobic symptoms in OCD are more generalized (e.g. bacteria and dirt).
- **Depressive disorder.** Obsessional symptoms follow the depression in depressive disorders and precede it in obsessional disorder.
- **Schizophrenia.** When obsessional thoughts have a peculiar content, the clinical picture may suggest schizophrenia. Assess if the patient realizes his beliefs are unreasonable or if they fit criteria for a delusion.
- **Organic cerebral disorders.**

Aetiology

An overview of the aetiology of OCD is shown in Table 24.8.

Table 24.8 Causes of obsessive–compulsive disorder

Predisposing factors	Precipitating factors	Maintaining factors
Genetics • 10-fold increased risk of OCD in first-degree relatives.	Stressful events: • Relationship problems • Unemployment • Financial difficulties • Puberty • Bullying at school • Physical illness	Checking and rituals Cycle of anxiety (see Fig. 24.1) Continuing stressful life events Depressive disorder
Neurobiological mechanisms 1 Structural: increased rate of minor non-localizing signs and functional MRI shows increased activity in caudate and cingulum 2 Neurotransmitters: likely dysregulation of 5-HT pathways due to efficacy of SSRIs in treating OCD. 5-HT antagonists reliably cause an increase in obsessionality. Involvement of the dopaminergic pathways is suggested by obsessionalism seen in basal ganglia disorders 3 Autoimmune: autoantibodies to the caudate nucleus (Sydenham's chorea) are associated with OCD in two-thirds of cases and there is a link between group A *Streptococcus* and OCD/tics (box 24.1).		
Early experiences • Exposure to obsessionality in the home has been linked to OCD via social learning theory • Psychological: obsessions are a conditioned response to an anxiety-provoking event. The patient develops avoidant behaviours to try and avoid experiencing the anxiety-provoking event. Freud's psychoanalytic approach considers the symptoms of OCD as unsolved conflicts or impulses of a violent or sexual nature. These impulses create anxiety, which is avoided by the use of defence mechanisms • Obsessive–compulsive personality		

Prognosis

About two-thirds of obsessional disorders improve within a year; the remaining one-third run a prolonged and usually fluctuating course with periods of partial or complete remission lasting a few months to several years.

Treatment

Making a diagnosis of OCD is not difficult—some useful screening questions are shown in Box 24.11. Guidance for the management of OCD is outlined in Box 24.12. Most of the measures can be initiated in primary care, but more severe cases or non-responders should be referred to a mental health specialist. The provision of information is the important first step in treatment. Patients with an OCD find their thoughts and actions so strange and irrational that they often fear that they are 'going mad' and could act on the impulses they are resisting. It is important to explain that OCD does not progress in this way. There is good evidence for a specialized form of CBT which includes 'exposure with response prevention'. This helps the patient to be able to relax when in situations they would usually use compensatory compulsive thoughts/behaviours and start to be able to resist doing them.

Psychopharmacology

There is robust evidence that 5-HT reuptake inhibitors suppress obsessive–compulsive symptoms, and

Box 24.11 Screening questions for obsessive–compulsive disorder

> Do you wash and clean a lot?
> Do you check things a lot?
> Are there any thoughts that keep bothering you that you would like to get rid of but can't?
> Do your daily activities take a long time to finish?
> Are you concerned about putting things in a special order or are you very upset by mess?
> Do these problems trouble you?

Box 24.12 Management of obsessive–compulsive disorder

Assessment
- Make a diagnosis and detect any co-morbidities
- Risk assessment (including self-harm and suicide)

General measures for all patients
- Psychoeducation
- Problem-solving techniques and relaxation
- Self-help books or websites

Mild functional impairment
- Offer brief CBT (including exposure with response prevention)

Moderate functional impairment
- SSRI or
- Full course of CBT (including exposure with response prevention)

Severe functional impairment
- Combined treatment with SSRI and CBT
- Clomipramine
- Treatment-resistant patients: consider adding an atypical antipsychotic
- High-risk patients: consider inpatient admission (e.g. risk of suicide, self-neglect, severe co-morbid depression, or eating disorder)

the action is independent of their antidepressant effect. Effective drugs include the SSRIs and the tricyclic drug clomipramine, which is a non-specific inhibitor of 5-HT uptake. The efficacy of all SSRIs is similar and clomipramine is probably slightly superior. SSRIs are the usual first choice because clomipramine has to be given in high dosage, which increases the risk of anticholinergic and cardiac side effects. There is some evidence for the adjunctive use of atypical antipsychotics in severe treatment-resistant OCD; the most efficacious choices seem to be risperidone or quetiapine (see Science box 24.1 and Case study box 24.2).

SCIENCE BOX 24.1

Obsessive–compulsive disorder in adults: an autoimmune disease?

Sydenham's chorea is the archetypical condition demonstrating molecular mimicry; in response to streptococcal infection, the body produces antineuronal antibodies, which attack the streptococci but cross-react with the basal ganglia producing choreoathetoid movements. It has been suggested that some cases of childhood OCD and tic disorders may be a similar autoimmune disease, now termed **paediatric autoimmune neuropsychiatric disorders associated with streptococcal infections (PANDAS)**.[1] This is further discussed on p. 501. However, the majority of patients who present with OCD are adults. Could there be an autoimmune basis to (at least a subset of) these cases? Several small trials have been done including a case–control study which found a significantly greater proportion of adults with OCD had positive antistreptolysin O titres (ASOT) or antineuronal antibodies than controls with depression or schizophrenia.[2] Pozzi et al. performed a meta-analysis of 13 studies investigating the association of ASOT with OCD and tic disorders.[3] There was insufficient data to quantitatively assess OCD (suggesting minimal evidence in this domain currently for the aetiology of OCD as an autoimmune condition) but a positive association between ASOT and tic disorders was found. The hunt for novel approaches to treating OCD continues.

1 Swedo SE, Leonard HL, Garvey M, et al. Pediatric autoimmune neuropsychiatric disorders associated with streptococcal infections: clinical description of the first 50 cases. *American Journal of Psychiatry* 1998;155:264–271.

2 Nicholson TR, Ferdinando S, Krishnaiah RB, et al. Prevalence of anti-basal ganglia antibodies in adult obsessive-compulsive disorder: cross-sectional study. *British Journal of Psychiatry* 2012;200:381–386.

3 Pozzi M, Pellegrino P, Carnovale C, Perrone V. On the connection between autoimmunity, tic disorders and obsessive-compulsive disorders: a meta-analysis on anti-streptolysin O titres. *Journal of Neuroimmune Pharmacology* 2014;9:606–614.

CASE STUDY BOX 24.2

Obsessive–compulsive disorder

Fiona, a 32-year-old woman who was 28 weeks pregnant was referred to psychiatry by her GP. Since becoming pregnant, Fiona had become excessively concerned that she might be harming her baby by letting germs enter her body. This had led to her washing her hands over 50 times per day, and showering ten times daily. When finishing washing, she was never quite sure she had done it adequately, and would repeat the process multiple times. Fiona described having visions of her baby covered in bacteria popping uncontrollably into her mind, and the urge to cut herself to release any germs in her blood. Fiona frequently requested for an ultrasound to be done to check she had not harmed the baby. The GP had given her self-help materials and offered an SSRI, which had been refused on the grounds that drugs might cause the baby damage. The psychiatrist organized a psychiatric nurse to support Fiona at home and an intensive course of individual CBT, which helped her to reduce the behaviours slightly. She gave birth to a healthy girl at 39 weeks, after which her symptoms improved greatly. She continued to receive CBT for another 6 months, after which she was able to return to work.

Further reading

Butler G, Grey N, Hope T. *Manage Your Mind: The Mental Fitness Guide.* 3rd ed. Oxford: Oxford University Press; 2018. [A useful account of self-help methods for anxiety disorders and other conditions.]

Connor KM, Kobak KA, Churchill LE, Katzelnick D, Davidson JR. Mini-SPIN: a brief screening assessment for generalized social anxiety disorder. *Depression and Anxiety* 2001;14:137–40.

Gale C, Davidson O. Generalised anxiety disorder. *BMJ* 2007;334:579–581.

National Institute for Health and Care Excellence. Generalised anxiety disorder and panic disorder in adults: management. Clinical guideline [CG113]. Published January 2011. http://nice.org.uk/guidance/cg113.

National Institute for Health and Care Excellence. Obsessive-compulsive disorder and body dysmorphic disorder: treatment. Clinical guideline [CG31]. Published November 2005. http://guidance.nice.org.uk/cg31/.

National Institute for Health and Care Excellence. Social anxiety disorder: recognition, assessment and treatment. Clinical guideline [CG159]. Published May 2013. http://nice.org.uk/guidance/cg159.

Parmentier H, Garcia-Campayo J, Prieto R. Comprehensive review of generalized anxiety disorder in primary care in Europe. *Current Medical Research and Opinion* 2013;29:355–367.

Soomro GM, Altman DG, Rajagopal S, Oakley BM. Selective serotonin reuptake inhibitors versus placebo for obsessive-compulsive disorder. *Cochrane Database of Systematic Reviews* 2008;1:CD001765.

Veale D, Roberts A. Obsessive-compulsive disorder. *BMJ* 2014;348:g2183.

Concern about physical symptoms is a common reason for people to seek medical help. Many of these symptoms, such as headache, chest pain, weakness, dizziness, and fatigue, remain unexplained by identifiable disease even after careful medical assessment. Several general terms have been used to describe these types of symptom—somatoform, medically unexplained, and functional. We prefer the terms 'medically unexplained physical symptom' or 'functional symptom', because they imply a disturbance of some kind in bodily functioning without implying that the symptom is psychogenic. Patients and doctors often assume that a physical symptom implies that a physical pathology exists. However, commonly experienced and often severe, distressing, and disabling symptoms, such as menstrual pain or 'tension headache', indicate that this is not always the case. By assuming that a physical symptom is explained by physical disease/pathology, we may be subjecting the patient to unnecessary tests and hospital visits, adding to patient distress, and failing to deliver the integrated management required.

There are many kinds of these symptoms (Box 25.1), presenting across healthcare settings. They are considered in this psychiatry textbook because (1) psychological factors (including, at times, psychiatric disorder) are important in aetiology and (2) psychological and behavioural interventions have a fundamental role in treatment

A major obstacle to effective management of patients with functional symptoms is that they feel their doctor does not believe them. They are concerned that they may be thought to be 'putting it on'. Note that the deliberate manufacture or exaggeration of symptoms or signs (malingering) is quite different (see p. 359).

Diagnosis

Diagnoses of three kinds may be given:

- **Descriptive physical syndromes.** These include fibromyalgia, chronic fatigue syndrome, non-cardiac chest pain, chronic pain syndrome, and irritable bowel syndrome (IBS). Although the specific terms

Box 25.1 Some common physical symptoms that are often 'functional'

- Pain syndromes:
  - Abdominal pain
  - Non-cardiac chest pain
  - Headache
  - Atypical facial pain
  - Muscular pain
  - Low back pain
  - Pelvic pain
- Fatigue
- Non-ulcer dyspepsia
- Irritable bowel/food intolerance
- Palpitations
- Dizziness
- Tinnitus
- Dysphonia

are useful in everyday medical practice, there is substantial overlap, and many patients with, for example, fibromyalgia will also have IBS.

- **Psychiatric syndromes as the primary cause of the functional symptoms.** Psychiatric disorders, such as depression, anxiety, and adjustment, are common *primary* causes of functional symptoms, and commonly present via the general hospital's emergency department or cardiology clinic. For example, a patient with generalized anxiety disorder has multiple autonomic symptoms of anxiety (which are an integral part of the diagnostic criteria), including palpitations; the palpitations are themselves alarming, and trigger negative automatic thoughts about possible cardiac illness and its outcomes, thereby maintaining anxiety, autonomic arousal, and physical symptoms. The physical symptoms may resolve with effective treatment of these psychiatric disorders. Psychiatric disorders such as anxiety disorder may also be *secondary* to functional symptoms, which are then exacerbated and maintained by the psychiatric disorder.
- **Psychiatric syndromes comprising health concern and functional symptoms.** The appropriate

psychiatric diagnosis is of a somatoform disorder (ICD-10). These are conditions characterized by (1) *persistent abnormal concern* about physical health, and (2) one or more *physical symptoms unexplained by physical pathology*. Within the somatoform disorders, there are several specific disorders (see Box 25.2) of which you should

Box 25.2 The somatoform disorders

Somatoform autonomic dysfunction

Common. A large, ill-defined, category of patients who present repeatedly with one or more unexplained physical symptoms, attributable to a system under autonomic control (cardiovascular, gastrointestinal, respiratory, urogenital), which persist in spite of negative investigation and reassurance.

Somatization disorder

Uncommon. *Multiple*, recurrent, and changing unexplained physical symptoms, with multiple presentations to medical care, often over a period of many years. Chronic and often fluctuating course.

Hypochondriasis

Severe persistent anxiety about ill health and conviction of disease, with repeated presentation of concern about the possibility of one or more *specific* diseases (such as cancer or heart disease), despite negative medical investigations and appropriate reassurance.

Body dysmorphic disorder

Persistent, inappropriate concern about the appearance of the body (e.g. about the shape and size of the nose or breasts), despite reassurance. Some patients demand cosmetic plastic surgery, which is helpful only in those with clear and reasonable expectations.

Persistent somatoform pain disorder

The intensity and duration of pain cannot be accounted for by any primary physical or mental disorder.

Dissociative disorder

Partial or complete loss of the normal integration between (1) memories of the past, (2) awareness of identity and immediate sensations, and (3) movement, in the absence of a medical explanation.

be aware. The draft ICD-11 proposes replacing somatoform disorder and somatization disorder with 'bodily distress disorder' (see 'Further reading') and moving hypochondriasis to the group of 'anxiety and fear-related disorders'.

Epidemiology

Functional symptoms are common: about one-fifth of the population in all countries and communities. In primary care, only a small proportion of people with functional symptoms ever receive a specific physical diagnosis (Fig. 25.1). Most functional symptoms are transient, and are therefore not usually brought to medical attention. However, a sizeable minority persist and are disabling. Up to half of patients remain disabled after 12 months.

Functional symptoms may occur alone, or may accompany serious physical illness. For example, following a heart attack or cardiac surgery, minor muscular chest aches and pains in the chest may be misinterpreted as evidence of angina, and lead to unnecessary worry and disability. It is, therefore, important not to assume that all chest pain in someone with chest pathology is due to that pathology. Explanation and advice about how to respond to pain, perhaps via a psychologically informed cardiac rehabilitation programme, improve quality of life.

Aetiology

Functional symptoms are often put down to *either* physical *or* psychological causes. This 'mind–body dualism' is unhelpful, as it prevents us using more effective, integrated models to explain aetiology or to plan treatment. It is also often unacceptable to patients. By implication, in the absence of physical pathology, a symptom is 'all in the mind', and, in the presence of physical pathology, a symptom is not influenced at all by psychological or social factors.

An alternative approach uses an integrated model in which *physical, psychological*, and *social* factors all

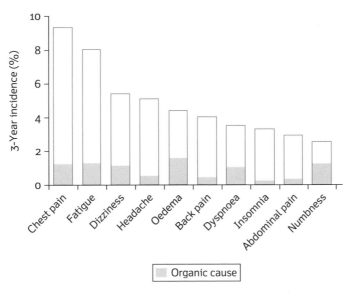

Fig. 25.1 Three-year incidence of ten common presenting symptoms and proportion of symptoms with a suspected organic cause in US primary care attenders.

Reprinted from *The American Journal of Medicine*, 86, 3, Kroenke K., A. D. Mangelsdorff, Common symptoms in ambulatory care: Incidence, evaluation, therapy, and outcome, pp. 262–266. Copyright © 1989 Published by Excerpta Medica Inc.

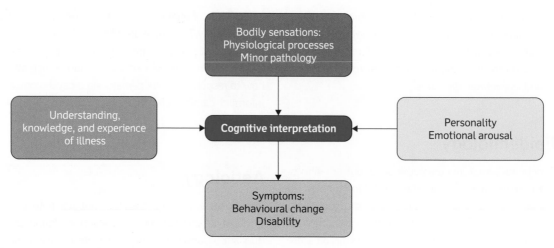

Fig. 25.2 Aetiology of medically unexplained symptoms.

contribute to the formation of functional symptoms, in three stages (see Fig. 25.2):

1 Initially, minor bodily sensations are triggered, by usually benign causes. These include hangover, autonomic effects of anxiety, minor musculoskeletal pathology, lack of sleep, inactivity, overeating, fatigue, sinus tachycardia, or minor arrhythmias.

2 The next, and key, step is *attribution*: the process of assigning a putative cause to the symptom. Attributions may be *normalizing*—assigning benign causes such as the effects of a hangover, or tiredness; *psychologizing*—assigning causes such as stress or depression; or *somatizing*—assigning more serious physical causes such as tumour, endocrine disease, or cardiac disease. Whether an individual normalizes, psychologizes, or somatizes is influenced by several factors, including:

   (a) *the person's usual 'attributional style,'*—which may be seen as a feature of their personality, that is, it is relatively static through time;

   (b) *their personal situation at that time*—if they are undergoing a period of interpersonal stress, or excessive demands at work, they may be distressed and more likely to somatize;

   (c) *their family medical history*—a middle-aged man with a family history of heart disease

may be understandably concerned about the implications of a chest pain which is, in fact, of musculoskeletal origin;

   (d) *their personal medical history*—including experience of illnesses and their management, whether successful or unsuccessful;

   (e) *their knowledge of relevant illnesses*—derived from multiple sources including healthcare professionals, family, friends, and media coverage, whether accurate or inaccurate;

   (f) *their family and friends' response to the physical sensation*;

   (g) *their doctor's (or other healthcare professionals') response.*

3 Finally, patients' understandable attempts to alleviate their symptoms may paradoxically exacerbate them. For example, excessive rest to reduce pain or fatigue may prolong it, by leading to physical deconditioning, and by increasing patient focus on their symptoms and disability, rather than on their abilities and opportunities. Furthermore, they may devote great energy to seeking 'the answer' on the Internet, to the extent that their life becomes defined by their illness. Disability benefits may be an understandable disincentive for some patients to return to productive employment. Ongoing litigation can maintain the patient's focus

on their disabilities rather than their abilities. Finally, doctors may unintentionally maintain symptoms by failing to address patients' concerns, or by excessive investigation or multiple referrals within secondary care, as they seek a physical explanation.

Management

Although it is always essential to consider physical disease as the cause of the patient's symptoms, an approach exclusively devoted to this can lead to difficulties if no disease is found. It is better to adopt a more integrated, biopsychosocial approach from the start. Explain that physical symptoms are often only fully explained by considering physical, psychological, and social factors relating to the individual's health, and use examples to illustrate this—a stressed businessman facing a deadline who presents with chronic, debilitating headache, for example; or a head teacher with chronic bowel symptoms which worsen as the school's annual inspection looms. This keeps open the option of a wider discussion of causes, either initially or in due course, and allows psychological treatment to be presented as a part of *usual* medical care rather than as an *alternative* that the patient may feel does not take his physical symptoms seriously.

Assessment

A thorough physical assessment is essential, to both exclude the possibility of physical disorder, and to emphasize to the patient that you are taking their concerns seriously. This should include:

- listening carefully to the patient;
- conducting a focused physical examination;
- organizing any medically indicated physical investigation. Tests should be justified in terms of the likelihood and value of new information. Investigations that cannot be medically justified may increase anxiety, increase disease conviction, and reinforce illness behaviours.

In addition, a more psychological approach should be taken, from the start, to include:

- identifying the patient's concerns—about the symptoms and belief of their cause;
- reviewing any previous history of 'unexplained' symptoms;
- investigating how the patient reacts to and attempts to cope with the symptoms—for example, activity avoidance or work sickness absence; are these behaviours likely to help or hinder?
- screening—for depression, anxiety, and alcohol and substance misuse;
- interviewing a corroborant—to ascertain their views on the cause of the symptoms, and possible ways forward.

Treatment

A thorough, patient-focused, integrated assessment, as previously described, is the first step in effective management, and should be followed by careful explanation and reassurance.

Provide explanation and reassurance

Most patients are reassured by being told that the symptoms they have:

- are common;
- are rarely associated with serious disease;
- are real, and their doctor is familiar with them;
- often settle with time;
- need not be an impediment to an active life;
- can be reviewed again should the symptoms persist.

A positive explanation for symptoms is more helpful than a statement that no disease is present. This explains how behavioural, psychological, and emotional factors may exacerbate physiologically based physical symptoms. Most patients accept integrated explanations, which include psychological and social factors as well as physiological ones, provided they feel the symptoms are accepted as real. The explanation can usefully show the link between these factors—for example, how anxiety leads to physiological changes, which are experienced as somatic symptoms, which, if attributed to disease, lead to increased anxiety.

Simple advice on self-help techniques can then be given, including how to control negative thoughts (see p. 163), use physical relaxation techniques (see p. 160), and increase activity levels. A self-help book which uses evidence-based, cognitive behavioural approaches should be recommended.

Reassurance needs to be given carefully. It is essential to elicit the patient's specific concerns before offering reassurance and to target this appropriately. Reassurance that fails to address a patient's concerns is ineffective. When anxiety about disease is severe (hypochondriasis), repeated reassurance is not only ineffective but may perpetuate the problem.

Communicate effectively

Effective communication is crucial to success. Tips include:

- discuss and agree the treatment plan with the patient;
- agree follow-up arrangements, and be specific—when, who, why;
- involve key carer(s) in your communication;
- involve primary care—they have an important 'gate-keeper' role;
- communicate the treatment summary clearly in writing—to patient, carer, and key clinician(s).

Encourage graded return to normal activity

Reduced activity levels are both a consequence and a cause of functional symptoms. Graded increase in activity is not only a goal of treatment but also a part of treatment. The patient can make a list of activities which they used to undertake, but which they no longer engage in, or which they engage in less frequently. They then choose one or two and formulate a realistic and phased return to those activities. A diary can help plan and record activities.

Identify and treat any psychiatric disorder

In particular, consider the possibility of anxiety, depression, and alcohol and substance misuse. Explain to the patient how the psychiatric disorder is contributing to the maintenance of their physical symptoms. Offer simple treatments as part of a stepped care approach.

Review medicines

Medicines should be reviewed, and consideration should be given to reducing or stopping those that do not have a clear medical indication.

Consider prescribing antidepressants

Antidepressants may be appropriate for two different reasons. The first is because of their *antidepressant* function—depressive illness is common in patients with functional symptoms. The second is because of their *neuromodulating* function—antidepressants may help people with functional symptoms by modifying nerve action and, thereby, the extent to which physiological disturbance in the 'soma' is manifest in the 'psyche'. There is good evidence, for example, for the role of antidepressants in some pain syndromes and in IBS.

Refer—if appropriate

It is often tempting to refer challenging patients to another doctor but this can worsen outcomes. When there is a clear reason for further medical or psychiatric referral, this should be discussed with the patient. The referral letter should clearly explain what is required of the specialist, for example confirmation, or negation of the diagnosis or advice on management.

Address social factors

These may include, for example, marital disharmony, financial problems, and unemployment or under-employment, and may be potent maintaining factors.

Consider further psychiatric treatment

Help from psychiatric services might include:

- advice on more complex antidepressant drug regimens;
- management of complex associated social and psychological problems;
- specialist psychological interventions, including:
  - *CBT*. Cognitive elements include modification of thoughts and beliefs, by reducing catastrophization, and promoting normalizing attributions. Behavioural elements include increased physical and other activity, and reduced illness-related behaviours such as symptom monitoring and searching for medical evidence. CBT has been shown to be effective in RCTs for hypochondriasis, and for a variety of functional syndromes;
  - *illness-specific interventions*, such as graded exercise therapy to treat physical deconditioning in chronic fatigue syndrome.

Some common clinical problems

Irritable bowel syndrome

In primary care, about half of the patients seen with gastrointestinal complaints have functional disorders, the most common being IBS. Most have mild symptoms and can be managed in primary care by providing self-help information including (1) dietary advice (assess and modify fibre intake; probiotics), (2) lifestyle advice (increase physical activity; limit caffeine, alcohol), and (3) first-line, symptom-targeted medication (e.g. antispasmodic agents as required; laxatives for constipation; loperamide for diarrhoea; and educate the patient to modify dosing according to response) (current NICE advice). One-third of patients seen in primary care are referred to gastrointestinal specialists for further assessment and treatment. Other treatment options:

- **Antidepressants.** Tricyclic antidepressants are indicated at low dose as second-line agents, and SSRI antidepressants as third-line agents. Here, these medications are not being used as antidepressants, but as modifiers of nerve function and, thereby, of intestinal motility and pain sensation.
- **Psychological interventions.** There is evidence to support the use of CBT and hypnotherapy, but not acupuncture or reflexology.
- **Management of associated psychiatric disorder,** such as anxiety and depression.

Musculoskeletal pain and chronic pain

Musculoskeletal symptoms (e.g. neck pain, limb pain, low back pain, joint pain, and chronic widespread pain) are frequent reasons for consultation in primary care. Most patients can be effectively managed by:

- *explaining the difference between 'hurt' and 'harm'* (or pain vs pathology) using, for example, menstrual pain or tension headache (where there can be very severe pain without disease) as examples;
- *reassuring patients* about the benign nature of their symptoms;
- *helping patients regain control* over the pain, rather than the pain controlling them;
- *encouraging early mobilization*, and early return to work, with small graded increases in activity;
- *advice that analgesics should be taken regularly* rather than a pain contingent basis;
- *setting realistic goals*, and encouraging rewards for success.

The treatment of severe chronic pain is difficult, and patients are often referred to specialist pain clinics. Many have physical disease, but experience more pain, distress and disability than is explained by the pathology. Analgesia should be optimized and patients should be encouraged to try new approaches to coping including:

- *distraction*—by engaging in non-pain-related activities;

- *reducing any behaviour that focuses attention on the pain*—for example, repeatedly rubbing or checking the area;
- *cognitive approaches*—such as identifying and challenging negative thoughts and beliefs relating to the pain;
- *antidepressant medication*—as an antidepressant or as an analgesic/neuromodulator;
- *intensive multidisciplinary pain management programmes*—which integrate physical therapies, graded rehabilitation, medication, psychological techniques, and active involvement of patients and their families in care.

Chronic fatigue syndrome/myalgic encephalomyelitis

Fatigue and malaise are common following influenza, hepatitis, infectious mononucleosis, and other viral infections, but usually improve over days and weeks. Chronic fatigue syndrome (often known as myalgic encephalomyelitis, and shortened to CFS-ME), is characterized by (1) more persistent fatigue, and aching limbs with muscle and joint pains; and (2) the absence of physical or mental disorder sufficient to explain the symptoms. Mild physical exertion is often followed by increased fatigue and pain so that patients alternate brief periods of activity with prolonged rest, in a 'stop–start' pattern. Many patients are convinced that their symptoms are caused by a chronic virus infection or another undetected medical condition. However, after thorough physical assessment, few cases are found to have a specific medical cause (e.g. anaemia, persistent infection, or endocrinopathy).

In most cases of fatigue, the causes of the syndrome are neither wholly psychological nor wholly physical, but a mixture of the two, with psychological factors becoming increasingly common over time. A common triad at the outset is:

- **physical**—a viral illness;
- **social**—presenting at a time of personal stress;
- **psychological**—in an individual with a driven personality.

In such cases, recovery from the viral illness is often slow, and inactivity and resultant physical deconditioning start to play an important role. As the person senses that they are recovering, they may suddenly return to their former lifestyle, only to relapse quickly because their physical condition is still impaired. Morale may well suffer and, in some, a depressive syndrome may emerge, which may merit antidepressant treatment.

The treatment of this disorder is challenging, not least because it arouses passionate feelings among sufferers and their carers. The clinician should explain that the syndrome is real, common, and familiar, and that, although there is no specific medical treatment, there are effective treatments. A graded programme of slowly increasing activity should be started with regular monitoring. Emphasize that patients should exercise progressively rather than alternating erratically between excessive activity and resting in bed. CBT and graded exercise therapy have both been shown to be helpful in RCTs. The role of pacing, in which patients adapt their lifestyle to the energy that they have available, is less certain, following a controversial trial (see 'Further reading').

Multiple chronic functional symptoms

Patients who have multiple functional symptoms over long periods are said to have somatization disorder. They are difficult to treat and management is often focused on 'coping' (limiting distress and unnecessary investigation) rather than 'curing'. The general approach already described for the treatment of functional symptoms is used, with an emphasis on avoiding inappropriate investigation and ensuring a consistent approach. If possible, this should be by a single doctor, usually based in primary care, who can act as 'gatekeeper' to ensure that specialist care is accessed appropriately.

Management may include the following:

- Review the (often large) medical notes, and discussion with the (often many) doctors currently involved.
- Negotiate with other doctors to simplify healthcare by:

- limiting the number of healthcare staff involved;
- agreeing who has primary responsibility;
- minimizing the use of psychotropic and other drugs;
- ensuring that referrals and investigations are arranged only in response to a clear medical indication.
- Arrange brief, regular appointments with the lead clinician (proactive vs reactive appointments).
- Avoid repeated reassurance about the symptoms.
- Focus on enabling coping.
- Encourage/plan a graded return to normal activities.
- Involve relatives in the treatment plan.
- Be realistic about outcomes.

Dissociative disorders

These are fascinating disorders. The Greeks coined the term *hysteria* ('disease of the womb') for these disorders, and the term persisted until recently. However, its use is clearly inappropriate now that we know that both sexes suffer from these disorders, and that the cause is embedded in the brain, and not the female reproductive system! Symptoms vary widely, and include unexplained sensory and motor symptoms; unexplained amnesia, with or without fugue (wandering); stupor; and identity disorder. Crucially, a dissociative symptom is one that suggests physical illness but occurs in the *absence* of relevant physical pathology and is produced through unconscious psychological mechanisms. Note that there are two obvious practical difficulties here: (1) it is seldom possible to exclude physical pathology completely when a patient is first seen, and (2) it is difficult to be certain that the symptoms are produced by unconscious mechanisms rather than consciously and deliberately (the latter is known as malingering).

The *prevalence* of dissociative disorder varies between countries, being higher in lower-income countries. In higher-income countries, the prevalence is typically between 3 and 6 per 1000 for women, and rather less for men. Most dissociative disorders of recent onset—seen in general practice or hospital emergency departments, for example—recover quickly. Those that persist for longer than a year are likely to continue for many years more. Occasionally, organic disease may be present but undetectable when these patients are first seen, becoming obvious later. For this reason, patients should receive a thorough physical assessment, and should be followed up most carefully.

Although dissociative symptoms are not produced deliberately, they are nevertheless shaped by the patient's concepts of illness. Sometimes, the symptoms resemble those of a relative or friend who has been ill. Sometimes they originate in the patient's previous experience of ill health; for example, dissociative memory loss may appear some years after head injury. Usually there are obvious discrepancies between signs and symptoms of dissociative disorder and those of organic disease; for example, a pattern of sensory loss that does not correspond to the anatomical innervation of the part. These discrepancies are important in diagnosis.

Dissociative motor symptoms include paralysis of voluntary muscles, tremor, tics, and abnormalities of gait. *Dissociative sensory symptoms* include anaesthesiae, paraesthesiae, hyperaesthesiae, pain, deafness, and blindness. In *dissociative amnesia,* patients are unable to recall long periods of their lives and sometimes deny any knowledge of their previous life or personal identity. In *dissociative fugue*, the patient loses his memory and wanders away from his usual surroundings. In *dissociative stupor*, the patient is motionless and mute and does not respond to stimulation, but he is aware of his surroundings. *Multiple personality dissociative disorder* is a rare condition, in which there are sudden alterations between the patient's normal state and another complex pattern of behaviour, which constitutes a 'second personality'.

Diagnosis depends partly on the exclusion of physical causes, but also on psychological assessment to identify psychological reasons for the onset and course of the symptoms. A vital differential diagnosis is from physical disease. This depends on careful physical assessment highlighting any unusual physical signs that are unlikely to have a physical basis. Dissociative symptoms are common accompaniments to physical

Box 25.3 Management of acute dissociative disorder

- Medical and psychiatric history from patient and informants.
- Full examination and appropriate investigation to exclude physical causes.
- Sympathetic but positive reassurance that the patient is suffering from a temporary condition, with which the doctor is familiar, and which is not a serious medical disorder.
- Discussion of the expected rapid recovery.
- Avoidance of reinforcement of disability or symptoms.
- Offer continuing assessment and treatment of related psychiatric or social problems.

disorder, that is, it is not necessarily an 'either/or' diagnosis.

Acute disorders seen in general practice or hospital emergency departments often respond to simple measures (Box 25.3). For *persistent cases*, the general approach is similar, although the results are less satisfactory. Attention is directed away from the symptoms and towards problems that have provoked the disorder. Staff should show sympathetic concern for the patient, but at the same time encourage self-help and avoid reinforcing the disability. For example, a patient who complains of paralysis of the legs should be encouraged to return to walking, via physiotherapy, with strengthening and walking exercises.

Self-inflicted and simulated illness

Factitious disorder

The term factitious disorder refers to the intentional production of physical pathology or the feigning of physical or psychological symptoms, with the apparent aim of being diagnosed as ill. Factitious disorder differs from malingering in that it does not bring any external reward such as avoidance of military or other occupational duties, or financial compensation.

Box 25.4 Some ethical issues in the management of factitious disorders

Confidentiality
- Disclosure of diagnosis to other parties (e.g. employers such as the NHS).
- Circulation between hospitals of details of patients with suspected factitious disorder.

Privacy
- Searching patients' belongings for evidence to support the diagnosis.
- Covert videotaping to provide evidence to support the diagnosis.

Common symptoms include skin lesions ('dermatitis artefacta') and pyrexia of unknown origin. Sometimes the patient deliberately worsens an existing physical disorder, for example, preventing the healing of varicose ulcers or neglecting the care of diabetes. At other times the whole condition is induced, for example, by self-inflicted damage to the skin.

There is no specific treatment. Supportive counselling is often offered, and helps some patients but many do not take up the treatment. If deliberate feigning of symptoms and signs is established, patients should be told sympathetically what has been discovered and offered help with whatever problems might have led to the behaviour. This should be part of a sympathetic plan that also offers psychological help. Box 25.4 summarizes the ethical issues.

Munchausen syndrome is an extreme and uncommon form of factitious disorder in which a patient gives a plausible and often dramatic history of an acute illness, with feigned symptoms and signs. Symptoms may be of any kind, including psychiatric symptoms. These patients often attend a series of hospitals, giving different names to each. Frequently, strong analgesics are demanded for pain. Patients may obstruct efforts to obtain additional information about them and may interfere with diagnostic investigations. It has a poor prognosis.

Munchausen syndrome by proxy refers to a form of child abuse in which a parent (or occasionally another adult, such as a nurse) gives a false account of symptoms in a child, and may fake physical signs (see p. 195).

Malingering

Malingering is the fraudulent simulation or exaggeration of symptoms with the intention of gaining financial or other rewards. It is the obvious external gain that distinguishes malingering from factitious disorder. When cli
nically significant malingering occurs it is most often among prisoners, the military, and people seeking compensation for accidents. However, more minor malingering, such as feigning illness to secure extra holiday from work, is common.

Malingering should be diagnosed only after a full investigation of the case. When the diagnosis is certain, the patient should be informed tactfully of this conclusion and encouraged to deal more

appropriately with any problems that contributed to the behaviour.

Further reading

Gureje O, Reed GM. Bodily distress disorder in ICD-11: problems and prospects. *World Psychiatry* 2016;15:291–292.

National Institute for Health and Care Excellence. Irritable bowel syndrome in adults: diagnosis and management. Clinical guideline [CG61]. Published February 2008, updated April 2017. https://www.nice.org.uk/guidance/cg61.

White PD, Goldsmith KA, Johnson AL, et al. Comparison of adaptive pacing therapy, cognitive behavior therapy, graded exercise therapy, and specialist medical care for chronic fatigue syndrome (PACE): a randomized trial. *Lancet* 2011;377;823–826. [The objection in some quarters to this trial is exemplified by the following letter: Shepherd C. Patient reaction to the PACE trial. *Lancet Psychiatry* 2016;3:e7–e9.]

Introduction

Organic psychiatric disorders result from brain dysfunction caused by organic pathology inside or outside the brain. Dementia is the most common condition, with Alzheimer's disease alone affecting 1 per cent of the population at 60 years, rising to 40 per cent over 80 years. Many of the rarer organic psychiatric disorders tend to affect a wider age range, but present in similar ways. Given the changing demographics of most developed countries, disorders producing cognitive impairment in older adults are becoming increasingly important for provision of healthcare services and in daily clinical practice. This chapter will cover the more common causes of cognitive impairment, and there is additional information in Chapters 18 and 20 on psychiatry of older adults in psychiatry and medicine.

There are three common clinical presentations of organic psychiatric disorders:

1 **Delirium**—an acute generalized impairment of brain function, in which the most important feature is impairment of consciousness. The disturbance of brain function is generalized, and the primary cause is often outside the brain; for example, sepsis due to a urinary tract infection.

2 **Dementia**—chronic generalized impairment, in which the main clinical feature is global intellectual impairment. There are also changes in mood and behaviour. The brain dysfunction is generalized, and the primary cause is within the brain; for example, a degenerative condition such as Alzheimer's disease.

3 **Specific syndromes**—which include disorders with a predominant impairment of isolated areas; for example, memory (amnesic syndrome), thought, mood, or personality change. These include neurological disorders that frequently result in organic psychological complications; for example, epilepsy.

Table 26.1 lists the main categories of psychiatric disorder associated with organic brain disease. The

Table 26.1 Classification of organic psychiatric disorders causing brain disease

Global syndromes	• Delirium • Dementia
Specific syndromes	• Amnesic syndrome • Organic mood disorder • Organic delusional state • Organic personality disorder

Table 26.2 Clinical features of delirium

Impaired consciousness	• Disorientation • Poor attention and concentration • Loss of memory
Behaviour	• Overactive • Underactive
Thinking	• Muddled (confused) • Ideas of reference • Delusions
Mood	• Anxious, irritable • Depressed • Perplexed
Perception	• Misinterpretations • Hallucinations, mainly visual • Acute onset, fluctuating course, worse in the evening

following sections describe these syndromes and the psychiatric consequences of a number of neurological conditions. Organic causes of other core psychiatric conditions (e.g. anxiety and psychosis) are covered in the relevant specific chapters.

Delirium

Delirium is characterized by an acute impairment of consciousness producing a generalized cognitive impairment. The word delirium is derived from the Latin, '*lira*', which means to wander from the furrow. Delirium is a common condition, affecting up to 30 per cent of patients in general medical or surgical wards, with the primary cause often being a systemic illness. The term '**acute confusional state**' is a synonym for delirium.

Clinical features

The features of delirium differ widely between patients, but there are eight main themes within the presentation (Table 26.2).

1 **Impairment of consciousness** is the most important sign, and is seen as a deficit of attention, concentration, and awareness. Often the patient will not be able to follow or engage in a logical conversation. The features *fluctuate in intensity* and are often *worse in the evening*.

2 **Disorientation**—uncertainty about the time, place, and identity of other people.

3 **Behaviour** may be either overactive, with noisiness and irritability, or underactive. Sleep is often disturbed.

4 **Thinking** is slow and confused but the content is often complex. Ideas of reference and delusions are common.

5 **Mood** may be anxious, perplexed, irritable, or depressed and is often labile.

6 **Perception** may be distorted with misinterpretations, illusions, and visual hallucinations. Tactile and auditory hallucinations occur but are less frequent.

7 **Memory.** Disturbance of memory affects registration, retention, and recall, as well as new learning.

8 **Insight** is impaired.

The diagnostic criteria for delirium are shown in Box 26.1.

Prevalence

Delirium is an extremely common condition and may occur in all age groups. Those at the extremes of age, with pre-existing dementia, or who have a serious

Box 26.1 ICD1-10 F05 Delirium

Main features

An aetiologically non-specific organic cerebral syndrome characterized by concurrent disturbances of consciousness and attention, perception, thinking, memory, psychomotor behaviour, emotion, and the sleep–wake schedule.

Associated features

Degree of severity ranges from mild to very severe.

Duration

Variable.

Exclusions

Delirium caused by alcohol or substance intoxication or withdrawal, delirium superimposed on pre-existing dementia (NB: coded as F5.01), sleep–wake disorder.

ICD-11 beta draft: key changes 7D90 Delirium

As above, plus added specification that the condition develops over a short period of time and shows fluctuating severity across the day.

Source data from *International Classification of Diseases*, 10th Revision (ICD-10), World Health Organization 2016, and *International Classification of Diseases*, 11th revision (ICD-11), World Health Organization Beta draft 2016.

physical illness make up the majority. Prevalence is positively correlated with severity of physical illness: on a general medical or surgical ward, one-third of patients will experience delirium during their hospital stay, while in intensive care units, up to 70 per cent of patients meet the criteria, including many young people. The prevalence of delirium in the community is unknown.

Co-morbidity

Half of all cases of delirium occur in patients with an underlying (diagnosed or undiagnosed) dementia syndrome. Delirium is also more common in those with neurological conditions (e.g. stroke or Parkinson's disease) and primary mood or anxiety disorders.

Differential diagnosis

The key differentials of delirium are dementia, depression, and non-organic psychoses. Table 26.3 outlines the key differences between these conditions.

Aetiology

There are many causes of delirium, the most important of which are listed in Box 26.2. However, most episodes of delirium are multifactorial, each of which may with different causes being relevant at different points in the illness. The neuropathology of delirium is poorly understood, partly as it is very challenging to conduct research (e.g. cerebral imaging and neurotransmitter assays) in such extremely unwell patients. A diffuse slowing is seen upon the EEG, and there are global changes in the cerebral circulation. Neuroimaging suggests involvement of the prefrontal cortex, thalamus, posterior parietal lobe, and subcortical regions. It is unclear currently why some functions (e.g. speech, motor, or sensory) remain intact in delirium, while others are badly deranged. Acetylcholine plays an important role—anticholinergic drugs significantly increase the risk of delirium in the elderly, while cholinesterase inhibitors are protective, but the mechanism of this is unknown.

Delirium is more frequent in children and older adults, among people with previous brain damage of any kind, in conditions of low sensory input (such as deafness and poor vision), or in malnutrition. Isolation, immobility, stress, use of restraints, and the intensive care environment have also been shown to be risk factors.

Assessment

Assessment should aim to identify the underlying physical cause of delirium, and to place this in the context of the patient's premorbid level of cognition and functioning. The diagnosis is clinical and is usually obvious upon talking to the patient. Typically, a standard medical and surgical history is taken, rather than a formal psychiatric interview. Often little history can be obtained directly, so it is essential to contact relatives, carers,

Table 26.3 Differential diagnosis of delirium

Characteristic	Delirium	Dementia	Depression	Psychosis
Onset	Acute	Gradual (often insidious)	Usually gradual	Variable
Level of consciousness	Impaired	Normal	Usually normal	Normal
Attention	Poor	Intact	Mildly impaired	Poor
Memory	Impaired	Impaired (primary problem)	Inconsistent (pseudodementia)	Intact
Mood	Variable	Normal	Low and flat	Incongruous
Hallucinations[a]	Usually visual	Visual or auditory	Auditory	Auditory
Delusions	Persecutory, but fleeting	Paranoid, fixed	Mood congruent	Complex, systematized, often paranoid
Reversibility	Usually	Not usually	Usually	Sometimes
Course	Fluctuating	Progressive	Diurnal variation	Chronic relapsing and remitting

[a] Hallucinations may be experienced in any of the five senses for all diagnoses; the table above merely gives the mostly commonly encountered for comparison.

friends, and other clinicians in order to gather the story. Include a comprehensive list of medications, including over-the-counter remedies, alcohol, and smoking. A full examination of all physical systems should be undertaken, including a detailed neurological examination. Physical investigations should include:

- blood for full blood count, urea and electrolytes, liver function tests, thyroid function tests, calcium, phosphate, magnesium, glucose, lactate, troponin, albumin, paracetamol and salicylate, and haematinics;
- blood and urine cultures;
- arterial blood gas;
- ECG;
- urinalysis;
- chest X-ray;
- consider further tests, for example, CT head, lumbar puncture, and EEG.

Complex cognitive investigations are usually not needed, but the following are useful simple tests to quantify the level of impairment:

- Abbreviated Mental Test Score (AMTS)—out of 10 points, a score of 6 or less is taken as delirium (Box 26.3).

Box 26.2 Some causes of delirium

- Systemic infection: for example, urinary tract, chest, cellulitis, and intravenous lines
- Neurological infection: meningitis or encephalitis
- Stroke or myocardial infarction
- Trauma or head injury
- Metabolic failure: cardiac, respiratory, renal, or hepatic
- Hypoglycaemia
- Electrolyte abnormalities
- Nutritional deficiencies: vitamin B_{12}, thiamine, and nicotinic acid
- Drug intoxication or withdrawal
- Alcohol withdrawal
- Raised intracranial pressure or space-occupying lesions
- Post-ictal states or status epilepticus

Box 26.3 Abbreviated Mental Test Score questions

What is your age? (1 point)

What is the time to the nearest hour? (1 point)

Give the patient an address, and ask him or her to repeat it at the end of the test, for example, 42 West Street. (1 point)

What is the year? (1 point)

What is the name of the hospital or number of the residence where the patient is situated? (1 point)

Can the patient recognize two persons (the doctor, nurse, carer, etc.)? (1 point)

What is your date of birth (day and month sufficient)? (1 point)

In what year did World War 2 begin? (1 point) (Other dates can be used, with a preference for dates sometime in the past)

Name the present monarch/dictator/prime minister/president. (1 point)

Count backwards from 20 down to 1. (1 point)

- Mini Mental State Examination (MMSE)—30 points, with more than or equal to 25 taken as normal, mild dementia 21–24, moderate 10–20, and severe less than 10 points.

The AMTS is often used sequentially to monitor for improvement or decline in functioning. The MMSE is primarily used for dementia, but may be helpful in delirium.

Management

Treatment of delirium is directed both to dealing with the underlying physical cause and with measures to treat the patient's anxiety, distress, and behavioural problems.

1 **Treat the underlying cause.** This obviously depends on the exact aetiology, but frequently involves giving oxygen, fluids, antibiotics, and pain relief, as well as any specific treatments. Intravenous access (and other invasive procedures) should only be undertaken if there is a valid indication.

2 **Reassurance and reorientation.** Patients need reassurance to reduce anxiety and disorientation; this should be repeated frequently. A clock should be visible at all times, and the patient reminded of the time, place, day, and date regularly.

3 **Predictable, consistent routine.** On the ward the patient should be nursed either in a quiet side room or next to the nursing station. It should be reasonably dark at night and light during the day. Meals and activities should occur at standard times each day. Relatives and friends should be encouraged to stay or to visit frequently.

4 **Avoid unnecessary medications.**

5 **Explain to relatives and friends** what delirium is and what has caused it. This helps them to reassure and reorientate the patient.

6 **Sleep** is often disturbed, and it is reasonable to give small doses of hypnotics (e.g. zopiclone 3.75 mg) or benzodiazepines (e.g. temazepam 10 mg) at night to promote sleep. Benzodiazepines should be avoided during daytime as their sedative effects may increase disorientation. The exception to this is in alcohol withdrawal or in order to treat seizures.

7 **Disturbed, violent, or distressed behaviour** may be treated with carefully monitored antipsychotic medications. There is some high-quality evidence supporting the use of antipsychotics in delirium, with a consistent two-thirds of patients experiencing clinical improvement. Haloperidol is the traditional choice (given orally, intramuscularly, or intravenously), although atypical antipsychotics are becoming more commonly used. High-dose haloperidol has a greater risk of extrapyramidal effects than atypicals, so a maximum dose of 5 mg/24 hours should be aimed for. Olanzapine and quetiapine have the most evidence for efficacy and tolerability in delirium, but can be sedating. If possible, benzodiazepines should be avoided as they risk worsening confusion and sedation. If a patient is acutely distressed or agitated, an intramuscular dose is usually needed,

Delirium

As a general hospital duty doctor you are called in the middle of the night to see a 79-year-old man who has become disturbed and distressed 3 days after major abdominal surgery. The nursing staff, who have not known the patient before, say the patient has been attempting to pull out his drip, has been shouting incoherently, and seems frightened. He has accused them of being guards in a prison. You look at the case notes, which contain routine medical information, but find that in the nursing notes the patient has been intermittently rather drowsy and that during the day his relatives reported that he seemed confused.

You find it difficult to interview the patient, who seems unable to concentrate on your questions and makes disconnected comments about being in prison and having been attacked by people who want to kill him. He is unable to say where he is or to tell you the date. You diagnose delirium. You notice that he has pyrexia and the nurses tell you that he appears to be developing a wound infection. You examine the wound, and find it red, hot, and painful. You continue intravenous fluids, start antibiotics, and take a swab for culture from the wound.

You arrange for the patient be moved to a quiet, well-lit side room. You explain to the patient that he is safe in hospital and that you will be able to help him feel better. One of the nurses takes responsibility for looking after the patient and for repeatedly reassuring him that all is well. Despite reassurance, the patient remains very agitated. Your prescribe 1 mg of haloperidol, which the patient is willing to take as syrup.

In the morning you review the patient, who is calmer. You discuss a consistent, reassuring regimen with the day nursing staff, explain to the relatives what has happened, and encourage them to spend time with the patient explaining and reassuring him about what is going on. You also discuss the response of the patient and your treatment with the responsible medical team so that they are able to continue with a consistent long-term plan.

with follow-on treatment orally for as long as necessary. This should be regularly reviewed, and never used unless other methods of management have been exhausted.

Delirium has an acute onset but the typical course, even treated, can be much longer. It is not unusual for it to take several weeks for a full recovery (see Case study box 26.1).

Dementia

Overview of dementia

Dementia is *a generalized decline of intellect, memory, and personality, without impairment of consciousness, leading to functional impairment.* It is a clinical syndrome, rather than a diagnosis in itself, which may be caused by a variety of pathologies. This section will outline common features of the dementias, and further information on specific diagnoses follows in the latter part of the chapter.

Dementia is an acquired disorder, as distinct from learning disability in which impairments are present from birth (see Chapter 19), although the onset may be at any age. Onset before the age of 65 is called pre-senile dementia. Although most cases of dementia are irreversible, small but important groups are remediable, meaning that the assessment process must aim to exclude reversible causes before making a diagnosis of a progressive condition. Dementia is on the increase, largely due to an ageing population, and managing patients effectively is a large part of a junior doctor's job in general medical and surgical rotations.

Clinical features

Dementia usually presents with impairment of memory. In some cases, the main presenting feature may be a change in behaviour or a psychiatric symptom (Box 26.4). The clinical picture depends in part on the patient's premorbid personality; for example, neurotic and paranoid traits may become

Box 26.4 Clinical features of dementia

Cognition

- **Memory problems:** usually an insidious onset, although it may be noticed after a sudden decline due to a change in social circumstances or physical illness. Memory loss is more obvious for recent than for remote events. Forgetfulness usually appears early and is prominent; difficulty in new learning is a conspicuous sign. Confabulation may occur
- Impaired attention
- Aphasia, agnosia, and apraxia
- Disorientation in time (early), place, and person (later)
- 'Personality change'

Behaviour[a]

- Odd and disorganized
- Restless, wandering (especially in the evenings)
- Self-neglect
- Disinhibition
- Loss of initiative, reduction in interests, and social withdrawal

Mood[a]

- Anxiety

- Depression (be sure to distinguish between true dementia and pseudodementia)
- Irritability or agitation
- Catastrophic reactions: a sudden change to tears or anger when patients are stretched in their abilities or upset

Thinking[a]

- Slow and impoverished
- Reduction in abstract thought, reduced flexibility, and increased perseveration
- Impaired judgement
- Delusions—paranoid
- Speech echoes disturbed thinking and shows syntactical errors and nominal dysphasia

Perception[a]

- Illusions
- Hallucinations—often visual

Insight

- Impaired

[a] Together these symptoms are known as the 'Behavioural and Psychological Symptoms of Dementia (BAPS).

exaggerated. People who are socially isolated or deaf may be less able to compensate for failing intellectual abilities. On the other hand, a person with good social skills may maintain a social facade despite severe intellectual deterioration. There are no generic criteria in the ICD-10 for dementia as a clinical syndrome; specific criteria for the common and important pathologies are included in the following subsections.

Prevalence

Dementia currently affects about 45 million people worldwide, with the numbers set to increase dramatically as life expectancy increases further. Table 26.4 gives an idea of the prevalence of dementia at different ages. It is four times more common in men than in women.

Table 26.4 Global prevalence of dementia

Age (years)	Prevalence (%)
40–59	0.01
60–64	1.6
65–69	2.6
70–74	4.3
75–79	7.4
80–84	12.9
85–89	21.7
≥90	43.1

Source data from *Alzheimer's and Dementia*, 9, 1, Prince MB, Albanese E, Wimo A et al, The global prevalence of dementia: a systematic review and metaanalysis, pp. 63–75. 2013 The Alzheimer's Association.

Differential diagnosis

The main differentials are those shown in Table 26.3, including the key differences between delirium and dementia. However, always consider that symptoms (especially isolated forgetfulness) may be a feature of normal ageing or, in a young person, that the diagnosis could be a learning disability.

A common diagnostic problem is presented by so-called depressive pseudodementia. In this syndrome, a depressed patient complains of poor memory and appears intellectually impaired because poor concentration leads to inadequate registration. Depressed mood may lead to slowness and self-neglect. Characteristic features are:

- the depressed mood preceded the memory problems;
- memory testing shows that the poor performance improves when interest is aroused;
- the patient is psychomotor retarded and may be unwilling to cooperate in the interview; by contrast, patients with dementia are usually willing to reply to questions but make mistakes.

Conversely, an organic disorder can present with a mood disorder or a behaviour change that suggests a functional disorder. The points in favour of an organic cause are:

- the cognitive disorder preceded the mood or other disorder;
- cognitive defects occur in specific areas of intellectual function;
- neurological signs;
- the presence of symptoms seldom found in functional disorders, such as visual hallucinations.

It is important to consider a possible organic cause in every case of acute psychological or behavioural disturbance, especially when there are atypical features. The diagnosis of functional disorder is partly by exclusion of organic causes but also by the finding of positive evidence of psychological aetiology, since organic causes may be undetectable in the early stages of disease.

Aetiology

Dementia has many causes, of which the most important are listed in Table 26.5. Among older patients, the majority of cases are caused by Alzheimer's disease (55 per cent), vascular dementia (20 per cent),

Table 26.5 Causes of dementia

Irreversible causes	Potentially reversible causes
Primary degenerative conditions:	Neurological:
• Alzheimer's disease (55%)	• Normal-pressure hydrocephalus
• Lewy body dementia (15%)	• Intracranial tumour
• Frontotemporal dementia (Pick's disease)	• Chronic subdural haematoma
• Huntingdon's disease	Vitamin deficiencies:
• Wilson's disease	• Vitamin B_{12}
• Multiple sclerosis	• Folic acid
• Motor neuron disease	• Thiamine
Vascular: multi-infarct dementia (20%)	Endocrine:
Toxins: alcohol	• Hypothyroidism
Traumatic head injury	• Cushing's syndrome
Infections: HIV, encephalitis, Creutzfeldt–Jakob disease	
Anoxia: cardiac arrest, carbon monoxide poisoning	
Metabolic: hepatic encephalopathy, diabetes mellitus	

and Lewy body dementia (15 per cent). Although these and many other causes are irreversible, when assessing a patient the clinician needs to keep in mind the whole range of causes so as not to miss any that might be partly or wholly treatable, such as an operable cerebral neoplasm.

Assessment

Patients may present to primary care with symptoms of dementia, or a suspicion may arise while they are being treated for another health problem. Memory assessment clinics are the single point of access to services in the UK. The aim should be to perform the minimum of investigations to reveal the cause of the disorder, whether acute or chronic. Basic assessment should include the following:

1 **Detailed history taking.** Any suspicion of dementia should lead to detailed questioning about intellectual function and neurological symptoms. It is important to interview other informants, since patients are often unaware of the extent of the change in themselves. An assessment of mood should be made.

2 **Full physical examination,** focusing on the neurological system and including vision and hearing.

3 **Cognitive testing.** The MMSE is used widely in assessment; it tests orientation, registration, attention and calculation, recall, and language and has high sensitivity and specificity. A clock drawing test may be added to examine executive function.

4 **Laboratory investigations.** Basic haematology, biochemistry, liver function, thyroid function, vitamin B_{12}, folate, thiamine, calcium, and erythrocyte sedimentation rate should be carried out.

5 **Imaging.** A CT or MRI brain scan is recommended, as they are valuable in the diagnosis of both focal and diffuse cerebral pathology. More specialized imaging, for example, a single-photon emission computed tomography/positron emission tomography (SPECT/PET) scan or DaTSCAN (for

Alzheimer's or Lewy body dementia respectively) may be requested by secondary care.

Management of dementia

The initial step in the management of dementia is to treat any physical disorder, be it causal or co-morbid. After this, treatment aims to reduce disability and provide support. Specific attention should be paid to behavioural and psychological symptoms, as these are associated with high morbidity in patients and carers. Whenever possible, care is community based with admission to hospital being reserved for the few patients at risk of harming themselves or others, or those with complex physical or psychiatric co-morbidities. A summary of treatment approaches is shown in Box 26.5.

Medications do not yet play a prominent role in the treatment of dementia. There are four main groups of drug used in dementia:

1 **Acetylcholinesterase inhibitors** (donepezil, galantamine, rivastigmine) increase the concentration of and duration of action of acetylcholine in the central nervous system. There is evidence that in moderately severe Alzheimer's disease, these drugs improve cognitive function and behaviour for up to a year. There is no current evidence that these drugs halt or delay the progression of disease. In the UK, acetylcholinesterase inhibitors are licensed for use in patients with mild to moderate Alzheimer's disease, or those with agitation not controlled by non-drug measures or antipsychotics. These drugs should only be prescribed by specialists, and should be stopped after 6 months if there is no clinical benefit. Common adverse effects include nausea, diarrhoea, dizziness, and insomnia. Acetylcholinesterase inhibitors are not recommended for non-Alzheimer's dementia with the exception that rivastigmine has recently been licensed for dementia associated with Parkinson's disease.

2 **Memantine** is a glutamine NMDA receptor antagonist which improves cognition, mood, and

Box 26.5 Management of dementia

General measures	Psychological
<ul><li>Treat any physical disorders.</li><li>**Psychoeducation** of patient, family, and carers. This should include information on symptoms of dementia, course and prognosis, treatments, local support opportunities, and financial and legal considerations (e.g. capacity and driving).</li><li>Provide a personalized, multidisciplinary care plan.</li><li>Appropriate setting of care and social/healthcare package.</li><li>Refer to occupational therapy, physiotherapy, or dieticians as needed.</li><li>Advance decision-making: end of life care, resuscitation, and power of attorney.</li><li>Support for carers: training, voluntary sector support groups, and respite care.</li><li>Palliative care input.</li></ul>	(Includes evidence-based options recommended in the UK.)<ul><li>Structured group cognitive stimulation programme—evidence that this improves MMSE scores in the medium term.</li><li>Reminiscence therapy.</li><li>For agitation and challenging behaviour: aromatherapy, dance/music therapy, animal therapy, and massage.</li><li>Psychological support for carers—counselling or CBT.</li></ul>**Pharmacological**<ul><li>Acetylcholinesterase inhibitors.</li><li>Memantine.</li><li>For agitation: antipsychotics and benzodiazepines.</li><li>For depression: antidepressants.</li></ul>

behaviour in moderate to severe Alzheimer's disease. Memantine is a second-line treatment for moderate to severe Alzheimer's disease.

3 **Antipsychotics should generally be avoided whenever possible** and only have a role in patients with severely distressing symptoms or agitation causing risk to self or others. They should be avoided in those with mild–moderate dementia, as there is a slight increase in mortality. Before using an antipsychotic, the above-mentioned non-pharmacological methods should be used, and the patient nursed in a safe, low-stimulation environment. Oral medications should be offered before parenteral drugs are given. The recommended drugs are risperidone and olanzapine. A few patients need long-term oral antipsychotics to manage their behaviour at home (see Science box 26.1).

4 **Benzodiazepines should be avoided wherever possible,** especially during the day. Intramuscular lorazepam is a suitable alternative to an antipsychotic for extreme agitation, and should be tried if antipsychotics do not relieve the symptoms.

Depression is common in patients with dementia, and should be treated along usual guidelines (see Chapter 21).

Specific dementia syndromes

The most common causes of dementia are Alzheimer's disease, vascular dementia, and Lewy body dementia. The main clinical features of less common causes are outlined in Table 26.6, more detail on which can be found in the 'Further reading' section. The previous section on management is relevant to all causes of dementia.

Alzheimer's disease

Alois Alzheimer, a German psychiatrist and neuropathologist, described the salient features of what is now known as Alzheimer's disease in 1906. Alzheimer's disease is the most common cause of dementia, accounting for 50–60 per cent of cases worldwide. Prevalence at age 65 is about 5 per cent, rising to 40 per cent of those aged over 85 years; Alzheimer's therefore represents high morbidity and a significant financial burden on healthcare systems. About 80 per

SCIENCE BOX 26.1

Are antipsychotics safe and effective to use in dementia?

Ninety per cent of patients with Alzheimer's disease experience behavioural and/or psychiatric problems, the most common being psychosis, agitation, and aggression. These can make managing the patient challenging, and are psychologically difficult for both patient and carer. Non-pharmacological interventions should be the first-line approach, but is there evidence for the use of antipsychotics in this situation?

First-generation antipsychotics have been used for several decades, and are probably at least partly effective, but run a high risk of sedation and extrapyramidal side effects. The use of atypical antipsychotics has increased, but their use has been controversial. The best evidence comes from the Clinical Antipsychotic Trials of Intervention Effectiveness–Alzheimer's Disease (CATIE-AD).[1] This was a randomized controlled trial of olanzapine, risperidone, quetiapine, or placebo for up to 36 weeks in 421 patients with aggression or agitation. The authors report that olanzapine and risperidone showed greater clinical improvement than the comparison groups but all drugs were poorly tolerated, with high levels of sedation and confusion.

The Cochrane Collaboration reviewed this question in 2008.[2] They identified 16 randomized controlled trials, primarily using olanzapine and risperidone. They reported risperidone and olanzapine reduced aggression in Alzheimer's disease, but that for psychosis, only evidence for risperidone reached significance.

One problem has consistently arisen in this area. Atypical antipsychotics seem to be associated with a greater risk of stroke and all-cause mortality when used in Alzheimer's patients. The US Food and Drug Administration and European Medicines Agency have both issued warnings regarding the significant increase in mortality (odds ratio 1.7) for patients with Alzheimer's taking atypical antipsychotics.[3, 4] Several studies have now confirmed an association between stroke and antipsychotics (both first and second generation)—the risk being greatest in the first 3 months of treatment.[5] At present there is no evidence for differing risks between the atypical antipsychotic group.[6]

1 Schneider LS, Dagerman KS, Insel P. Risk of death with atypical antipsychotic drug treatment for dementia: meta-analysis of randomised placebo-controlled trials. *JAMA* 2005;294:1934–1943.

2 Ballard CG, Waite J, Birks J. Atypical antipsychotics for aggression and psychosis in Alzheimer's disease. *Cochrane Database of Systematic Reviews* 2008;1:CD003476.

3 Food and Drug Administration. Information on conventional antipsychotics—FDA Alert 2008. http://www.fda.gov.

4 European Medicines Agency. CHMP Assessment report on conventional antipsychotics. Published November 2008. https://www.ema.europa.eu/documents/report/chmp-assessment-report-conventional-antipsychotics-procedure-under-article-53-regulation-ec-no-726/2004_en.pdf.

5 Douglas IJ, Smeeth L. Exposure to antipsychotics and risk of stroke: self controlled case series study. *BMJ* 2008;337:a1227.

6 Ballard C, Hanney ML, Theodoulou M, et al. The dementia antipsychotic withdrawal trial (DART-AD): long term follow up of a randomised placebo-controlled trial. *Lancet Neurology* 2009;8:151–157.

cent of patients live in the community rather than residential settings.

Pathology

Postmortem and neuroimaging data have shown that a brain affected by Alzheimer's is significantly smaller than age-matched controls, with widened sulci and enlarged ventricles. There is cell loss, shrinkage of the dendritic tree, proliferation of astrocytes, and increased gliosis. There are two key histological findings:

1 **Amyloid plaques** are extracellular areas of dense, insoluble beta-amyloid peptide surrounded by neuronal injury and dystrophic neurones and filled with highly phosphorylated tau protein.

2 **Neurofibrillary tangles** are made up of helical filaments of the microtubule-associated protein,

Table 26.6 Rare degenerative neurological diseases causing dementia

Condition	Pathology	Epidemiology	Clinical features
Frontotemporal dementia (group of conditions including Pick's disease)	Preferential atrophy of the frontal and temporal lobes Ubiquitinated inclusion bodies, loss of cortical neurons, gliosis, and spongiform change	20–60/100,000 Onset 45–60 years Male = female 50% have a family history	Abnormal social behaviour/conduct Change in personality Reduction of speech Mood symptoms Dietary changes Stereotyped behaviour Hallucinations, delusions
Huntington's chorea	Autosomal dominant degenerative disorder of frontal lobes and caudate nucleus	70 per million in Europe Onset 35–44 years Male = female	Choreiform movements Dysarthria Ataxia Dementia Persecutory delusions
Prion disease (includes CJD, vCJD, Kuru)	Deposits of prion protein throughout the brain causing a spongiform encephalopathy. Majority sporadic, may be acquired or iatrogenic	Sporadic CJD: 1 per million per year Onset 15–60 years Male = female	Rapidly progressive dementia Myoclonus Focal neurological signs Death within 6 months
HIV-associated dementia (AIDS–dementia complex)	Metabolic encephalopathy caused by the HIV lentivirus, and activation of macrophages in the brain which secrete neurotoxins	10–20% of patients with untreated AIDS Recent decline in numbers following widespread use of HAART	Insidious onset, memory loss, poor attention and concentration Apathy and social withdrawal Depression or psychosis Focal neurology (motor), ataxia, and tremor Myoclonus and seizures

CJD, Creutzfeldt–Jakob disease; HAART, highly active antiretroviral therapy; vCJD, variant Creutzfeldt–Jakob disease.

tau, in a highly phosphorylated state. These are found throughout the cortical and subcortical grey matter (Fig. 26.1).

Other common histopathological features include cerebral amyloid angiopathy, Lewy bodies (see later), hippocampal sclerosis, and vascular injuries. The occipital lobe and cerebellum tend to remain relatively unscathed.

Beta-amyloid is derived from a larger protein, APP, which is encoded by the *APP* gene on chromosome 21. Mutations in this gene have been found which produce an early-onset autosomal dominant form

of Alzheimer's, although this is exceptionally rare. Mutations in the presenilin genes, which encode proteins involved in the cleavage of APP to beta-amyloid, also cause an autosomal dominant form of the disease. The exact method by which plaques and tangles are formed is poorly understood, and a large amount of research at the molecular and cellular levels is currently under way.

It has been shown that the neurons lost tend to be primarily cholinergic, leading to the 'cholinergic hypothesis', which suggests that the cognitive impairment in Alzheimer's is due to a deficit of cholinergic

(a)

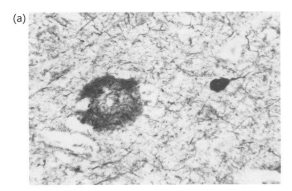

(b)

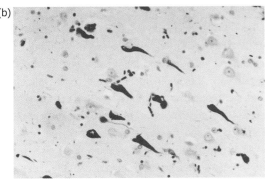

Fig. 26.1 (a) Amyloid plaque and neurofibrillary tangle from the brain of a patient who died of Alzheimer's disease. The plaque shows denser outer staining with an inner core. (b) Characteristic flame-shaped neurofibrillary tangles from the brain of a patient who died from Alzheimer's disease. The tangles are stained with an antibody to hyperphosphorylated tau protein.

Courtesy of Professor Margaret Esiri.

neurotransmission. This is what has led to the development of the acetylcholinesterase inhibitors.

Aetiology

The cause of Alzheimer's disease is unknown, except for some rare genetic types accounting for less than 1 per cent of cases. Some of the known risk factors are shown in Box 26.6. A family history of Alzheimer's is the single most important risk factor; first-degree relatives of those with late-onset Alzheimer's disease have a threefold risk of developing the condition. A small number of families with mutations in the *APP*, presenilin, and *APOE4* genes have inherited autosomal dominant forms of the disease, but most cases are thought to be sporadic.

Box 26.6 Risk factors for Alzheimer's disease

- Age
- Family history
- Male gender
- *APP*, presenilin, or *APOE4* gene mutation carrier
- Previous head injury
- Down's syndrome
- Hypothyroidism
- Parkinson's disease
- Cardiovascular disease (including hypertension)

Clinical features

Alzheimer's disease represents the 'classic' presentation of dementia, so the descriptions of clinical features on p. 367 are all relevant. The diagnostic criteria for Alzheimer's disease are shown in Box 26.7.

Typical early symptoms:

- **Memory impairment.** Episodic amnesia for recent events occurs before more remote memories are lost. Onset is usually insidious and progression steady. Semantic and procedural memory tends to be lost later.

- **Abnormalities in executive function.** Disorganization, lack of ability to reason, and lack of insight.

- **Disorientation** is usually an early sign of visuospatial difficulties and may be evident for the first time when the person is in unfamiliar surroundings; for example, on holiday.

Box 26.7 ICD-10 F00 Alzheimer's Disease

Alzheimer's disease is a primary degenerative cerebral disease of unknown aetiology with characteristic neuropathological and neurochemical features. The disorder is usually insidious in onset and develops slowly but steadily over a period of several years.

ICD-11 beta draft: key changes 9A61

No significant changes are expected.

Adapted from *International Classification of Diseases*, 10th Revision (ICD-10), Copyright (2016) World Health Organization.

- **Olfactory dysfunction.**

  Later onset symptoms:

- **Mood variations.** Mood may be predominantly depressed, euphoric, flattened, or labile.
- **Poor sleep,** with multiple awakenings and wandering.
- **Social behaviour declines** and self-care may be neglected, although some patients maintain a good social facade despite severe cognitive impairment.
- **Personality change** may occur, often with an exaggeration of less favourable traits.
- Signs of **parietal lobe dysfunction**—such as dysphasia, dyspraxia, and agnosia.

Course

There is a progressive decline, the rate of which is not necessarily steady. Incidental physical illness may cause a superimposed delirium resulting in a sudden deterioration in cognitive function from which the patient may not recover fully. Death occurs usually within 3–10 years of the first signs of the disease, and is most frequently from bronchopneumonia.

Vascular dementia

Vascular dementia (also known as **multi-infarct dementia**) is the second most common cause of dementia, accounting for 15–20 per cent of cases. It is a clinical syndrome caused by a variety of different cerebrovascular pathologies, including but not confined to infarctions.

Pathology

Vascular dementia is associated with ischaemic, haemorrhagic, and other vascular pathology (e.g. cerebral amyloid angiopathy) in the brain. Both large and small blood vessels may be involved. Neuroimaging has identified that in patients with vascular dementia the following typically occur:

- Multiple infarctions and ischaemic lesions in the white matter.
- Atrophy of old infarcted areas.

- Bilateral pathology.
- Lesions involve the full thickness of the white matter.
- Changes in blood flow in unaffected regions.
- The entire brain is smaller and the ventricles expanded.

Clinical features

Vascular dementia usually presents in the late sixties or early seventies, with a more sudden onset than Alzheimer's disease (Table 26.7). Patients may present after a stroke, or due to a sudden unexplained decline in function. Unlike Alzheimer's, executive dysfunction, emotional changes, and personality changes tend to occur early, before memory loss becomes apparent. The symptoms are characteristically fluctuating, and episodes of confusion are common, especially at night. Depression and apathy are prominent features. On examination there may be focal neurology, often upper motor neuron deficits, and signs of cardiovascular disease elsewhere. Life expectancy is usually 3–5 years, with the majority dying from ischaemic heart disease or stroke.

Diagnosis

The differential diagnosis from Alzheimer's disease is difficult to make with certainty without neuroimaging (Table 26.7). Suggestive features

Table 26.7 Clinical features of Alzheimer's disease and vascular dementia

Alzheimer's disease	Vascular dementia
Insidious decline	Stepwise progression
Poor memory	Patchy impairment of cognitive function
Progressive disorientation	
Mood change variable	Poor memory
Restless activity	Executive dysfunction
Insomnia	Depression or apathy
Decline in social behaviour	Episodes of confusion
Personality change	Personality change
Dysphasia, dyspraxia	Neurological signs

Box 26.8 ICD-10 F01 Vascular Dementia

Vascular dementia is the result of infarction of the brain due to vascular disease, including hypertensive cerebrovascular disease. The infarcts are usually small but cumulative in their effect. Onset is usually in later life.

Subtypes: multi-infarct dementia, subcortical dementia

ICD-11 beta draft: key changes 9A62 Vascular Dementia

As for ICD-10 plus: speed of information processing, complex attention, and/or frontal-executive functioning are usually affected

Source data from *International Classification of Diseases*, 10th Revision (ICD-10),World Health Organization 2016, and *International Classification of Diseases*, 11th revision (ICD-11), World Health Organization Beta draft 2016.

are patchy defects of cognitive function, stepwise progression of the condition, and the presence of hypertension or peripheral signs of cardiovascular disease. The diagnostic criteria for vascular dementia are shown in Box 26.8.

Aetiology

Risk factors include:

- vascular risk factors (male, family history, hypertension, diabetes mellitus, hyperlipidaemia, smoking);
- specific risk factors for stroke: atrial fibrillation, coagulopathies, polycythaemia, sickle cell disease, carotid disease;
- late life depression;
- lower educational levels.

Lewy body disease

Frederick Lewy was a German neuropathologist who worked with Alzheimer, and in 1912 described the spherical neuronal inclusion bodies found in some patients with dementia that are now known as 'Lewy

bodies'. The nomenclature in this area is rather confusing:

- Lewy body dementias: umbrella term encompassing all dementias with Lewy bodies and parkinsonism.
- Dementia with Lewy bodies: dementia occurring before, concurrently or within a year of parkinsonism.
- Parkinson's disease dementia: dementia starting over 1 year after the onset of parkinsonism.
- Lewy body disease: pathological description of presence of Lewy bodies.

However, for non-specialists, general knowledge of typical features is perfectly adequate. Lewy body dementias are more common in men and those with a family history of parkinsonism.

Pathology

There is usually a mixture of Lewy bodies and Alzheimer-type amyloid plaques and tangles. Lewy bodies are dense, intracytoplasmic inclusions made of phosphorylated neurofilament proteins, associated with ubiquitin and alpha-synuclein. These are primarily found in the basal ganglia, and later spread into the cortex. Neuronal loss is prominent, and there is a slight reduction in total brain volume. The significance of the Alzheimer's-like pathology is unknown.

Clinical features

- **Dementia**—relative sparing of memory, with *fluctuating* cognitive ability and level of consciousness is typical. Significant deficits in attention, executive function, and visuospatial abilities are seen.
- **Parkinsonism**—tremor, bradykinesia, rigidity, and postural instability.
- **Visual hallucinations.**
- **Falls.**
- **Depression.**
- **Hypersensitivity to psychotropic medications,** especially antipsychotics.

Aetiology

The cause of Lewy body dementia is unknown, but once again family history is a key risk factor, and rare familial types have been found. No environmental risk factors have been identified.

Course and prognosis

Life expectancy for Lewy body dementia is 4–10 years, with the rate of cognitive decline similar to that in Alzheimer's. Frequently, the early stages are only recognized in retrospect, but function can be much more impaired than in other dementias due to pronounced parkinsonism affecting movement. Perceptual and behavioural disturbance can be severe in the later stages of the illness, and a high proportion of patients need residential care.

Treatment

The principles of treatment remain as previously outlined, but there are a couple of specific points relating to Lewy body dementia. Parkinsonism should be treated with l-dopa and other antiparkinsonian medications if they are tolerated. Anticholinergics should be avoided as there is evidence that they can increase confusion and visual hallucinations in these patients. There is modest evidence for efficacy of rivastigmine in the early stages. Patients tend to tolerate antipsychotics extremely poorly; if other options fail, the best evidence is for use of small doses of quetiapine. Risperidone should be avoided.

Other organic psychiatric syndromes

Transient global amnesia

This syndrome is an occasional but important cause of episodes of unusual behaviour, which may present as emergencies. Doctors who are not familiar with the syndrome may misdiagnose it as a dissociative disorder (see p. 357). The condition occurs in middle or late life, and more commonly in men. There are abrupt episodes, lasting several hours, of global loss of recent memory. The patient apparently remains alert and orientated, and usually asks repeated questions about what is going on. There is complete recovery, although there may be amnesia for the episode. The cause is unknown, but there is some evidence that episodes may be associated with migraines or acute physical or emotional stress. There is no specific treatment but the usual investigation for delirium, plus a CT/MRI scan of the head are usually needed to exclude other diagnoses.

Amnesic syndrome

The amnesic syndrome is characterized by a prominent disorder of recent memory, in the absence of the generalized intellectual impairment observed in dementia or the impaired consciousness seen in delirium. The condition usually results from lesions in the posterior hypothalamus and nearby midline structures, but occasionally results from bilateral hippocampal lesions. It is often described as **Korsakov's syndrome**, after the Russian neurologist who first described the clinical features, or as the **Wernicke–Korsakov syndrome**, because the amnesic syndrome may accompany an acute neurological syndrome described by Wernicke (**Wernicke's encephalopathy**). This is characterized by impairment of consciousness, memory defect, disorientation, ataxia, and ophthalmoplegia. The prominent causal factor in most cases appears to be thiamine deficiency. The central feature of the amnesic syndrome is a profound **impairment of recent memory** (Box 26.9).

Box 26.9 Clinical features of amnesic syndrome

- Recent memory severely impaired
- Remote memory spared
- Disorientation in time
- Confabulation (to fill gaps in memory)
- Other cognitive functions preserved

Aetiology

Alcohol abuse is the most frequent cause, and seems to act by causing a deficiency of thiamine. Another cause of thiamine deficiency is malnutrition. Other causes include carbon monoxide poisoning, vascular lesions, encephalitis, and tumours of the third ventricle.

Treatment

For cases that may be due to **thiamine deficiency**, this vitamin should be prescribed in the hope of limiting further damage. Oral thiamine is sufficient in non-urgent situations, but patients admitted to hospital should be given parenteral B vitamins (Pabrinex®). Oral thiamine, vitamin B complex, and multivitamins should be continued lifelong. Otherwise, there is no specific treatment and the general measures are those described previously for dementia.

Neurological syndromes

A variety of primary neurological conditions may also cause cognitive decline and/or other neuropsychiatric symptoms. The details are beyond the scope of this book, but a few important facts are given here, and a useful reference can be found in the 'Further reading' section.

- Psychiatric symptoms are extremely common after cardiovascular events. Depression occurs in up to 50 per cent in the year after a stroke, and personality change may occur even outside of those who develop dementia.

- Cerebral tumours may present with frontal executive dysfunction, delirium from raised intracranial pressure, or cognitive decline.

- Normal pressure hydrocephalus is a rare reversible cause of dementia. It presents with a triad of ataxia, dementia, and urinary incontinence. Definitive treatment requires surgical insertion of a ventriculoperitoneal shunt to improve the circulation of cerebrospinal fluid.

- Multiple sclerosis: 70 per cent experience depression or mood lability. Cognitive decline is extremely common in the later stages.

- Head injuries: these may present acutely with amnesia (around the time of the accident or retrograde), delirium, or emotional symptoms. Longer-term severe injuries are associated with cognitive impairment and personality change. The latter is especially common after frontal lobe damage.

Psychiatric manifestations of epilepsy

Epilepsy is a very common condition, with a lifetime risk of 3.4 per cent for males and 2.8 per cent for females. People with epilepsy suffer from the misconceptions and prejudices of other people about epilepsy as well as from the condition itself. The prevalence of psychiatric disorders in people with epilepsy is four times greater than in the general population, but there is a wide variation depending upon the type of epilepsy. Epilepsy can be restricting; for example, the inability to drive or to go swimming unsupervised. This may lead to depression or other minor psychiatric presentation. There are several ways in which epilepsy predisposes to psychiatric disturbance:

- Effects of stigma and social restrictions.

- Brain injury as a cause of epilepsy may directly cause psychiatric symptoms.

- Behavioural disturbances associated with a seizure—a prodrome, automatic behaviours during a seizure, and post-ictal delirium. Rarely, post-ictal psychosis is seen.

- Psychiatric disorders occurring between seizures—these are shown in Box 26.10 and should be treated along usual guidelines. Many mood stabilizers also have anticonvulsant properties so may be particularly useful.

Box 26.10 Associations between epilepsy and psychological problems of epileptic individuals

Depression

- Lifetime risk of a major depressive episode is 20 per cent, but subclinical symptoms are seen in around half of epileptics.
- Risk factors: right-hand side epileptic focus, complex partial seizures, temporal lobe epilepsy, and difficult-to-control seizures.

Suicide and deliberate self-harm

- Five-fold increase risk of suicide in those with a diagnosis of epilepsy.
- Increase in DSH.
- Strongest risk factor is depression, rather than epilepsy-related factors.

Anxiety disorders

- Very common, 15–20 per cent prevalence.

Psychosis

- Associated with a left-hand sided focus.
- High risk with greater than 10 years of poorly controlled seizures.

Sexual problems

- Reduced libido, erectile dysfunction, and disinhibition are all reported.
- Medications may be to blame, but the location of the epileptic focus is also relevant.

Forensic psychiatric presentations

- Men with epilepsy are three times more likely to receive a criminal conviction than those without. The mechanism of this remains unclear.

Further reading

David A, Fleminger S, Kopelman M, et al. *Lishman's Organic Psychiatry: A Textbook of Neuropsychiatry*. 4th ed. Oxford: Blackwells; 2012. [This is a useful reference for all topics within this chapter, and for primary neurological conditions causing psychiatric presentations.]

Gelder MG, Andreasen NC, López-Ibor JJ, Geddes JR, eds. Chapter 4.1: Delirium, dementia, amnesia, and other cognitive disorders. In: *New Oxford Textbook of Psychiatry*. 2nd ed. Oxford: Oxford University Press; 2012:325–412.

Kales HC, Gitlin LN, Lyketsos CG. Assessment and management of behavioral and psychological symptoms of dementia. *BMJ* 2015;350:h369.

National Institute for Health and Care Excellence. Dementia: assessment, management and support for people living with dementia and their carers. NICE guideline [NG97]. Published June 2018. https://www.nice.org.uk/guidance/ng97.

O'Brien JT, Thomas A. Vascular dementia. *Lancet* 2015;386:1698–1706.

Robinson L, Tang E, Taylor JP. Dementia: timely diagnosis and early intervention. *BMJ* 2015;350:h3029.

27 Eating disorders

Classification of eating disorders

The term 'eating disorder' describes a range of conditions characterized by abnormal eating habits and methods of weight control which lead to a significant impairment of psychological, social, and physical functioning. Eating disorders are serious, complex conditions; they are not simply a problem of eating too much or too little, or an attempt to achieve the perfect physique. Anorexia nervosa has the highest mortality of any psychiatric disorder, and it is notoriously difficult both to engage eating-disordered patients, and to treat them successfully. There is a positive association between early diagnosis and prognosis, so the skills to recognize an eating disorder—whether they present with psychological or physical symptoms—are essential for all clinicians.

At the time of writing, the description of eating disorders within diagnostic classification systems has been undergoing considerable change. Under the ICD-10 and DSM-IV classification systems, three main eating disorders were recognized (Fig. 27.1):

1 anorexia nervosa;

2 bulimia nervosa;

3 eating disorder not otherwise specified (EDNOS).

However, this classification has been shown to have various difficulties:

- The majority of cases were attracting an 'EDNOS' label, whereas it was supposed to be a residual category (Fig. 27.1).

- EDNOS contained within it the subdiagnosis 'binge eating disorder' (BED). Recent research has demonstrated BED accounts for approximately 10 per cent of eating disorders in clinical cohorts.

- The categorical nature of the system does not allow for the fact that most eating disorders change over time, and frequently move back and forth along the spectrum of presentations.

- The DSM-5 classification system (see 'Further reading') has tried to tackle the first two of these difficulties, and the upcoming ICD-11 will echo these changes (Table 27.1) There is now a separate category for BED, and three other defined conditions. This is a positive change, but has only reduced the 'NOS/unspecified' percentage to some extent, and has not considered the changeable nature of eating disorder symptomatology. Hopefully in the future a solution to the difficulty of turning a spectrum of pathology into a categorical system will emerge.

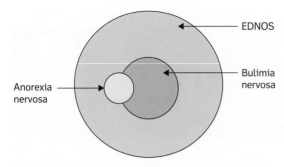

Fig. 27.1 Venn diagram illustrating the relationship between the diagnoses of anorexia nervosa, bulimia nervosa, and eating order not otherwise specified (EDNOS).

Reproduced from *International Journal of Eating Disorders*, 13, 5, C. G. Fairburn, S. L. Welch, P. J. Hay, The classification of recurrent overeating: The "binge eating disorder" proposal, pp. 155–159. Copyright (2006) with permission from John Wiley and Sons.

Epidemiology of eating disorders

Many patients with eating disorders, especially those of a normal weight, never come to medical attention. This makes gathering accurate epidemiological data challenging. Large household surveys in the USA/ Europe have suggested that approximately 30 per cent of eating-disordered patients seek help; these tend (but are not always) to be the more severe end of the spectrum, pointing to a 'tip of the iceberg' effect. In clinical practice, the ratio of females with anorexia nervosa to males is 10:1, although it is likely many cases of anorexia nervosa in men go unrecognized or have fitted less neatly into the diagnostic categories and so attracted an EDNOS label. Table 27.2 gives an overview of epidemiology; the newer diagnostic categories do not yet have a reliable research database to quote.

Anorexia nervosa

Anorexia nervosa is a clinical syndrome characterized by abnormally low body weight, an intense fear of gaining weight, and a distorted perception of body weight and shape. The term 'anorexia nervosa' was first used by William Gull in 1874, and his original description of the essence of the condition contains all of the core elements of the diagnostic criteria that we use today. At the same time, the French physician Charles Lasègue published a similar work, and while Gull and Lasègue

Table 27.1 Classification of eating disorders

DSM-IV	ICD-10	DSM-5	ICD-11 beta draft
Anorexia nervosa	Anorexia nervosa	Anorexia nervosa	Anorexia nervosa
Bulimia nervosa	Bulimia nervosa	Bulimia nervosa	Bulimia nervosa
Eating disorder not otherwise specified (EDNOS)	Atypical anorexia nervosa	Binge eating disorder	Binge eating disorder
	Atypical bulimia nervosa	Avoidant–restrictive food intake disorder	Avoidant–restrictive food intake disorder
	Overeating associated with psychological disturbance	Rumination–regurgitation disorder	Rumination–regurgitation disorder
	Eating disorder unspecified	Pica	Pica
		Feeding and eating disorders not otherwise specified	Feeding and eating disorders unspecified

Table 27.2 Epidemiology of eating disorders

	Anorexia nervosa	Bulimia nervosa	Binge eating disorder[a]
Lifetime risk	Females: 1% Males: <0.5%	1–4% Females > males	2–3% Females > males
Prevalence	Females: 0.5–1% Males: 0.3%	1%	1–2%
Median age of onset	16 years	20 years	23 years

[a] Data for BED is in its infancy due to being a relatively new separate diagnostic category.

were very explicit in their descriptions of the physical findings in anorexia nervosa, both were cautious about extrapolating to describe the psychopathology underlying it, and how to fit this into the classification of other psychiatric conditions (see 'Further reading'). Our understanding has improved in the last century, but there are still many unanswered questions.

Clinical features and diagnostic criteria

The core clinical features of anorexia nervosa are shown in Box 27.1 and Fig. 27.2. Anorexia nervosa may present as primarily restrictive or with binge–purge behaviours. On the whole, anorexia nervosa is an easy

Box 27.1 Features of anorexia nervosa

Core clinical symptoms

- Restriction of food intake leading to an abnormally low body weight
- Behaviours designed to prevent weight gain or continue loss
- Purging via vomiting, use of laxatives, emetics, or diet medications
- Excessive exercise
- A fear of weight gain
- Disturbance in perception of body weight and shape and/or self-evaluation based primarily upon weight and shape

Associated behavioural symptoms

- Obsessional behaviours around food (e.g. restricted types of foods consumed, food-related rituals, persistent cookery for others, hoarding of food, and preference for eating alone)
- Episodes of binge eating followed by purging (*binge–purge subtype*)

- Exercise-related rituals
- Body checking (e.g. repeatedly looking in mirrors or touching specific areas)
- Use of appetite suppressants (e.g. cigarettes or chewing gum)
- Hyperactivity
- Frequent weighing (often multiple times per day)

Associated psychological symptoms

- Preoccupation with thoughts of food
- Low mood and anxiety
- Low self-esteem
- Social withdrawal
- Inflexibility of thought and behaviour
- Perfectionism
- Thoughts of self-harm or suicide
- Insomnia
- Poor insight into or denial of having any problems

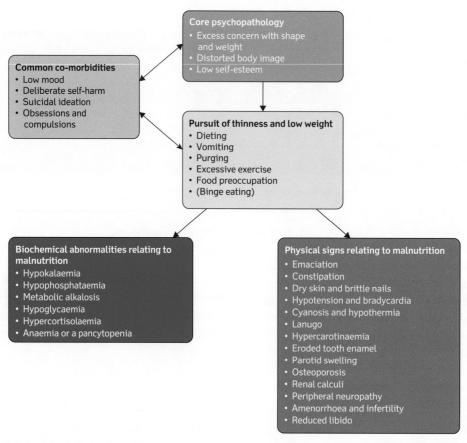

Fig. 27.2 Clinical features of anorexia nervosa.

diagnosis to make; the majority of cases concern a young female who has reduced her food intake and lost weight over the preceding few months, and who is brought to medical attention by a concerned member of the family. It is also relatively common for patients to present to primary care with physical symptoms (e.g. amenorrhoea, dry skin, constipation) or to hospital as an emergency (e.g. fainting, complications of electrolyte abnormalities or low mood with suicidal thoughts).

Core psychopathology

Patients with anorexia nervosa universally have very low self-esteem. They tend to value themselves based on their weight and body shape, rather than by the usual values of the society they live in. Due to their body image disturbance, an emaciated patient typically believes (despite all evidence to the contrary) that they are overweight. This, plus a fear of weight gain or 'fatness', leads to the complex and exhaustive schedule of exercise behaviours seen in patients to avoid an upwards trend in weight. The abnormal thoughts surrounding weight and shape in anorexia nervosa are conventionally described as an **overvalued idea** rather than a delusion, although there is debate around this topic.

Physical consequences of starvation

Low weight that is abnormal for the patient's age, height, and development is essential for the diagnosis; a BMI of less than 18.5, weight less than 85 per cent of expected, or below the 5th centile for children/adolescents are arbitrarily used cut-offs for diagnosis (see Box 27.6 on p. 391 for how to calculate BMI). Common sense should be used in managing cases where other features suggest anorexia nervosa but weight remains at a normal level.

Medical complications of anorexia nervosa include the following:

- Amenorrhoea—primary or secondary. Amenorrhoea may occur before weight loss is significant, and represents a global impairment of the hypothalamic–pituitary–gonadal axis. In the undernourished state, concentrations of follicle-stimulating hormone, luteinizing hormone, and oestrogen in the blood are very low or even undetectable. Pelvic ultrasound in an underweight woman will show small ovaries, with no sign of the heterogeneity of follicles seen during a typical menstrual cycle. This almost always reverses with weight gain. In males, testicular function is reduced, with a decreased level of testosterone production. There is a loss of libido.
- Constipation (may be due to poor intake or secondary to laxative misuse).
- Dry skin and hair loss.
- Lanugo (fine downy hair covering much of the body).
- Cardiovascular complications: poor circulation with cold blue extremities, hypotension, and bradycardia.
- Myopathy: proximal muscle groups are affected first, with the patient having trouble climbing stairs or rising unaided from a squatting position.
- Osteoporosis: a consequence of a combination of low calcium and vitamin D intake, low weight, and low circulating oestrogen levels. Bone density is reversible with weight restoration.
- Consequences of self-induced vomiting: damage to dental enamel, swelling of parotid gland, calluses on backs of fingers (Russell's sign), peripheral oedema.

- Renal calculi.
- Peripheral neuropathy—especially in those following vegan diets.

Biochemical abnormalities

Patients who vomit, use laxatives, or take diuretics are at high risk from dehydration and electrolyte disturbances. Vomiting produces a loss of gastric acid, leading to a metabolic alkalosis and hypokalaemia. Cardiac arrhythmias are not uncommon in this situation, and can lead to sudden death. Laxative abuse can cause dehydration, hypokalaemia, hyponatraemia, and a metabolic acidosis. Diuretics produce dehydration and hyponatraemia. Hypoglycaemia is rare, but is another recognized cause of sudden death. Reduced levels of haemoglobin, leucocytes, or platelets can occur, but they are not nearly as common as the electrolyte disturbances, and are a marker of severe starvation. Hypercortisolaemia and low thyroxine levels may also be seen, and are adaptive measures to reduce metabolic rate and deal with the stress of malnutrition. Vitamin D deficiency is also common.

Peripheral oedema is a relatively frequent occurrence in severely emaciated patients. It is unclear currently what leads to the retention of fluid in starvation, but it can lead to pulmonary oedema and congestive cardiac failure, and therefore should be taken seriously. The exception to this is refeeding oedema, seen in inpatients on very high-calorie diets—this is usually benign.

Co-morbidity

Depressive disorder (and/or deliberate self-harm) is seen in 40–60 per cent of patients with anorexia nervosa. Other frequently occurring conditions include obsessive–compulsive disorder, body dysmorphic disorder, sleep disorders, anxiety disorders, and chronic fatigue syndrome. Co-morbid personality disorders or traits are common in anorexia nervosa, especially obsessive–compulsive, avoidant, or borderline features.

Differential diagnosis

- **Bulimia nervosa** (see p. 387).

- **Avoidant–restrictive food intake disorder (AFRID)** (see p. 389).

- **Eating disorder unspecified.** Patients with disordered eating that is clinically significant, but which does not fit the criteria for a specific eating disorder.

- **Mood disorder.** Core features include low mood, fatigue, and anhedonia. Loss of appetite and weight loss are common, but the patient will not show the specific psychopathology and other weight control behaviours seen in anorexia nervosa

- **Substance abuse.** Patients with chemical dependencies (especially intravenous opioid users) may present as extremely underweight, but do not show the other characteristics of an eating disorder.

- **Iatrogenic drugs.** Many drugs may cause weight loss, through either loss of appetite or a direct effect on metabolism; for example, antidepressants (SSRIs, bupropion), stimulants, topiramate, orlistat, and sibutramine.

- **Organic disorders.** These can usually be identified by a clear history and lack of associated core psychopathology, but specific investigations may need to be done:
  - **Gastrointestinal disorders:** inflammatory bowel disease, coeliac disease, chronic pancreatitis.
  - **Endocrine disorders:** hyperthyroidism, diabetes mellitus, insulinoma.
  - **Neurological disorders:** brain tumours affecting the hypothalamus, dementia, chronic degenerative conditions (e.g. motor neuron disease).
  - **Cancer.**

Aetiology

Like most psychiatric disorders, there is no one cause of anorexia nervosa. A multidimensional model including biological, psychological, and social factors is the best explanation at the current time. It is likely that factors interact with one another, such that, at a specific point, a vulnerable individual becomes ill. Table 27.3 outlines the major predisposing factors known for anorexia nervosa.

Course and prognosis

Anorexia nervosa is a very difficult condition to treat; severity of malnutrition is the most robust prognostic sign. Approximately 50 per cent of patients have a good outcome (including return to normal weight), 25 per cent make a partial recovery, and 25 per cent remain severely ill. The aggregate mortality rate from anorexia nervosa has been shown in meta-analyses to be 0.5 per cent per year. Complications of starvation account for 50 per cent of deaths, with suicide making up the majority of the remaining half. Box 27.2 shows the main factors associated with a poor prognosis.

Why exactly anorexia nervosa is such a persistent condition is unknown, but maintaining forces include the following (see also Fig. 27.3):

1 Starvation itself causes many of the symptoms of anorexia nervosa. Odd eating behaviours, an obsession with food, and excessive exercise are all seen in starved individuals in other contexts.

2 The precipitating factors in the illness may be ongoing; for instance, dealing with the sequelae of sexual abuse.

3 Denial is common in anorexia nervosa, patients often recognize at some level there is a problem but minimize its importance. It is impossible for the illness to recede unless the patient accepts that there is a problem.

4 Anorexia nervosa becomes part of the patient, and they may not be able to envisage themselves without it. It may be that this is due to abnormal brain circuitry or habit forming—this is poorly understood—but it makes it very hard for patients to initiate recovery.

See Case study box 27.1 for an example case.

Table 27.3 Aetiology of anorexia nervosa: predisposing factors

Biological factors	Psychological factors	Social factors
Genetics: • Heritability 50–70% • First-degree relatives have an eightfold increased risk • May be subclinical eating disorders within the family • Twin studies show 65% monozygotic concordance	**Personality traits:** • Obsessive, anxious, and perfectionistic traits are seen in the majority of patients from early childhood	**Upbringing and environment:** • Strong link between high parental expectations and anorexia nervosa • Overprotective parents • Parents with rigid inflexible patterns of thought and behaviour • Poor conflict resolution skills within the family
Cerebral abnormalities: • Neuroimaging shows widening of sulci and ventricular enlargement in patients (may reverse with weight gain) • Hypoperfusion of temporal lobes on functional MRI	**Influence of family or the home environment:** • Parents with eating disorders tend to extend their abnormal concerns onto their children • Emotional enmeshment within the family	**Societal pressures:** • Fashion for abnormal thinness and a 'size zero' culture • Popularity of exclusion diets in Western countries • Occupation that values specific body shapes (e.g. ballet, modelling)
Serotonin dysregulation: • Serotonin activation leads to appetite suppression in controls and animal models • Underweight patients have reduced levels of serotonin metabolites in the CSF	**Previous adverse experiences:** • Bereavement • Abuse in childhood (30%) • Parental divorce • Family illness • Change of home or school • Bullying at school	
Loss of weight for other reasons: • Subgroup of patients develop anorexia nervosa after losing weight due to organic illness (more common in children)		

Source data from: *International Classification of Diseases*, 10th Revision (ICD-10), World Health Organization 2016; *International Classification of Diseases*, 11th revision (ICD-11), World Health Organization Beta draft 2016; *Diagnostic and Statistical Manual of Mental Disorders*, 4th Edition (DSM-IV), American Psychiatric Association, 1994; *Diagnostic and Statistical Manual of Mental Disorders*, 5th Edition (DSM-5), American Psychiatric Association, 2013.

Box 27.2 Poor prognostic factors in anorexia nervosa

• Long length of illness at first presentation
• BMI less than 14 at diagnosis
• Older age of onset
• Bulimic features (bingeing and purging)
• Presence of anxious, obsessive, or dependent traits in childhood
• Personality disorder
• Relationship difficulties within the family
• Anxiety when eating with others
• Male sex

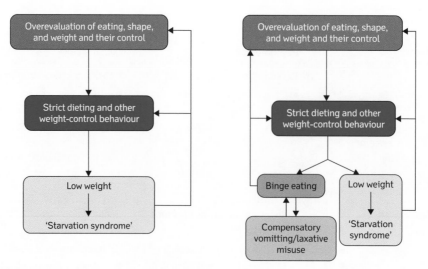

Fig. 27.3 A schematic representation of the maintenance of eating disorders.

Reprinted from *Behaviour Research and Therapy*, 41, C. G. Fairburn, Z. Cooper, R. Shafranwith, Cognitive behaviour therapy for eating disorders: A transdiagnostic theory and treatment, pp. 509–28. Copyright © 2003 Elsevier Science Ltd. All rights reserved.

CASE STUDY BOX 27.1

Anorexia nervosa

Susan, a 21-year-old law student, presents to her GP with low mood. She is clearly emaciated, and admits to keeping to less than 500 kcal/day and spending 2 hours in the gym each evening. The GP examines Susan, finding her to have a BMI of 15.8 with dry cracked skin, lanugo, and bradycardia. He suspects anorexia nervosa and while Susan is unsure, she agrees to blood tests and urgent referral to secondary care. Susan is assessed 48 hours later at the eating disorders service, where she gives a history of straight A grades at school, playing clarinet with the university orchestra, and has parents who are both barristers. Susan feels under pressure to achieve well in her degree and says her mother and sister are both constantly 'on a diet'. With support, Susan agrees she has anorexia nervosa and to come for outpatient therapy. She feels she cannot take time out from her degree for more intensive treatment. Susan starts weekly CBT and manages to gain some weight and her periods restart. However, she refuses to go above a BMI of 17.6, saying she wants to focus on her degree and disengages from further treatment.

Six months later, Susan is taken to hospital after fainting at orchestra practice. Susan's BMI is 12.3, heart rate 38, and potassium 2.9 mmol/litre. She is admitted to the general hospital for medical stabilization, but refuses to eat. Susan denies any problem and asks to discharge herself. Due to the medical risks Susan is detained under the MHA on Section 3. When stable, she is transferred to an eating disorder inpatient unit. Here the team gradually reintroduce oral feeding, initially alongside nasogastric feeds. Susan is reluctant to start eating, and takes several weeks to comply with the programme but eventually does so. She makes good progress and is discharged back to the care of her parents at a BMI of 19 after 5 months in hospital, with the plan to not return to university until the following year. Susan works hard to continue her recovery and the family attend family therapy together. Two years later, Susan completes her degree with first class honours. She tells her GP that in retrospect, the use of the MHA was very beneficial, as it gave her permission to start eating again, and from there she was able to start working on her underlying problems.

Bulimia nervosa

Bulimia nervosa is an eating disorder characterized by frequent recurrent episodes of uncontrolled excessive eating ('binges'), compensatory methods of weight control, and a fear of becoming fat. The term 'bulimia' refers only to the episodes of uncontrollable excessive eating, and may also be present in other forms of eating disorder. Unlike anorexia nervosa, for which there are historical accounts dating back to medieval times, bulimia nervosa was first described as a distinct clinical entity in 1979. Gerald Russell, a British psychiatrist, published a case series of 30 patients with bulimia nervosa and used them to describe the defining features of the condition. Since Russell's initial work, it has been realized that bulimia nervosa is a common condition, and unlike anorexia nervosa, effective treatments have since been developed to treat it.

Clinical features

The clinical features of bulimia nervosa are shown in Box 27.3. A 'binge' is defined by the ICD as '*a distinct period of time during which the individual experiences a subjective loss of control over eating, eating notably more or differently than usual, and feels unable to stop eating or limit the type or amount of food eaten*'. Bulimia nervosa can be divided into two subtypes, purging and non-purging (<10 per cent), of which the former carries greater medical risk. It is not unusual for patients with bulimia nervosa to have a history of anorexia nervosa. The typical pattern is that a patient will diet or fast for a period, at the end of which the patient 'loses control' and binges. A binge may be triggered by certain stimuli (e.g. if the calorie limit for the day is exceeded, when at home alone, or after an emotionally charged situation) or occur unprovoked. The foods eaten during a binge are usually high in carbohydrate and fats and are usually foods the patient avoids at other times. The majority of binges occur when the patient is at home and alone, as they tend to be embarrassed and disgusted by their behaviour. After a

binge, the patient feels guilty and concerned they will gain weight, and tries to rid themselves of the food by purging. The cycle then starts again with a new period of strict control of food intake. Unlike in anorexia nervosa, the patient is usually aware of the limitations the condition is having on their life (e.g. poor concentration, unable to eat out with friends, and physical complications), and feels guilty about this. This guilt, and the feelings of hopelessness that tend to accompany it, predispose to low mood and suicidal ideation.

Box 27.3 Clinical features of bulimia nervosa

Core clinical symptoms

1 Frequent, recurrent episodes of binge eating (at least once per week over at least 1 month).
2 Inappropriate compensatory behaviours used to prevent weight gain (e.g. fasting, vomiting, use of laxatives, emetics, diuretics or diet medications, and exercise).
3 Preoccupation with body weight and shape and/or self-evaluation based primarily upon weight and shape.
4 The patient is not underweight and therefore does not have all the features needed for a diagnosis of anorexia nervosa.

Associated behavioural symptoms

- Strict dietary rules surrounding food (restricted diet in terms of quantity or food types, food-related rituals, preference for eating alone).
- Excessive exercise.

Associated psychological symptoms

- Preoccupation with thoughts of food.
- Cravings for specific foods.
- Low self-esteem.
- Perfectionistic or emotionally unstable personality traits.
- Low mood (80 per cent).
- Anxiety disorders.
- Thoughts of self-harm or suicide.
- Misuse of substances or alcohol (~30 per cent).

Physical consequences

Body weight is normal in the majority of patients, as dieting and purging compensates for the binges. However, repeated vomiting can lead to serious complications. Hypokalaemia is particularly serious, resulting in weakness, cardiac arrhythmia, and renal damage. Metabolic alkalosis and hypochloraemia may also occur. Regular vomiting may cause swelling of the parotid glands, erosion of dental enamel by stomach acid, and calluses on the back of the fingers which are used to induce emesis. Occasionally, patients present to the emergency room vomiting blood, often due to a Mallory–Weiss tear. Menstrual abnormalities are common, although these reverse if normal eating is resumed. Use of laxatives and diuretics may cause fluid shifts, hyponatraemia, and metabolic acidosis. It is important to explain to the patient that these substances do not cause weight loss, merely fluid and electrolyte shifts within the body.

Differential diagnosis

- **Anorexia nervosa** can be differentiated from bulimia nervosa principally by a low body weight.
- **BED** (see p. 389).
- **Eating disorder unspecified.**

- **Kleine–Levin syndrome** is a sleep disorder seen in adolescent males, characterized by recurrent episodes of binge eating and hypersomnia.
- **Mood disorder.** Weight gain and binge eating may occur, but the patient will not show the specific psychopathology and other weight control behaviours seen in bulimia nervosa.
- **Organic disorders.** These can usually be identified by a clear history and lack of associated core psychopathology, but specific investigations may need to be done; for example, upper gastrointestinal disorders with associated vomiting, and brain tumours.

Aetiology

The main risk factors for bulimia nervosa are shown in Table 27.4.

Course and prognosis

As many people with bulimia nervosa never present for treatment, the natural course of the disorder is not completely understood. It seems to be a chronic illness; cohort studies suggest 30 per cent of patients still meet criteria for bulimia nervosa 10 years after onset. Anorexia nervosa is a very rare outcome. See Case study box 27.2 for an example case.

Table 27.4 Risk factors for bulimia nervosa

Biological	Psychological	Social
Genetics: • Heritability 50–70% • Family history of eating disorders is common • Female gender • Age (15–40 years) • Endocrine abnormalities • Type 1 diabetes • Early menarche • Obesity in childhood	• Critical comments in early life about eating, shape, or weight • Family environment with a focus on shape and dieting • Sexual or physical abuse in childhood • Low self-esteem • Perfectionism • Ongoing family conflicts	• High parental expectations • Living in a developed country • Cultures that encourage dieting and value thinness • Occupation (e.g. ballet dancer)

CASE STUDY BOX 27.2

Bulimia nervosa

Charlie, a 25-year-old type 1 diabetic, was referred to psychiatry from the endocrine services. Her consultant was concerned that Charlie had recently lost 10 kg in weight, and her HbA1c had increased to 11 per cent. He suspected she was omitting her insulin with the aim of losing weight. At the assessment, Charlie admitted she had been reducing her insulin, and had been bingeing regularly and making herself sick after meals. She felt self-conscious that she was not thin like her non-diabetic friends, and that she had not achieved as well as her siblings, who had all been to university. Charlie's BMI was 22.3, and there were no physical abnormalities on examination. She agreed to start fluoxetine, titrating up to 60 mg daily, see a dietician, and to have outpatient CBT. Over the next 4 months, Charlie

managed to reduce her bingeing and purging, but was unable to give herself adequate insulin due to fears of excessive weight gain, and lost more weight. A joint meeting between the eating disorder and endocrine teams was arranged, where it came to light that Charlie now had proliferative diabetic retinopathy and would need pan-retinal photocoagulation therapy. Charlie found the idea she might lose her sight terrifying, as this acted as a motivator for change. She continued CBT and by the end of her sessions her weight had stabilized at a BMI of 21.5, she had stopped purging completely, and was able to take her daily insulin. At 1-year follow-up, Charlie had maintained these changes, and although she occasionally binged and purged, was managing her diabetes appropriately, and had applied to go to university.

Binge eating disorder

BED is a condition characterized by binge eating, but without the compensatory behaviours to prevent weight gain that are seen in anorexia nervosa or bulimia nervosa. It is a common condition (see p. 381) but rarely seen in clinical practice as the medical complications are fewer and patients typically feel very ashamed of their behaviour and are embarrassed to ask for help.

Clinical features

Clinical features of BED include:

- episodes of binge eating larger than normal quantities of food during which the patient experiences a lack of control over the amount they are eating;
- during binges the patient typically eats faster than usual and eats until they feel uncomfortably full;
- eating alone due to embarrassment and shame over bingeing behaviour;
- low self-esteem and guilt due to bingeing behaviours.

The main physical consequence of BED is that 50 per cent of patients are overweight or obese. The remainder are typically in the upper half of the normal weight range. Patients may have wide fluctuations in weight over time, as the severity of their bingeing waxes and wanes. There is strong evidence to suggest an association between BED and diabetes, but as BED is a fairly recent diagnostic entity, the epidemiology and aetiology of the association is as yet unclear.

Co-morbidities

The majority of patients with BED have psychiatric co-morbidities, most commonly depression (30–40 per cent) or anxiety disorders (30–40 per cent). There is some association with alcohol misuse. Avoidant and emotionally unstable personality traits are more common than in the general population.

Course and prognosis

Observational studies suggest that like other eating disorders, BED is a chronic condition, typically lasting for more than a decade. Over that period it is usual for the severity to vary over time, frequently relating to changing stresses in the individual's life. Factors associated with a poorer outcome include abnormal perception of weight and shape, impulsive personality traits, and a history of childhood abuse.

Avoidant–restrictive food intake disorder

ARFID is a condition in which the patient eats an insufficient quantity or variety of food that leads to them not being able to meet their nutritional needs. It is a disorder primarily seen in children, but that can continue into adult life or even develop in later life. The prevalence of ARFID is unknown.

Clinical features

Patients with ARFID are unable to eat certain foods/food groups, or only eat foods which are deemed 'safe' according to some applied rule. If they are asked to eat foods outside the safe range, they may become anxious and may experience vomiting or gagging. The majority of patients are underweight or fail to gain weight appropriately as they develop, and may have nutritional deficiencies.

Typical examples of restrictive eating include:

- only eating foods based on colour, size, or shape;
- only eating foods with a specific smell, taste, or texture;
- only eating hot or cold foods;
- refusing foods related to a negative experience in the past (e.g. a near-choking incident, a food they were eating when bad news was delivered or an accident occurred). This is more common in adult-onset cases.

ARFID sufferers do not show the typical abnormalities in perception of body weight and shape, or concern about weight gain, as those with anorexia nervosa, bulimia nervosa, or BED. The restrictive eating typically leads to social withdrawal and problems with psychosocial functioning.

It is important to exclude other causes of poor nutrition, for example, an organic illness, lack of food availability, or the side effects of medication.

Assessment of an eating disorders patient

Assessment of a patient presenting with any eating problem has three primary aims:

1 To make a diagnosis.

2 To make an assessment of physical and psychological severity, and therefore associated risks.

3 To start the process of gaining the patient's trust and identifying their level of insight and motivation for change.

Screening

Screening in primary care is a helpful strategy when a patient presents with suggestive features of an eating disorder (perhaps a physical symptom) or common co-morbidities. The high-risk groups that should be especially targeted include:

- adolescent females;
- ballet dancers;
- gymnasts;
- models and modelling students;
- type 1 diabetic patients;
- medical students and doctors.

A specific and quick method of screening in primary care is the SCOFF questionnaire (Box 27.4). The questionnaire is valid for both anorexia nervosa and bulimia nervosa, and a score of at least 2 should lead to further assessment

History

In primary care or an emergency setting, only information needed to make a probable diagnosis and assess

Box 27.4 The SCOFF questionnaire

- Do you make yourself **Sick** because you feel uncomfortably full?
- Do you worry that you have lost **Control** over how much you eat?
- Have you recently lost more than **One** stone (14 lb) in a 3-month period?
- Do you believe yourself to be **Fat** when others say you are thin?
- Would you say that **Food** dominates your life?

Box 27.5 Areas to cover when assessing a patient presenting with an eating disorder

General psychiatric assessment

(See Chapter 17)

Past history

- Previous diagnoses of eating disorders
- Past treatment for eating disorder and how successful it was
- Changes in weight over time (if relevant, ask about rate of recent weight change)
- Physical complications in the past relating to the eating disorder (e.g. osteoporosis)
- Previous psychiatric conditions (mood, OCD, anxiety)
- History of self-harm or suicidal ideation
- Personal history: ask about childhood eating difficulties, abuse, bullying, educational achievement, age of menarche/pubertal onset, family history of eating disorders
- Personality traits: anxious, avoidant, obsessive, emotionally unstable

Current behaviours

- Current eating pattern (what, when, how much, specific rules, periods of fasting)
- Fluid consumption (amount and type)
- Bingeing
- Purging (of all types)
- Exercise routine
- Medications (prescribed, illicit, over-the-counter, alcohol, caffeine, nicotine, diet pills, and supplements)

Current psychological symptoms

- Feelings about food, weight, and shape
- Mood and anxiety symptoms
- Ideas of self-harm or suicide

Current physical complications

- Ask about all physical symptoms (include menstrual abnormalities and those shown on p. 382)

acute risks is likely to be feasible. In secondary care, a full assessment should be taken. This would include general psychiatric assessment (Chapter 5) and gathering of specific eating disorder-related information as shown in Box 27.5. It is important to try and get a clear idea about the personal and social context of which the eating problems have developed as well as an account of current behaviours.

Physical examination

As the physical consequences of starvation can be very dangerous, it is important to undertake a full physical examination. The following should be undertaken (or if appropriate facilities are unavailable immediately, arranged to be done in primary care as soon as possible):

- Measurement of weight and height, and calculation of BMI (Box 27.6). For children, it is helpful to use percentage of expected weight and to look at their weight on a growth chart, or use a BMI centile chart (preferably referencing to their own chart if available) as BMI alone is less accurate. If possible, weigh the

patient in light clothing after they have used the toilet. Be aware of the propensity of patients to hide weights in their clothes, or water-load before

Box 27.6 Calculation of body mass index (BMI) using the World Health Organization Classifications (2016)

$$BMI = \frac{weight \ (kg)}{height \ (m)^2}$$

- BMI ≥25: overweight
- BMI 18.5–25: ideal body weight range
- BMI <18.5: underweight

Level of risk in underweight patients:

- BMI 17–18.49: mild
- BMI 16–16.9: moderate
- BMI 15–15.9: severe
- BMI <15: extreme and life threatening

© World Health Organization 2018 http://www.euro.who.int/en/health-topics/disease-prevention/nutrition/a-healthy-lifestyle/body-mass-index-bmi [accessed 18/10/2018].

being weighed. The latter can be tested for using urine specific gravity on a urinalysis stick. Try to be neutral but sensitive during the weighing process, which can be very distressing for patients.

- Full general physical examination to look for complications of starvation, vomiting, or other eating disorder behaviours. Include pulse rate, blood pressure, and temperature. If possible, do an ECG.
- Watch the patient walking, climbing stairs, and rising from a chair. Next, ask them to squat down on the floor and then get up without using their hands: the **'stand and squat test'**. Patients with proximal myopathy will struggle to do this and it is a sign of dangerous emaciation.

Psychological tests

The most widely used questionnaire for detecting an eating disorder is the **EDE-Q questionnaire**). There are many others, but as the diagnosis is clinical, they are mainly used in research. It is also worth testing all patients with the **Beck Depression Index** and **Hospital Anxiety and Depression Scale**, to pick up any significant co-morbidities.

Investigations

An eating disorder is a clinical diagnosis, and investigations are done merely to pick up and treat complications, and to help risk stratify (Table 27.5).

Table 27.5 Investigations in eating disorders

Investigation	Typical abnormalities in severe starvation
Blood tests	
FBC	Anaemia, thrombocytopenia, leucopenia
U&Es	Increased urea and creatinine if dehydrated
	Low potassium, phosphate, magnesium, and chloride
TFTs	Increased T3 and T4
LFTs	Increased bilirubin and hepatocellular markers
Lipids	Increased cholesterol
Cortisol	Increased levels
Sex hormones	Decreased LH, FSH, oestrogens, and progestogens
Arterial blood gas	Metabolic alkalosis (vomiting), metabolic acidosis (laxatives)
ECG	Prolonged QTc interval
	Relating to hypokalaemia—flattened T-waves
Urinalysis	Reduced specific gravity in water loading
	Increased specific gravity in dehydration
Blood glucose	Low
DXA scan	Osteopenia or osteoporosis

FBC, full blood count; DXA, dual energy X-ray absorptiometry; FSH, follicle-stimulating hormone; LFTs, liver functions tests; LH, luteinizing hormone; TFTs, thyroid function tests; U&Es, urea and electrolytes.

Risk assessment

The main risks in anorexia nervosa are the effects of starvation (self-neglect) and deliberate self-harm or suicide. All patients should be considered at high risk of these. Driving is a particular issue in those with a very low BMI, poor concentration, or episodes of hypoglycaemia or hypokalaemia. The main medical risks are arrhythmias, electrolyte disturbances, anaemia, heart failure, and gastrointestinal bleeds (rare). Patients with any of the characteristics shown in Box 27.7 are at

Box 27.7 Criteria for admission to hospital in eating disorders

- BMI less than 14 (NB: BMI is unreliable in children and those with oedema)
- Rapid weight loss (>1 kg/week)
- Electrolyte imbalances or hypoglycaemia
- Bradycardia, arrhythmias
- Hypotension or a postural drop
- Hypothermia
- Suicidal ideation or deliberate self-harm
- Psychosis or another change in mental state
- Refusal to engage with treatment
- Failure of outpatient treatment
- Patients with bulimia nervosa may need a short admission to break a binge–purge cycle, or for medical risks relating to another condition (e.g. diabetes or pregnancy).

It is important that if a patient is admitted to hospital that there is good communication between different specialties. Inpatient or day-patient care (which is usually for anorexia nervosa, occasionally bulimia nervosa) typically includes the following elements:

- Supported meals (see 'Nutritional rehabilitation (refeeding)') and dietary advice.
- Psychoeducation including the nature of eating disorders and the physical risks associated with eating-disordered behaviours. This is a helpful intervention to try and motivate the patient towards change.
- Individual and group psychotherapy.
- Physical monitoring.
- Monitoring of activity levels and re-establishment of a healthy exercise routine.
- Management of medications.
- Support and advice for carers plus family therapy if appropriate.

extremely high risk, and admission to hospital should be considered. The MARSIPAN guidelines (see 'Further reading') are a helpful guide.

Management of eating disorders

Successful treatment of eating disorders is possible, but like other mental disorders requires hard work on the part of the patient, their carers, and the professionals treating them. Success largely depends on creating a good relationship with the patient, and gaining their collaboration. An overview of treatment is shown in Table 27.6. The vast majority of patients will be treated as outpatients, but most need input from specialists in the treatment of eating disorders. Admission to hospital (general, psychiatric, or a specialist eating disorders unit) may be needed if there is high medical or psychiatric risk, or if lower-intensity treatments fail (Box 27.4).

Nutritional rehabilitation (refeeding)

It is important to negotiate a reasonable dietary plan with the patient and to set this out clearly, together with a medically acceptable, but not over-ambitious, target weight. The aim for underweight patients should be to increase weight gradually via a balanced meal plan of three meals and three snacks per day. It is reasonable to aim for 0.5–1 kg gain per week in inpatients, and 0.5 kg gain per week in outpatients. Refeeding is usually started at 1200–1500 kcal/day (to avoid refeeding syndrome) (Box 27.8), and titrated up to achieve the required gain. Supplements may be used to increase caloric intake once a normal food intake has been achieved. Occasionally, nasogastric tube feeding may be required for severely unwell patients. Eating should be supervised, either by a nurse while in hospital or by a parent/carer at home. They have three important roles:

1 To reassure the patient that she can eat without the risk of losing control over her weight.

2 To be firm about the agreed targets.

Table 27.6 Management of eating disorders

	Anorexia nervosa	Bulimia nervosa	Binge-eating disorder
Choose appropriate setting of care	Outpatient (95%) Day-patient Inpatient care Admission to general hospital for medical stabilization	Outpatient (98%) Day-patient (rare) Inpatient care (rare) Admission to general hospital for medical stabilization	Primary care Secondary care outpatients
General aspects of care	Psychoeducation Self-help resource	Psychoeducation Self-help resource	Psychoeducation Self-help resources
Nutritional rehabilitation	Dietary advice and support for regain of weight and normalization of eating habits Aim for weight gain of 0.5 kg/week (outpatients) and 1 kg/week (inpatients) Nasogastric feeding may be used if oral refeeding in not tolerated or risk is high	Dietary advice to normalize eating habits Weight maintenance diet	Dietary advice to normalize eating habits
Psychological therapies	Consider CBT or IPT Family therapy (especially for adolescents)	CBT for bulimia nervosa Family therapy (especially for adolescents)	CBT for binge eating disorder
Pharmacological treatments	Daily multivitamins Consider need for and antidepressant or antipsychotic (see text)	Antidepressant: best evidence for SSRIs, e.g. fluoxetine 60 mg daily	Consider antidepressant (first line SSRI)
Miscellaneous	Monitoring for and treatment of refeeding syndrome		

Box 27.8 Refeeding syndrome

Refeeding syndrome is a metabolic disturbance that occurs in the first few days of starting to refeed a severely malnourished patient. It occurs when carbohydrate is suddenly provided, and metabolism shifts from fat to carbohydrate. Insulin increases, which leads to increased uptake of phosphate, and an increased metabolic rate can cause excessive cellular uptake of electrolytes. The main biochemical features include:

- hypophosphataemia;
- hypokalaemia;
- hypomagnesaemia;
- hypoglycaemia;
- thiamine deficiency.

Hypophosphataemia is common and may cause confusion, coma, fits, and sudden death. Shift of fluids may increase cardiac work and precipitate acute heart failure. Patients should be monitored for peripheral and pulmonary oedema daily.

Electrolytes should be checked regularly, and supplements given as appropriate. Prescribing daily thiamine, a vitamin B complex, multivitamins, and minerals is sensible. In severe malnutrition, a course of Pabrinex® is helpful.

3 To ensure that the patient does not hide food, induce vomiting, or take purgatives.

For patients already at a healthy weight, the focus is on re-establishing a normal eating pattern and consumption of a maintenance diet (typically 1800–2500 kcal/day depending on sex, age, and activity levels).

Psychological therapies

The success of a therapeutic intervention depends highly on the motivation of the patient for change, and the relationship between the therapist and patient. It may be helpful for the patient to have motivational interviewing to help them be ready to make behavioural changes before active treatment begins. It is usually helpful if the patient considers the pros and cons of their eating disorder, and looks at the impact it is having upon their life.

For bulimia nervosa and BED, there is strong evidence that specialized forms of CBT or guided self-help are highly effective. These are therefore the first-line interventions, although other forms of therapy may be chosen in some cases. CBT aims to provide psychoeducation about the illness and its effects, help re-establish regular eating, and examine the factors behind and that maintain the eating disorder. For both conditions, specialized enhanced CBT leads to 50–75 per cent of patients achieving a lasting recovery, and a further 25–30 per cent make significant improvements.

In anorexia nervosa, research evidence for specific psychotherapies is less strong, and there is no good evidence that one type is more effective than another. Enhanced CBT has some evidence for efficacy in adults, and is the typical first choice, with the emphasis being on changing the dysfunctional cognitions relating to weight and shape and helping the patient make behavioural changes. In the UK, guidelines also recommend IPT, cognitive analytic therapy, or family therapy as first- or second-line options.

For children and adolescents, family-based therapy ('the Maudsley method') has a strong evidence base and is the first-line approach. Family therapy sessions and individual therapy for the young person run alongside a three-phase programme in which the parents take complete control of refeeding their child and helping them to develop normal eating habits again.

Phase 1. The parents are urged to take control of the patient's eating, and help them to gain weight. The patient has no input in meal planning, shopping, food preparation, cooking, or serving meals. The expectation is that all food is consumed, and no eating-disordered behaviours are undertaken. There will be much confrontation at this stage, and many tears may be shed.

Phase 2. The parents help their child to take more control over their eating again, while general family issues and relationship problems are dealt with.

Phase 3. This starts when the patient is able to maintain their weight in the healthy range, and has normal eating habits. Treatment then focuses on helping them to develop a normal relationship with their body, working on issues such as perfectionism and low self-esteem, and adjusting family life back to normality.

Pharmacotherapy

The main treatment for all eating disorders is a combination of nutritional rehabilitation and psychotherapy. However, there is good evidence that antidepressants are effective adjuncts in bulimia nervosa and BED. For bulimia nervosa, SSRIs, tricyclics, MAOIs, and atypical antidepressants are equally effective. **SSRIs** (specifically 60 mg fluoxetine in the morning) are the first-line drugs, as they have the best cost, side effect, tolerability, and safety record. High doses are required for the effect, which is not dose dependent. BED also responds to antidepressants, with an SSRI being the first-line choice.

For anorexia nervosa, there is little evidence that any psychotropic medication improves the underlying psychopathology. Medication is used for co-morbidities or if standard treatment approaches do not lead to improvement. In bulimia nervosa, high-dose SSRIs are effective at reducing binge–purge behaviours in the short term. There is some emerging evidence that low-dose atypical antipsychotics (especially olanzapine) may be helpful with regaining weight and in reducing anxiety levels to allow the patient to start eating again. The risk of excessive weight gain is extremely low. Low doses should be used in underweight patients, to avoid excessive sedation or other adverse effects. All patients should take a multivitamin/multimineral supplement daily.

Compulsory treatment

In the UK, approximately 20 per cent of inpatient admissions to specialist eating disorders units are for compulsory treatment. They are usually patients with severe emaciation, a long-standing illness, and poor engagement with treatment. If a patient is at medical risk but is not consenting to treatment, and is shown to lack capacity, they may be detained under the MHA. The MHA allows for the treatment of physical problems that are a direct result of a mental disorder (e.g. emaciation in anorexia nervosa), so a patient may be refed under this legislation. The least restriction option for treatment should always be used, but in extremely ill patients, compulsory treatment may be necessary (see Science box 27.1).

Obesity

Obesity is defined by the WHO as the accumulation or presence of excess body fat to the extent that it may impair health. The WHO has also defined obesity in terms of BMI: 'overweight' is a BMI of 25–30, and 'obesity' a BMI of greater than 30. The rationale behind this is based on mortality statistics; lowest mortality is found among individuals with a BMI of 19.5–24.9. Obesity is not an eating disorder, and it does not feature in the DSM-5 or in the Mental Health section of the ICD. However, binge-eating is an eating disorder and it is becoming increasingly recognized that the most effective treatment is a behavioural approach similar to that used in other eating disorders, and that adding a cognitive dimension to the therapy can significantly reduce the rate of relapse. It may therefore fit into the wider transdiagnostic approach to eating disorders, and this, combined with the epidemiological significance, is the reason why obesity is included in this chapter.

Epidemiology

Data from Public Health England (2014) reported that 24 per cent of UK men and 26 per cent of women were obese. Slightly higher figures have been published for the USA. In the UK, almost 20 per cent of 10-year-olds are above the 95th centile for weight on standard growth charts. Over the period 1990–2010, the rates of obesity rose significantly, but have plateaued in the past 6 years. Unfortunately, there is strong evidence to show that obese children are highly likely to remain obese into adult life.

Aetiology

Most obesity can be attributed to genetic predisposition exacerbated by social factors that encourage overeating. However, the following may all contribute:

Biological risk factors

Genetics. The heritability of obesity is estimated to be approximately 75 per cent, meaning the vast majority of the cause of obesity is genetic. In greater than 99 per cent of cases this is a complex polygenic risk, but there are rare single gene defects (e.g. lack of the *ob/ob* gene for leptin) and other genetic syndromes (e.g. Prader–Willi syndrome and Down's syndrome) in which obesity is a frequent or ubiquitous characteristic. Obesity is more common in some ethic groups.

Organic and psychiatric causes:

- **Organic:** hypothyroidism, Cushing's syndrome, polycystic ovary syndrome, hypogonadism, growth hormone deficiency, pseudohypoparathyroidism, and low birth weight.
- **Psychiatric:** depression, BED, and Klinefelter syndrome.
- **Drugs:** antipsychotics, antidepressants, mood stabilizers, insulin, steroids, oral contraceptives, and steroids.

SCIENCE BOX 27.1

Atypical antipsychotics and anorexia nervosa

Since the 1960s, it has been suggested that antipsychotics could be of value in anorexia nervosa (AN). The rationale behind the use is that severe AN has features in common with psychotic disorders, as the irrational cognitions surrounding weight and shape are held strongly despite evidence to the contrary, is egosyntonic, and encompasses lack of insight. There is strong evidence from systematic reviews that atypical antipsychotics reduce anxiety and agitation and promote weight gain; could they therefore be a useful adjunct in AN?

Evidence on this topic has only started emerging in the past decade, and the majority of RCTs have used olanzapine in relatively small sample sizes.[1,2] Lebow et al. have conducted the largest meta-analysis to date focusing primarily on atypical use in AN. They compared the effect of an atypical antipsychotic (for at least 4 weeks) to no treatment or placebo on BMI and psychopathology in AN (N = 198). Almost all the studies used olanzapine in both inpatient and outpatient settings. They found no significant change in BMI or core psychopathology at a median of 8 weeks of follow-up. The authors concluded that, while longer-term studies using a wider range of antipsychotics are needed, it appears that antipsychotic-induced hunger is not enough to override the drive for thinness in AN.

A systematic review from 2015 which examined various aspects of inpatient treatment in AN has also looked at this question.[3] It also reported no significant increase in weight gain with atypical antipsychotics compared to placebo. A sub-analysis of adolescents did show a statistically significant increase in weight compared to placebo, but this was not at a clinically significant level. A recent study of 187 inpatients looked at the efficacy of adding olanzapine or aripiprazole to an SSRI in AN.[4] Between admission and discharge, the patient group showed significant improvements in BMI, but there was no significant difference between those on an SSRI alone or with addition of either atypical. Aripiprazole was more effective at reducing bingeing and purging episodes than olanzapine.

Animal studies have investigated the role of dopamine blockade on hyperactivity in a murine model of AN.[5] These suggest that dopamine antagonists that primarily block D_2/D_3 receptors are the most effective at reducing hyperactivity and weight loss in these mice. This may translate into clinical use in the future, but further studies are needed.

There is currently insufficient evidence to advise sensibly on the use of atypical antipsychotics in AN. One hindrance to obtaining good evidence is the difficulty of recruiting patients into clinical trials and the high drop-out rates (typically ~20 per cent) observed. At present, the best option is to make a risk/benefit analysis for an individual patient if other treatment methods have been ineffective. As in any patient starting an atypical, there is the risk of extrapyramidal symptoms, sedation, and diabetes. Some atypicals are associated with prolongation of the QT interval, which can be particularly dangerous in underweight patients. The potential risks and benefits should be carefully considered, but the current evidence base suggests that atypicals are usually well tolerated in AN, even if their efficacy is unclear.

1 McKnight RF, Park RJ. Atypical antipsychotics and anorexia nervosa: a review. *European Eating Disorders Review* 2010;18:10–21.

2 Lebow J, Sim LA, Erwin PJ, Murad MH. The effect of atypical antipsychotic medications in individuals with anorexia nervosa: a systematic review and meta-analysis. *International Journal of Eating Disorders* 2013;46:332–339.

3 Suarez-Pinilla P, Peña-Pérez C, Arbaizar-Barrenechea B, et al. Inpatient treatment for anorexia nervosa: a systematic review of randomised controlled trials. *Journal of Psychiatric Practice* 2015;21:49–59.

4 Marzola E, Desedime N, Giovannone C, Amianto F, Fassino S, Abbate-Daga G. Atypical antipsychotics as augmentation therapy in anorexia nervosa. *PLoS One* 2015;10:e0125569.

5 Klenotich SK, Ho EV, McMurray MS, Server CH, Dulawa SC. Dopamine 2/3 receptor antagonism reduces activity based anorexia. *Translational Psychiatry* 2015;5:e613.

Psychological risk factors

Psychological aspects. Obesity is more common in those with significant levels of anxiety, depression, and low self-esteem.

Social risk factors

Diet. The availability of food has increased gradually over the last 100 years, so that the average person in a developed country has access to an abundance of food. There has been an increasing trend towards buying preprepared foods, eating outside the home and snacking between meals, all of which are associated with obesity. The recommended UK daily requirements are 1940 kcal/day for women and 2550 kcal/day for men.

Sedentary lifestyle. The change in our lifestyles towards sedentary work, routine use of motorized transport, screen-based entertainment, and a reduction in easy access to open spaces have meant that the population as a whole does inadequate exercise. The recommended 30-minute sessions of cardiovascular exercise three times per week are only done by 20–30 per cent of the population, mostly under 35 years. Obesity is higher in urban areas.

Social class. There is a clear correlation between social class and obesity in almost every culture. In developed countries, people in lower social classes are more likely to be obese, whereas in developing countries the reverse is true. It is unclear why this occurs, as explanations such as cost of food or fashions do not hold true in research. Smoking tends to keep people's weight low; on average, 5 kg is gained when someone stops.

Assessment

The aim of assessing an obese patient is threefold;

1 To detect any underlying physical or psychological cause.
2 To detect any adverse consequences of being obese.
3 To assess the patient's motivation for changing their weight and behaviour.

A full history should be taken, including current medications and use of alcohol and nicotine. It is helpful to get an idea of weight changes over time, previous weight loss attempts, and current diet and exercise routine. The following measurements and investigations should be undertaken during assessment:

- Weight, height, and calculation of BMI. Note that BMI is less accurate in those who are extremely muscular, children, and the very elderly (the latter due to loss of muscle mass with age).
- Measurement of waist circumference: greater than 102 cm in men or greater than 88 cm in females is associated with increased cardiovascular risk.
- General physical examination. Look for signs of secondary causes of weight gain (e.g. hypothyroidism, Cushing's syndrome, polycystic ovary syndrome). Measure blood pressure and pulse. Do an ECG.
- Blood tests: U&Es, FBC, LFTs, TFTs, $Ca/PO_4/Mg$, lipid profile, HbA1c, fasting glucose.

Consequences of obesity

Obesity is associated with significant mortality and morbidity, and some of the conditions it predisposes to are shown in Table 27.7. Smoking rates are higher in obese patients than in the general population, and the combined risk of most associated conditions is greater than the two separate risks added together.

Individuals who are obese are less likely to have good psychosocial function than those of a healthy weight. They are more likely to drop out of education and be unemployed and to access mental health services than those at healthy weights.

Management

The most important aspect of management is for the patient to be well informed about their situation, and to be motivated towards weight loss and a healthier lifestyle. The options for treatment are shown in Box 27.9, but for the majority the basis will be the establishment of a diet and regular exercise leading to weight loss, together with behavioural modification interventions

Table 27.7 Mortality and morbidity of obesity

	Conditions associated with obesity
Mortality	Life expectancy is reduced on average by 3 years for men and women with a BMI of 30–34.9
	Life expectancy is reduced on average by 8 years for men and 6 years for women with a BMI ≥35
	Standardized mortality index for a BMI of 30 = 118
Cardiovascular	Ischaemic heart disease, hypertension, hyperlipidaemia, heart failure, thromboembolic disease
Endocrine	Diabetes mellitus
	Menstrual disorders, infertility, polycystic ovary syndrome, erectile dysfunction
Obstetric	Perinatal complications, gestational diabetes
Neurological	Stroke, carpal tunnel syndrome, idiopathic intracranial hypertension
Psychiatric	Depression
Musculoskeletal	Gout, osteoarthritis, back pain
Dermatological	Cellulitis, stretch marks, hirsutism
Gastrointestinal	Gastro-oesophageal reflux disease, gallstones, fatty liver
Respiratory	Obstructive sleep apnoea, asthma
Anaesthetic	Complications during anaesthesia
Oncology	Association between obesity and most gastrointestinal cancers, plus cervical, thyroid, ovarian, and breast cancer

Box 27.9 Management options for obesity

Psychoeducation

- This should cover the benefits of a balanced diet and exercise plus the risks of substance misuse and obesity.

Dietary modifications

- There is no evidence that one particular type of diet is more efficacious than another. A diet containing all major food groups and essential vitamins and minerals is recommended; a deficit of 500 kcal/day will lead to approximately 0.5 kg weight loss per week.
- Five per cent weight loss is associated with significant cardiovascular benefits and is a good initial goal.

Establishing regular exercise

- Recommendation is for 30 minutes of cardiovascular exercise five times per week.

- A combination of moderate calorie restriction and exercise leads to more weight loss than severe caloric restriction alone.

Psychological therapy

- Self-help book and online programmes based on CBT principles.
- Group behavioural therapy programmes.
- CBT for obesity.

Pharmacological treatment

- Antiobesity medication: orlistat.
- Bariatric surgery.

Surgical treatment

- Bariatric surgery.

designed to lead to continuation of a healthy lifestyle in the long term.

Behavioural programmes

Behavioural programmes were first advocated as a means of treating obesity in the 1960s. There are currently three main methods of providing a behavioural programme for obesity:

1 Individual or guided self-help (only effective in the highly motivated patient).

2 Group programmes; for example, Weight Watchers and Slimming World.

3 CBT.

Group programmes

Organized group programmes are found all over the world and despite usually involving a membership fee are very popular. Patients can either join a local group which meets weekly or have an online membership. The programme helps with determining goal weight, devising a meal plan, and educating the patient about food, exercise, and healthy living. The members are weighed at each meeting, and give feedback to one another on their progress. There is an opportunity to discuss feelings around weight, shape, and food, and so the programme effectively works by using members to motivate one another, and combines this with elements of CBT.

Cognitive behavioural therapy for obesity

In the last decade, it has become increasingly recognized that an approach similar to that used for other eating disorders is effective in treating obesity. Specialized CBT is now available, which involves a two-phase approach:

Phase 1: achieving a healthy weight and lifestyle:

- Weight goals (setting realistic goals for particular reasons).
- Education around nutrition.
- Weight loss (based on a personalized balanced daily meal plan).
- Increasing exercise.
- Working on any body image difficulties.

- Identifying and overcoming problems that might threaten weight maintenance.

Phase 2: long-term maintenance of a healthy weight and lifestyle. This phase helps the patient to acquire the skills and motivation for long-term weight maintenance. This includes appropriate cognitive responses to changes in weight, and how to adapt behaviours to cope with this.

Short-term studies have shown this treatment to be effective in producing weight gain and maintenance, but the long-term effects are currently unknown.

Medications

Drug treatment should be considered only once dietary, exercise, and behavioural approaches have been tried, and the patient has failed to reach their target weight or achieved less than 5 per cent loss. Orlistat is the only drug licensed in the UK at present. Orlistat should only be used in adults with a BMI greater than 30, or BMI greater than 28 plus cardiovascular risk factors, and only continued for longer than 3 months if the patient has lost at least 5 per cent of body weight. It acts by inhibiting lipase in the gut, and reduces absorption of fat by about a third. Orlistat has significant side effects, typically abdominal cramps, flatus, oily faecal incontinence, and poor absorption of fat-soluble vitamins. Patients should take a vitamin supplement daily.

Bariatric surgery

Bariatric surgery refers to any surgical technique in which the aim is to treat obesity. It is only recommended for severely obese patients (BMI >40) or those with a BMI of 35–39.9 with co-morbidities relating to obesity who have not lost weight using behavioural and pharmacological treatments and who are fit for anaesthesia and surgery. The surgery generally involves reducing the size of the stomach (to increase early satiety) or decreasing the length of bowel through which food may be absorbed. Gastric banding is a reversible procedure, whereas gastrectomy or gastric bypass is not. Weight loss is usually rapid, with vast amounts being lost in the 2 years following surgery.

Complications from the operations are common, and patients are usually unable to eat 'normally' again. They may experience gastrointestinal symptoms in the long term, and need to take multivitamin supplements to avoid deficiencies.

Further reading

American Psychiatric Association. *Diagnostic and Statistical Manual of Mental Disorders*. 5th ed. Arlington, VA: American Psychiatric Publishing; 2013.

Brumberg J. *Fasting Girls: The History of Anorexia Nervosa*. 2nd ed. New York: Vintage Books; 2001.

Fairburn C, Cooper Z. Eating disorders, DSM-5 and clinical reality. *British Journal of Psychiatry* 2011;198:8–10.

Fairburn CG, Cooper Z, Shafran R. Cognitive behaviour therapy for eating disorders: a 'transdiagnostic' theory and treatment. *Behaviour Research and Therapy* 2003;41:509–528.

National Institute for Health and Care Excellence. Eating disorders: recognition and treatment. NICE guideline [NG69]. Published May 2017. https://www.nice.org.uk/guidance/ng69.

National Institute for Health and Care Excellence. Obesity: identification, assessment and management. Clinical guideline [CG189]. Published November 2014. https://www.nice.org.uk/guidance/cg189.

McKnight RF, Boughton N. A patient's journey with anorexia nervosa. *British Medical Journal* 2009;399:46–51.

Royal College of Psychiatrists, Royal College of Physicians. MARSIPAN: management of really sick patients with anorexia nervosa. 2nd ed. Published 2014. http://www.rcpsych.ac.uk/usefulresources/publications/collegereports/cr/cr189.aspx.

Schmidt U, Treasure J. *Getting Better Bit(e) by Bit(e): A Survival Kit for Sufferers of Bulimia Nervosa and Binge-Eating Disorder*. 2nd ed. London: Routledge; 2015.

Treasure J. A guide to medical risk assessment for eating disorders. South London & Maudsley NHS Foundation Trust. Published 2009. http://www.kcl.ac.uk/ioppn/depts/pm/research/eatingdisorders/resources/GUIDETOMEDICALRISKASSESSMENT.pdf.

28 Sleep disorders

The term sleep disorder (**somnipathy**) simply means a disturbance of an individual's normal sleep pattern. Doctors typically see patients in whom the disturbance is having a negative effect upon physical, mental, or emotional functioning, but subclinical disturbances of sleep are common and something almost everyone will suffer at some point in their life. Sleep disorders are a heterogeneous group, ranging from the frequently experienced insomnia to the extremely rare hypersomnias such as Kleine–Levin syndrome. However, there are many shared characteristics and this chapter will concentrate mainly on providing a framework for assessment, diagnosis, and management in the generic sense, with some guidance on specific disorders in the latter sections.

A good working knowledge of basic sleep disorders is essential in all specialties of clinical medicine. As a general rule, sleep disorders within the general hospital environment tend to be poorly managed, with great detriment to the patient. There are a variety of reasons why it is important to be able to diagnose and treat sleep disorders:

- Epidemiology: sleep disorders are very common and affect all ages.

- Co-morbidities: sleep disturbances may be a primary disorder or secondary to a mental or physical disorder. They are often prodromal symptoms of psychiatric conditions.

- Impact upon physical health: poor sleep is linked to increased mortality and morbidity from many pathologies (see 'Consequences of inadequate sleep', p. 405).

- Medications (not just psychotropics) often affect sleep.

- Sleep disturbance is an important part of many primary psychiatric conditions (e.g. mood disorders, psychosis, anxiety disorders); further information on these can be found in the chapter relating to each disorder.

What is normal sleep?

Sleep is a natural state of bodily rest seen in humans and many animals and is essential for survival. It is different from wakefulness in that the organism has a decreased ability to react to stimuli, but this is more easily reversible than in hibernation or coma. Sleep

Box 28.1 Proposed functions of sleep

- Recovery of physical and psychological strength
- Restoration: repair, wound healing, immune system function, correction of metabolic disturbances, and temperature regulation
- Energy conservation
- Preservation: allows animals to remain silent and hidden when at risk from predation
- Discharge of emotions
- Memory consolidation

is poorly understood, but it is likely that it has several functions relating to restoration of body equilibrium and energy stores. There are a variety of theories regarding the function of sleep, which are outlined in Box 28.1.

The state of sleep can be identified by electroencephalography (EEG), which records the net electrical activity of the brain. Two distinct sleep states have been defined according to their EEG patterns, muscle tone, and various physiological parameters: **non-rapid eye movement** (**NREM**) and **rapid eye movement** (**REM**) sleep. NREM sleep is divided into four stages, and REM sleep typically precedes them: stage 1 → stage 2 → stage 3 → stage 4 → stage 3 → stage 2 → REM, which repeats in cycles throughout the night (Fig. 28.1).

NREM sleep

Stage 1 occurs at sleep onset, or when aroused from another stage of sleep. Sudden twitches or hypnagogic jerks may occur at the onset of sleep. The EEG shows theta waves at 4–7 Hz, some muscle tone is lost, and consciousness reduced. Stage 1 accounts for 4–16 per cent of total overnight sleep.

Stage 2 is characterized by high-frequency bursts on the EEG (**sleep spindles**) and accounts for 45–55 per cent of overnight sleep. Muscle tone is lost, and there is complete loss of conscious awareness of the environment.

Stage 3 only accounts for 4–6 per cent of total sleep, and shows delta waves (**slow wave**).

Stage 4 shows the slowest activity on the EEG (0.5–4 Hz), and is the deepest stage of sleep. This is when parasomnias, such as night terrors, sleep walking, and bed wetting, occur. It accounts for 12–15 per cent of sleep.

The combination of stages 3 and 4 is also known as **slow-wave** or **delta sleep**.

REM sleep

REM sleep accounts for approximately a quarter of normal sleep time in healthy adults, and shows an EEG pattern very similar to the awake state. Muscle tone is completely lost except for spontaneous movements of the extraocular and middle ear muscles. Respiration rate, heart rate, blood pressure, and core temperature regulation all become irregular. People who are awoken from REM sleep usually say they were dreaming, but unless the content of dreams is recalled they are quickly forgotten.

During a typical night, cycles of sleep lasting approximately 90 minutes occur. They start with NREM sleep for 80 minutes, followed by 10 minutes of REM sleep. As the night progresses, the REM stage tends to lengthen, with subsequent shortening of NREM. The quantity of stage 3 and 4 sleep is reduced gradually throughout the night. Total sleep time varies between individuals, but is usually somewhere between 5 and 9 hours. This pattern can be seen on a hypnogram (see Fig. 28.1).

Circadian sleep–wake rhythms

The timing of when sleep occurs is regulated by the suprachiasmatic nucleus (SCN) in the anterior hypothalamus, whose neurons fire in a sinusoidal pattern across approximately 24 hours. Environment cues (**zeitgebers**) entrain the intrinsic rhythm of the SCN and include light, exercise, work schedules, and social interactions. The SCN controls temperature, cortisol, and growth hormone secretion, which it links into the sleep–wake cycle. The pineal gland secretes the hormone melatonin, which is related to the light–dark cycle rather than the sleep–wake cycle. Melatonin is secreted into the blood during

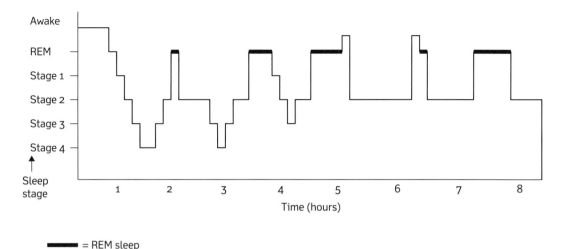

Fig. 28.1 An example of a normal hypnogram from an adult.

darkness, so duration of melatonin secretion is a proxy measure of day length. Melatonin is transported across the blood–brain barrier to act upon the SCN, thereby linking the light–dark and sleep–wake cycles.

Consequences of inadequate sleep

Prolonged sleep deprivation inevitably leads to death—usually due to loss of temperature regulation and overwhelming sepsis—clear evidence that sleep is essential to survival. There is increasing high-quality evidence that inadequate or disturbed sleep has a myriad of negative consequences (Table 28.1); for example, being implicated in one-quarter of road traffic accidents and increasing the risk of developing type 2 diabetes mellitus by 22 per cent. It is worth keeping these in mind when considering the general hospital patient complaining of poor sleep.

Table 28.1 Consequences of sleep disturbance

Short-term consequences	Long-term consequences
• Fatigue (mental, emotional, physical)	• Depression
• Poor concentration and attention	• Anxiety disorders
• Increased reaction time, inaccuracy	• Memory problems
• Impaired judgement	• Decreased cognitive function
• Yawning, aches, tremors, shivers	• Worsening of primary psychiatric conditions
• Irritability	• Increased risk of physical health conditions:
• Hallucinations, disorientation, persecutory ideas (*extreme sleep deprivation*)	• Overall increased mortality
	• Type 2 diabetes
	• Cardiovascular disease
	• Obesity
	• Reduced immune function
	• Reduced growth (children)

Classification of sleep disorders

There are approximately 90 sleep disorders, many of which are poorly understood and subject to regular change in definition as research progresses. The result is that attempting to classify sleep disorders is challenging, and ultimately very confusing. A simple way to approach it is to consider what can go wrong with sleep patterns; this reduces the field to four basic categories:

1 Not enough sleep (**insomnia**).

2 Sleeping too much (**hypersomnia**).

3 Disturbed episodes during or related to sleep (**parasomnias**).

4 Inappropriate timing of sleep, or the sleep–wake cycle loses synchrony with the rest of society (**circadian rhythm disorders**).

Making this distinction is adequate to allow most simple management strategies to be tried, but a thorough history and examination will usually allow you to be more specific as to the diagnosis if specialist help is likely to be needed.

Sleep disorders are covered by all classification systems, but the array of confusing terminology has led to the development of a third classification system. The **International Classification of Sleep Disorders** is now in its third edition (**ICSD-3**), published by the American Academy of Sleep Disorders based on international collaboration. It is not necessary for nonspecialists to have more than a working knowledge of clinically useful groupings, but Table 28.2 is included as a reference guide.

Screening

It is very quick and simple to screen for sleep disorders; suggested questions are shown in Box 28.2. If any of the questions produce positive answers, a full assessment should be carried out. It is important to target the following high-risk groups:

- Any patient presenting with psychiatric symptoms.
- Patients with a psychiatric history.
- General hospital inpatients.
- Patients with neurological, endocrine, or respiratory disease.
- Patients with any other chronic disease.

Assessment of sleep disorders

As with any patient, take a full history (relevant to your clinical setting but including both psychiatric and physical symptoms if possible) and try to speak to the patient's room or bed partner to get a collateral view.

Sleep history

- Precise nature of the sleep complaint (including onset, duration, course, frequency, and severity). Were there any significant events or stressors around the time of the onset of the problem?
- Pattern of symptoms, timing, and exacerbating or relieving factors (e.g. does it vary at weekends or during holidays?).
- Behaviour while asleep, dreams/nightmares, episodes of awakening, and perceived quality of sleep.
- Effect of symptoms upon mood, behaviour, work, social life, school, and bed partner or other family members.
- Previous sleep problems and treatments.

Daily routine

- Time and mode (natural, alarm) of waking; ease of getting up.
- Activities and level of alertness during the day.
- Daily naps.
- Preparations for bed.
- Time of going to bed.
- Activities in bed (reading, TV, sex, eating).
- Time of falling asleep.
- Night-time awakenings.

Table 28.2 Classification of sleep disorders: simplified comparison of the three main classification systems. Bullet points show commoner conditions subclassified within a category of disorders

ICSD-3	DSM-5	ICD-10/ICD-11 (beta draft 2016)
Insomnia: • Primary • Secondary	**Insomnias:** • Primary • Secondary • Related to another mental health disorder	**Insomnias:** • Short term • Chronic
Sleep-relating breathing disorders: • Obstructive sleep apnoea • Central apnoea	**Breathing-related sleep disorders:** • Obstructive sleep apnoea • Central apnoea	**Sleep-relating breathing disorders:** • Obstructive sleep apnoea • Central apnoea
Hypersomnias: • Primary • Narcolepsy • Kleine–Levin syndrome	**Hypersomnias:** • Primary • Narcolepsy • Hypersomnia related to another mental health problem	**Hypersomnias:** • Idiopathic • Narcolepsy • Kleine–Levin syndrome • Hypersomnia secondary to medication
Circadian rhythm sleep–wake disorder: • Delayed sleep phase disorder • Advanced sleep phase disorder • Non-24-hour sleep disorder • Irregular sleep–wake disorder • Shift work disorder • Jet lag disorder	**Circadian rhythm sleep disorder:** • Delayed sleep phase disorder • Advanced sleep phase disorder • Non-24-hour sleep disorder • Irregular sleep–wake disorder • Shift work disorder • Jet lag disorder	**Disorders of sleep–wake schedule:** • Circadian rhythm sleep–wake disorder—subtypes: advanced; delayed; non-24-hour; irregular; shift work; jet lag
Parasomnias: • Disorders of arousal • REM sleep behaviour disorders • Nightmares	**Parasomnias:** • Non-REM sleep arousal disorders • REM sleep behaviour disorders • Nightmares	**Parasomnias:** • Parasomnia • Sleep talking
Sleep-related movement disorders: • Restless leg syndrome • Periodic limb movement disorder	**Sleep-related movement:** • Restless leg syndrome • Periodic limb movement disorder	**Sleep-related movement disorders:** • Restless leg syndrome • Periodic limb movement disorder
Other sleep disorder related to physical health problem	Sleep disorder due to a general medical condition	
Substance-induced sleep disorder	Substance-induced sleep disorder	

Source data from: *International Classification of Sleep Disorders*, Third Edition (ICSD-3), World Health Organization 2014; *International Classification of Diseases*, 10th Revision (ICD-10), World Health Organization 2016; *International Classification of Diseases*, 11th revision (ICD-11), WHO, Beta draft 2016; *Diagnostic and Statistical Manual of Mental Disorders*, 5th Edition (DSM-5), American Psychiatric Association, 2013.

Box 28.2 Screening for sleep disorders

- Do you sleep long enough and well enough?
- Are you very sleepy during the day?
- Do you do unusual things or have strange experiences at night?

- Consumption of caffeinated drinks, nicotine, alcohol, or stimulating drugs—how much and at what time?

Physical examination. A full physical examination should be undertaken, focusing specifically on the respiratory, neurological, and endocrine systems.

Further investigations

The majority of patients presenting with sleep problems will need no investigations other than those just listed. However, in complex cases the following may be useful:

1 **Sleep diaries**. The patient records activities, sleep, mealtimes, caffeine intake, and sleep-related symptoms over a 2-week period. These are often extremely revealing as to the cause of the problem.

2 **Video recordings** (home or hospital) can be very useful in demonstrating parasomnias.

3 **Actigraphy**. This is the monitoring of sleep–wake cycles and/or body movements via a unit worn as a wristwatch.

4 **Polysomnography** (sleep study) involves the monitoring of various physiological parameters during sleep. Basic polysomnography includes the recording of EEG, electro-oculography (EOG), and electromyography (EMG), but often ECG, pulse oximetry, oesophageal pH, and respiratory monitoring are added. This is combined with audio and video recording of the patient overnight, and is the most definitive method of diagnosing a specific sleep disorder. The downside is that it has to be done in a special sleep laboratory, which is expensive and may not be suitable for very young, acutely disturbed patients, or disabled patients.

5 **The Multiple Sleep Latency Test** (MSLT) is the gold standard for diagnosis of hypersomnia. The patient is put to bed at intervals throughout the day, and the length of time it takes them to fall asleep is recorded.

General principles of management

For sleep disorders that are secondary to another diagnosis, the emphasis should always be on treating the primary condition. Most other sleep disturbances can be treated using behavioural regimes: prescribing hypnotics should be avoided unless necessary.

Sleep education

Providing accurate information about normal sleep and the effects of external factors on sleep reduces the patient's feeling of being out of control. Irrespective of the underlying diagnosis, the following should be discussed with the patient:

- Functions of sleep.
- How sleep changes with age.
- Sleep as an active process with different stages.
- Factors adversely affecting sleep (physical symptoms, mental health, behaviour, drugs, work patterns, etc.).
- The effects of sleep loss (Table 28.1).
- How to keep a sleep diary.
- Different types of sleep problems.

Sleep hygiene

Sleep hygiene refers to the behavioural and environmental factors preceding sleep that may interfere with it. Establishing appropriate sleep habits is a vital part of the treatment of sleep disorders. Components of good sleep hygiene are shown in Box 28.3, and again should be discussed with all patients. Box 28.4 shows the various treatment options available for sleep disorders.

Box 28.3 Sleep hygiene

- Ensure the bedroom is comfortable; control light, temperature, and noise.
- Relax for at least 1 hour before bed.
- Avoid caffeinated drinks (and other stimulants) after 4 pm.
- Avoid smoking for an hour before bed.
- Have a milky (or other tryptophan-containing) snack before bed.
- Avoid activities other than sleeping or having sex in bed (e.g. TV, using a computer, eating).
- Avoid daytime naps.
- Keep to a regular daily schedule for waking and going to bed.
- Ensure regular exercise (although not late at night).
- Eat a stable, regular, suitable diet.
- Moderate alcohol consumption.

Box 28.4 Treatment strategies for sleep disorders

General measures

- Treat the underlying cause of the problem (medical or psychiatric)
- Psychoeducation
- Ensure good sleep hygiene
- Advise on safety measures (e.g. driving, around the home if sleepwalking)
- Relaxation, mindfulness, and/or problem-solving training

Psychological treatments (mainly used for insomnia)

- CBT
- Sleep restriction therapy

Pharmacological treatments

- Hypnotics (short term)
- Stimulants (narcolepsy, hypersomnias)
- Melatonin (sleep–wake disturbances)
- Antidepressants (underlying depression, narcolepsy)

Physical measures

- Continuous positive airway pressure (CPAP) (obstructive sleep apnoea)
- Light therapy (circadian rhythm disturbances)
- Chronotherapy (circadian rhythm disturbances)

Specific sleep disorders

Insomnia

Insomnia is usually a symptom rather than a disorder, and refers to an unsatisfactory quantity and/or quality of sleep, which persists for a considerable period of time, including difficulty falling asleep, difficulty staying asleep, or early final wakening. It is extremely common and may be a primary disorder, but is more often secondary to another medical or psychiatric condition.

The patient may present with either or both of the following:

1 **A complaint relating to sleep:** trouble getting to sleep; repeated awakenings; early morning awakening; perceived poor quality of or unrefreshing sleep or inadequate quantity of sleep.

2 **Symptoms secondary to the sleep problem:** daytime sleepiness, irritability, fatigue, poor attention and concentration, and substandard performance at daily activities.

Epidemiology

Insomnia affects one-third of adults occasionally, and approximately 10 per cent on a clinically significant basis. Insomnia is more common in females, the elderly, shift workers, and those with medical or psychiatric co-morbidities.

Aetiology of insomnia

Table 28.3 contains an overview of the main causes of insomnia. This is not an exhaustive list, and more detailed information can be found in the 'Further reading' section. Secondary causes of insomnia constitute 98 per cent of cases, so take a careful history. A list of drugs that interfere with sleep can be found on p. 420.

Course and prognosis

There has been little research into the natural course of insomnia, as the wide range of aetiologies makes it difficult to generalize. However, it is known that untreated primary insomnia is usually lifelong and that untreated insomnia of any cause tends to gradually worsen with time. Although some cases of insomnia

Table 28.3 Aetiology of insomnia

Secondary causes (common)	Primary causes (rare)
• Medical disorders	• Primary (idiopathic) insomnia
• Psychiatric disorders	• Sleep apnoea syndromes
• Substance use or misuse	• Restless leg syndrome
• Poor sleep hygiene	• Periodic limb movement syndrome
• Environmental	• Central alveolar hypoventilation syndrome (*Ondine's curse*)
• Hormonal	• Ekbom's syndrome (delusional parasitosis)
• Circadian rhythm disturbance	
• Pain	
• Jet lag or shift work	
• Rebound insomnia from overuse of hypnotics	

will run a prolonged course, the prognosis of an ad-equately treated episode of secondary insomnia is very good.

Management

The most important aspects of the management of insomnia are:

1 identifying and treating the secondary cause(s) of the insomnia;

2 a clear explanation of what is causing the problem and how it will be treated;

3 ensuring good sleep hygiene (Box 28.3).

A general outline of management options is shown in Box 28.5. Psychological interventions should be used as a first-line treatment, as they are more effective and provide longer-term benefit than medications.

CBT is the most effective treatment for chronic insomnia. Around 70 per cent of patients with insomnia will benefit from CBT, and the effects are maintained in the long term. It acts by identifying thoughts that prevent sleep from occurring, and finds ways to challenge these and alter behaviour. Components of CBT for insomnia include:

• identifying intrusive thought patterns;

• addressing misconceptions about sleep;

• establishing a daily review and planning session in the early evening;

• relaxation training;

Box 28.5 Management of insomnia

General measures

• Identification and treatment of the cause of insomnia
• Psychoeducation
• Improve sleep hygiene

Psychological treatments (first line)

• **CBT**—*high-quality evidence for efficacy*
• Stimulus control therapy
• Sleep restriction
• Relaxation therapy

Pharmacological treatments (second line)

• Hypnotics:
  • Benzodiazepines
  • Non-benzodiazepines
• Antihistamines
• Antidepressants

• distraction and thought blocking;

• challenging negative thoughts;

• motivation to maintain cognitive and behavioural change.

Stimulus control therapy. This form of treatment plays on the natural instinct to become sleepy when presented with a familiar pre-bedtime routine and environment. Stimulus control involves removing everything from the bedroom that might hinder sleep, and then reconditioning the person to associate the room with sleep.

Sleep restriction therapy. This is especially helpful for patients who spend long periods in bed, but are awake for much of the time. Reducing the time spent in bed helps to consolidate the sleep, providing higher-quality rest. This treatment is hard work, and requires a highly motivated patient.

Pharmacotherapy

There are a large number of prescription and over-the-counter medications available that are designed to help people sleep. Many of the latter do not have a psychoactive component or it is at a low dose and are safe but relatively ineffective, whereas prescribed drugs are more likely to be helpful but often cause tolerance and dependence. Avoid using any hypnotic in patients with hepatic encephalopathy or severely impaired respiratory function. A quick guide to prescribing 'sleeping tablets' is shown in Box 28.6.

Benzodiazepines are the most commonly used class of hypnotic, and are highly effective at inducing sleep. Unfortunately, tolerance and dependence occur within 14 days, and they may cause rebound insomnia if used regularly. Shorter-acting drugs are better for those with difficulty dropping off to sleep and longer-acting for patients with frequent or early morning awakening. There is a higher risk of 'hangover' with longer-acting hypnotics.

Non-benzodiazepine hypnotics ('Z-drugs'— zopiclone, zolpidem, and zaleplon) are as effective as benzodiazepines, but with a slightly lower risk of tolerance and dependence. However, they do cause morning sedation and are not currently licensed for long-term use.

Box 28.6 Prescribing sleeping tablets

Safest starting choices include:
- temazepam 10 mg at night
- zopiclone 3.75–7.5 mg at night
- zolpidem 10 mg at night

Note: halve doses in the elderly or those with liver disease.

Sedating antihistamines are widely available as off-prescription sleeping aids. Diphenhydramine (Benadryl®, Nytol®) and promethazine are the most common. Antihistamines are effective hypnotics, but the effects do tend to wear off with time and often cause drowsiness the next day. The most frequent side effect is headache.

Antidepressants have traditionally had a role in the treatment of insomnia. A low dose of trazodone or mirtazapine is a good choice, but runs the risk of a number of side effects. SSRIs are typically slightly stimulating.

Atypical antipsychotics are being used more frequently for night sedation but there is a minimal evidence base. Quetiapine is the most researched and has the best risk–benefit ratio when given at doses of 50–200 mg (the antipsychotic dose being 300–900 mg) at night.

See Case study box 28.1 for an example.

Hypersomnias

Hypersomnia means **excessive daytime sleepiness** but may also simply refer to excessive time spent asleep, and is a term used to cover a heterogeneous group of sleep disorders. The epidemiology of hypersomnias is hard to ascertain due to difficulty detangling subjective fatigue from objective excessive sleepiness but the prevalence of clinically significant sleepiness is approximately 5 per cent. Many of the syndromes can be effectively treated, so they are important conditions to diagnose and manage. The generalist only needs a working knowledge of the commoner and/or more severe hypersomnias.

General clinical features

Excessive daytime sleepiness manifests itself in a variety of different ways. Patients may present with:

1 a complaint about sleep:
   - daytime sleepiness;
   - irresistible, unrefreshing episodes of sleep during the day;
   - abnormally long length of night-time sleep;

Insomnia

A 46-year-old man, Peter, presented to his GP complaining of poor sleep. He described difficulty in getting to sleep, frequent awakenings during the night, and waking up at 5–6 am daily. He had tried over-the-counter sleeping tablets and milky drinks at bedtime, but found them of no use. Peter's wife said she had noticed him snoring extremely loudly at night and stopping breathing sometimes, which worried her. She also felt that Peter had become withdrawn and was smoking more after being made redundant 6 months previously. The GP examined Peter, and apart from finding him to be rather overweight (BMI = 38), there were no abnormalities. She also took a full psychiatric and sleep history, and decided that the causes of the insomnia were threefold: a depressive disorder, OSA, and poor sleep hygiene. Peter chose to try an SSRI for his mood, understood he should avoid hypnotics as they cause respiratory depression, and accepted a referral to the sleep apnoea clinic. Over the next few months, Peter had a good response to the SSRI and his sleep improved slightly. Later that year he received a CPAP machine which increased his sleep quality immensely and allowed him to feel ready to look for another job.

- prolonged difficulty in waking up, often with disorientation ('sleep drunkenness');
- recurrent periods of almost continuous sleep for days on end, which occur every few months.

2 symptoms secondary to the sleep problem.

Often the patient may not be fully aware of their condition, and it is brought to medical attention by a family member, employer, or after an accident.

The Epworth Sleepiness Scale is a self-completed questionnaire which asks the patient to rate their chance of dozing off in eight daily situations. It has a high sensitivity and is therefore a good screening tool for hypersomnia.

Aetiology

The major causes of hypersomnia are shown in Table 28.4. In an adult with new-onset sleepiness, the most common causes are an underlying psychiatric or medical condition, or the effects of substances.

Table 28.4 Aetiology of hypersomnia

Hypersomnia secondary to a psychiatric condition	Hypersomnia due to substances	Hypersomnia related to a breathing disorder	Hypersomnias of central origin	Hypersomnias related to a general medical condition
Mood disorders	**Alcohol**	Obstructive sleep apnoea	Narcolepsy—with or without cataplexy	**Neurological diseases:** brain tumours, raised intracranial pressure, Parkinson's disease
Somatoform disorders	**Prescribed drugs:** hypnotics, antidepressants, antipsychotics, antihistamines, antiparkinson drugs		Idiopathic hypersomnia	
Personality disorders			Kleine–Levin syndrome	
Dementia or delirium	**Recreational drugs:** opiates			**Endocrine diseases:** hypothyroidism, acromegaly
	Toxins: arsenic, bismuth, carbon monoxide, vitamin A, copper			Infectious diseases
				Post-traumatic hypersomnia

Narcolepsy

Narcolepsy is characterized by excessive daytime sleepiness, irresistible episodes of sleep, and cataplexy. Cataplexy is a sudden loss of skeletal muscle tone, usually trigger by emotion or surprise. There are three subtypes.

1 **Type 1.** Narcolepsy with cataplexy.

2 **Type 2.** Narcolepsy without cataplexy.

3 **Narcolepsy secondary to another condition.** This is rare—examples include hypothalamic tumours, Prader–Willi syndrome, or a paraneoplastic phenomenon.

Narcolepsy is not particularly rare; the majority of cases are with cataplexy, and have a prevalence of 0.2–0.5 per 1000. Males and females are equally affected. Narcolepsy tends to present in the teenage years and is usually lifelong.

Clinical features

There is a classical tetrad of excessive sleepiness, cataplexy, sleep paralysis, and hypnagogic hallucinations but it is actually very rare. Typical presenting symptoms include the following:

1 Daytime sleepiness: this is present every day, and tends to worsen gradually until there is an irresistible, uncontrollable, and refreshing short episode of sleep. These are uncontrollable, and may occur at inappropriate times.

2 Cataplexy: triggered by specific emotional, stressful, or surprising stimuli in the environment and all voluntary muscles except the respiratory and extraocular musculature are involved. The patient may fall to the ground, or merely become suddenly very weak. Consciousness is preserved during the attack, and there is rapid recovery.

3 Sleep paralysis: the inability to move on going to or waking up from sleep.

4 Hypnagogic (at the onset of sleep) or hypnopompic (upon waking up) hallucinations.

5 Parasomnias.

6 There is an association with obesity.

7 Consequences of the narcolepsy: for example, depression, anxiety, and problems at school or work.

It is a clinical diagnosis and no investigations are needed. **Reduced hypocretin-1 (orexin) concentration** in the CSF is a highly sensitive and specific marker for narcolepsy. Similarly, the human leucocyte antigen HLA-DR2 haplotype is found in 80–90 per cent of patients with narcolepsy.

Management

As well as general measures (Box 28.4), there are a few specific management strategies for narcolepsy:

- **Practical support.** Psychoeducation and support at work/school are important. This is especially the case if cataplexy limits activities that can be undertaken (e.g. driving).

- **Avoid sedative medications.**

- **Scheduled naps.** Short 20-minute naps should be built into the daily timetable to reduce the likelihood of irresistible sleeps.

- Pharmacotherapy. Stimulants have the best evidence and **modafinil** is the first-line choice. It is relatively good at controlling sleepiness and has a lower tolerance and illicit marketplace than methylphenidate or methamphetamine. Side effects include headache, hypertension, and diarrhoea. Noradrenergic and serotonergic reuptake inhibitors are helpful for cataplexy; venlafaxine and fluoxetine are most effective.

Kleine–Levin syndrome (recurrent hypersomnia)

This is a rare condition, almost exclusively affecting adolescent males, which is characterized by recurrent episodes of hypersomnia and binge eating. Periods of excessive sleepiness last for days to weeks, during which there is rapid weight gain. It may be accompanied by hypersexuality, irritability, odd behaviours, and psychosis. The latter may lead to an erroneous diagnosis of schizophrenia. Between attacks the patient recovers completely. Kleine–Levin syndrome is a clinical diagnosis, which usually lasts for the adolescent years and then gradually burns out. Treatment is similar to that for narcolepsy, with stimulants and behavioural modification being the first-line approaches. Occasionally, lithium may be helpful if there is severe functional disruption during episodes.

Idiopathic hypersomnia (primary hypersomnia)

Idiopathic hypersomnia is a state of daily excessive sleepiness of unknown aetiology. It has three characteristic features:

1 Prolonged night-time sleeping (more than 10 hours)—the person sleeps very soundly and cannot be woken by alarms, telephones, etc.

2 Sleep drunkenness on waking—there is often difficulty in waking up, confusion, and irritability for an hour or more.

3 Excessive daytime sleepiness with frequent, unrefreshing naps.

Diagnosis is made on exclusion of other hypersomnias, usually by polysomnography. Treatment is as for narcolepsy, but without the scheduled naps, as these are unrefreshing and therefore unhelpful.

Sleep apnoea

Sleep apnoea is a group of conditions in which there are pauses in breathing during sleep. The pause must last at least 10 seconds to meet diagnostic criteria, during which there is a measurable desaturation in blood oxygen levels. Frequent awakenings when breathing resumes lead to unrefreshing sleep and daytime sleepiness. A clinically relevant level of sleep apnoea is thought to be more than five episodes per hour. Obstructive sleep apnoea (OSA) is very common (see 'Further reading'), whereas central sleep apnoea syndromes are extremely rare.

Obstructive sleep apnoea

Obstruction of the upper airways occurs during sleep if there is a combination of low muscle tone and excessive soft tissue around the airway. The major risk factor is obesity, but it is also more common in certain anatomical neck variants, men, and the elderly. OSA has a prevalence of 4 per cent and 2 per cent in adult men and women, respectively. It usually presents from 40 to 60 years.

Symptoms include:

- snoring;
- apnoeic episodes ending with loud resumption of breathing;
- nocturia;
- severe fatigue upon waking up;
- daytime headaches;
- excessive daytime sleepiness;
- poor concentration, irritability, and loss of libido.

Diagnosis is made by polysomnography, including audio-video recording of a night's sleep.

Treatment of OSA

- **Weight loss.** Even loss of only 5 per cent of body weight can reduce symptoms dramatically.
- **Avoidance of alcohol and sedatives.**
- **CPAP** at night is the most effective treatment. It involves wearing a large, heavy mask in bed, which is difficult to get used to. However, good compliance leads to excellent results and many patients do persevere.
- **Surgery** is occasionally used to reconstruct the nose or upper airways if the cause is an anatomical aberration.

Parasomnias

The word parasomnia literally means *around sleep*, and refers to undesirable, abnormal skeletal muscle activity, behaviours, or emotional–perceptual events that occur during sleep. Parasomnias may happen at sleep onset, during sleep, during transition between stages of sleep, or when going from sleep to wakefulness. A simplified classification is shown in Table 28.5, along with some epidemiology to demonstrate that these are conditions frequently seen in clinical practice. Diagnosis is usually clinical but polysomnography

Table 28.5 Classification and epidemiology of (common) parasomnias

	Prevalence	Male:female	Typical age of presentation	Associations
Non-REM sleep arousal disorders				
Confusional arousal	15–17% children 2–4% adults	1:1	Prepubertal	Family history of parasomnias Other sleep disorders
Sleepwalking	15% children 4% adults	1:1	4–12 years	Family history
Sleep terrors	3% children 1% adults	1:1		Family history
REM sleep behaviour disorders				
REM sleep behaviour disorder	0.3–0.5%	>1:1	50–60 years	Neurological disease
Nightmares	1% clinically significant	Unknown	All ages	
Restless leg syndrome	2–3% (increases with age)	1:2	All ages	Family history Pregnancy Anaemia

can be useful in those presenting with multiple sleep problems or an unclear history.

Sleepwalking (somnambulism)

Sleepwalking is characterized by complex, automatic behaviours occurring during sleep. Typical activities include wandering around the house, rearranging objects, eating, and urinating. Very rarely, more dangerous activities such as carrying weapons, driving, and homicide have occurred. The person's eyes are usually wide open, and they stare into space. It is not possible to communicate with the person, although they may mumble to themselves. The person usually returns to bed easily, and the episode is not remembered in the morning. There are a variety of risk factors and associations with sleepwalking, which are shown in Box 28.7.

Sleep terrors (parvor nocturnes, incubus)

Sleep terrors are characterized by a sudden awakening in which the patient sits upright, screams loudly, and has marked autonomic activation (sweating, mydriasis,

Box 28.7 Factors associated with sleepwalking and sleep terrors

- Alcohol
- Anticholinergic drugs
- Family history
- Febrile illness
- Lithium carbonate
- Menstruation
- Neurological disorders
- Nocturnal seizures
- OSA
- Periodic limb movements
- Pregnancy
- Sleep deprivation
- Stress
- 'Z-drugs'

tachycardia, tachypnoea). Occasionally there may be frantic motor activity, which can lead to falling out of bed and injury. The episode occurs early in the night and usually lasts 10–15 minutes. The patient soon quietens and goes back to sleep, and is unable to remember the events in the morning.

Confusional arousal ('sleep drunkenness')

Confusional arousal refers to periods of mental or behavioural confusion upon waking, either at night or after a daytime nap. It represents an incomplete transition from the deep stages of NREM sleep to wakefulness. During the period, the person may undertake goal-directed behaviours, but these are very slow and inaccurate. There is no specified treatment, but all the supportive and general measures for managing sleep disorders may be helpful.

Treatment

In the majority of cases of NREM sleep arousal disorders no specific treatment is necessary:

- Provide reassurance and psychoeducation.
- Exclude (or treat) other physical and mental health conditions.
- Encourage good sleep hygiene and regular sleep–wake cycles.
- Avoid sleep deprivation, alcohol, and other precipitating factors.
- Make environmental changes to avoid injury.
- Benzodiazepines: occasionally needed and reasonably effective, try clonazepam 0.5–1.0 mg at night (see Case study box 28.2).

REM sleep behaviour disorder (RSBD)

REMD is a condition in which patients exhibit motor activity during REM sleep due to a loss of atonia. Typically the patient acts out a vivid, terrifying dream with complex movements and vocalizations. Sleep injury (of both patient and bed partner) is common. Sleep for both the patient and bedroom companion is disrupted, and can lead to relationship problems. The majority of cases of RSBD are associated with neurological disease (especially Parkinson's disease or neurodegenerative conditions), narcolepsy, or antidepressants.

Treatment

- Ensure a safe sleeping environment for the patient and their bed partner.
- Eliminate or treat any predisposing or aggravating factors.
- Clonazepam 0.5–1.0 mg at night is very effective at controlling the symptoms in most patients.

Nightmares

Nightmares are frightening dreams that cause the patient to wake up, usually feeling slightly confused. The patient may be distressed, and can take time to get back to sleep. Nightmares frequently occur after a stressful event, high fever, or occasionally after eating certain foods. There are a large number of drugs that are associated with nightmares; these are

---

CASE STUDY BOX 28.2

Sleepwalking

Sarah, an 8-year-old girl, was taken to see her paediatrician by her mother, Claire. Claire said that she had been keen for Sarah to attend a weekend away with her Brownie Pack, but was worried about her going due to Sarah's frequent sleepwalking. From the age of three, Sarah had got up almost every night and wandered about the house in a daze. Claire was concerned that Sarah would hurt herself at night if she was in an unfamiliar environment, or that the other girls would tease her. Sarah had no previous medical history or other symptoms, and physical examination was normal. The paediatrician reassured Claire that sleepwalking is common in children, and that Sarah would probably grow out of it. He stressed that Claire should be safety conscious and discuss the problem with the adults supervising the Brownie trip. Claire did so, and Sarah went on the trip as planned. She did sleepwalk, but the hall had been made safe for her, and there were no adverse consequences.

Box 28.8 Drugs associated with nightmares

- Antimuscarinics
- Beta-blockers
- Clonidine
- Digoxin
- Indomethacin
- Methyldopa
- Nicotine patches
- Pergolide
- Reserpine
- Verapamil
- Withdrawal from alcohol, benzodiazepines, or opiates

shown in Box 28.8. Treatment is rarely needed, but infrequently sleep will be adversely affected enough for the patient (or their bed partner) to seek medical attention. In that situation, the patient should consider their sleep hygiene, try relaxation techniques, avoid precipitating drugs, or try a low-dose antidepressant.

Restless legs syndrome (RLS, Willis–Ekbom's disease)

This is a common condition characterized by an unpleasant, uncomfortable urge to move the legs in the evening or at night. Patients use many terms to describe the feeling but universally say the sensation is temporarily relieved by movement. RLS is a frustrating disorder and may cause insomnia, night awakenings, depression, or anxiety. It is probably caused by a dopamine system dysfunction and is highly associated with abnormalities in iron levels and handling. The majority of patients have a family history of RLS, but the symptoms are often triggered or worsened by caffeine, alcohol, fatigue, and stress. RLS is associated with iron deficiency, renal failure, diabetes, pregnancy, psychotropic medications, and peripheral neuropathies.

Treatment

Investigate for associated conditions and take a detailed drug history. Replace iron if ferritin is low

and recommend good sleep hygiene. Heat, massage, and stretching may provide minimal relief and there is some evidence that evening exercise is helpful. For severe cases, non-ergot dopamine agonists (e.g. rotigotine, pramipexole, and ropinirole) or gabapentin are usually efficacious.

Circadian rhythm disorders

Circadian rhythm disorders are chronic sleep difficulties due to a disruption of the patient's circadian rhythm and/or a difference between an individual's sleep–wake cycle and that of the society around them. If left to their own timetables, patients with circadian rhythm disorders usually achieve adequate normal-quality sleep. However, if they are trying to function in line with other people, they often suffer severe insomnia and/or hypersomnia, which can interfere with normal social and occupational activities. The major types of circadian rhythm disorders are outlined in Table 28.6.

Treatment

General measures. It is very important to explain the nature of a normal sleep pattern, appropriate sleep hygiene, and the usefulness of a regular daily routine.

Chronotherapy. Depending on the nature of the sleep–wake aberration, attempts should be made to retrain the patient into a normal routine by manipulating bedtime. A regular sleeping and waking time must be established, with no more than 7–8 hours of total sleep. If necessary, a phase-delay approach can be used. This involves going to bed 2 or 3 hours later than usual until the desired bedtime is reached, and then staying at this time. These are difficult strategies, and require cooperation from the patient and their family/cohabitants.

Light therapy. Phototherapy is given with a 10,000 lux lamp for 30–90 minutes before the patient's usual spontaneous awakening. The timing of the light can be gradually altered until a

Table 28.6 Circadian rhythm disorders

Disorder	Essential characteristics
Delayed sleep phase syndrome	Patients naturally fall asleep much later than conventional, often about 1–3 am. Sleep is then normal, but enforced awakening at socially convenient times produces excessive morning sleepiness. Common in young adults
Advanced sleep phase syndrome	This is the opposite of delayed sleep phase syndrome, with early sleep onset (6–8 pm) and very early awakening. This rarely comes to medical attention
Irregular sleep–wake pattern	A completely chaotic sleep pattern. It is associated with Alzheimer's disease, hypothalamic tumours, and developmental disorder
Non-24-hour sleep–wake disorder ('*free-running disorder*')	The patient's intrinsic circadian clock is not entrained to 24 hours; sleeping and waking often occur 1–2 hours later each day, continually going around the full 24-hours cycle. It is more common in blind individuals, and those with a history of severe head injury
Shift-work sleep disorder	This condition can affect those who work night shifts, or are on frequently changing rotas. Often patients complain of physical symptoms (e.g. gastrointestinal upset, headaches, and aches) rather than sleep difficulties
Time-zone change syndrome ('jet lag')	This occurs in people who frequently travel between different time zones. Symptoms include insomnia, daytime fatigue, apathy, depression, reduced daytime alertness, and physical complaints (e.g. diarrhoea, headache)

satisfactory waking time is reached. Light restriction may be necessary in the evenings, especially during summer. For those with advanced wakening, the light should be used in the evening to delay sleep.

Melatonin is a hormone secreted from the pineal gland, which is under the influence of the hypothalamic SCN. It is secreted during darkness, linking the sleep–wake and light–dark cycles and inducing sleep. Some patients find taking melatonin 1–2 hours before bedtime can promote sleepiness (see Science box 28.1).

Sleep problems related to psychiatric disorders

Characteristic patterns of sleep disturbance are a part of many psychiatric conditions and may also be caused by psychotropic medication. The diagnostic criteria of several psychiatric conditions (e.g. depression, mania) include sleep disturbance as an essential component. Table 28.7 gives an overview of common presentations and some strategies for management.

Sleep problems related to general medical conditions

It is impossible to cover the sleep disturbance related to all pathologies; this section merely aims to highlight general principles and some common conditions (see Table 28.8). It is important to take a sleep history from all patients—especially those in hospital—as simple measures can often improve the situation. This can have a big impact on the patient's ability to cope with their other problems. The following points should be borne in mind:

- Treatment of the underlying medical condition should be the first priority.
- Take a full drug history, including over-the-counter medications. Some off-prescription drugs affect

SCIENCE BOX 28.1

Melatonin and jet lag

Jet lag is the response of the body struggling to adjust to moving across time zones and is a miserable experience. It is worse travelling eastwards compared to westwards. Symptoms include sleep disturbance, fatigue, irritability, and poor concentration. This can impact significantly on those travelling for business. It was claimed in the early 1990s that short-term use of melatonin could reduce the length and severity of jet lag and it is now widely used by travellers. Has this claim been substantiated?

In 2003, a Cochrane review was published on this topic and it remains the highest quality evidence to date.[1] The review found melatonin to significantly reduce jet lag compared with placebo, but the effect was non-dose dependent. The authors calculated the NNT as 2.

More recently, a systematic review including 35 trials (although the majority of participants were young, male, military personnel) reported a less significant effect of melatonin on jet lag.[2] It only found the effect for journeys eastwards and for when crossing more than two time zones.

Melatonin is available over the counter in several countries, including the USA, but at the time of writing is not licensed for use in jet lag in the UK.[3] It is increasingly prescribed off-licence and appears to be well tolerated.

1 Herxheimer A, Petrie KJ. Melatonin for the prevention and treatment of jet lag. *Cochrane Database of Systematic Reviews* 2002;2:CD001520.

2 Costello RB, Lentino CV, Boyd CC, et al. The effectiveness of melatonin for promoting healthy sleep: a rapid evidence assessment of the literature. *Nutrition Journal* 2014;13:1–17.

3 Jackson G. Come fly with me: jet lag and melatonin. *International Journal of Clinical Practice* 2010;64: 135–141.

Table 28.7 Sleep problems in psychiatric disorders.

Condition	Characteristic sleep pattern	Management strategies
Depression	**Very common:** Early morning waking Insomnia **Less common:** Excessive daytime sleepiness Frightening dreams Frequent awakenings	• Treat the underlying mood disorder assertively • Ensure good sleep hygiene • Regular routine of activities, meals, and bedtime • Use a sedating antidepressant, e.g. mirtazapine, tricyclics, or trazodone • For mania, try a sedating antipsychotic, e.g. olanzapine or quetiapine • For hypersomnia, choose SSRIs or bupropion
Mania	Reduced need for sleep Chaotic sleep patterns	
Anxiety disorders	Insomnia **Less common:** Frequent awakenings, early morning waking, reduce sleep time, panic attacks	• Treat the anxiety disorder or PTSD, including reassurance and psychoeducation • Teach some relaxation and mindfulness techniques • Use a sedating antidepressant • Short-term benzodiazepines if necessary
PTSD	Nightmares relating to the traumatic event Insomnia Frequent awakenings	

(continued)

Table 28.7 Continued

Condition	Characteristic sleep pattern	Management strategies
Eating disorders	**Anorexia nervosa:** Insomnia Frequent awakenings Early morning waking NB: ask about waking in the night to eat or exercise **Bulimia nervosa:** Lack of sleep due to night time binges Excessive daytime sleepiness	• Treat the eating disorder aggressively • Restoring weight to healthy range usually improves the insomnia significantly • Planning regular evening meals and breakfast often reduces night-time awakening to eat • In bulimia nervosa, try to break the binge–purge cycle. Ask household members to support the patient in not getting up at night • Use a sedating antidepressant, e.g. mirtazapine
Psychosis (especially those with persecutory delusions)	Insomnia Chaotic sleep patterns Excessive daytime sleepiness	• Try to detangle the effects of substances, psychosis, and disorganized behaviour from a primary or underlying sleep disorder • Promote good sleep hygiene • Use a sedating or more activating antipsychotic as appropriate • Short-term hypnotics if floridly psychotic or upon first starting an antipsychotic
Dementia	Sleep problems are common but variable in presentation; may be insomnia or hypersomnia Total sleep time often reduced Day-night reversal is common in Alzheimer's: patients get up at night and wander about Associated with evening confusion and agitation	• General principles of treating sleep disorders should be followed • Ensure good sleep hygiene and safety • Reinforce 24-hour cycle with environmental cues and regular routine • Try low-dose sedating antidepressants (e.g. trazodone) for evening agitation • Avoid hypnotics
Alcohol and substance misuse (use of and withdrawal)	Any sleep disturbance may occur but insomnia and/or an abnormal sleep–wake cycle is commonest Withdrawal from alcohol, opiates, or benzodiazepines causes agitation and insomnia.	• Manage addiction and withdrawal along usual guidelines • Promote good sleep hygiene measures • Avoid use of sedatives and hypnotics

sleep adversely (e.g. nasal decongestants and slimming pills) or the patient may have tried sleeping aids. If additional treatment for sleep is required, consider the patient's co-morbidities and interactions with other medications. Ask for advice from other specialties or the pharmacist.

• Avoid hypnotics wherever possible, especially in respiratory disorders, due to the risk of respiratory depression.

Drugs and sleep

Substances, be they prescription, over-the-counter, or recreational, are a common cause of sleep disturbance. It is imperative to always take a full drug history (including all three categories of alcohol, caffeine, and nicotine) in all patients you see. Boxes 28.9 and 28.10 show some of the more common culprits causing insomnia and hypersomnia, but these are

Table 28.8 Sleep disorders related to general medical conditions

Medical condition	Sleep disturbance	Specific treatment strategies
Respiratory disease: • COPD • Asthma	Nocturnal dyspnoea Frequent awakenings Insomnia (*often secondary to dyspnoea-induced anxiety*)	• Tackle anxiety • Theophylline and salbutamol can cause insomnia: reduce doses if possible • Avoid hypnotics
Cardiovascular disease: • Cardiac failure • Angina	Orthopnoea Nocturnal angina Paroxysmal nocturnal dyspnoea	• Lie more upright at night • Choose antihypertensives less likely to cause insomnia • Beta-blockers cause nightmares
Gastro-oesophageal reflux disease (GORD) and peptic ulcers	Nocturnal awakenings related to reflux	• Treat GORD • Avoid reflux-inducing foods, caffeine, and alcohol in the evenings
Iron deficiency	Restless leg syndrome Periodic limb movements in sleep	Iron supplements; treat underlying condition
Endocrine disease	Diabetes: insomnia, snoring, frequent awakenings Hyperthyroidism: insomnia Hypothyroidism: hypersomnia	• Treat underlying condition • Screen for OSA in diabetes • Screen for goitre in thyroid disease
Parkinson's disease	Progressive insomnia Parasomnias Periodic limb movements in sleep	• Review antiparkinsonian medications • Behavioural modifications • Clonazepam
Epilepsy	Disrupted night-time sleep combined with daytime sleepiness	• Control seizures • Choose sedating antiepileptic drugs
Conditions causing chronic pain (*including rheumatological conditions and cancer*)	Insomnia, disrupted sleep	• Corticosteroids and NSAIDs disrupt sleep • Optimize pain relief; many strong analgesics are sedatives
Chronic renal failure	Disrupted sleep, OSA, restless leg syndrome	• Improves with dialysis • Avoid medications or use lowest doses possible

COPD, chronic obstructive pulmonary disease; GORD, gastro-oesophageal reflux disease; OSA, obstructive sleep apnoea.

not comprehensive lists and it is worth always looking up individual drugs. When prescribing psychotropics, consider interactions with other medications which might potentiate or reduce their effects on sleep.

Alcohol is a highly effective sedative, and is commonly used by patients with mental health difficulties to self-medicate insomnia. Acute use of alcohol causes an increased total sleep time, but also vivid dreams and nightmares. Chronic alcoholism and withdrawal from alcohol are both associated with insomnia. Use of a long-acting benzodiazepine (e.g. chlordiazepoxide or diazepam) to treat withdrawal usually potentiates sleep.

Box 28.9 Drugs commonly causing insomnia

- Antidepressants (SSRIs, MAOIs, venlafaxine, bupropion)
- Antiparkinsonian medication
- Bronchodilators
- Cardiovascular medication (beta-blockers, digoxin, verapamil)
- Chemotherapy drugs
- Corticosteroids
- NSAIDs
- Stimulants (methylphenidate, methamphetamine, dexamphetamine, cocaine, caffeine, nicotine)
- Thyroxine
- Withdrawal (hypnotics, opiates, alcohol, cannabis)

Nicotine is a stimulant, and smoking in the evenings can disrupt sleep patterns. High-dose nicotine patches may have the same effect, so the 16-hour (rather than 24-hour) patches may be preferred by patients.

Box 28.10 Drugs commonly causing hypersomnia

- Antidepressants (mirtazapine, trazodone, tricyclics)
- Antiemetics
- Antiepileptic drugs
- Antihistamines
- Antiparkinson drugs
- Antipsychotics
- Anxiolytics
- Hypnotics
- Methyldopa
- Progestogens

Opiates tend to cause sedation and improved sleep quality when used at therapeutic doses, but produce profound insomnia when associated with misuse. Insomnia and increased alertness are important features of withdrawal, and are often difficult for patients to manage.

Further reading

American Academy of Sleep Medicine. *International Classification of Sleep Disorders*. 3rd ed. Darien, IL: American Academy of Sleep Medicine; 2014.

Anderson SL, Griend JPV. Quetiapine for insomnia: a review of the literature. *American Journal of Health-System Pharmacy* 2014;71:394–402.

Falloon K, Arroll B, Raina EC, Antonio F. The assessment and management of insomnia in primary care. *BMJ* 2011;342:d2899.

National Institute for Health and Care Excellence. Continuous positive airway pressure for the treatment of obstructive sleep apnoea/hypopnoea. Technology appraisal guidance [TA139]. Published March 2008. http://guidance.nice.org.uk/TA139/.

Schwartz JR, Roth T. Neurophysiology of sleep and wakefulness: basic science and clinical implications. *Current Neuropharmacology* 2008;6:367–378.

Trauer J, Qian MY, Doyle J, Rajaratnam SM, Cunnington D. Cognitive behavioural therapy for chronic insomnia: a systematic review and meta-analysis. *Annals of Internal Medicine* 2015;163:191–204.

Zeman A, Britton T, Douglas N, et al. Narcolepsy and excessive daytime sleepiness. *BMJ* 2004;329:724–728.

29 Problems due to use of alcohol and other psychoactive substances

Overview of issues relating to psychoactive substance misuse

Archaeological evidence has demonstrated that for at least the past 10,000 years humans have been using psychoactive substances. From the chewing of coca leaves in Ancient Peru (*c.*4000–3000 bce) to the popular use of laudanum in Victorian England, the recreational, cultural, and medicinal use of 'mind-altering' substances has been widespread. As of 2016, alcohol and other psychoactive substances remain a leading cause of medical and social problems world-wide: humans are clearly vulnerable to their attraction. Although a myriad of substances are available, only a few are commonly used, and all tend to produce similar harms upon the individual and society. This chapter will provide a general approach to managing a patient presenting with a problem stemming from substance misuse.

Epidemiology

It is extremely difficult to gather accurate data on the use of substances in the general population, especially if they are illegal. It is therefore likely that most figures are underestimations of the true incidence. The WHO estimates that tobacco, alcohol, and illicit drugs are a factor in 12.4 per cent of all deaths worldwide. This is a stark reminder of the severity that problems associated with substance usage can reach, but the morbidity surrounding them affects a much wider section of society.

Table 29.1 Epidemiology of psychoactive substance misuse

Substance	Prevalence
Alcohol	5.9% deaths worldwide attributable to alcohol
	13–18% of UK adults regularly drink over recommended limits
	4% of UK adults have alcohol dependency
Tobacco	19% of UK adults, >1.5 billion users globally
Cocaine	2–5% lifetime prevalence in Europe
Opioids	Estimated 3 million IV users worldwide
Hallucinogens	3% aged 16–30 years report lifetime use
Cannabis	30% of those aged <30 years have tried cannabis at least once; 6% used it regularly for at least 3 months (UK)
Ecstasy	15% of young people report lifetime use

In the UK, 80 per cent of adults drink alcohol, 19 per cent smoke tobacco, and 30 per cent admit to having used an illegal drug at least once in their lifetime. Worldwide, the highest prevalence of drug misuse is found in the 16- to 30-year age group, with males outnumbering females at a ratio of 4 to 1. Table 29.1 shows a selection of epidemiological figures associated with commonly used substances.

Terminology related to the use of psychoactive substances

Substance misuse is associated with an array of confusing terminology, the majority describing different disorders that may occur due to use of any substance. The following terms are internationally agreed and appear in major classification systems:

- **Intoxication** is the direct psychological and physical effects of the substance that are dose dependent and time limited. They are individual to the substance and typically include both pleasurable and unpleasant symptoms.
- **Harmful use.** A pattern of psychoactive substance use that is causing damage to health. The damage may be physical (e.g. abscesses due to the self-administration of injected substances) or mental (e.g. memory loss secondary to heavy consumption of alcohol).
- **Dependence.** When the body develops a physical and/or psychological 'need' for persistent use of a substance. Typical features are shown in Box 29.1.
- **Tolerance** is the state in which repeated administration leads to decreasing effect.
- **Withdrawal** is a set of symptoms and signs occurring when a substance is reduced or stopped

Box 29.1 Characteristics of the dependence syndrome

1 A **strong desire** or sense of compulsion to take the substance.
2 **Difficulties in refraining** from using the substance.
3 A physiological **withdrawal state** when substance use has stopped or been reduced. Withdrawal symptoms may be avoided by further use of the substance.
4 Evidence of **tolerance**.
5 Progressive **neglect of alternative pleasures or interests** due to the use of the psychoactive substance and the time needed to obtain supplies, or to recover from its effects.
6 **Persistent use of the substance despite clear evidence of harm.**

after persistent usage. The nature, time to onset, and course of the symptoms vary for different substances and may include convulsions or delirium.

- **Substance-induced psychosis.** Hallucinations and/or delusions directly due to substance misuse. Psychosis may occur during intoxication or withdrawal, or as a chronic aspect of dependency.
- **Amnesic syndrome** is the chronic prominent impairment of recent and/or remote memory. Immediate recall is usually preserved and recent memory is characteristically more disturbed than remote memory. Disturbances of time sense and ordering of events are usually evident, as are difficulties in learning new material. Confabulation may be marked but is not invariably present. Other cognitive functions are usually relatively well preserved and amnesic defects are out of proportion to other disturbances. It may be caused by intoxication or chronic use of alcohol, solvents, benzodiazepines, and possibly cannabis.

Why do people use substances?

There are a multitude of reasons why someone might take a substance at a given time; however, some general reasons apply and are listed here. The initial reason for taking a substance is often straightforward, but may become more complex and change over time.

Pleasurable experiences. About one-fifth of drug use is primarily to gain pleasure, usually in the form of a buzz or high, numbness, dissociation, drowsiness, or comfort. Those who experience energy and confidence will often use to try and relive the initial experience they encountered.

Peer pressure is unfortunately prevalent among young people. Personal vulnerability—a lack of personal resources needed to cope with the challenges of life—is a cause of the success of peer pressure.

Self-medication for psychiatric and physical symptoms is extremely common. Alcohol and benzodiazepines are widely used for anxiety, depression, and stress-related disorders. Individuals with psychosis, chronic pain, or neurological conditions are the greatest users of 'medicinal' cannabis.

Availability. The availability of most psychoactive substances is limited in one way or another. If a substance is easily available, people are more likely to use it; however, illegal substances also hold a particular fascination to some individuals. Psychoactive substances are usually obtained in one of three ways:

- Purchased legally (e.g. nicotine, alcohol).
- Prescribed by doctors (e.g. benzodiazepines).
- Purchased illegally: this category includes most of the other substances discussed in this chapter or substances with age limits for purchase. Control of the availability of such drugs depends on political action and requires extensive activity by the police and other enforcement agencies to detect and control the importation and distribution of drugs.

Attitudes of the community. Some social, cultural, and religious groups disapprove of drug taking, and this shared value helps to restrain its members. In other groups, drug taking is condoned or even encouraged and it gives a person status among his peers.

Dependence and tolerance develop as time progresses, and a physical and psychological 'need' for the drug will take over from previous reasons for use.

The law

In the UK, the legal framework for managing people who take psychoactive substances is defined by the **Misuse of Drugs Act of 1971** and the **Psychoactive Substances Act 2016**; most other countries have similar legislation. The Misuse of Drugs Act segregates illegal drugs into three classes (A, B, and C) according to the relative dangers of each drug to both an individual and the socioeconomic effects on society. Some common drugs in each category are shown in Box 29.2. There is therefore some debate as to the validity of the current system. The classification of a particular substance is not set in stone; for example, cannabis was changed from a class B to a class C drug in 2004, and then back to class B in 2009. Punishable offences include:

- possession of a controlled substance unlawfully;
- possession of a controlled substance with intent to supply it;

Box 29.2 Classification of illegal drugs under the UK Misuse of Drugs Act 1971

Class A

- Ecstasy
- LSD
- Heroin and methadone
- Cocaine and crack
- Magic mushrooms (whether prepared or fresh)
- Methamphetamine and other amphetamines if prepared for injection
- Any class B drug that is injected

Possession—up to 7 years' imprisonment and/or an unlimited fine.

Supply—up to life imprisonment and/or an unlimited fine.

Class B

- Cannabis
- Amphetamines (excluding methamphetamine)
- Methylphenidate (Ritalin®)
- Ketamine
- Codeine
- Cathinone derivatives—including mephedrone

Possession—up to 5 years' imprisonment and/or an unlimited fine.

Supply—up to 14 years' imprisonment and/or an unlimited fine.

Class C

- Minor tranquillizers and sedatives
- Benzodiazepines
- Khat
- GHB (gamma hydroxybutyrate)
- Anabolic steroids

Possession—up to 2 years' imprisonment and/or an unlimited fine.

Supply—up to 14 years' imprisonment and/or an unlimited fine.

Contains public sector information licensed under the Open Government Licence v3.0, http://www.nationalarchives.gov.uk/doc/open-government-licence/version/3/.

- supplying or offering to supply a controlled drug;
- allowing premises you occupy or manage to be used unlawfully for the purpose of producing or supplying controlled drugs.

The field of substance misuse is ever changing, with new psychoactive compounds appearing on the market with increasing frequency. The **Psychoactive Substances Act 2016** has been passed to try and control the widespread use of these novel psychoactive substances or 'legal highs'. The Act has made it an offence to produce, supply, or offer to supply *any* psychoactive substance if the substance is likely to be used for its psychoactive effects and regardless of its potential for harm. The only exemptions from the Act are those substances already controlled by the Misuse of Drugs Act: nicotine, alcohol, caffeine, and medicinal products. The act has not made individual possession of a psychoactive substance illegal (except in custodial institutions), but it covers importation, supply, and production with the aim of reducing availability of these compounds, and sentences range from 1 to 7 years' imprisonment.

The penalties do not relate to individuals holding a valid prescription or licence for the drug (e.g. heroin as diamorphine may be prescribed by a doctor). In the UK, it is the patient's responsibility to inform the Driver and Vehicle Licensing Agency (DVLA) of 'any disability likely to affect safe driving', which includes drug misuse. Since 2000, legislation called Drug Testing and Treatment Orders allow a court to order a person with a drug problem to undergo treatment and follow-up in the community for up to 3 years. This includes urine drug toxicology.

The harms associated with taking psychoactive substances

There are a variety of potential problems associated with taking substances. These are discussed in further detail under the specific sections for each substance, but Table 29.2 shows the general types of problems that commonly occur. It is rare for one negative effect of a drug to occur in isolation; frequently if the person is being physically affected by their drug usage, it is likely they will be dependent upon the substance and that it will be having social consequences too.

The stages of change model in relation to substance misuse

Much of the way in which we approach the treatment of problems relating to drug usage is based upon the

Table 29.2 Categories of harm associated with taking substances

Physical damage	Relating to dependence	Social harm
Acute: harms following a single dose of the drug (e.g. respiratory depression from opioids)	**Intensity of pleasure:** highly pleasurable drugs tend to fetch a higher street value. Smoking or IV injection of drugs creates the fastest effects but requires stronger, more dangerous formulations	**Intoxication:** harm or damage to property and people due to a single drug use (e.g. violence or car accidents due to alcohol)
Chronic: harms due to long-term or regular drug use (e.g. lung cancer caused by tobacco)		**Social harms:** destruction of the individual's social circle, family, and personal achievements
IV drug use: highest risk of acute toxicity and secondary harms; (e.g. blood-borne viruses (HIV, hepatitis) or abscesses)	**Physical dependence and tolerance:** needing drugs in ever higher doses to avoid withdrawal	**Cost to the economy:** unemployment or poor productivity, the police, and the cost to health service providers can be very high
	Psychological dependence: intense cravings	

concept that there are stages of change. It is therefore helpful to understand this idea before moving on to the descriptions of managing specific substance problems. The stages of change model was developed in the late 1970s by DiClemente and Prochaska and was based on work studying how cigarette smokers could give up the habit. It relates to any behaviour on which humans become dependent, but is most commonly used in alcohol and opioid misuse or weight loss/eating disorder programmes. The premise is that deciding to stop using the substance is a behavioural change, and that behavioural change only occurs via a series of steps rather than one leap. Each person progresses through these steps (or stages) at their own pace. The five stages of change (shown in Fig. 29.1) are as follows:

- **Precontemplation.** Not yet acknowledging that there is a problem behaviour that needs to be changed. At this stage the person is not interested in any form of help, and any imposed treatment will not be successful.
- **Contemplation.** Acknowledging that there is a problem but not yet ready or sure of wanting to make a change. These individuals are usually open to receiving more education about the risks of their behaviour, and will consider the advantages and disadvantages of making a change.

- **Preparation.** Getting ready to change. The person has made a commitment to change, and will research methods of doing so.
- **Action.** Changing behaviour. This is the time when people are usually open to receiving help, and may seek support in doing so.
- **Maintenance.** Maintaining the behaviour change, and successfully avoiding any temptation to return to old habits.
- **Relapse.** Returning to older behaviours and abandoning the new changes. This may then link back into precontemplation to complete the cycle.

The majority of individuals with a substance misuse problem will go around the cycle many times before entering a stable state. They may learn to recognize the pitfalls that led them to relapse on a previous occasion, and reduce their chance of doing so again. Understanding what stage your patient is at is essential for determining if they are likely to engage with treatment, deciding what support is appropriate, and having realistic expectations of the outcome.

Alcohol-related problems

There are at least 2 billion users of alcohol worldwide, making it a major global public health concern.

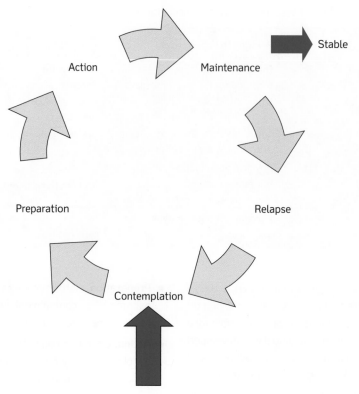

Fig. 29.1 The stages of change model.

What is a safe level of alcohol consumption?

There is probably no safe level of alcohol intake. The current recommendation is that all adults should limit themselves to **up to 14 units per week**. This amount should not be drunk all in one go, and there should be occasional drink-free days. One 'unit' of alcohol represents 8 g of ethanol, and corresponds to:

- half a pint of beer (3–4 per cent);
- a wine glass of wine (125 ml);
- a sherry glass of sherry or other fortified wine (50 ml);
- a standard measure of spirits (25 ml).

Alcohol consumption in the population

Reliable epidemiological data are difficult to obtain because people tend to underestimate both the amount they drink and the consequences of their drinking. Since 1945, the absolute quantity of alcohol consumed in Britain has increased threefold, although in the past 10 years there has been an increase in the percentage of adults who consume no alcohol (15 per cent). In 2014, approximately 14 per cent of the UK adult population drank above recommended limits, and 5 per cent were alcohol dependent. Overall problems relating to alcohol are more common in men than in women, although the gap is gradually closing. Excessive binge-drinking is most likely in young males, but alcohol problems are most common in those aged 30–50 years.

The rates of dangerous consumption of alcohol are much increased among people working in occupations that provide easy access to alcohol; for example, bar workers, brewery workers, and kitchen porters. They are also higher among executives, salespeople, journalists, actors, and others whose work is associated with social drinking. Doctors also have high rates of dangerous consumption.

There is marked international variation in alcohol consumption. Mediterranean countries frequently have higher rates of consumption than the UK (although this tends to be taken as regular daily drinks rather than as 'binges') whereas almost 50 per cent of adults globally— often in developing countries or for religious beliefs reasons—have never drunk any alcohol. Generally the wealth of a nation is proportional to the percentage of adults that drink alcohol. Typically the amount of alcohol consumed in a population is normally distributed, therefore population-based interventions to reduce intake should decrease both the amount individuals are drinking and the number of drinkers at dangerous levels.

Terminology

Although the term **alcoholism** is widely used in everyday speech, it has too vague a meaning to be clinically useful. The following terms constitute more useful categories:

- **Intoxication.** The immediate physical and mental effects of drinking alcohol.
- **Hazardous drinking** is a level or pattern of drinking that will eventually cause harm. It applies to anyone drinking above the recommended limits, but without current alcohol-related problems.
- **Harmful use** refers to a pattern of drinking that has already caused acute or chronic physical, mental, or social damage to the user.
- **Dependence syndrome.** There are seven characteristics of dependence upon alcohol, at least three of which must have been present in the previous year to make a diagnosis:
  1 Tolerance, as defined by either of the following:
     (a) a need for markedly increased amounts of alcohol to achieve intoxication or the desired effect;
     (b) a markedly diminished effect with continued use of the same amount of alcohol.
  2 Withdrawal, as defined by either of the following:
     (a) the characteristic withdrawal syndrome for alcohol;

  (b) alcohol is taken to relieve or avoid withdrawal symptoms.
  3 Alcohol is often taken in larger amounts or over a longer period than was intended.
  4 There is a persistent desire for or there are unsuccessful efforts to cut down or control alcohol use.
  5 A great deal of time is spent in activities necessary to obtain alcohol, use alcohol, or recover from its effects.
  6 Important social, occupational, or recreational activities are given up or reduced because of alcohol use.
  7 Alcohol use is continued despite knowledge of having a persistent or recurrent physical or psychological problem that is likely to have been caused or exacerbated by the alcohol.

Alcohol-related harm

Consumption of alcohol can lead to three types of harm: physical, neuropsychiatric, and social. There is potential for harm at any level of drinking.

Acute intoxication. Symptoms of alcohol intoxication relate jointly to the level of alcohol in the blood and the tolerance of the individual. Increasing blood alcohol levels lead to elated or unstable mood, impaired judgement, disinhibition, cognitive impairment, ataxia, slurred speech, incoordination, nystagmus, and eventually coma. This state leads to an increased risk of accidents (especially road traffic accidents), violence, and public order offences.

Physical effects of alcohol abuse

The main physical consequences of dangerous use of alcohol are shown in Table 29.3. From these, the overall **mortality rate** of subjects consuming dangerous levels of alcohol is at least twice the expected level.

Fetal alcohol syndrome

It was recognized that alcohol could adversely affect the developing fetus in the mid 1960s. Heavy

Table 29.3 Physical effects of the excessive use of alcohol

Gastrointestinal	• Gastritis and peptic ulcers
	• Acute pancreatitis
	• Chronic pancreatitis—*5% of dependent drinkers, presents with weight loss, steatorrhoea, and diabetes mellitus*
	• Fatty liver, hepatitis, and cirrhosis—*80% of cirrhosis deaths are due to alcohol*
	• Oesophageal varices
	• Malnutrition and vitamin deficiencies (B_1 (thiamine), A, D, B_6, E, and folate)
	• Carcinomas: hepatocellular, oesophageal, and oropharyngeal
Neurological	• Wernicke's encephalopathy
	• Korsakoff's syndrome
	• Peripheral neuropathy
	• Cerebellar degeneration
	• Dementia
	• Epilepsy
	• Fetal alcohol syndrome
Other	• Cardiovascular: hypertension, dilated cardiomyopathy
	• Metabolic: episodic hypoglycaemia, obesity or emaciation
	• Haematological: anaemia, thrombocytopenia, and leucopenia; haemochromatosis
	• Musculoskeletal: myopathy, osteoporosis, osteomalacia, gout
	• Skin: facial erythema, exacerbation of psoriasis

drinking during pregnancy may cause a syndrome of facial abnormality, growth retardation, muscular incoordination, low intelligence, and hyperactivity known as **fetal alcohol syndrome**. It is unclear if the risk is exactly dose dependent or partly idiosyncratic. It is prudent to advise pregnant women to abstain from alcohol throughout pregnancy.

Neuropsychiatric disorders due to alcohol abuse

See Table 29.4.

Intoxication and withdrawal

Alcohol-induced amnesia (memory blackouts). This is loss of memory for events that occurred during a period of intoxication. Such episodes can occur after a single episode of heavy drinking in people who do not habitually abuse alcohol. When they occur regularly they indicate frequent heavy drinking; when they are prolonged, affecting the greater part of a day or whole days, they indicate sustained excessive drinking.

Idiosyncratic intoxication (or pathological drunkenness) is a marked change of behaviour occurring within minutes of taking alcohol in amounts that would not induce drunkenness in most people. Often, the behaviour is aggressive.

Alcohol withdrawal

Withdrawal symptoms characteristically appear on waking, after the fall in blood alcohol concentration

Table 29.4 Neuropsychiatric effects of the excessive use of alcohol

Intoxication states	• Memory blackouts
	• Idiosyncratic intoxication
Withdrawal states	• Simple and complex withdrawal
	• Delirium tremens
Toxic and nutritional states	• Korsakov's syndrome
	• Wernicke's encephalopathy
	• Alcoholic dementia
Perceptual disturbances	• Transient hallucinations
	• Alcoholic hallucinosis
Neurological conditions	• Cerebellar degeneration
	• Marchiafava–Bignami syndrome
Associated states	• Depressive disorder
	• Anxiety symptoms
	• Suicide and deliberate self-harm
	• Personality change
	• Pathological jealousy
	• Sexual dysfunction

during sleep. The earliest and commonest feature is acute tremor ('the shakes'). The person may be agitated and easily startled, suffering nausea, retching, and sweating. If more alcohol is drunk, these symptoms are usually relieved quickly; if not, they may last for several days. As withdrawal progresses, misperceptions and hallucinations may briefly occur. Objects appear distorted in shape, or shadows seem to move; disorganized voices, shouting, or snatches of music may be heard. Later there may be epileptic seizures, and finally, after about 48 hours, **delirium tremens** may develop.

Delirium tremens

This is a severe form of withdrawal syndrome that occurs when the patient is physically dependent on alcohol. The features are as follows:

1 **Delirium:** clouding of consciousness, disorientation in time and place, impairment of recent memory, illusions and hallucinations, fearfulness, and agitation.

2 Physical symptoms: **gross tremor** of the hands (which gives the condition its name), **ataxia**, **autonomic disturbance** (sweating, tachycardia, raised blood pressure, dilation of the pupils), and marked **insomnia**. There may also be fever.

3 **Hallucinations** are characteristically visual and often frightening, involving Lilliputian people or animals. Auditory and tactile hallucinations also occur.

4 **Dehydration and electrolyte disturbance** are characteristic. Blood testing shows leucocytosis, raised erythrocyte sedimentation rate, and impaired liver function.

Delirium tremens usually lasts 3–4 days. As in other kinds of delirium, the symptoms are characteristically worse at night. It has a mortality rate of up to 5 per cent. Treatment should be with a reducing regimen of benzodiazepine (see p. 448) combined with the general measures for treating delirium on p. 365.

Toxic and nutritional conditions

There are three neuropsychiatric disorders of this kind: (1) **Wernicke's encephalopathy**, (2) **Korsakoff's syndrome**, and (3) **alcoholic dementia**.

Wernicke's encephalopathy

Wernicke's encephalopathy is an acute-onset degenerative encephalopathy due to thiamine deficiency. The deficiency results from a combination of poor nutritional intake, reduced absorption, decreased hepatic storage, and impaired usage. It is occasionally seen in non-alcoholics; for example, anorexia nervosa, hyperemesis gravidarum, starvation, or post-gastric resection. Wernicke's is characterized by haemorrhages and secondary gliosis in the periventricular and periaqueductal grey matter, which causes damage to the structures surrounding them. The worst affected areas are the hypothalamus, midbrain, and cerebellar peduncles. Clinically, Wernicke's presents

Box 29.3 Treatment of Wernicke's encephalopathy

- Admit as an inpatient to a general hospital setting with resuscitation facilities.
- Give high-dose parenteral B vitamins for 3–7 days. Typically two ampoules of Pabrinex® (500 mg thiamine) are given IV three times daily.
- There is a high risk of anaphylaxis with Pabrinex® IV, reduced by giving intramuscularly. The patient should be closely monitored.
- Treat withdrawal with a benzodiazepine reducing regimen.
- If the patient responds, continue Pabrinex® until the improvement ceases. If there is no response, stop the treatment.
- Continue oral thiamine 100 mg three times daily for at least a month.

as a tetrad of **acute confusion**, **ophthalmoplegia**, **nystagmus**, and **ataxia**. The patient may also develop an acute peripheral neuropathy, and tachycardia. This is an emergency presentation, the treatment of which is shown in Box 29.3. Prevention of Wernicke's is simple: adequate provision of thiamine. Patients with an alcohol problem should be advised to take vitamin B supplements, and those undergoing detoxification prescribed high-dose prophylaxis.

Korsakoff's syndrome (amnesic syndrome)

About 80 per cent of people who have Wernicke's encephalopathy go on to develop Korsakoff's syndrome, but it may also occur independently. The central features of Korsakoff's syndrome are retrograde and anterograde amnesia, especially a profound impairment of recent memory. The patient can recall events immediately after they have occurred, but cannot do so even a few minutes afterwards. Thus, on the standard clinical test of remembering an address, immediate recall is good, but grossly impaired 10 minutes later. One consequence of the profound disorder of memory is an associated disorientation in time. Gaps in memory are often filled by **confabulation**. The patient may give a vivid and detailed account of recent activities that, on checking, turn out to be inaccurate.

Such a patient is often suggestible and therefore vulnerable. Other cognitive functions are relatively well preserved. Unlike the patient with dementia, the patient with an amnesic syndrome seems alert and able to reason or hold an ordinary conversation, so that the interviewer may at first be unaware of the extent of the memory disorder. The aetiology is not clear, but may be partly due to thiamine deficiency. Long-term thiamine replacement is therefore recommended. About 75 per cent of patients will have static memory impairment, while the other 25 per cent are split equally into those who slightly improve and those who decline in a stepwise process.

Alcoholic dementia

Alcoholic dementia can arise after prolonged, heavy intake of alcohol. Intellectual impairment is often associated with enlarged ventricles and widened cerebral sulci, as seen on a CT scan. After prolonged abstinence, some gradual improvement occurs in these changes, suggesting that the shrinkage is not wholly due to the loss of the brain cells. The causes of the dementia are uncertain but probably include a direct toxic effect of alcohol on the brain, and secondary effects of liver disease.

Perceptual disturbances

Transient hallucinations of vision or hearing are reported by some heavy drinkers, generally during withdrawal, but without all the features of delirium tremens or alcoholic hallucinosis.

Alcoholic hallucinosis is a rare condition characterized by distressing auditory hallucinations (usually of voices uttering threats) occurring in clear consciousness. Some patients argue aloud with the voices, others feel compelled to follow instructions from them. Delusional misinterpretations may follow, often of a persecutory kind, so that the clinical picture can resemble schizophrenia. The condition can arise while the person is still drinking heavily, or when intake has been reduced. It is of variable duration and if chronic needs to be distinguished from a primary schizophrenic disorder. It usually responds to antipsychotics and has a good prognosis. The symptoms may reoccur if drinking resumes.

Cerebellar degeneration

Alcohol is directly toxic to the Purkinje cells of the cerebellar cortex. Destruction of these cells leads to a chronic cerebellar atrophy in about 40 per cent of chronic alcoholics. Patients present with severe limb ataxia, dysarthria, poor coordination, slurred speech, and occasionally nystagmus.

Associated psychiatric disorders

- **Depressive disorder** may be induced by drinking as alcohol is a central nervous system depressant. However, depressed patients sometimes drink heavily to relieve their symptoms, so care needs to be taken to find out the sequence of changes. In alcohol dependence, 80 per cent of patients fit diagnostic criteria for depression. Many will recover without treatment if they remain abstinent, otherwise an antidepressant may be beneficial.

- **Anxiety symptoms** occur frequently, especially during periods of partial withdrawal. However, some patients with a primary anxiety disorder use alcohol to relieve their symptoms, so, as with depression, care is needed to determine the sequence.

- **Suicidal behaviour and deliberate self-harm** are more frequent among people who use alcohol heavily. Estimates of the proportion of harmful users of alcohol who eventually kill themselves vary from 6 to 20 per cent.

- **Personality change** in heavy users of alcohol often includes self-centredness, lack of concern for others, and a decline in standards of conduct (particularly honesty and responsibility).

- **Pathological jealousy (Othello's syndrome)** is an infrequent but serious complication of heavy alcohol use.

- **Sexual dysfunction** is common, usually as erectile dysfunction or delayed ejaculation. The causes include the direct effects of alcohol and a generally impaired relationship with the sexual partner as a result of heavy drinking.

Social damage due to alcohol

Excessive drinking can cause serious social damage, including:

- poor work performance and sickness absence;
- unemployment;
- violence and aggressive behaviour;
- accidental damage;
- road accidents: in the UK about a third of drivers killed on the road have blood alcohol levels above the statutory limit;
- crime, mainly social disorder and petty offences, but also fraud, sexual offences, and crimes of violence including murder;
- emotional and conduct problems in the patient's children;
- healthcare costs tend to be extremely high: alcohol is implicated in 50–70 per cent of emergency room admissions and 16 per cent of total hospital admissions.

Co-morbidities

The majority of psychiatric disorders are more common in patients with alcohol problems, and the issue is clouded by alcohol being a causative factor in many of them too. Frequent co-morbidities include:

- depression;
- anxiety disorders;
- suicide (4 per cent lifetime risk in harmful use, 15 per cent in dependency) and deliberate self-harm;
- schizophrenia (plus 20 per cent of those with schizophrenia have an alcohol problem);
- substance misuse: people may take substances either to enhance the positive aspects of alcohol or reduce the unpleasant side effects; benzodiazepines are a particular risk, especially

given the relative ease of obtaining them on prescription to avoid withdrawal;

- eating disorders: up to half of patients with an eating disorder misuse alcohol, especially those with bulimia nervosa.

Aetiology

As with most psychiatric conditions, the cause of an alcohol problem in a given individual is likely to be multifactorial and highly related to the time and context. Some of the simple social reasons why people may drink alcohol were discussed in the introductory section on p. 425. The best way to consider the aetiology of alcoholism is via the biopsychosocial model (Box 29.4).

Assessment and treatment of people with alcohol problems

Screening for alcohol use problems

In the UK, 20 per cent of patients attending primary care appointments and up to 30 per cent of hospital inpatients drink more than the recommended weekly limits of alcohol. The simplest method of screening is to ask the patient how much alcohol they drink per week, and try to calculate the units consumed from this. Given the answer to this question, and considering the high-risk groups for alcohol misuse (Box 29.5), further screening questionnaires can then be used.

Questionnaires are the standard method for identifying alcohol use disorders. In primary care,

Box 29.4 Aetiology of alcohol use problems

Biological

- Genetic factors:
  - Heritability of 40–60 per cent
  - Concordance between monozygotic twins of 48 per cent and dizygotic twins of 32 per cent
  - Gene linkage studies have identified genes that are associated with alcohol problems, for example, alcohol dehydrogenase, monoamine oxidase, the serotonin transporter, and $GABA_A$ receptor. Polymorphisms in genes that metabolize alcohol (e.g. aldehyde dehydrogenase, *ALDH2*) tend to carry a lower risk of alcohol problems than the wild type
- Variations in alcohol metabolism:
  - Metabolism is primarily by alcohol dehydrogenase (ADH) and aldehyde dehydrogenase (ALDH). There are polymorphisms and variants of ADH which produce a quicker breakdown.
  - An inactive form of ALDH (*ALDH*2*) is carried by about half of Asian people; this leads to a build-up of aldehyde on ingestion of alcohol. Vomiting, flushing, and tachycardia ensue, which tend to cause homozygous individuals to avoid alcohol.

- Individual responses to alcohol:
  - Those who are more sensitive to alcohol tend to drink less
  - There may be an association between alcohol dependence and the D_2 receptor
- Family history of substance abuse
- Intrauterine exposure to drugs and alcohol

Psychological

- Risk taking or anxious personality traits
- Psychiatric problems in childhood (e.g. conduct disorder and abuse)
- Co-morbid psychiatric disorders: anxiety disorders, depression, or ADHD

Social

- Laws affecting availability and price of alcohol
- Cultural attitudes and practices
- Peer pressure and/or role models
- Economic situation and employment
- Level of education
- Behaviour within the family unit
- Divorce or relationship problems

Box 29.5 High-risk groups for alcohol problems

- Patients with psychiatric co-morbidities
- Personal or family history of alcohol misuse
- History of conduct disorder, ADHD, or antisocial personality disorder
- Relationship or sexual problems
- Legal difficulties
- Unemployment or repeated absences from work
- Emotional or behavioural issues with the patient's children
- Patients presenting with gastritis, peptic ulcer, liver disease, peripheral neuropathy, seizures (especially those starting in middle life), and repeated falls among the elderly

the **Alcohol Use Disorders Identification Test** (**AUDIT**) can be used (Box 29.6). A cut-off score of five on this questionnaire has a sensitivity of 84 per cent, a specificity of 90 per cent, and a likelihood ratio for a positive result of 8.4. The briefer **CAGE Questionnaire** is probably less sensitive but more specific; a score of three or more has a specificity of almost 100 per cent. If the screening questions raise the possibility of an alcohol problem, a full assessment of the patient should be made. This can usually be managed in primary care if there are no physical or significant psychiatric complications arising at that time.

Assessment

A full psychiatric history should be taken to screen for co-morbidities as well as details of alcohol intake.

History that is suggestive of alcohol dependence syndrome includes:

- drinking upon waking (relief drinking) to stave off withdrawal symptoms;
- secrecy over amount of alcohol consumed;
- preference for cheap forms of alcohol (e.g. cider);
- stereotyped pattern of drinking: minimal variation in amount and type of alcohol consumption day-to-day;

- if the person has become abstinent but then takes a drink, they quickly return to their old drinking patterns (reinstatement after abstinence).

Find out about the impact of alcohol upon physical health, work performance, family life, and any current legal problems. Always ask about dependent children. Record any previous treatments and how successful they were. Assess the patients' willingness for change.

A detailed physical examination is essential, both to identify harm already caused by alcohol and to predict future problems. It should concentrate on looking for signs of liver disease, malnutrition, neurological signs, and problems with cognition.

Appropriate basic investigations should be carried out. The most simple and useful are blood tests for markers that change in the context of heavy alcohol intake. Markers may also be used to monitor response to treatment. In addition, it is worth checking a full blood count, U&Es, creatinine, haematinics, and lipid profile.

1 **Blood alcohol** concentration estimation using a breathalyser is the most direct measure, although this does not distinguish between a single recent episode of heavy drinking and chronic abuse.

2 **Gamma-glutamyltranspeptidase** levels are raised in about 80 per cent of people with drinking problems. It has a sensitivity and specificity of about 60 per cent.

3 **Mean corpuscular volume** is increased in about 60 per cent of people with drinking problems.

4 **Carbohydrate-deficient transferrin.** Transferrin is a glycoprotein that binds iron tightly for transportation. The proportion of carbohydrate on the transferrin structure varies with alcohol intake. A value of greater than 20 units per litre indicates heavy drinking, and has a sensitivity of 75 per cent and a specificity of 90 per cent.

5 **Urate levels** are raised in about half of all people with drinking problems, but they are only useful as screening tests for men as they are poor discriminators in women.

Box 29.6 Alcohol Use Disorders Identification Test (AUDIT)

1 How often do you have a drink containing alcohol?
   (0) Never
   (1) Monthly or less
   (2) 2–4 times a month
   (3) 2 or 3 times a week
   (4) 4 or more times a week

2 How many drinks containing alcohol do you have on a typical day when you are drinking?
   (0) 1 or 2
   (1) 3 or 4
   (2) 5 or 6
   (3) 7 to 9
   (4) 10 or more

3 How often do you have six or more drinks on one occasion?
   (0) Never
   (1) Less than monthly
   (2) Monthly
   (3) Weekly
   (4) Daily or almost daily

4 How often during the past year have you found that you were not able to stop drinking once you had started?
   (0) Never
   (1) Less than monthly
   (2) Monthly
   (3) Weekly
   (4) Daily or almost daily

5 How often during the past year have you failed to do what was normally expected of you because of drinking?
   (0) Never
   (1) Less than monthly
   (2) Monthly
   (3) Weekly
   (4) Daily or almost daily

6 How often during the past year have you needed a first drink in the morning to get yourself going after a heavy drinking session?
   (0) Never
   (1) Less than monthly
   (2) Monthly
   (3) Weekly
   (4) Daily or almost daily

7 How often during the past year have you had a feeling of guilt or remorse after drinking?
   (0) Never
   (1) Less than monthly
   (2) Monthly
   (3) Weekly
   (4) Daily or almost daily

8 How often during the past year have you been unable to remember what happened the night before because you had been drinking?
   (0) Never
   (1) Less than monthly
   (2) Monthly
   (3) Weekly
   (4) Daily or almost daily

9 Have you or has someone else been injured as a result of your drinking?
   (0) No
   (2) Yes, but not in the past year
   (4) Yes, during the last year

10 Has a relative or friend or a doctor or other health worker been concerned about your drinking or suggested that you cut down?
   (0) No
   (2) Yes, but not in the past year
   (4) Yes, during the last year

The score is the number in brackets for each answer; more than 5 suggests an alcohol use disorder, and more than 8 suggests alcohol dependence.

6 **Liver function tests.** Alanine and aspartate aminotransferases increase in heavy drinking, and represent hepatocellular damage.

Treatment of people with alcohol problems

Alcohol use disorders should be viewed as a chronic relapsing and remitting condition; success may not come first time around. An initial first step for all is a thorough enquiry into drinking habits and related problems. This is not only a way of detecting the harmful user of alcohol, but also a first step in treatment because it helps the patient to recognize the extent and seriousness of their problem. This recognition is needed as a means of motivating the patient to control their drinking. Without such motivation, treatment will fail.

There are four steps in the basic approach to managing alcohol problems (Box 29.7):

1 Assessment.

2 Psychoeducation and motivational therapy.

3 Safe withdrawal from alcohol.

4 Relapse prevention and treatment of underlying issues.

When to obtain specialist help

Most problem drinkers can be treated in primary care. The main reasons for referral to a specialist are:

1 severe withdrawal symptoms, especially fits or delirium tremens, which should be treated as emergencies;

2 planned withdrawal from alcohol when home withdrawal is inappropriate;

3 medical or psychiatric complications requiring specialist assessment;

4 complex personal or interpersonal problems requiring more intensive psychological treatment than simple counselling.

Box 29.7 Treatment options for a patient with an alcohol problem

Assessment
- Extent of drinking, evidence for dependence, alcohol-related disabilities, and co-morbidities
- Arrange medical treatment for physical complications
- Arrange psychiatric treatment for mental health problems

Psychoeducation
- Safe drinking advice
- Education for patient and family
- Help with 'SMART' goal-setting

Motivation for change
- Brief interventions
- Motivational interviewing (extended brief interventions)
- Self-help materials

Safe withdrawal
- Community based: benzodiazepines and oral thiamine
- Inpatient based: benzodiazepines and parenteral thiamine, and management of complications

Relapse prevention and treatment of underlying issues
- Outpatient follow-up or CBT
- Residential or day-patient programmes
- 12-step programmes (e.g. AA)
- Marital or family therapy
- Medications: disulfiram, acamprosate, naltrexone, and nalmefene
- Ongoing vitamin supplementation (including thiamine)
- Antidepressants for depression or anxiety disorders
- Assistance with employment, accommodation, and legal issues

Abstinence versus controlled drinking

It is important to decide whether to aim for total abstinence from alcohol or for controlled drinking. Abstinence is the most appropriate goal for people with harmful use of alcohol, including dependence. However, not all such patients will accept this goal; they either refuse treatment or report abstinence while continuing to drink alcohol. Controlled drinking is **not** a suitable goal for those patients who:

- have previously been alcohol dependent;
- had a previous failure of controlled drinking;
- have serious psychiatric co-morbidity;
- have incurred serious physical consequences of drinking that require abstinence;
- are in a job (such as heavy goods vehicle driving) that carries a risk to others;
- are pregnant.

Reduction to the recommended 14 units per week should be in achievable stages, say 5 or 10 units a week, but the process should not be so prolonged that motivation is lost. If it becomes obvious that this technique is not working, abstinence should be aimed for immediately.

Psychoeducation for the patient and family

The patient and family should be fully informed of the dangers of alcohol and the impact that alcohol has already had on the patient and family. It is important to avoid confrontation and aggression during treatment, so some interpersonal skills may need to be taught. Occasionally, family members are unable to help in the patient's recovery; in this case, it may be necessary to ask the family to step back and allow other people to help in the short term. Self-help materials based on motivational techniques, CBT, and 12-step programmes are frequently helpful for all concerned.

Motivation for change

There are a variety of techniques for helping to move a precontemplative or contemplative patient into

Box 29.8 FRAMES: a brief intervention for alcohol use disorders

- Structured **feedback** about personal risks
- Emphasis on it being the patient's **responsibility** to make changes
- **Advice** to cut down or cease drinking
- **Menu** of options for making changes to the drinking pattern
- Being **empathetic** in interviewing
- Reinforcing a patient's **self-efficacy** for change

Reproduced from *Behavioural and Cognitive Psychotherapy*, 21, 4, Bein TH, Miller WR, and Boroughs JM, Motivational interviewing with alcoholic outpatients, pp. 347–56. © British Association for Behavioural and Cognitive Psychotherapies 1993.

the next part of the cycle of change. It may be that the discussion in the earlier sections is adequate to motivate change, but frequently another intervention is needed. In systematic reviews, motivation enhancement techniques alone have similar outcomes to CBT and Alcoholics Anonymous (AA) programmes.

The simplest intervention is called a **brief intervention** and can be delivered easily by any trained health professional in a few minutes. It involves giving simple, structured advice that aims to reduce alcohol intake to less dangerous levels.

Extended brief interventions take approximately 30 minutes, and are based on motivational interviewing. They use the FRAMES acronym to provide the tools for change and strategies for making changes dealing with underlying issues (Box 29.8). They are best administered by a trained alcohol support worker.

Withdrawal from alcohol: detoxification

When the patient is dependent on alcohol, a sudden cessation of drinking may cause severe withdrawal symptoms (including delirium tremens or seizures), so detoxification should be carried out under medical supervision. The treatment is a combination of long-acting benzodiazepines and B vitamins.

Benzodiazepines work in two ways: firstly by reducing the risk of complications, and secondly by decreasing the cravings, tremor, anxiety, insomnia, and nausea that occur during withdrawal. Chlordiazepoxide is the drug of choice, because it has a long half-life and less ability to be abused than diazepam.

Withdrawal in the community

RCTs have shown that in less severe cases, and where there is no significant physical illness or history of previous withdrawal seizures, withdrawal can be done safely at home provided that there is support. The GP should supply benzodiazepines according to a reducing regimen (see next subsection) and oral thiamine plus a multivitamin.

Withdrawal in hospital

Patients with severe dependence, previous withdrawal seizures or delirium tremens, failed outpatient detoxification, or no social support need hospital admission for detoxification. They should be treated with a reducing regimen of chlordiazepoxide, such as:

- day 1: 20 mg chlordiazepoxide four times daily;
- day 2: 15 mg chlordiazepoxide four times daily;
- day 3: 10 mg chlordiazepoxide four times daily;
- day 4: 5 mg chlordiazepoxide four times daily;
- day 5: 5 mg chlordiazepoxide twice daily;
- 'as needed' doses may be added up to a maximum of 200 mg per day.

Patients with seizures or delirium tremens may need higher doses for longer, with a course of about 2 weeks in total. Metoclopramide is the most effective antiemetic in withdrawal. All patients should receive high-dose B vitamins, following local guidelines, either oral thiamine or parenteral Pabrinex®. Seizures are best treated by giving 10 mg diazepam, which may need to be doubled in those who are already taking benzodiazepines. Starting an anticonvulsant is not recommended. Patients with delirium tremens may need parenteral benzodiazepine and an antipsychotic.

Relapse prevention and treatment of underlying problems

There is little point in detoxification if it is not followed up with support to maintain abstinence and work upon the reasons behind the alcohol problem. The options available for further treatment divide into two main groups:

1 Psychological treatments:
   (a) Outpatient follow-up or CBT.
   (b) Residential or day-patient programmes.
   (c) 12-step programmes (e.g. AA).
   (d) Marital or family therapy.
2 Pharmacological treatments:
   (a) Medications to prevent relapse: disulfiram, acamprosate, and naltrexone.
   (b) Ongoing vitamin supplementation.
   (c) Antidepressants (or other medications) for psychiatric co-morbidities.

Psychological treatments

A range of different psychological therapies and interventions are available; there is no evidence that one is consistently superior in efficacy. Individual CBT can be effective in maintaining changes in behaviour. Anger management and relaxation therapy can also be beneficial. All of these types of therapy can also be administered in a group setting, as this provides the opportunity to learn through role play and role models.

If a more intensive form of treatment is required to prevent relapse, then a day-patient or residential rehabilitation programme may be indicated. In the UK, such treatment is rarely available because residential programmes have not been shown to be cost-effective, or to have a higher success rate at maintaining long-term abstinence than community-based programmes. In other countries, and in the private sector, these therapeutic programmes and communities may be accessible. The advantage of this treatment is that it removes the opportunity to drink in the early stages, and provides intensive individual and group therapy. Often working with a peer group who support one another to work through problems can be very helpful. Residential treatment may also be indicated if the patient has complex psychiatric co-morbidities (e.g. severe anorexia nervosa or depression).

There are a variety of self-help groups for people with alcohol-related problems, which can be very useful in helping to maintain motivation. Patients with alcohol problems often find it easier to talk to others who have had similar problems. **AA** is the largest organization, with 90,000 groups worldwide, and holds group meetings based on a 12-step programme. The programme views alcoholism as a chronic condition only cured by total abstinence. At the meetings, members will introduce themselves to one another, talk about their problems, and gain support from other members. Individuals work through the 12 steps at their own pace, discussing their progress with the group each week. Those who remain in the organization are usually helped, and anyone with a drink problem should be encouraged to try it.

Doctors have higher than average rates of alcohol problems, and they too often have difficulty in admitting their problems and seeking help, especially from colleagues working in the same area. In some countries, including the UK, arrangements exist for doctors to obtain help outside their area of work, through a national scheme for sick doctors (their website is http://www.sick-doctors-trust.co.uk).

Pharmacological treatments

Disulfiram (Antabuse®: 100–200 mg/day) is used, usually in specialist practice, as a deterrent to impulsive drinking. It interferes with the metabolism of alcohol by irreversibly blocking acetaldehyde dehydrogenase. As a result, when alcohol is taken acetaldehyde accumulates with consequent flushing, headache, choking sensations, rapid pulse, and anxiety. These unpleasant effects discourage the patient from drinking alcohol while taking the drug. Treatment with disulfiram carries the occasional risks of cardiac complications so the drug should not be started until at least 12 hours after the last ingestion of alcohol. Disulfiram has unpleasant side effects, including a persistent metallic taste in the mouth, gastrointestinal symptoms, dermatitis, urinary frequency, impotence, peripheral neuropathy, and toxic

confusional states (extremely rare). It should *not* be used in patients with recent heart disease, severe liver disease, or significant suicidal ideation. The main use of disulfiram is to provide the patient with time to recover confidence that they can manage life without alcohol; 6 months is the recommended prescription time. Single-blind studies (the patient must know they have taken the drug for it to work) show disulfiram to be effective in preventing relapse, and more so than acamprosate or naltrexone.

Acamprosate is a drug that enhances GABA transmission in the central nervous system. RCTs have shown it to reduce cravings for alcohol in patients with alcohol dependence. The usual dose is 666 mg three times daily, and is started 2–7 days after cessation of drinking. Patients who benefit from it should continue for 6 months to a year.

Naltrexone is an opiate antagonist, which inhibits the action of endogenous endorphins released when alcohol is drunk. It reduces the urge to drink, reduces the pleasurable 'high' produced by alcohol, and reduces the loss of control it causes. Short-term usage seems to reduce the risk of relapse, but is less effective than disulfiram. It is started once abstinence is achieved at 50 mg once daily. There is a small risk of hepatic toxicity if overused.

Nalmefene (Selincro®) is another opiate antagonist which was developed in the 1970s but has only recently accrued an adequate evidence base to be used widely for alcohol dependence. It has a similar effect to naltrexone but has a longer half-life and no hepatic toxicity. Side effects include nausea, dizziness, insomnia, and headache but are usually mild. Treatment is one 18 mg tablet daily, taken if the person if feeling the urge to drink.

Prognosis and the results of treatment

Alcohol misuse is associated with a 3.6-fold increased all-cause mortality rate when compared with age-matched controls. The risk of suicide is 10–15 per cent in patients with alcohol dependency for more than 5 years. For the majority of problem drinkers, brief interventions are as effective as more intensive treatments and a good proportion of patients improve or are cured. The results of treatment for patients with serious drinking problems are poor and the aim should therefore be the early detection and treatment of alcohol problems. It is important to maintain a helpful and non-judgemental attitude. Relapses should be viewed constructively and further help offered. Characteristics related to good outcome include strong motivation, good insight, and a supportive social and occupational structure.

Preventing alcohol-related harm

There are seven main ways in which alcohol problems in society may be reduced:

1 **Educate people,** effectively persuading them not to misuse alcohol. School-age education programmes are particularly important. Television and billboard adverts showing the harm alcohol may cause can deliver a striking message.

2 **Deter** harmful drinking with penalties. Laws on driving while intoxicated have massively reduced the number of road traffic accidents due to alcohol.

3 **Provide alternatives** to drinking alcohol and engaging in drink-related activities.

4 **Instigate harm-reduction strategies.** For example, the mandatory use of seatbelts, airbags, and low speed limits has reduced driving-related morbidity and mortality.

5 **Regulate the availability** of alcohol and its price. Increasing taxation on alcohol, limiting the hours it may be sold, and having a minimum age for purchase are all effective methods.

6 **Promote social, cultural, and religious movements** to reduce alcohol consumption.

7 **Treat individuals** who have alcohol-related problems.

Problems due to the use of psychoactive substances

In this chapter, we focus on the harmful effects of psychoactive substances to the user's health. The use of some of these substances is illegal in many countries. The use of others (e.g. nicotine) is legal despite the harmful medical consequences of smoking. It is important to distinguish between **harmful** use and **illegal** use of substances. The clinician's role should be directed at the former—to help the user overcome dependence and to avoid the adverse health consequences of psychoactive substance use. An explanation of the UK law surrounding illegal substance use is given on p. 425.

Epidemiology of psychoactive substance use

The extent of supply and consumption of drugs is often concealed because the possession of many drugs is illegal or socially unacceptable. Therefore, there are no reliable estimates of the extent of drug consumption in the population and it is hard to compare between countries. Some statistics are shown in Table 29.1 on p. 424.

In the UK, surveys of the general public suggest one-third of adults have used an illegal substance at least once in their lifetime, 25 per cent by the age of 16. The ratio of males to females using all substances is 3–4:1. Cannabis is the most commonly used illegal substance, accounting for about 80 per cent of those who admit to having used substances. Apart from alcohol, tobacco (nicotine) is the most frequently used legal substance, although its use has been declining in many developed nations. Unfortunately, worldwide the extent of psychoactive substance use seems to be increasing.

Patterns of substance misuse

There are a variety of different patterns of substance misuse seen in society:

• **Experimentation** is common among teenagers and students. Accessibility to substances and peer pressure promote usage, which aims to discover how the substance makes one feel. Cannabis, stimulants, and 'legal highs' are commonly taken, opioids and other 'harder' substances more rarely.

- **Use limited to particular situations.** Cannabis is frequently taken at house parties and as part of experimental sexual experiences, ecstasy and lysergic acid diethylamide (LSD) at nightclubs and raves.

- **Recreational use.** These groups of individuals regularly use substances (often a variety), but are not dependent upon them. A classic example would be the use of cannabis during university, which ceases once a career is begun and family life established.

- **Dependence.** A dependence syndrome develops, and substance use continues more to avoid the withdrawals than for the positive effects of the substance. The majority of the time only the dependent substance will be taken, but others may be substituted if the primary one is unavailable or the user is looking for a new experience. Opioids and benzodiazepines typically fall into this category.

- **Substance misuse combined with mental illness.** There are a group of individuals with substance problems who have a co-morbid psychiatric disorder. They may be using the substance to reduce their unwanted psychiatric symptoms or be particularly vulnerable to peer pressure.

Types of dependence

Not all people who use psychoactive substances become dependent on them. Dependence may be pharmacological or psychological, and the two may be mutually exclusive.

1 **Pharmacological dependence** is caused by changes in the receptors and other cellular mechanisms affected by the substance. Substances vary in the degree to which they cause pharmacological dependence: opioids and nicotine readily cause it; cannabis and hallucinogens are less likely to do so.

2 **Psychological dependence** operates partly through conditioning. Some of the symptoms experienced as a substance is withdrawn (e.g. anxiety) become conditioned responses that reappear when withdrawal takes place again. Cognitive factors are also important—patients expect unpleasant symptoms and are distressed by the prospect. For this reason, reassurance is an important part of the treatment of patients who are withdrawing from drugs. Drugs such as hallucinogens and stimulants frequently cause psychological dependence.

Harm related to the use of substances

Substance-related harm (Table 29.2) may be due to:

1 the toxic properties of the substances themselves (see following subsections on individual substances);

2 the method of administration (e.g. problems due to the intravenous (iv) use of substances; see Box 29.9);

Box 29.9 The harmful effects of intravenous drug taking

Some drug abusers administer drugs IV in order to obtain an intense and rapid effect. The practice is particularly common with opioids.

Local complications include:
- thrombosis of veins;
- wound infection or abscesses at the injection site;
- cellulitis;
- deep venous thrombosis—repeated injection into the femoral veins damages the valves and reduces venous return, which promotes clotting;
- damage to arteries;
- emboli—these may cause gangrene if within arteries, or a pulmonary embolus if from the veins.

Systemic effects are due to transmission of infection, especially when needles are shared. They include:
- sepsis;
- bacterial endocarditis;
- blood-borne infections: hepatitis B and C, HIV, and syphilis;
- increased risk of overdose.

Box 29.10 Social harm due to the use of psychoactive substances

There are various reasons why drug abuse has undesirable social effects:

1 **Acute intoxication** can lead to harm or damage to people or property. Violence and aggression may be a particular problem.
2 **Chronic intoxication** may affect behaviour adversely, leading to a poor work record, unemployment, motoring offences, failures in social relationships, and family problems including the neglect of children.
3 **The need to finance the habit.** Most illicit drugs are expensive and the abuser may cheat or steal to obtain money. Women may adopt prostitution, putting themselves at risk of sexually transmitted diseases and other problems.
4 **The creation of a drug subculture.** Drug users often keep company with one another, and those with previously stable social behaviour may be under pressure to conform to a group ethos of antisocial or criminal activity.
5 **Stigmatization.** Many social communities do not welcome those who have had substance problems, even after successful treatment. The individual may find it hard to reintegrate into society.

3 the social consequences of regular use of substances (Box 29.10).

How do patients with substance use problems present?

Dependent people may come to medical attention in several ways:

1 They may declare that they are dependent on or using a substance during a consultation, at health screening, or while in hospital for another reason.
2 They may request drugs for medical reasons. Some patients conceal their dependency, asking instead for opioids to relieve pain or for hypnotics to improve sleep. GPs and emergency department staff should be wary of such requests from patients who they have not met before, and if possible should obtain information about previous treatment (if necessary by telephone) before prescribing.
3 They may ask for help with the complications of substance use such as cellulitis, pneumonia, hepatitis, HIV/AIDS, or accidents, or for the treatment of a drug overdose, withdrawal symptoms, or an adverse reaction to a hallucinogenic drug.
4 Their dependence might be detected during treatment of an unrelated illness. A common scenario is the patient admitted to hospital for another reason, who then develops withdrawal symptoms.

Assessment and treatment of problems due to psychoactive substance misuse

History taking

A full psychiatric history should be taken, as well as a focused substance misuse history, covering current, past, and future usage:

1 Current use—TRAP (Type, Route, Amount, Pattern):
   - What type of drug(s) do you use? Always clarify any street names used. Include alcohol, tobacco, and cannabis. Then work through the following questions for each substance.
   - How do you use it? Smoking, snorting, IV, intranasal, orally, etc. Ask about needle sharing in IV use.
   - How much do you use? Ask how much of each drug they buy (e.g. heroin is sold in grams, cannabis in eighths of an ounce).
   - How often do you use it? Get them to describe a typical daily usage.
2 Evidence of dependency and harms:
   - Ask about tolerance, withdrawal, craving, and feelings of being out of control. Is there a restricted pattern of usage?
   - Why do you use (the substance)?

- Ask about normal activities: employment, studying, family life, hobbies, etc. Try to decide if the substance taking has taken over from all other activities. Problem use is suggested by repeated absence from school or work, occupational decline, self-neglect, loss of former friends, petty theft, prostitution, and joining the 'drug culture'.
- Complications of drug use: overdoses (deliberate or accidental), history of cellulitis, abscesses, deep venous thrombosis, blood-borne virus. Always ask about HIV status.

3 Past use and general history:
- When was the first time you used (a substance)? Ask specifically about how usage has changed over time, if different substances have been tried, and why they were stopped.
- Determine what treatments have been tried, what happened during withdrawal, how long they were 'clean' for, and what the triggers for relapse were.
- It is important to find out about dependent children.

4 Future usage:
- Assess what stage of change the patient is in.

A clear risk assessment should be made as to mood state, risk of violence, risk of suicide, and dependent others.

A full physical examination should be done. Include weight, height, BMI, and dentition. Feel for hepatomegaly. Clinical signs that suggest that drugs are being injected include:

- needle tracks and thrombosis of veins, especially in the antecubital fossa;
- scars of previous abscesses;
- concealing the forearms with long sleeves even in hot weather.

IV drug use should be considered in any patient who presents with subcutaneous abscesses, hepatitis, or HIV/AIDS, whether or not the person is asking for help with substance use.

Useful investigations include the following:

- **Urine drug screening.** Most substances can be detected in the urine, the notable exception being LSD. Specimens should be examined as quickly as possible, with an indication of the interval between the last admitted drug dose and the collection of the urine sample.
- **Blood tests:** full blood count, including mean cell volume, U&Es, liver function tests, and gamma-glutamyl transferase. Hepatitis and HIV screening.

Principles of treatment and rehabilitation

Ideally, the long-term aim of treatment will be to achieve complete abstinence and a return to normal living. This goal may need to be reached via a step-wise process in many individuals, and therefore an individual plan of treatment needs to be designed. The aims of any treatment plan should be:

- to motivate the patient towards change, and involve them in treatment planning;
- to minimize harms related to taking substances (physical, psychological, and social);
- to improve physical and mental health;
- to reduce criminal activity;
- to reduce the rates of blood-borne infections in the community;
- to stop substance use, or to substitute a safer alternative to provide maintenance in the short to medium term.

An outline of the treatment options is shown in Box 29.11. The majority of dependent substance users (except for nicotine and sometimes cannabis users) will need referral to a specialist addictions service.

Withdrawal strategies

Withdrawal of a substance can be done in several different ways, depending on the substance involved and the wishes of the patient. For opioids and benzodiazepines, it is usual to begin by replacing

Box 29.11 Treatment plan for a person using substances harmfully

- Assessment:
  - Type of drug(s) and amounts taken, IV usage and its dangers, evidence of dependence, and consequences of drug taking
- Psychoeducation of patient and family:
  - Pharmacology and psychology of dependence
  - Harms related to substance misuse
  - Self-help strategies and materials
- Clarification of treatment goals:
  - Production of a written treatment plan
- Treat urgent medical or psychiatric complications
- Harm reduction strategies:
  - Use of oral rather than IV preparations
  - Free contraception and sexual health services
  - Needle exchange programmes
- Arrange withdrawal of the substance(s)
- Substitute prescribing for maintenance
- Address underlying needs:
  - Individual counselling, CBT, or other therapies
  - Treatment of depression or anxiety
  - Marital or family therapy
  - Help dealing with social issues: accommodation, employment, and legal problems
  - Help establishing new interests
- Relapse prevention and longer-term support

the substance with an equivalent dose of a longer-acting compound of the same type (which has less acute withdrawal effects), and then withdrawing that substance. As noted earlier, psychological factors contribute to dependence, and strong and repeated reassurance is an important part of treatment. In most situations, withdrawal can be done at home under close supervision. Patients who have a need for urgent medical attention, severe psychiatric co-morbidities, or a history of complex withdrawals may need to be admitted to hospital for detoxification. There are a number of different options for how detoxification can take place:

- **Supported without medication.** In this scenario, the patient undergoes a planned detoxification, without the use of any further drugs but with support from some form of medical services.

- **Supported with symptomatic medication.** In this case, withdrawal is assisted by prescribed medications to reduce the symptoms of withdrawal. For example, antidiarrhoeals, antiemetics, antipyretics, or lofexidine are helpful in opiate withdrawal.

- **Supported with substitute prescribing.** The patient is changed from the dangerous illegal substance (e.g. heroin) to a safer prescribed version (e.g. methadone), and then this substitute is gradually reduced.

Maintenance programmes

Maintenance refers to the continued prescribing of a substance, usually an opioid or benzodiazepine, for a person who is unwilling to withdraw, combined with help with social problems and a continuing effort to bring the person to accept withdrawal. Maintenance is therefore more than merely providing drugs. The rationale for this procedure is to minimize harm in the following ways:

1 **To remove the need to obtain 'street' drugs,** and thereby reduce the need to steal, engage in prostitution, or associate with other drug users.

2 **To stop IV use,** thus reducing the spread of blood-borne viruses.

3 **To provide social and psychological help** to bring the person to the point at which they will be willing to give up drugs.

4 **To provide an incentive** for the patient to remain in contact with addiction services.

Unfortunately, the available evidence does not suggest that these aims are achieved regularly; many patients continue in their previous way of life, many continue to take street drugs as well as prescribed methadone, and few become willing to give up drugs completely.

In the UK, any doctor can prescribe continuing scripts for methadone or buprenorphine for the treatment of opiate dependence, but it should be initiated by a specialist. Substitute prescribing should only be considered for patients who are actively trying to change their behaviour, and who the doctor thinks are likely to comply with the treatment plan. Prescriptions are dispensed daily and the patient must visit a pharmacy daily to receive them. Most patients have supervised doses, meaning a registered person at the pharmacy watches them take the substance.

Longer-term treatments

After a successful detoxification, it is important to provide support to prevent relapse, tackle the issues underlying the substance misuse, and mend or minimize problems related to harm caused by the substance use. Evidence-based interventions (depending on the individual's specific problems) include:

- individual counselling or CBT for low self-esteem, depression, and anxiety;
- group therapies teaching social skills, communication skills, relaxation, or assertiveness;
- peer support groups;
- marital or family therapy;
- psychiatric input for co-morbidities.

A social worker should be assigned to the patient to provide help in finding suitable accommodation and employment, and in managing money. There may be legal problems to contend with. There are a range of special forms of accommodation, back-to-work schemes, and educational courses designed for those recovering from substance misuse.

Principles of prevention

There are two main strategies for prevention of harm related to the use of psychoactive substances:

1 **Reducing use.** This includes:
   - limiting availability;
   - penalties for usage;
   - health education, especially in schools;
   - media campaigns;

- tackling social causes such as poor social conditions, unemployment among young people, and lack of leisure facilities.

   However, there is little evidence that any of these measures are effective.

2 **Reducing harm** associated with use of substances. The harm reduction approach became more accepted in the 1980s in response to the spread of HIV/AIDS through IV drug use and sexual intercourse. The main features of this approach include:

   - the *education* of drug users about the dangers of IV use; such advice is often more effective when given by ex-drug users than by doctors;
   - schemes for *providing clean syringes and needles* in exchange for used ones in the hope of reducing the sharing of contaminated ones;
   - the prescription of *oral maintenance drugs* to avoid the use of IV drugs;
   - free supply of *condoms* to reduce sexual transmission.

These approaches are controversial since some of the measures can be seen to condone drug taking, but the danger of HIV infection is now generally considered to be greater than that of increasing drug abuse.

Effects and harmful use of specific substances

Opioids

This group of drugs includes morphine, diamorphine (heroin), codeine, dihydrocodeine, and synthetic analgesics such as pethidine and methadone. Opioids are substances that mimic the effects of endogenous opioids (endorphins and encephalins) by acting as agonists at the opioid receptors. More recently, an extract of the southeast Asian tree *Mitragyna speciosa* known as Kratom has started to be used recreationally. Kratom is a mu-opiate agonist with similar effects to opioids; like all novel psychoactive substances it is a relative unknown but seems to behave similarly to morphine. Increasing numbers of users are attending hospitals seeking help after using Kratom.

As well as the desired euphoric effect of opioids, they also have a wide range of other effects upon the body (Table 29.5). The high risk of respiratory depression makes the uncontrolled use of opioids very dangerous.

Table 29.5 Physiological effects of opioids: intoxication and withdrawal

Opioid intoxication	Opioid withdrawal
Psychological/neurological	
• Tolerance and dependence	• Intense craving for the drug
• Euphoria	• Restlessness and insomnia
• Confusion or delirium	• Muscle and joint pain
• Drowsiness	• Yawning
• Analgesia	
• Muscle spasticity	
Cardiovascular	
• Bradycardia and hypotension	• Tachycardia
Respiratory	
• Respiratory depression and hypoventilation	
Gastrointestinal	
• Nausea and vomiting	• Vomiting and diarrhoea
• Dyspepsia	• Abdominal cramps
• Constipation	
Autonomic nervous system	
• Dry mouth	• Running nose and eyes
• Pupil constriction	• Pupil dilatation
• Urinary retention	• Piloerection
• Itching	• Instability of temperature control
	• Sweating

Route of administration

Opioids can be taken by mouth, IV, by inhaling, or by smoking. When diamorphine is taken orally it undergoes extensive first-pass metabolism, converting it to morphine and reducing the euphoric effects. IV use avoids this metabolism, and diamorphine crosses the blood–brain barrier quickly and produces a rapid powerful euphoria. IV use of heroin carries all of the risks discussed previously. The antecubital fossa is usually the site first used for injecting, but eventually the veins become damaged and the user moves elsewhere. When venous access becomes extremely difficult, users may inject either subcutaneously (**skin popping**) or intramuscularly. The form of heroin most commonly used in the UK will only dissolve if mixed with an acid and heated. The use of citric acid powder and lemon juice is typical, with heating occurring on a spoon over a heat source. The use of acids is particularly troublesome because it causes immense damage to the veins.

Tolerance and dependence

Although some people take heroin intermittently without becoming dependent, with regular usage dependence develops rapidly, especially when the drug is taken IV.

Tolerance develops rapidly, leading to ever increasing usage. When the drug is stopped, tolerance diminishes so that a dose taken after an interval of abstinence has a greater effect than it would have had before the interval. This loss of tolerance can result in dangerous—sometimes fatal—respiratory depression when a previously tolerated dose is resumed after a drug-free interval; for example, after a stay in hospital or prison.

Withdrawal (Table 29.5). With heroin, these symptoms usually begin about 6 hours after the last dose, reach a peak after 36–48 hours, and then wane. These symptoms cause great distress, which drives the person to seek further supplies but seldom cause represents medical danger.

Complications of opioid use

These are shown in Table 29.6. The most common cause of death among opioid users is opioid

Table 29.6 Complications of opioid use

Biological	Psychological	Social
Infections: • Abscesses and cellulitis • Sepsis • HIV • Hepatitis B or C • Bacterial endocarditis **Cardiorespiratory:** • Deep vein thrombosis or pulmonary embolism • Aspiration • Respiratory depression • Cardiac arrhythmias Complications of pregnancy Death from overdose	• Depression • Anxiety disorders • Deliberate self-harm • Suicide	• Unemployment • Loss of accommodation • Breakdown of relationships • Loss of friends • Criminal record

overdose, which most frequently occurs after a period of abstinence during which tolerance has decreased. However, the rate of suicide among those dependent upon opioids is 14 times the rate of the general population, usually because of co-morbid depression.

The babies of opioid-dependent women are more likely than other babies to be premature and of low birth weight. Withdrawal symptoms after birth include irritability, restlessness, tremor, and a high-pitched cry. Later effects have been reported, these children being more likely as toddlers to be overactive and to show poor persistence. It is uncertain whether these late effects result from the challenging family environment often provided by these mothers, or from a lasting effect of the exposure to the drug.

In those who use heroin for a long time, there is a small risk of developing a toxic leucoencephalopathy. It is unknown if this is a direct effect of the opioid itself, or caused by a contaminant (or 'cutting' agent) added to the drug during production. Symptoms include confusion, ataxia, and deteriorating neurological function over some weeks.

Treatment of opioid dependence

The general principles of assessment and management should be carried out as described on p. 443.

Treatment of an opioid overdose

The key clinical findings in a patient who has taken an overdose of opioids are:

1 respiratory depression—possibly leading to respiratory arrest;

2 unreactive pinpoint pupils;

3 bradycardia;

4 hypotension;

5 snoring or other upper airway sounds;

6 reduced level of consciousness.

Patients should be approached using the principles of *airway, breathing*, and *circulation* and treated with oxygen, respiratory support, fluids, and inotropes if necessary. The antidote to opioids is **naloxone**, which may be given IV (preferably) or intramuscularly. The usual dose is 400 micrograms IV. Naloxone has a short half-life and repeated doses will need to be given every few minutes. Once the acute effect of the opioids has been reversed, supportive management is given.

Planned withdrawal of opioids (detoxification)

The general principles of drug withdrawal have been outlined earlier in this chapter. When heroin is

Box 29.12 The planned withdrawal of opioids (detoxification)

- When the starting dose is very high, or there have been previously complicated or failed withdrawals, withdrawal should occur in hospital.
- It is often difficult to judge the starting dose because patients often take adulterated preparations of heroin (and may lie about the amount taken). For this reason, treatment should be discussed with, and often carried out by, a specialist in drug dependence.
- The starting dose of methadone is usually 10–20 mg daily, which is increased in 10–20 mg steps until there are no signs of intoxication or withdrawal. The usual daily dose is 60–120 mg.
- The initial dose is reduced by about a quarter every 2 or 3 days, but a slower rate may be needed.
- The regimen should be agreed with the patient as a contract that they will accept throughout the treatment.
- Urine tests for drugs should be carried out weekly after withdrawal until the doctor is confident that the patient is remaining drug free.

withdrawn, psychological support is particularly important to avoid immediate relapse. Withdrawal is usually undertaken by substituting methadone (a longer-acting drug) for heroin. The main steps are shown in Box 29.12.

Continued prescribing (maintenance)

Methadone is a synthetic opioid agonist which is active when given orally, and has a long half-life (36 hours), making it suitable for once-daily dosing. Methadone is prescribed and dispensed daily, usually in a liquid preparation formulated to discourage efforts to inject it. Consumption by the recipient is often supervised. The equivalent dosage is difficult to determine since street drugs are adulterated to a varying degree, but 60–120 mg per day is the usual range. There is good evidence that patients treated with doses higher in that range (80–120 mg) are less likely to restart using illicit opioids. The treatment should be initiated by a specialist, although care can be shared with the primary care physician.

In some European countries, there have been trials using supervised injection of methadone or diamorphine for maintenance therapy. The two drugs appear to be equally effective, and there is a higher chance of preventing the illicit use of IV heroin than when using oral methadone.

Other maintenance treatment options include buprenorphine or alpha-2 agonists (clonidine or lofexidine); all are equally effective. Buprenorphine is available in two forms:

- Buprenorphine (Subutex® or generic)—available as sublingual tablets, Once-daily dosing, which starts with 4 mg when the first withdrawal symptoms are experienced, typical dose needed 12–16 mg daily.
- Buprenorphine and naloxone combination (Suboxone®)—a sublingual tablet designed to reduce misuse of prescriptions. If tablets are crushed and injected, the naloxone will precipitate withdrawal due to its high bioavailability; if taken orally, this does not occur.

Psychological treatments

The most successful programmes are those which combine withdrawal/maintenance with psychological and social support. Motivational interviewing and relapse prevention are useful, and for those patients with psychiatric co-morbidities, CBT is an effective intervention. Narcotics Anonymous is a similar group programme to AA, based on a 12-step mantra, and has a growing evidence base.

Prognosis

Opioid dependence is a chronic relapsing–remitting condition. Although about 90 per cent of opioid-dependent patients can withdraw successfully, about 50 per cent will recommence use by 6 months following withdrawal. After 7 years, only one-quarter to one-third of opioid-dependent people will have become abstinent, and between 10 and 20 per cent will have died from causes related to drug taking. Deaths are from accidental overdose—often related to loss of tolerance after a period of enforced abstinence—and from medical complications such as infection with

HIV. When abstinence is achieved, it is often related to changed circumstances of life, such as a new relationship with a caring person.

Cannabis

Cannabis (marijuana) is derived from the plant *Cannabis sativa* and is by far the most commonly used illicit substance. It is a class B substance. The active constituent is delta-9-tetrahydrocannabinol (THC). Data from 2015 reported almost one-third of UK adults admit to having used cannabis at some point, with 15 per cent having had a period of occasional or regular usage. The latter groups are generally aged 16–30 years. Usage tends to 'burn out' as individuals settle down in life but there are pockets of continued users and a smaller group who use cannabis medicinally for pain relief. 'Heavy' or daily usage is relatively uncommon.

Cannabis is available in a variety of forms:

- Marijuana/grass/weed: dried leaves and flowering parts of the *Cannabis* plant. Looks like dried herbs and is usually smoked, but can be added to or baked in food.

- Hash: purified compressed product made from the resin glands on the stalks of the cannabis plant. It is much more potent than the leaves, containing THC in very high concentrations. Hash is typically brown and comes in little blocks. It is taken mixed with tobacco via smoking, often through a vaporizer.

- Skunk: form of marijuana made from any of a group of hybrid cannabis plants which have been bred to make higher concentrations of THC. It is smoked.

- Cannabis oil: a resin of cannabinoids obtained from the cannabis plant through extraction with solvents. Typically added to foods.

The effects of cannabis vary with the dose, the user's expectations, and the social setting. Like alcohol, cannabis seems to exaggerate the pre-existing mood, whether euphoria or dysphoria. Most users report being chilled out, relaxed, happy, and talkative. It produces a feeling of enhanced enjoyment of aesthetic experiences, and distorts experiences of time and space. Cannabis can make people very hungry, giving them 'the munchies'. Cannabis is often considered a benign substance by recreational users, but this is far from the case—a single usage can lead to anxiety, paranoia, panic, and psychotic symptoms which can last up to 24 hours. Long-term effects are shown in Table 29.7 and Science box 29.1. Cannabis does not produce a *withdrawal syndrome*, and although *psychological dependence* can develop, physical dependence does not seem to occur. Secondary to the risks of depression, anxiety disorders, and psychosis is the so-called amotivational syndrome. It is not uncommon that once high-achieving children decide not to go to university as it is 'too much effort' or that their academic work suffers due to poor attention and memory difficulties.

Occasionally people will present asking for help in reducing their cannabis usage but more usually the

Table 29.7 Risks associated with cannabis

Psychological effects	Physical effects
• Dependence	• Reddening of conjunctivae
• Depression	• Tachycardia and hypertension
• Paranoia	• Dry mouth
• Anxiety	• Lowering of fertility
• Sleep disturbance	• If pregnant: low birth weight
• Psychosis	• All the risks associated with tobacco if smoked together
• Reduced concentration and memory	• Increased risk of injuries, especially road traffic accidents
• Reduced motivation: 'amotivational syndrome'	

SCIENCE BOX 29.1

Cannabis and psychosis

Cannabis is such a widely used substance that the risks associated with it are particularly well documented. A key association is that between cannabis and psychosis. Increasing pressure in some places to legalize cannabis (especially for medicinal use) raise concerns that rates of psychotic illness may rise as well. Understanding the relationship between cannabis and psychosis has become an area of great research in the past decade. Various questions arise: does cannabis cause psychosis or is there merely a shared vulnerability for both among users? Is the risk dose dependant? Is the psychosis characteristic to cannabis? Are particular drugs or treatments particularly efficacious in this patient group? Most of these have yet to be answered.

What is clear is that individuals with schizophrenia or first-episode psychosis are more likely to report use of cannabis (current or historic) than the general population.[1] This appears to be a dose-dependent relationship, with an odds ratio of 3–4 for developing psychosis in heavy cannabis users versus non-users.[2] The illness tends to occur in cannabis users at a younger age, on average 2 years earlier than non-users.[3] The likelihood of psychosis appears to be highly linked to genetic vulnerability. Those who are at high risk of psychosis (primarily due to family history) are more likely to develop a full psychotic disorder if they are using cannabis than not.

However, there are confounders in the picture (many trials are naturalistic or have been uncontrolled retrospective analyses)—many heavy cannabis users also take other substances, use alcohol and nicotine, and have multiple social difficulties. In order to isolate cannabis use from the myriad of surrounding confounders, a RCT would be needed, including multiple dosage groups, variable levels of usage, and elimination of other substances. Given this would be a long-term study, the practicalities and ethics mean it is unlikely to happen. For the time being, advice to all patients should be to avoid starting to use cannabis, and support them with graded withdrawal if they are already using cannabis. Public education, especially targeted at those at high risk of psychosis, should be a priority.

1 Ksir C, Hart CL. Cannabis and psychosis: a critical overview of the relationship. *Current Psychiatric Reports* 2016;18:12.

2 Marconi A, Di Forti M, Lewis CM, Murray RM, Vassos E. Meta-analysis of the association between the level of cannabis use and risk of psychosis. *Schizophrenia Bulletin* 2016;16:1262–1269.

3 Large M, Sharma S, Compton MT, et al. Cannabis use and earlier onset of psychosis: a systematic meta-analysis. *Archives of General Psychiatry* 2011;68:555–561.

presenting complaint is depression, anxiety, or psychosis. A gradual reduction of cannabis usage, combined with psychosocial measures is the most appropriate treatment method.

Good-quality public education about the harms of cannabis smoking may have an important impact on use trends in the future.

Synthetic cannabinoids ('spice')

These are manufactured substances that have been developed to act like THC on cannabinoid receptors. These are now illegal in the UK. They act like cannabis, but tend to be more potent, meaning the unpleasant side effects and risks are considerable. Synthetic cannabinoids are usually sold as herbal-like mixtures to be smoked or liquids that can be used in e-cigarettes. The general effects are the same as natural cannabis but tend to be more extreme. Specific risks include a higher rate of psychosis, serotonin syndrome (there is a cross-over leading to serotonin agonism), and acute kidney injury.

Benzodiazepines

Benzodiazepines are effective anxiolytics, hypnotics, anticonvulsants, and muscle relaxants, acting via the enhancement of GABA transmission at the $GABA_A$ receptor. When they hit the market in the 1960s it was not recognized that they carried a risk of dependence so they were freely prescribed, but tolerance was quickly noticed and crosses between all benzodiazepines. Now it is recommended benzodiazepines are avoided, but if absolute necessary are prescribed at the lowest dose possible for a maximum of 2–4 weeks.

There are no reliable epidemiological statistics available, but many studies report 10–15 per cent of 15–25-year-olds have used benzodiazepines recreationally at least once. They are usually taken orally, but occasionally IV. There is another large group of patients who are dependent upon prescribed benzodiazepines; they may be seen in primary or secondary care services.

A variety of different benzodiazepines are available, varying in their length of action. Temazepam and oxazepam are short acting; lorazepam and alprazolam are medium acting; and nitrazepam, chlordiazepoxide, and diazepam are long acting. Flunitrazepam, a particularly short-acting and potent benzodiazepine, is no longer available legally in many countries. It is also known as Rohypnol®, and has been used as a 'date-rape' drug.

The **benzodiazepine withdrawal syndrome** is characterized by irritability and anxiety, disturbed sleep, nausea, tremor, sweating, palpitations, headache, and seizures.

Management of benzodiazepine misuse

A planned withdrawal of benzodiazepines is the usual method of managing benzodiazepine dependence. The withdrawal symptoms are less pronounced with long-acting (e.g. diazepam) than with short-acting benzodiazepines (e.g. lorazepam), so a short-acting drug should be replaced with a long-acting drug in the equivalent dose before starting withdrawal. The dose is reduced very slowly, typically by 10 per cent per fortnight. Where possible, if large doses are involved then these should be dispensed daily by a specified pharmacist. If withdrawal symptoms appear during withdrawal, the dose can be increased slightly, and then reduced again by a smaller amount than before. Occasionally, inpatient detoxification may be needed, especially if there are acute psychiatric or physical co-morbidities to be treated, or the patient has had seizures during previous withdrawals.

Prescribing benzodiazepines

All doctors should use the following guidance to avoid their patient becoming dependent on benzodiazepines:

- Be very cautious about initiating a prescription for benzodiazepines.
- Prescribe the lowest dose possible.
- Limit the prescription to 2–3 weeks.
- Do not have prescriptions available for routine repeat refills.
- Never re-prescribe if the patient reports losing or forgetting their tablets.
- Do not prescribe benzodiazepines for another doctor's patients; tell them to go to their usual prescriber.

Ketamine

Ketamine is a general anaesthetic and analgesic which has become a commonly used recreational drug in the past decade. It is a class B drug. Ketamine is usually taken orally, but can be injected IV or intramuscularly. Sometimes ketamine is mixed with cannabis and smoked. Currently there are no good statistics on ketamine usage, but data from the USA from 2016 suggested about 5 per cent of those aged 12–25 had used it at least once in the past year.

When taken recreationally, ketamine has the following effects:

- Feeling chilled out or relaxed.
- Dissociative feelings—derealization and depersonalization. Users have reported sometimes feeling unable to move, an experience known as the 'k-hole'.
- Hallucinations—auditory and visual.
- Confusion, agitation, and panic attacks.
- Depression in some people if used regularly.

Regular users of ketamine experience tolerance, and tend to report that the dissociative features reduce over time which drives use of larger doses. The main problems associated with regular ketamine use are depression, hypertension, tachycardia, abdominal cramps, memory loss, injuries (due to the analgesic effect), and hepatic damage. A big problem is the damage to the bladder (ketamine-induced vesicopathy) that is increasing being seen, leading to incontinence, detrusor overactivity, and haematuria.

At present, there is no evidence base for treatment of ketamine misuse or dependence; general guidelines as described previously should be followed. Overdoses need supportive care as there is no antidote.

Stimulant drugs

Stimulant drugs potentiate the effects of neurotransmitters (including serotonin, dopamine, and norepinephrine), causing increased energy, a state of alertness, and euphoria. Users also experience insomnia, anorexia, dilated pupils, failure of thermoregulation, and increased heart rate and blood pressure. There tends to be an increase in confidence and impulsivity and a decrease in judgement which can lead to risky behaviour. Large doses can lead to cardiac arrhythmias and myocardial infarction. Overactivity sometimes leads users to drink large amounts of water; however, occasionally this causes overhydration and electrolyte abnormalities. Ecstasy in particular is associated with arrhythmias, seizures, dehydration, renal failure, rhabdomyolysis, or liver failure due to dehydration.

Stimulant drugs do not readily induce *tolerance*. On stopping the drugs there is low mood, reduced energy, and increased appetite but it is unclear if this is a withdrawal syndrome or merely rebound symptoms. Prolonged use of stimulants can lead to perceptual abnormalities, typically a paranoid psychosis which may resemble schizophrenia.

Stimulants are most commonly used by young people, but cocaine has a secondary following in the upper middle classes among young professionals. They are often taken in clubs or at parties, giving people more energy to dance. UK statistics suggest 20–25 per cent of university students have used stimulants. After cannabis, stimulants are the most commonly used illegal drugs within Europe.

Commonly used stimulants

1 **Amphetamine sulphate.** Taken by mouth, snorted, or injected.

2 **Methamphetamine** ('crystal meth'). A powerful and addictive form of amphetamine whose effects last up to 12 hours. Unlike amphetamine sulphate it can be smoked.

3 **Cocaine** hydrochloride is taken by sniffing into the nose (where it is absorbed through the nasal mucosa) or by injecting. Frequent snorting of cocaine can lead to perforation of the nasal septum. Free-base cocaine ('crack') is usually smoked to give a rapid and intense effect—unfortunately it also has a quick and severe comedown.

4 **Ecstasy (MDMA).** A stimulant that also has some hallucinogenic properties. Typically taken at clubs and parties occasionally and not usually associated with regular use or the taking of other substances.

5 **Mephedrone** ('MCAT') comes as a powder (or tablet) which can be taken orally, snorted, or injected. It is appearing more commonly across Europe and is a UK class B drug. Characteristic features include teeth grinding and cold blue peripheries.

6 **Methylphenidate** (Ritalin®). A stimulant prescribed for ADHD which is popular among students to help improve their concentration for studying. Unfortunately users rarely understand the risks of stimulants, with a common belief that because methylphenidate is available on prescription it must be safe.

Treatment of misuse of stimulants

There is no specific management for stimulant misuse; the general principles of treating any substance problem apply. There is evidence that education, harm-reduction measures, and targeting treatments at high-risk groups are all effective. For individuals with a long-term cocaine problem, more intensive programmes are often needed. Inpatient rehabilitation is frequently undertaken, with a comprehensive detoxification and therapy programme over several months.

This can be very effective if the patient is motivated to change. For emergency situations (e.g. psychosis), the usual forms of treatment should be used. Antipsychotics are effective for psychosis induced by stimulants, and fluoxetine has the best evidence base if an antidepressant is needed.

Prognosis

Unlike opioid and benzodiazepine misuse, the majority of individuals using stimulants do so for recreation and not on a regular basis. Very few continue to do so in the long term, and less than 1 per cent suffers a complication of usage. Heavy use of cocaine has a less good prognosis, but if treatment is sought it is usually effective.

Hallucinogens

The latest UK data suggests that use of hallucinogens—a long-term big player in the recreational drugs scene—is slightly reducing. Hallucinogens typically refer to synthetic compounds such as **LSD** and naturally occurring substances found in species of mushroom (e.g. *Psilocybe semilanceata*). Dissociative drugs such as phencyclidine (PCP) and ketamine (see earlier subsection) are becoming increasingly popular. Synthetic and naturally occurring **anticholinergic drugs** are also abused for their hallucinogenic effects. These substances do not tend to show tolerance and dependence.

LSD becomes psychoactive in a drop of solvent, and dissolved into an aqueous solution. It is then placed on to small pieces of blotting paper with pictures on ('tabs') or on to sugar cubes. These are then eaten, and the drug induces a 'trip', which may last for up to 12 hours. Mushrooms may be eaten or drunk as a broth.

The drugs produce distortions or intensifications of sensory perception, sometimes with 'cross-over' between sensory modalities so that, for example, sounds are experienced as visual sensations. Objects may seem to merge or move rhythmically, time appears to pass slowly, and ordinary experiences may seem to have a profound meaning. The body image may be distorted or the person may feel as if they are outside their body. These experiences can be pleasurable, but at times they are profoundly distressing and lead to unpredictable and dangerous behaviour. The physical effects of hallucinogens are variable; LSD can cause a rise in heart rate and dilation of the pupils.

Complications of hallucinogen use tend to relate to the user experiencing terrifying experiences (a 'bad trip'). This can lead to panic attacks, outbursts of aggression, and violence. Occasionally, regular users of hallucinogens can develop a persistent perceptual disorder, in which hallucinations occur days or weeks after the last dose. These may be new experiences, or 'flashbacks' of experiences occurring originally during intoxication. These can intermittently occur for years afterwards even if no more drugs are taken, but they do usually eventually cease. Individuals may need some form of psychotherapy to help them live with these experiences long term.

PCP or 'angel dust' is a synthetic hallucinogen with particularly dangerous effects. It is occasionally used as a pure drug, but is frequently mixed with either cocaine or cannabis and may be taken orally, smoked, snorted, or injected. Intoxication with this drug can be prolonged and hazardous, with agitation, aggressive behaviour, and hallucinations together with nystagmus and raised blood pressure. With high doses, there may be ataxia, muscle rigidity, and convulsions, and in severe cases, an adrenergic crisis with heart failure, cerebrovascular accident, or malignant hypothermia. Treatment is supportive, but should include antihypertensives, diuretics, and neuroleptics.

Novel psychoactive substances (NPS)

In the past decade, a myriad of synthetically developed substances have flooded the market. These novel psychoactive substances—frequently known as 'legal highs'—a term that since the introduction of the Novel Psychoactive Substances Act 2016 (at least in the UK)—is incorrect. NPS are typically designed to mimic the effects of other popular substances (cannabis, cocaine, hallucinogens). It is estimated the about two new substances hit the streets within Europe every week. The popularity of NPS has been due to being cheaper, more widely available, undetectable in urine drug screens, and until recently mostly legal. Now that the production and supply of these substances is illegal, there is hope that the rise in use may be reduced.

Most NPS are designed to produce an experience similar to that obtained while using more 'traditional' substances. The symptoms are therefore similar to those previously described for each group. Common types of NPS include:

1 synthetic cannabinoids—e.g. spice, black mamba

2 stimulants—e.g. mephedrone (class B drug; miaow miaow, MCAT), 'Vanilla Sky', bath salts.

3 hallucinogens—e.g. NBOMe, AMT

4 'downers'—benzodiazepine-like substances—e.g. APB, benzo-fury.

The risks of NPS are extremely difficult to be precise about, because it is such an unknown field. Things to consider if presented with a patient who is intoxicated/has overdosed on a NPS:

- Studies have shown that NPS often contain a mixture of substances, which may be from different types of drug, meaning the effects produced can be unpredictable and complex. The person will have no idea what they have actually taken.

- Manufacturing of NPS is unregulated—there could be any form of contaminant within the 'drug' itself.

- The biological and psychological effects of most NPS are not fully characterized so there is a lack of clinical evidence to guide treatment. Symptomatic treatment is therefore the only option.

- Data from emergency departments across Europe suggest the commonest problems presenting to hospital related to NPS are gastrointestinal upset, aggression, paranoia, and the consequences of 'bad trips'. Many users report a severe comedown after taking the substances.

- The risks of tolerance and dependence are unknown.

- Serious adverse effects reported include arrhythmias and serotonin syndrome. UK statistics show a steep increase in number of deaths related to NPS for the past decade. Mephedrone is the single largest culprit at present, although it is an ever-changing field.

The only sensible approach to NPS is to treat a patient symptomatically if they present acutely, and follow the usual steps for assessment and treatment you would for any other substance. Most importantly, remember to ask about the use of NPS during all substance history taking.

Further reading

Alcoholics Anonymous. Northern American website: www.aa.org/. United Kingdom website: www.alcoholics-anonymous.org.uk/.

Andrade C. Cannabis and neuropsychiatry, 2: the longitudinal risk of psychosis as an adverse outcome. *Journal of Clinical Psychiatry* 2016;77:E739–E742

Day E, Copello A, Hull M. Assessment and management of alcohol use disorders. *BMJ* 2015;350:h715.

Gelder MG, Andreasen, NC, López-Ibor JJ, Geddes JR, eds. *New Oxford Textbook of Psychiatry*. 2nd ed. Section 4.2: Substance use disorders. Oxford: Oxford University Press; 2012:426–520.

Gilani F. Novel psychoactive substances: the rising wave of 'legal highs'. *British Journal of General Practice* 2016;66:8–9.

Kraan T, Velthorst E, Koenders L, et al. Cannabis use and transition to psychosis in individuals at ultra-high risk: review and meta-analysis. *Psychological Medicine* 2016;46:673–681.

Office of National Statistics (ONS). Drug misuse: findings from the 2014/15 Crime Survey for England and Wales. Statistical Bulletin 03/15. Published March 2015. https://www.gov.uk/government/uploads/system/uploads/attachment_data/file/462885/drug-misuse-1415.pdf.

30 Problems of sexuality and gender

Sexual problems are encountered commonly in medical practice. It is an area in which accurate epidemiological data is hard to gather, but recent systematic reviews have stated that 40–50 per cent of women and 10–20 per cent of men report 'a sexual difficulty' within the past year. Gender-related issues are classified alongside sexual problems in the ICD and DSM classification systems, and are presenting with increasing frequency to mental health services. A working knowledge of how to manage these patients is therefore increasingly important for clinicians. It is helpful to think of sexual- and gender-related problems in three areas (Table 30.1):

1 Disorders of sexual function.

2 Disorders of sexual preference.

3 Gender identity disorders. These are discussed in detail in Chapter 32, p. 480 as they tend to present in childhood or adolescence.

Some knowledge of normal sexual behaviour may help you to assess a patient's presenting problem. Always remember there is enormous variation in the quantity and type of sexual behaviour considered 'normal' within a population, and a diverse range of views about the importance of sexual activity among individuals. Cultural norms and religious views are the greatest influences on an individual's sexual behaviour: it is helpful to get an idea of what is important to a patient when taking the history.

The age of first intercourse dropped steadily in the second half of the last century but has since stabilized. This was probably due to the relaxation of social attitudes towards sexuality that occurred in the post-war decades. At present, about 20 per cent of females and about 30 per cent of males experience heterosexual intercourse before the age of 16. More than 80 per cent of both sexes have experienced sexual intercourse by the age of 20 years. Earlier age of first intercourse is associated with lower social class, lower levels of education, and lack of religious affiliation. The earlier first intercourse occurs, the less likely it is to be accompanied by adequate contraceptive use and the more it is felt by the subject, in retrospect, to have been too early.

Data from the UK and USA in 2015 reported that 94 per cent of adults report mostly or exclusively heterosexual (erotic thoughts and feelings are directed towards a person of the opposite sex) experience and attraction. The remainder report homosexual (lesbian/gay), bisexual, or 'other' as

Table 30.1 Problems of sexuality and gender

Disorders of sexual function	Disorders of sexual preference	Gender identity disorders
Lack of sexual desire *(Rarely, excessive sexual desire may be reported)* Men: • Erectile impotence • Ejaculatory dysfunction Female: • Failure of genital arousal • Anorgasmia • Vaginismus • Dyspareunia	• Exhibitionism • Fetishism and fetishistic transvestism • Paedophilia • Voyeurism • Sadomasochism	• Gender identity disorder/gender dysphoria

their sexual orientation. All of these types of sexual orientation are part of the normal human spectrum of behaviour.

Problems of sexual function

It is difficult to establish the prevalence of sexual problems in the population because of the challenges involved in carrying out surveys of people's sexual behaviour. The commonest kinds of problems presenting to primary care are shown in Table 30.2. Frequent causative factors are listed in Table 30.3.

Low sexual desire

This problem may occur in both sexes but is commoner in women. In some cases, sexual desire has always been low (**primary low sexual desire**); this may be within the range of biological variation, or it may be due to biological or psychological aetiology. In other cases, sexual desire has been normal in the past but has become impaired (**secondary low sexual desire**); the causes then include general problems in the relationship between the partners,

Table 30.2 Relative frequency of sexual problems

	Frequency (%)
Women	
Low sexual desire	50
Orgasmic dysfunction	20
Vaginismus	20
Dyspareunia	5
Men	
Erectile dysfunction	60
Premature ejaculation	15
Delayed ejaculation	5
Low sexual desire	5

physical disorders, psychological problems, or substances (Table 30.3). It is worth noting that after an episode of depression, it can take some time for normal sexual desire to return.

Erectile dysfunction is the inability to reach erection or sustain it long enough for satisfactory coitus. Primary erectile dysfunction is rare and usually has a physical basis, such as neurological damage or

Table 30.3 Causes of sexual dysfunction

Physical disorders	Psychological factors and mental disorders	Drugs
• Hypogonadism	• Anxiety about performance	• Antidepressants[a]
• Hyperprolactinaemia	• Previous adverse sexual experiences	• Hypnotics
• Autonomic neuropathy[a]	• Lack of privacy	• Anxiolytics
• Cardiovascular disease (especially previous myocardial infarction)[a]	• Anxiety disorders	• Antipsychotics[a]
• Diabetes mellitus[a]	• Low mood	• Antihypertensives[a]
• Epilepsy	• Mania	• Beta-blockers[a]
• Renal failure and dialysis	• Psychosis	• Diuretics[a]
• Pelvic inflammatory disease[b]		• H_2-receptor blockers
• Endometriosis[b]		• Alcohol
• Previous rectal surgery		
• Previous breast surgery		
• Pain		

[a] Factors particularly related to erectile dysfunction.
[b] Factors particularly related to vaginismus/dyspareunia.

leakage from the penile cavernous bodies. Secondary erectile dysfunction is extremely common, and is typically multifactorial. The commonest factors involved are performance-related anxiety, mental disorders, and drugs. Assessment of erectile dysfunction should identify whether it is invariable (suggesting a physical or drug cause) or present only in some circumstances (suggesting a psychological cause). Questions should be asked about erections on waking from sleep, and during masturbation; if they are present, a physical cause is unlikely.

Orgasmic dysfunction

In men, orgasmic dysfunction is seen as premature ejaculation or delayed ejaculation; in women it is usually known as 'anorgasmia'.

Premature ejaculation

Premature ejaculation is habitual ejaculation earlier than the man would like it to happen, usually before penetration or shortly afterwards. It is common among young men during first sexual encounters, and usually improves with increasing sexual experience. The partner can assist by interrupting foreplay whenever the man feels himself becoming highly aroused (**stop–start technique**). This process prolongs the period during which the man can be highly aroused, but not ejaculate.

Delayed ejaculation

Delayed (or complete lack of) ejaculation is typically due to general psychological factors surrounding sexual activity. It can also be caused by drugs, notably antipsychotic drugs, SSRIs, and MAOIs.

Female anorgasmia

Lack of female orgasm during intercourse is frequent although most women can achieve it through clitoral stimulation. Surveys suggest that a small proportion of women never experience orgasm, so it should not necessarily be considered abnormal. Typical causes include psychological factors and drugs.

Conditions with discomfort or pain

Pain on intercourse occurs mainly among women, either as vaginismus or as dyspareunia. Vaginismus is painful spasm of the vaginal muscles during intercourse. This spasm may be due to aversion to intercourse or from a physical cause such as post-episiotomy scars or pelvic disease. The condition may be made worse by an in-experienced or inconsiderate partner. Generally, the spasm begins when the man attempts penetration, but in severe cases it occurs even if the woman attempts to insert her own finger into the vagina. In such severe cases, no intercourse can take place.

Dyspareunia is pain on intercourse. When the pain arises after even partial penetration of the vagina, it may result from impaired lubrication with vaginal se-cretions or from painful scarring. When pain is felt only during deep penetration, it may be due to pelvic path-ology, so should be fully investigated.

Assessment

Patients with sexual problems initially often complain about other symptoms because they feel too embar-rassed to reveal a sexual problem directly. For example, a patient may ask for help with anxiety, depression, poor sleep, or gynaecological symptoms. It is there-fore important to ask routinely a few questions about sexual functioning when assessing patients with non-specific psychological or physical symptoms.

In a full assessment, the interviewer should begin by explaining why it will be necessary to ask about in-timate details of the patient's sexual life, and should then ask questions in a sympathetic, matter-of-fact way (Box 30.1). Whenever possible, both sexual part-ners should be interviewed, separately and together. Do a full physical examination to exclude physical causes of sexual problems (Box 30.2). It may be ne-cessary to refer females for specialist gynaecological examination.

Treatment

Treatment begins by dealing with any remediable cause. If no such cause is found, psychological factors

---

Box 30.1 Assessment of a sexual problem

- Define the problem, including:
  - its nature;
  - recent or long-standing;
  - whether with this partner only;
  - does it occur during masturbation.
- Assess sexual drives of both partners (frequency of sexual arousal, masturbation, and intercourse) and their sexual orientation.
- Assess fears relating to sexual activity (e.g. pregnancy, HIV).
- Enquire about the marital relationship and social relationships in general.
- Sexual development including traumatic experiences.
- Previous and present psychiatric and medical illness and treatment; pregnancy, childbirth and abortion(s); alcohol and drug use.
- Assess the mental state, especially for depressive disorder.
- Assess motivation for treatment.
- Physical examination and any relevant laboratory tests.

Box 30.2 Physical examination of men with sexual dysfunction

1 Is there evidence of diabetes mellitus or adrenal disorder?
   - Hair distribution, gynaecomastia
   - Blood pressure, peripheral pulses
   - Fundi for retinopathy
   - Reflexes, especially ankle
   - Peripheral sensation
2 Are there any abnormalities of the genitalia?
   - Penis: congenital abnormalities, foreskin, pulses, tenderness, plaques, infection, urethral discharge
   - Testicles: size, symmetry, texture, sensation

Table 30.4 Treatment options for disorders of sexual function

General measures	• Treat underlying physical or mental health conditions • Psychoeducation • General reassurance and support
Psychological	• Couples therapy • Individual psychotherapy (to explore underlying fears, memories, or difficulties)
Specific disorders	
Erectile dysfunction	• Stop or reduce dose of causative drugs • CBT • Pharmacological options: phosphodiesterase inhibitors (sildenafil), intracavernosal injections of smooth muscle relaxants (e.g. papaverine or prostaglandin E_1), • Surgical insertion of semi-rigid rods (rare)
Vaginismus	• Behavioural therapy: psychoeducation and graded exercises to overcome the muscle spasm. Graded dilators can be very useful
Dyspareunia	• Psychotherapy or CBT are the most effective options if physical causes have been excluded

should be explored and therapeutic approaches considered (see Table 30.4).

Psychological treatment of sexual dysfunction

Some patients will present with more than one disorder of sexual function, or have a broader difficulty with sexual interactions. In these cases, specialized sexual therapy is the most effective intervention, especially if the couple can be treated together. There are three stages: (1) improving communication, (2) education, and (3) 'graded activities'.

1 **Improving communication** has two main aims: (a) to help the couple to talk more freely about their problems and (b) to increase each partner's understanding of the wishes and feelings of the other. This will help the couple to achieve a general relationship that is more affectionate and satisfying.

2 **Education** focuses on important aspects of the male and female sexual responses; examples are the longer time needed for a woman to reach sexual arousal, and the importance of foreplay, including clitoral stimulation, in bringing about

vaginal lubrication. Psychoeducation is often the most important part of the treatment of sexual dysfunction, and it may need to be repeated when the couple have made some progress with the graded activities described next.

3 **Graded activities** begin by negotiating with the couple a mutually agreed ban on full sexual intercourse. The couple are encouraged instead to explore the pleasure that each can give the other by tender physical contact. The partners are encouraged to caress each other but not to touch the genitalia at this stage. When they can achieve caressing in a relaxed way that gives enjoyment to each partner, the next stage is genital foreplay without penetration. When genital foreplay can be enjoyed by both partners, the next stage is the resumption of full intercourse in a gradual and relaxed way. At each stage, each partner is encouraged to find out and provide what the other enjoys. The couple are advised to avoid checking their own state of sexual arousal. Such checking is common among people with sexual disorder, and has the effect of inhibiting the natural progression of sexual arousal to orgasm. Each partner should be encouraged to allow feelings and physical

responses to develop spontaneously while thinking of the other person.

The overall results of sex therapy are that about a third of cases have a successful outcome and another third have worthwhile improvement. Patients with primary low sexual drive generally have a poor outcome.

Disorders of sexual preference

Disorders of sexual preference are sometimes known as **paraphilias**. A sexual preference can be said to be abnormal by three criteria:

1 Most people in a society regard the sexual preference as abnormal.

2 The sexual preference can be harmful to other people (e.g. sadistic sexual practices).

3 The person with the preference suffers from its consequences (e.g. from a conflict between sexual preferences and moral standards—it is 'egodystonic').

In the current classification systems, changes are underway to try and separate those individuals who engage in behaviours that might be seen as abnormal in society as a whole but are not causing the individual or others distress or harm, and those whose behaviour is risky or distressing to self or others. The phrases 'paraphilic behaviours' and 'paraphilic disorder' can be used to distinguish between the two groups.

There are three common circumstances in which doctors see patients with abnormal sexual preferences: they may be asked for help by the person with the abnormal sexual preference; they may be approached by the sexual partner; or they may be asked for an opinion when a person has been charged with an offence against the law—for example, exhibitionism or a sexual act with a child. (These offences, and others unrelated to abnormal sexual preference, are considered in Chapter 12.)

Disorders of sexual preference can be divided into (1) abnormalities of the sexual 'object' and (2) disorders of the sexual act (Box 30.3). The aetiology of these conditions is not known, and the various theories will not

Box 30.3 Abnormalities of sexual preference

1 Abnormalities of the sexual object:
   - Sexual fetishism
   - Fetishistic transvestism
   - Paedophilia
2 Abnormalities of the sexual act:
   - Exhibitionism
   - Voyeurism
   - Sexual sadism
   - Sexual masochism

be discussed. They may, however, be associated with the presence of other disorders, including depression, alcohol abuse, and dementia. Treatment is described after the descriptions of the disorders, on p. 463.

Disorders of preference of the sexual object

Fetishism

In this condition, an inanimate object is relied upon to achieve sexual excitement. Among the many objects that can evoke arousal in different people, common examples are rubber garments, women's underclothes, and high-heeled shoes. The smell and texture of these objects is often as important as their appearance in evoking sexual arousal. Some fetishists buy the objects, but others steal them and may come to the notice of the police. The individual may use the object with a partner (e.g. they wear it), but often it is a solitary accompaniment of masturbation. Almost all fetishists are men and most are heterosexual.

Fetishistic transvestism

In this condition, the person wears clothes of the opposite sex as a means of sexual arousal. They may also want to temporarily look like the opposite gender. It can be thought of as a special kind of fetishism. Nearly all transvestites are men. The clothing varies from a single garment to a complete set of clothing. Cross-dressing nearly always begins after puberty. At first, the clothes are worn only in private; a few people, however, go on to wear the clothes in public, usually hidden under male outer garments, but occasionally without precautions against discovery. A few transvestites wear a complete set of female garments; the condition then has to be distinguished from gender dysphoria (see p. 480). The essential difference is that transvestites are sexually aroused by wearing the clothing (this is typically the primary motivation) while those with gender dysphoria are not.

Paedophilia

Paedophilia is the sexual preference for children, typically those who are prepubertal or in early puberty. The child is usually above the age of 9 years but prepubertal, and may be of the same or opposite sex to the paedophile. The sexual contact may involve fondling, masturbation, or full coitus with consequent injury to the child. Epidemiology suggests most paedophiles are men. Few paedophiles seek the help of doctors; those who do are mostly of middle age although the behaviour has often started earlier. Given the volume of pornographic material depicting sex with children available, it is likely that paedophilic fantasies are not rare, although paedophilia as an exclusive form of sexual behaviour is infrequent.

Disorders of preference of the sexual act

The second group of disorders of sexual preference involves variations in the behaviour carried out to obtain sexual arousal. Generally, the acts are directed towards other adults but sometimes towards children (e.g. by some exhibitionists or sadists).

Exhibitionism

In this condition, sexual arousal is obtained repeatedly by exposure of the genitalia to an unprepared stranger. The act of exposure is usually preceded by a period of mounting tension which is released by the act. Nearly all exhibitionists are men who typically expose themselves to females. Most exhibitionists fall into two groups. The first consists of men with inhibited temperament who generally expose a flaccid penis and feel

much guilt after the act. The second consists of men with aggressive personality traits who expose an erect penis while masturbating, and feel little guilt afterwards. In Britain, exhibitionists who are arrested are charged with the offence of **indecent exposure**.

When exhibitionism begins in middle or late life, the possibility of organic brain disorder, depressive disorder, or alcoholism should be considered since these conditions occasionally 'release' this pattern of behaviour. In other people, the exhibitionism may start during a period of temporary stress.

Voyeurism

Voyeurism is observing others as the preferred and repeated way of obtaining sexual arousal. Most voyeurs are inhibited heterosexual men. Some voyeurs spy on couples who are having intercourse, others on women who are undressing or naked.

Sexual sadomasochism

Sadomasochism is a preference for sexual activity that involves bondage or inflicting pain on another person. If the individual prefers to receive such stimulation, the disorder is called **masochism**. If the individual prefers to administer such stimulation, the disorder is called **sadism**. Beating, whipping, and tying are common forms of such activity. Sometimes the acts are symbolic and cause little actual damage, but occasionally the acts cause serious injuries.

Mild sadomasochistic behaviour is common and is considered to be part of the range of normal sexual activity, especially if it is consensual.

Management of disorders of sexual preference

A basic guide to assessment is shown in Box 30.4.

Treatment

Management of a patient presenting with a disorder of sexual preference will be highly dependent upon their circumstances. For sex offenders, they may be undergoing treatment as part of their court-defined treatment

Box 30.4 Assessment of abnormalities of sexual preference

- Identify the problem. Clearly identify any distress and/or harm(s) being caused to the patient or others.
- Assess normal sexual functioning and treat any difficulties identified.
- Consider the 'role' of the abnormal sexual behaviour (is the patient using this as a way of coping with loneliness or anxiety?).
- Exclude associated mental disorder (depression, alcoholism, and dementia)—especially in older patients with onset of new behaviours.
- Exclude associated or causative organic disorders (including intracranial pathology, Parkinson's disease, and other basal ganglia lesions).
- Assess motivation for treatment.

plan (this may be under the mental health act), for others it may be a more typically outpatient situation. It is very important to treat any co-morbidities, especially depression, aggressively. The following may be considered:

Pharmacological treatments

- SSRIs have a reasonable evidence base in the paraphilias. Pro-serotonergic drugs appear to reduce the sexual urges and compulsions experienced by those with paraphilias; this may be akin to their effect in obsessive–compulsive spectrum conditions. SSRIs also have a high rate of sexual side effects due to their effect on the $5-HT_2$ receptor which some patients actually find therapeutic.

- Antiandrogen treatments. These are extensively used in sex offenders to decrease sexual drive, although the evidence base at reducing recidivism is not strong. Options include gonadotropin-releasing hormone (GnRH) analogues, cyproterone, and other synthetic steroidal agents.

Psychological treatments

Often motivational interviewing may be a helpful start, usually followed by CBT-based approaches. Evidence suggests that psychological therapies are not very effective at reducing reoffending in sex offenders, but there is no real evidence base in the wider population who experience paraphilic behaviours. If the individual is in a relationship, involving the partner in therapy or having some specific relationship counselling is very valuable.

Disorders of gender identity

Gender identity disorder/gender dysphoria is discussed in Chapter 32.

Further reading

Bancroft JHJ. *Human Sexuality and its Problems*, 3rd ed. Edinburgh: Churchill Livingstone; 2009. [A comprehensive account of normal and abnormal sexual behaviour.]

Hawton K. *Sex Therapy: A Practical Guide*. Oxford: Oxford University Press; 1985. [Although dated, this still provides a clear and practical account of simple kinds of therapy suitable for use by the non-specialist.]

Holoyda BJ, Kellaher DC. The biological treatment of paraphilic disorders: an updated review. *Current Psychiatric Reports* 2016;18:19.

Johnson AE, Wadsworth J, Field J. *Sexual Attitudes and Lifestyles*. Oxford: Blackwell; 1994. [A very interesting large UK survey of sexual experience and attitudes in the general population.]

McCabe MP, Sharlip ID, Lewis R, et al. Incidence and prevalence of sexual dysfunction in women and men: a Consensus Statement from the Fourth International Consultation on Sexual Medicine 2015. *Journal of Sexual Medicine* 2016;13:144–152.

31 Personality and its disorders

CHAPTER CONTENTS

Personality

Personality is a difficult concept to define: it is extremely hard to encapsulate what makes a person '*who they are*' in general terms. Personality is typically thought of as the set of characteristics which make us think, feel, and act in our own unique way. Personality is pervasive; people tend to behave in similar ways throughout life and across differing social and interpersonal contexts. The characteristics of personality, called **traits**, are a set of common features which are observed in variable degrees in different people. Traits provide a useful structure in which to describe a personality: Box 31.1 shows some common personality traits. Some traits may be perceived as an asset to the individual, while others are more of a nuisance. We all have a little more or a little less of any given trait.

The word 'temperament' rather than personality is used to describe the behavioural characteristics displayed by young children. This is because our personality takes time to develop; it is shaped by a multitude of environmental, biological, and factors which interact throughout early life. By our late teens or early twenties, the majority of individuals have the set of traits which define the personality we will have for the rest of our lives. Having an understanding of an individual's personality helps clinicians to predict their patients' response to illness and its treatment.

Personality disorder

The majority of us have some less favourable aspects to our personality, but we work around them and/or have more prominent favourable traits that allow us to get on with our lives. For a minority of people, their less favourable traits are so prominent that they cause problems for themselves or for those around them. It is these people who we think of as having a **personality disorder**. It is extremely difficult to draw a line between normal personality and personality disorder, so this simple pragmatic approach is helpful in clinical practice.

People with a personality disorder may:

- have difficulties with social situations and relationships;

Box 31.1 Common personality traits

(Note that many traits are on a continuum e.g. extra-version—intraversion, only one end of the spectrum is given for brevity.)

- Openness to experience
- Conscientiousness
- Extraversion
- Agreeableness
- Neuroticism
- Honesty and humility
- Self-esteem
- Harm avoidance
- Novelty seeking
- Perfectionism
- Ability to express emotions
- Rigidity
- Impulsivity
- Psychoticism
- Obsessionality

- have difficulties controlling their feelings and/or behaviour;
- react in unusual ways to illness or to treatment;
- behave in unusual ways when mentally ill;
- have more extreme or unusual reactions to stressful events;
- behave in ways that are detrimental to themselves or others
- be more prone to developing other types of mental disorder.

Personality disorder versus mental disorder

Are personality disorders a type of mental illness? This is a challenging question, and one which many mental health legislative systems across the world have not yet found a satisfactory answer for. Historically, it was argued that personality disorder is lifelong and stable across time and situation, whereas mental disorders tend to have a definable onset and variable, highly context-dependent course. This is a useful way of thinking about a patient's problems to make a formulation, but not a definitive answer. Recent research

suggests that many troublesome personality traits (e.g. impulsivity, affective instability) tend to reduce in prominence with age, so personality may be less stable than initially presumed. At present, UK law defines mental disorder as 'any disorder or disability of the mind'; this broad definition covers personality and mental disorders, so the patient can be treated according to the risks to self and others presented at that time, rather than entirely based on having mental illness rather than personality difficulties.

One point it is helpful to hold in mind is that there are a group of patients who, when not suffering from mental disorder, do not have troublesome personality traits. However, when they become depressed, anxious, or psychotic, those traits become more prominent. This frequently complicates treatment, but also diagnosis, especially if you are meeting the patient for the first time. It is best to avoid diagnosing a personality disorder during a clear episode of mental illness unless there is a clear collateral history pointing towards this.

Types of personality disorder

Classification of personality disorders has been a controversial area since the mid twentieth century. Personality is clearly a complex, multidimensional concept, but classification systems tend to be categorical, with numerical checklists leading to a diagnosis. The latest classification systems are moving towards a dimensional system, but are not there yet (Table 31.1). The DSM-5 has maintained a categorical system but included in the 'emerging methods' system a prototype dimensional system, which may be adopted in time. The current ICD-10 classification is categorical, but the upcoming ICD-11 is probably going to make a radical change towards asking clinicians to make a diagnosis of 'personality disorder: mild, moderate, or severe'. There will no longer be separate diagnostic categories. The idea of a severity rating (given that personality is supposed to lifelong) is acknowledging that in reality, the severity and form of personality disorders do fluctuate over time. The clinician will then be able to qualify the diagnosis further using domain traits, the details of which (at time of writing) are yet to be published.

Table 31.1 Classification of personality disorders in DSM-5 and ICD-10

DSM-5	ICD-10
Cluster A. 'Odd or eccentric'	
Paranoid	Paranoid
Schizoid	Schizoid
Schizotypal	(Schizotypal classified with schizophrenia)
Cluster B. 'Dramatic and emotional'	
Antisocial	Dissocial
Borderline	Emotionally unstable (borderline or impulsive subtypes)
Histrionic	Histrionic
Narcissistic	–
Cluster C. 'Anxious and fearful'	
Avoidant	Anxious (avoidant)
Dependent	Dependent
Obsessive–compulsive	Anankastic

Source data from *Diagnostic and Statistical Manual of Mental Disorders*, 5th Edition (DSM-5), American Psychiatric Association, 2013.

The following sections outline the typical characteristics seen in patients with each of the categorical personality disorders as they are currently defined. It is very common for patients to have features from several categories, which may be called a 'mixed' personality disorder, and is one of the reasons why the current classification systems are not perfect.

Anxious (avoidant) personality disorder

- Feelings of tension, worry, insecurity, and inferiority.
- Avoidance of interpersonal contact due to fears of rejection or criticism.
- Preoccupation with past criticism or rejection (or perception of criticism).
- Need to be liked and accepted.
- Tends to exaggerate risks in everyday situations.
- Tends to avoid new experiences.

Obsessive–compulsive (anankastic) personality disorder

- Perfectionism.
- Rigidity and inflexibility—in thoughts, beliefs, and actions.
- Focus on minutiae of detail.
- Tendency to overthink decisions and then worry about the consequences (this can lead to indecisiveness).
- Easily irritated by others who interrupt their routines or do not live up to their high personal standards.
- May experience unwelcome thoughts or impulses that are not severe enough to meet criteria for obsessive–compulsive disorder.

Dependent personality disorder

- Passive reliance on other people to make decisions (usually a partner, without whom they struggle to manage everyday life).
- Compliance with the wishes of others.
- Avoidance of responsibility.
- Fear of abandonment.
- Feelings of helplessness and incompetence.

Paranoid personality disorder

- Highly sensitive (may be excessively put out by small setbacks).
- Suspicious and mistrusting of others.
- Tendency to distort experiences by misconstruing actions of others as hostile.
- Prone to jealousy.

- Tendency towards irritability and being argumentative.
- May have feelings of undue self-importance, and feel that others let them down all the time.

Schizoid personality disorder

- Lack of emotions and very limited ability to express emotions towards others.
- Limited capacity to experience pleasure.
- Minimal interests in social contacts or the opinion of others.
- Preference for being alone and keeping detached.
- Highly introspective with a rich fantasy world.

Schizotypal personality disorder

Schizotypal personality disorder lies somewhere between psychosis and a personality disorder, hence the classification in different chapters of the DSM (personality) and ICD (psychosis) systems. It is most frequently found in first-degree relatives of patients with schizophrenia. There are odd ideas and ways of thinking which are abnormal, but do not reach the threshold of being a delusion or perceptual abnormality. The characteristics are lifelong and don't follow the typical course of schizophrenia:

- Eccentric behaviour.
- Unusual ideas or thoughts (that do not reach the status of a delusion or formal thought disorder) or ideas of reference.
- Quasi-psychotic experiences (usually with external provocation).
- Vague speech with minimal or odd content.
- Inappropriate or incongruent affect.
- Anhedonia.
- Tendency towards social withdrawal.

Emotionally unstable personality disorder

Patients with emotionally unstable personality disorder (EUPD) present frequently to healthcare providers, especially in emergency situations and so are one of the more familiar disorders. There are two subtypes of EUPD: impulsive and borderline. The term 'borderline' is a historical hangover, relating to the now abandoned idea that the condition was related to (on the borderline with) schizophrenia.

Typical features of EUPD-impulsive subtype include:

- impulsive actions without consideration of the consequences;
- unpredictable, unstable moods;
- outbursts of extreme emotion which the person finds difficult to control;
- difficult interpersonal relationships which are intense and unstable; tendency to initially idealize another only to denigrate them later when it falls apart.

EUPD-borderline subtype has the above-listed features, plus:

- disturbance in self-image;
- uncertainty about self-identity;
- chronic feelings of emptiness;
- actions to avoid abandonment by others;
- self-destructive behaviours, for example, deliberate self-harm, suicide attempts, reckless spending, promiscuity, eating disordered behaviours, substance misuse;
- episodes of dissociative symptoms or pseudo-hallucinations when under stress.

Histrionic personality disorder

- Very social, outgoing individual who likes to be centre of attention and is very theatrical.
- Tendency to manipulative and provocative behaviour.
- Shallow labile emotions which tend to be overexpressed.
- Self-indulgent.
- Lack of consideration for others.
- Constantly seeking approval and attention.

- Sexually provocative behaviour is common but long-lasting genuine love is unusual (this may not be appreciated by the patient).
- Highly suggestible.

Narcissistic personality disorder

The word narcissism refers to morbid self-admiration. This disorder is not included in the ICD-10, but the trait is referred to under 'other' personality disorders.

- Grandiose sense of self-importance.
- Preoccupation with fantasies of their own brilliance, power, intellect, success, etc.
- Craves attention from others to acknowledge their own superiority.
- Tendency to exploit others and never return a favour.
- Minimal empathy.
- May be envious of other people and/or believe others are envious of them.

Antisocial (dissocial) personality disorder

- Impulsive behaviours.
- Low tolerance of frustration.
- Lack of ability to consistently work towards a goal.
- Callous acts with no concern for the feelings of others.
- Disregard for social rules and obligations; this may lead to a forensic history starting in mid childhood.
- Tendency to violence and aggression.
- Lack of guilt and tendency to blame others.
- Failure to sustain close relationships: interpersonal problems leading to divorce are frequent, as are domestic violence and neglect or abuse of children.
- Failure to learn from experience, leading to behaviours that persist or escalate despite negative social consequences and legal penalties.

Impacts of personality disorder

Patients with personality disorders may present complaining about psychological symptoms, but more often they present with sequelae of their personality difficulties or co-morbidities (Box 31.2). Psychiatric co-morbidities are extremely common (especially anxiety and mood disorders) and tend to be difficult to treat. Research evidence shows that patients with personality disorders are less likely to respond to standard treatments than those with normal personality. Rates of completed suicide in those with personality disorders are high; 5–8 per cent of those with EUPD die by suicide. Interpersonal relationships are a key problem area for most patients with personality disorders—building a therapeutic rapport may therefore be difficult and is one reason why outcomes of treatment may be less good. In a minority of cases, individuals with personality disorders are aggressive, violent, or commit crimes: personality disorders can therefore pose significant risk to others.

Box 31.2 Morbidity and mortality related to personality disorders

- Reduced life expectancy—combination of suicide rates, increased physical health problems, and risky lifestyle choices
- High rates of suicide
- Higher risk of dying by homicide
- Increased risk of cardiovascular and respiratory disease
- Increased rate of serious accidental injuries
- Increased rate of deliberate injuries sustained by another person or by self
- Increased risk of sexually transmitted diseases and unwanted pregnancies
- Physical health conditions secondary to smoking, substance misuse, and harmful use of alcohol

Epidemiology

The overall prevalence of personality disorder in international studies is approximately 6 per cent. In the community, rates are marginally higher in men than women, but in outpatient settings this is reversed, probably as females are more likely to seek help than males. Personality disorders are seen across all countries, in all ethnic groups, and are more prevalent in urban than rural settings. In primary care, approximately 25 per cent of patients fit criteria for an ICD-10 personality disorder: in psychiatric outpatients it is 50 per cent, and in prisoners, 55–65 per cent. Antisocial personality disorder (ASPD) is more common in men, while the majority of those with histrionic and emotionally unstable disorders are female. Personality disorders often coexist with mental disorders. A particularly important association is between ASPD and alcohol and substance abuse. There is also a strong association between borderline personality disorder, self-harm, and eating disorders.

Aetiology

Personality and its disorders result from the interaction of genetic factors and upbringing. The relative contribution of these causes is uncertain: this is partly due to the complexity of the interaction and partly due to the challenge of identifying and recording experiences in early life and then being able to relate them to personality features assessed many years later. The heritability of most traits is very high, and many people can identify relatives who are 'similar' to them in personality. Early adverse effects—especially abuse, physical illness, or loss—and parenting received in childhood are very important in the development of personality.

The best understood condition is ASPD—known aetiological factors include the following:

- Genetics: 20 per cent of first-degree relatives of those with ASPD also have the disorder. Monozygotic concordance is 60–70 per cent.
- Brain abnormalities: 50 per cent have EEG abnormalities, high rates of minor facial and cranial anomalies, learning disorders, and hyperactivity disorders. Low levels of serotonin metabolites in

the CSF are associated with aggressive, violent behaviour.

- Adverse childhood experiences: early separation from parents, being raised within the social care system, childhood abuse, erratic parenting, or lack of supervision.
- Association with parents with personality disorders or severe mental health problems themselves.

Assessment of personality

It is helpful to include an assessment of personality as part of a full psychiatric history. To get an accurate description of an individual's personality, the clinician can gather information from:

1 a description of the person by someone who knows them well (e.g. a family member) or another professional (e.g. GP);

2 the patient's own account of their thoughts, feelings, and behaviour in the past and at present;

3 the patient's behaviour in the interview.

A useful method of getting relevant information is to ask 'How do you think your friends and family would … describe your personality?' or '… describe you as a person?'

Describing personality

Unless there is a personality disorder, personality can be described without using technical terms, for example:

- meticulous, but overcautious, and prone to worry excessively;
- precise and reliable, but irritable and easily offended;
- outgoing and generous, but highly emotional.

Note that these short descriptions include both 'favourable' and 'unfavourable' traits. Such brief descriptions are sufficient in most clinical situations, but sometimes it is helpful to refer to the traits listed in Box 31.1.

Systematic enquiries about personality

For patients whom you suspect of having personality difficulties, a standard approach to interviewing should be used. This is to ensure that all relevant aspects of personality have been considered. The areas to cover include the following:

- Current and past relationships: family, peers at school, work colleagues, and intimate relationships. Ask about ease of forming and keeping relationships, ability to confide in others, and levels of sociability.
- Usual mood: are they usually cheerful or gloomy? Does their mood tend to be stable, unstable, or volatile? If unstable, do mood changes occur spontaneously or in response to something? Do they show their feelings or try to hide them?
- Usual daily routine and activities and their ability to cope with changes in this.
- Use of substances, alcohol, and nicotine
- Attitudes to illness, beliefs (e.g. religious) and personal standards.
- Other traits that you think might be relevant, such as those listed in Box 31.1.

Is there personality disorder?

Having built up a picture of the personality, you can decide whether the personality is disordered. The criterion for disorder is suffering (distress or disability) by the patient or by others as a result of the patient's personality. This is ultimately a judgement about the extent to which the patient's problems have been caused by personality and how much by other factors.

Management of personality disorder

Since personality is by its nature unchanging, it is not surprising that personality disorders are difficult to treat. There are, nevertheless, ways of helping patients with personality disorder, usually by helping them acknowledge their difficulties and dealing with any factors that exacerbate the problems. Management includes:

1 diagnosing the personality disorder, communicating the diagnosis to the patient, and helping them take responsibility for their actions;
2 assessing the risk to self and others;
3 helping the patient to deal with or avoid situations that provoke problem behaviours;
4 identifying positive personality features and working on developing these, especially those which improve low self-esteem;
5 identifying and treating any co-morbid psychiatric disorder(s). It is frequently the case that problem behaviours increase when the patient becomes depressed, anxious, or has other psychopathology;
6 treating any associated substance misuse;
7 providing general support and psychoeducation to the patient and family.

Treatment for personality disorders is usually a long-term intervention, and there may be a number of set-backs and crises along the way. Patience is essential. It is very important to build a good relationship between the patient and professional. The patient should feel valued as a person, and be able to trust and confide in the healthcare professional. At the same time, the relationship should not be allowed to become too intense, nor should the patient become dependent or demanding. When more than one person is involved in treatment, their respective roles should be defined and made clear to the patient. Any attempt to 'split' a team should be discussed between the professionals and with the patient. It is usually helpful to have a very clear care plan, which is available to out-of-hours healthcare professionals.

Psychological interventions

The mainstay of treatment for personality disorders is psychological treatment. All patients should receive psychoeducation about personality disorders and any co-morbidities. Self-help materials may be useful in less severe personality disorders, or to help with specific problems such as low self-esteem.

Cognitive behavioural therapy

CBT is useful for people with low self-esteem and difficulties in social relationships.

It is a common choice for patients with Cluster C (anxious) personality disorders, and may be of some benefit for those with prominent paranoid or borderline traits. Specialized forms of CBT for psychosis have shown efficacy in schizotypal personality disorder.

Dialectical behavioural therapy

This is a variant on and specialized form of CBT that was developed for patients with an EUPD. It focuses on reducing self-destructive behaviours and helping the patient comply with treatment. It has both an individual psychotherapy element and a group skills training class, each of which last about a year. DBT is the best evidence-based treatment for EUPD at the present time.

Mentalization-based therapy

A relatively new therapy which combines elements of dynamic therapy and cognitive techniques. The focus is on helping the patient to recognize and deal with how they are feeling at that point in time and to become better at managing those feelings. It was developed for EUPD but has been found to be useful across a wide range of personality difficulties.

Psychodynamic therapy

This is a good choice for those with troubled early experiences and/or patients who need clear boundaries within therapy. A skilled therapist is needed to manage and interpret the transference, which can be intense. Paranoid, histrionic, and antisocial personalities do not usually engage well with dynamic approaches.

Therapeutic communities

Therapeutic communities are groups of patients and clinical facilitators (typically psychologists) who meet regularly to work together to try and overcome their personality-related problems. They are designed to help the patient overcome problematic behaviours by:

- learning more about personality disorders from others with similar problems;
- working in a closed confidential environment which promotes trust;
- exploring their problems in a 'safe' environment, with their peers providing a combination of supportive but challenging relationships;
- learning to take responsibility for their themselves and their actions.

Although traditionally the term 'therapeutic community' has been associated with group residential settings, it is increasingly being applied to more flexible arrangements including day programmes, such as the innovative Complex Needs Service in Oxfordshire (see Box 31.3).

Pharmacological interventions

The role of medications in the management of personality disorders is limited; they are mainly used to treat co-morbid mental illness. Conditions such as depression, anxiety, or eating disorders should be treated along usual guidelines. There is some evidence (almost entirely from treating patients with EUPD or ASPD) for using psychotropics to manage certain aspects of personality disorder, but psychological approaches should be the first approach where possible:

- Antipsychotics are useful for reducing impulsivity and aggression. There is some evidence that they may improve affective dysregulation in EUPD. Antipsychotics may be helpful to reduce stress in a 'crisis', and some patients find short-term use or 'PRN' ('as needed') doses beneficial.

Box 31.3 Oxfordshire's Complex Needs Service

The Oxfordshire Complex Needs Service provides treatment for those with personality disorders or complex needs which are not catered for within standard mental health services. Traditionally, this group of people has been regarded as difficult to help, with the result that services have been difficult to find, and, where they exist, often poorly organized and poorly evidence based. The Complex Needs Service emphasizes the person's own responsibility and they can, for example, self-refer to the service. They progress through several tiers, as follows:

- **Initial assessment and options group.** This provides informal support, and introduction to a group environment, while the person considers whether tier 2 is right for them.
- **Intensive group programme.** This comprises of a group therapy session for 3 hours weekly. The session starts and ends with a community meeting, chaired by a group member, and includes a therapeutic group using an integrative, multimethod psychotherapeutic model. Twenty-four-hour telephone support is available from other members throughout the week.
- **Intensive day programme.** This is an intensive (usually 2 or 3 days per week for at least 18 months) commitment to a therapeutic community which uses several psychotherapeutic approaches, including psychodrama, CBT, dialectical behaviour therapy, and activity groups.
- **Post-therapy programme.** This aims to support patients as they take on new responsibilities and opportunities in work, education, and relationships—aspects of life which many of us take for granted, but which may be new and challenging to many Complex Needs Service patients.

- Mood stabilizers are helpful in reducing mood instability, impulsivity, and aggression.
- Antidepressants are effective at reducing anxiety in Cluster C personality disorders, and have a small effect in stabilizing mood in EUPD. They are frequently used due to so many patients having co-morbid affective and anxiety disorders.
- Benzodiazepines should be avoided where possible, as there is good evidence that patients with personality disorders are highly prone to dependency.

Further reading

Gask L, Evans M, Kessler D. Personality disorder. *BMJ* 2013;347:f5276.

Royal College of Psychiatrists. Personality disorder. Published 2015. http://www.rcpsych.ac.uk/healthadvice/problemsdisorders/personalitydisorder.aspx. [This leaflet is a good resource for patients and carers, but also gives a simple clear description of personality difficulties for those first encountering them in clinical practice.]

Tyrer P, Reed GM, Crawford MJ. Classification, assessment, prevalence, and effect of personality disorder. *Lancet* 2015;385:717–726.

32 Child and adolescent psychiatry: specific disorders

Introduction

This chapter describes common and/or important mental health disorders seen in children and adolescents. More general information about classification, aetiology, assessment, and management is discussed in Chapter 17. Many of the psychiatric problems seen in adolescence are the common disorders of adulthood; in the latter part of the chapter, these are briefly covered, identifying adolescent-specific presentation or treatment with reference to the general information in relevant chapters on adults.

Epidemiology

Mental disorders are very common in childhood and adolescence; meta-analysis data from international studies suggest a prevalence of 10 per cent in 5–15-year-olds. It is difficult to get accurate epidemiology data for preschool-age children—partly as fewer studies have been done, but also because many behavioural and emotional problems are short-lived and the child 'grows out' of them. Boys tend to be more prone to hyperactive, disruptive, and autistic spectrum disorders, while girls predominant the emotional disorders. Table 32.1 gives an overview of epidemiology of common mental health disorders.

Problems of preschool children

Common problems in preschoolers are shown in Table 32.2. Most problems are short-lived and whether they are reported to doctors depends on the attitudes of the parents as well as on the severity of the issue. The aetiology of these conditions is primarily related to individual variations in development and temperament, but family problems can play a role in certain situations. In the UK, a health visitor is uniquely placed to assess the child and provide advice and support.

Table 32.1 Epidemiology of common mental health disorders in school-aged children

	Overall (%)	Females	Males
Overall prevalence of any mental disorder (5–16 years)	10		
Overall prevalence of any mental disorder (5–10 years)		5%	10%
Overall prevalence of any mental disorder (11–16 years)		10%	13%
Anxiety disorders	2–3		
Depression:			
Overall	0.9	1:1	
13–17 years	3.5	3:1	
Bipolar disorder	1	1:1	
Disruptive disorders	4	1:4	
Tic disorders	1	1:5	
Tourette's syndrome	0.5		
ADHD	3	1:4	
ICD-10 hyperactivity disorder[a]	1.5		
Autistic spectrum disorder	0.9	1:4	
Eating disorders	0.4		
OCD	0.5	>1:1	
Deliberate self-harm (11–16 years):			
Overall	1.2		
DSH in children with a mental disorder	10–18		

[a] ICD-10 criteria for hyperactivity disorder are significantly more stringent than the DSM-IV/5 criteria for ADHD.

Neurodevelopmental disorders

Neurodevelopmental disorders are conditions that arise due to abnormalities in growth or development of the central nervous system. Some of these disorders cause emotional and behavioural difficulties or are highly associated with other mental disorders; it is these conditions that tend to present to psychiatry. A summary is shown in Table 32.3. They tend to present in early to mid childhood.

Autistic spectrum disorders

Autistic spectrum disorders (ASD) are neurodevelopmental conditions characterized by deficits and delays in social and communicative development, which are associated with restricted patterns of interest and behaviour. As the name suggests, ASD are a spectrum of conditions, with individuals varying both in severity and form of the disorder. Due to this heterogeneity, the nomenclature and classification of ASD have been through various incarnations. Until recently they have been known as pervasive developmental disorders, with subtypes of childhood autism, atypical autism, Rett's syndrome, and Asperger's syndrome. However, these subtypes were not terribly helpful clinically, so the classification systems have now all moved towards a single diagnosis of ASD.

ASD are characterized by a triad of impairments:

Table 32.2 Common disorders of preschool children

Disobedience	• Common in children aged 2–5 years; usually improved with parenting skills training and behavioural reward strategies
Temper tantrums	• Normal for children aged 1–3 years, usually mild and improve with time • Usual triggers include frustration at not being able to make themselves understood, wanting independence, hunger, fatigue, or wanting attention • Management consists of helping parents to discipline consistently and avoid paying attention to the child during the tantrum
Breath holding	• Periods of breath holding occur in 5% of children aged 2–5 years • Breath-holding spells usually occur when a child is frustrated, angry, or upset • The child starts a tantrum but suddenly goes quiet. Usually they start breathing again quickly, but persistent children may turn blue or purple during the spell and pass out for a few seconds. This is alarming but the child recovers spontaneously. • Reassurance is very important, and helping parents to react calming to the breath-holding and avoid giving the child attention is usually an effective treatment strategy.
Sleep problems	• Sleep difficulties affect one-third of preschool children and are usually a temporary phenomenon • The role of the doctor is primarily to reassure, but also to exclude sleep disturbance secondary to another physical (e.g. asthmatic cough) or mental health problem • Common problems include insomnia, nightmares, and night terrors (see the section on sleep disorders)
Feeding problems	• Food fads and food refusal are frequently seen in preschoolers, but only rarely is it clinically significant • The great majority of children are healthy and growing well and there is no cause for concern • Behaviour is frequently reinforced unintentionally by parents, and parents can be helped by supporting them to reduce anxiety around food and ignore the behaviours while offering an appropriate, balanced diet • Child behaviour-reward strategies may be helpful—e.g. a star chart for trying new foods • Pica is the eating of items that are not foods (e.g. soil, paint, and paper) and is sometimes seen in toddlers. Pica is often associated with other behaviour problems, autism, or learning disability so a full assessment of the child is needed. Pica usually improves spontaneously with time
Attachment disorders	• Not a common problem, but important to diagnose • Attachment disorders occur when a child does not form a normal secure relationship with their caregiver(s). Children may also show inappropriate familiarity to unfamiliar adults • Risk factors: children raised in care or institutions, experience of abuse or neglect, prolonged separation from caregivers (e.g. due to hospitalization), mother with severe postnatal depression, one of a very large family so they get minimal attention

1 **Deficits in social interactions:**
- Difficulties in initiating and sustaining interactions with other people.
- Child may not respond to affection normally, and may not value the company of their parents over that of complete strangers. They frequently do not understand how to make or maintain friends, and have difficulty playing or sharing interests with others.
- Typical clinical features include babies who don't like being held, reduced eye contact, unusual facial expressions, lack of gestures, poor understanding of others' feelings, lack of empathy, and few peer relationships.

Table 32.3 Neurodevelopmental disorders

Disorders of intellectual development	See Chapter 19
Autistic spectrum disorders	See text
Developmental learning disorders: • Reading ('dyslexia') • Written expression • Maths	Persistent difficulties in learning specific academic skills leading to performance lower than would be expected for the child's age and general intellect. These conditions are usually picked up soon after a child starts school. Specialist teaching and support can help the child to make significant progress
Development disorder of motor coordination ('dyspraxia')	Delay in acquiring gross and fine motor skills. The child tends to be clumsy, slow, and inaccurate in their movements. There is a spectrum of severity, with the majority catching up with their development by adulthood
Chronic developmental tic disorders	See text
Attention deficit hyperactivity disorders	See p. 492

2 **Communication difficulties:**

- Speech may be absent (25 per cent), completely normal, or anywhere in between. (Note that the eponymous name Asperger's syndrome is commonly used to refer to children with ASD who have normal language abilities.)
- Common abnormalities of speech include unusual patterns or ways of speaking, echolalia, odd prosody (unusual pitch/stress/rhythm/ intonation), and pronoun reversal (referring to themselves as he or she).
- Autistic children have difficulty in two-way conversations, and some ask a string of questions instead.

3 **Restricted, repetitive inflexible interests and behaviours:**

- Very specific, fixed interests that are unusual in context, intensity, or focus are almost universal in ASD, for example, a special interest in front- loading washing machines or patterns in licence plates. The child may have no interest in the toys their peers play with.
- Stereotyped or repetitive movements, speech or use of objects, for example, lining up items, hand flapping, head rolling, and repeating words over and over.

- Fixed inflexible routines with an insistence on 'sameness'. Ritualized behaviours. Autistic children are frequently highly distressed by changes in their routine.
- Sensory hyper- or hyposensitivity. It is common that children over-react or are indifferent to sensory inputs, for example, loud noises, sensation of specific fabrics, temperate, and strong odours.

The clinical features of ASD must develop early in life and cause distress or impairment to the child. It is important to exclude other potential causes of the symptoms, for example, deafness, poor vision, learning disability, or specific speech and language deficits. Sixty to seventy per cent of those with ASD also have a learning disability.

Aetiology

The pathogenesis of autism is poorly understood, but is likely to be multifactorial with a strong polygenic genetic component. The phenotypic variation in ASD is consistent with a polygenic aetiology, which is then further modified by environmental exposures.

Genetic factors. Twin studies indicate that autism has 90 per cent heritability. The risk of autism in a sib- ling of an affected child is 10–20 per cent, a massive increase over the general population risk. There are also higher rates of social, language, and learning problems in relatives, suggesting that autism may represent the severe end of a general predisposition to developmental difficulties.

Organic brain disorder. There is evidence that children with ASD have faster brain growth in early childhood, and increased brain size overall (2–10 per cent) by adulthood. Functional imaging has shown differences in connectivity and metabolic activity in multiple areas compared to normal controls. Twenty per cent of those with ASD have epilepsy.

Cognitive abnormalities involve, in particular, symbolic thinking and language. An important deficit, present in many but not all of these children, is the inability to judge correctly what other people are thinking and to use this knowledge to predict their behaviour (lack of a 'theory of mind'). It is proposed that this deficit is the core abnormality underlying ASD.

Environmental factors. Meta-analysis data including more than 50 potential environmental risk factors have found no significant evidence to link ASD to any specific factor. There is no evidence that abnormal parenting or childhood vaccinations are associated with ASD. There is limited evidence that adverse events in the perinatal period and increased parental age predispose to ASD.

Course and prognosis

About two-thirds of the children who meet the criteria for ASD have useful speech, although serious impairments usually remain. Most of the abnormal behaviours continue into adulthood, but may improve and become less socially impairing with time, especially with behavioural interventions. Worldwide, about 20 per cent of children with ASD attend a mainstream school, but in the UK it is 70 per cent. This is because specialist ASD centres have been set up within certain schools in each area to provide the extra support to allow children with milder deficits to be with their neurotypical peers but still receive some extra help. At present, evidence suggests that for the less impaired end of the ASD spectrum, this approach gives better outcomes. Those individuals with a normal IQ usually go on to live independently and work, while those with learning disabilities may need help throughout life.

Assessment

An appropriate assessment of the child and their family should be carried out, including all of the general points outlined on p. 190. The gold standard diagnostic tools are the **Autism Diagnostic Interview** and **Autism Diagnostic Observation Schedule**, which are interviews carried out with the parents and child, respectively. A full examination should be undertaken to exclude an organic cause for the symptoms.

Management

Treatment of ASD will never be curative; it is therefore a question of providing appropriate skills and an environment in which the child can learn to interact with the rest of society in the best way possible. Box 32.1 shows

Box 32.1 Treatment options for autistic spectrum disorders

General

- Psychoeducation for the child and their family
- Finding an appropriate educational setting
- Mainstream school
- Mainstream school with special provision for ASD
- Specialist school for learning disability and/or ASD
- Education in the home
- Treating psychiatric and physical co-morbidities
- Parental training courses—to help teach behavioural modification techniques
- Parental support (e.g. respite care and carers groups)

Biological

- Atypical antipsychotics
- Stimulants
- Antidepressants
- Melatonin

Psychological

- Speech and language therapy
- Social skills training
- Behavioural modification programmes

an outline of the various treatment options. Most children will need input from a variety of professionals; for example, paediatrician, psychiatrist, neurology, psychologist, speech and language therapist, or occupational therapist.

Psychological treatments

The mainstay of treatment in any ASD is intensive, focused behavioural training programmes. Usually, the aim is to reduce troublesome behaviours, while promoting more socially acceptable and productive ones. Children with ASD cannot transfer skills easily, and need to be taught how to do this, although this is not always successful. Social skills training classes are of help for higher-functioning children, especially as this provides them with a sheltered opportunity for social interaction. Speech and language therapists are invaluable in the early years; they can help the child to achieve their verbal potential, which then to some extent defines what they can later achieve.

Biological treatments

Pharmacological treatments are only indicated in ASD to help reduce symptoms that have not responded to behavioural and psychological interventions. Several RCTs have demonstrated that atypical antipsychotics (especially risperidone) are effective in reducing aggression, tantrums, stereotypies, and self-injury. The side effects may be significant, so they are reserved for use after behavioural modifications have failed. Stimulants or atomoxetine are effective in children with co-morbid ADHD, and SSRIs can decrease repetitive or obsessive behaviours. Recently, there has been much debate as to the worth of melatonin in affecting sleep cycles; some parents advocate the use of it in their autistic children who suffer from severe sleep–wake cycle disturbances.

Gender identity disorder

Gender identity disorder (GID) is a condition in which a person experiences discomfort with the biological sex with which they were born to such an extent that it becomes clinically significant. The nomenclature in this area is confusing: at present the main classification systems use different names:

- ICD-10: gender identity disorder.
- ICD-11 beta draft: gender incongruence.
- DSM-5: gender dysphoria.

However, they specify almost identical clinical criteria for the diagnosis. The individual needs to have a desire to live and be accepted as a member of the opposite gender, and usually would like to make their body congruent with that gender. These feelings should present for at least 2 years and not due to another mental disorder.

Typical clinical features of GID include:

- repeatedly stating a desire to be a member of the other gender;
- a desire to look like the other gender—for example, to dress as the opposite sex do or alter their genitals/secondary sex characteristics;
- a preference for games, toys, or activities typically associated with the other gender;
- a preference for associating with members of the other gender;
- use of verbal and physical mannerisms more typical of the opposite sex.

The prevalence of GID is unknown. The mean age of presentation to psychiatric services is 7–8 years, typically when parents become concerned their child's behaviour is not just a passing phase. There is a second peak in mid adolescence, when those who were 'unsure' become clearer in their mind as they start to go through puberty.

Aetiology

The cause of this disorder is unknown. A number of factors have been shown to influence psychosexual development, but their relationship to GID is currently unclear:

- **Hormones.** Female children with congenital adrenal hyperplasia produce an excess of androgens, leading to virilization. These children tend to engage in more masculine games and behaviours from a young age, and often have male friends. However, they do not have the psychological wish to be the other sex. There have been several cases of male children who have undergone penectomy secondary to trauma and were reassigned to female before 2 years of life. These children, although brought up as females, tend to revert to their original sex in early adulthood, or become homosexual in orientation. This suggests a prenatal influence on gender identity.

- **Early differences in behaviour.** Children as young as 10 months are thought to be able to distinguish between those who are the same and those who are the opposite sex from themselves. By 12 months, children start to show a preference for toys associated with their sex, and start to prefer the company of the same-sex parent. Boys begin to be more assertive and physically aggressive at about 18 months, while girls are more passive. At about this age, children become aware of sex stereotypes, believing that boys like to play with trucks and building things, whereas girls cook and play with dolls.
- **Parental influences.** There is robust evidence that parents tend to buy toys for their child that are gender related—dolls for girls and soldiers for boys. When mothers are presented with a young child call John and dressed as a boy, they treat them as a boy, even if the child is actually a dressed-up girl.

Assessment and management

Assessment of a child with GID should include a full psychiatric assessment. It is important to identify any other mental disorders and exclude an intersex condition or other physical cause for the symptoms.

Psychoeducation is a key part of treating GID. Educating the whole family about gender identity, normal and abnormal, is very important and helps to establish that it is not necessary for boys to behave in one specific way, and that variation is normal.

Wait-and-see approaches. For some children, especially the very young, it can be appropriate to support the family in general terms, but just wait to see how the child's identity changes as they get older.

Behaviour modification techniques can be used to help the child in adapting to who they are and fitting in with other children. Finding other children of their biological sex who are less stereotypical in their behaviours (e.g. sporty girls, non-physical more home-orientated boys) can assist the child in widening their peer group and interests. Individual CBT can be used in older children, to address abnormal thought paths and associated psychological issues.

Social transition. Some families decide to allow the child to live as the opposite sex. This is not a decision to be made lightly, and involves considerable discussion with all concerned, including the child's school. The child can change their hair, clothes, pronoun, and even name. As these are reversible changes, a trial run can be done before a final decision is made. The child, and those they come into contact with (e.g. peers at school, siblings, and teachers) need education and support during the process.

Physical transition. Puberty is universally a very distressing time for patients with GID. Physical changes are unwanted, and problems such as facial hair and menses are particularly difficult to contend with. It is possible to use GnRH analogues to block puberty in the early stages, and later (depending on the child's preferences) to either give cross-sex steroids or stop the GnRH to allow normal puberty to continue. However, these should be initiated by specialists after very careful consideration. At present, surgical interventions are not recommended in children.

Prognosis and outcome

At present, the factors which determine if children with GID will continue to have gender dysphoria into adulthood are unknown. A proportion of them do become comfortable with their biological sex, but the figures are unclear. Approximately two-thirds of these children with GID have a homosexual or bisexual orientation in adulthood. Some children with GID make the decision to change to the other sex, and spend the rest of their life living as the other gender. GID is strongly associated with other psychiatric disorders, especially depression, anxiety disorders, and poor self-esteem.

Disorders of school-age children and teenagers

Disorders in older children and adolescents are shown in Table 32.4; those of adolescence are fundamentally the same as the adult disorder and are discussed in their relevant chapters.

Anxiety disorders

It is normal for children to have worries, and to feel apprehensive about new people, situations or activities. For some children, those worries can become more prominent, distressing and start to interfere with their daily life: these are anxiety disorders. Anxiety disorders are common, especially in girls. Anxiety disorders tend vary with age; separation anxiety and phobic disorder usually start in preschool years, while social anxiety starts later. Panic disorder is usually only seen in adolescents. The general symptoms and co-morbidities associated with anxiety are shown in Box 32.2; features

Box 32.2 Symptoms of childhood anxiety disorder

- Separation anxiety
- Fearfulness
- Timidity
- Excessive worrying
- Poor concentration
- Poor sleep
- Avoidance behaviours (school, parties, sleepovers, etc.)
- Physical symptoms: headache, nausea, vomiting, abdominal pain, or bowel disturbance
- Overdependence on adults
- Decline in school performance
- Co-morbidities: mood disorders, eating disorders, or substance abuse

of specific anxiety disorders are similar to those seen in adults (see Chapter 24).

Separation anxiety disorder

Separation anxiety disorder occurs when the child fears that harm will occur to an attachment figure if they are apart, and is severe enough to interfere with daily activities and social development. It occurs in 3–5 per cent of primary school-age children, and is more common in girls. Children with separation anxiety cling to their parents and are extremely distressed when parted from them. In severe cases, it may present as school refusal, or avoidance of leaving the house. The condition may be initiated by a frightening experience such as admission to hospital, or by insecurity in the family; for example, when the parents are contemplating divorce. Separation anxiety is often maintained by overprotective attitudes of the parents and treatment is directed to changing these attitudes and reassuring the child. The majority of children will 'grow out' of it, even without intervention from professionals.

Aetiology

1 **Genetics.** Children with parents who have anxiety disorders are two to four times more likely to develop one than the general population.

Table 32.4 Psychiatric disorders in older children and adolescents

Children aged 5 to (approximately) 13 years	Adolescents
- Anxiety disorders	- Depression
- OCD	- Bipolar disorder
- Mood disorders	- Anxiety disorders and OCD
- Attachment disorder	- Eating disorders
- Somatization disorders	- Schizophrenia and other psychoses
- Enuresis and encopresis	- Deliberate self-harm and suicide
- Eating disorders	- Somatoform disorders
- Tics and Tourette's syndrome	- Substance abuse
- ADHD	- Conduct disorder
- Conduct disorder	
- Sleep disorders	

Heritability for anxiety disorders is estimated to be 40–50 per cent.

2 **Personality.** The child's temperament plays a large role—if they are shy or hesitant and fearful in new situations, they are at higher risk of an anxiety disorder.

3 **Parent–child attachment.** An insecure attachment to either parent is linked to anxiety disorders, as is a lack of reassurance and support being provided from parent to child. Overly strict parenting can also promote anxiety, as the child tends not to develop confidence to explore their environment.

4 **Parental anxiety disorder.** If parents or other people in the home are anxious, then (independent from the genetic risk) the child may also learn anxious behaviour from them.

Course and prognosis

The episode of anxiety itself is likely to remit, but leaves the child at high risk of developing anxiety-related problems or depression in adulthood; 50 per cent of adults with depression have had an anxiety disorder in childhood or adolescence.

Treatment

The stages of treatment are summarized in Box 32.3. Psychological treatments—specifically CBT—are the first-line approach, as there is good evidence for their efficacy. If therapy does not provide an adequate response, an SSRI can be tried, but the NNT for a clinically positive response is three in adolescents and four in children. Usually, a combination of a supportive approach, education, and CBT will be effective. Benzodiazepines are not recommended.

Somatic symptoms of emotional disorder

Children often communicate distress by complaining repeatedly of physical symptoms for which no physical cause can be found. The terms **functional** or **medically unexplained symptoms** are sometimes used, and the process is called somatization. The symptoms are usually associated with stressful circumstances or with parental anxiety. Common complaints are of abdominal pain, headache, limb pains, and sickness. Of these, abdominal pain is particularly frequent.

Treatment. The steps in treatment are summarized in Box 32.4. The doctor explains to the child and parents that the physical symptoms are undoubtedly real, and are treatable. The relationship to stress and anxiety is explained; the analogy with headache is often helpful. When the symptom is pain, the parents are advised to convey sympathy but not to focus attention on the pain. The child and parents are helped to find ways of reducing the experience of pain without taking analgesics, such as having distracting activities or relaxing music available.

Box 32.3 Treatment of childhood anxiety disorder

General measures

- Psychoeducation: explain the nature of the problem to the parents and child
- Provide self-help materials
- Help the child to talk about their worries
- Reduce or avoid stressors

Psychological treatment

- CBT
- Relaxation therapy

Pharmacological treatment

- SSRIs

Box 32.4 Treatment of somatic symptoms of emotional disorder

- Explain that the symptoms are real but have psychological rather than physical causes
- Help the child to talk about the symptoms and worries
- Reduce or avoid stressors
- Psychoeducation for family members
- Family therapy if there is unresolved conflict or relationship problems
- CBT or behavioural therapy to modify the child's illness behaviour
- Avoid using analgesics and anxiolytics

Selective mutism

Selective mutism is a condition in which a person who is normally capable of speech is unable to speak in certain situations, or to specific people. It is classified as an anxiety disorder, and is a condition almost exclusively found in children. The person has a normal understanding of language and can often speak fluently at home with familiar people, but refuses to do so in some situations, for example, at school or in the presence of strangers. Selective mutism is reported to be present in 4 in 1000 children, but there have been no large epidemiological studies to date. The age of onset is usually 2–5 years, but it often does not become evident or a problem until the child starts school. It is more common in girls. A history of a speech disorder or abuse are the main risk factors.

Assessment and management

A general assessment of the child should be carried out, as on p. 190. It is important to exclude ASD or another developmental disorder. It may be necessary to assess the child in a variety of settings—for example, home, school, or outpatients—and with and without their carers. Treatment at an early age is important, as children with selective mutism rarely improve spontaneously.

Behavioural therapy is an effective treatment. The premise is that the mutism is a learnt behaviour. Stimulus fading is a common technique, where the patient is brought into an environment with someone else they are comfortable with, then gradually (in small steps) another person is introduced to the group, and the process continues slowly as the child gets used to it.

Play or art therapy is often used to try and examine the reasons underlying the child's mutism.

Family therapy helps to identify difficulties in family relationships that are contributing to the mutism, and to help the rest of the family cope with the mutism.

Speech and language therapy is often helpful, even if the child has no specific speech disorder.

There is currently no evidence for the use of medications in children with selective mutism.

Obsessive–compulsive disorder

Obsessive–compulsive disorder (OCD) is a condition characterized by obsessions and/or compulsions that the person feels driven to perform in order to prevent an imagined dreaded event. The general features of OCD in children are very similar to those seen in adults and are described on p. 342. The only diagnostic difference between adults and children is that while adults must realize that their thoughts are unreasonable or excessive to meet diagnostic criteria for OCD, in children this is not required. It is common for younger children not to have a clear idea of what they are trying to avoid while performing a ritual, and they may not be able to fully describe the obsessions they are experiencing. OCD is highly associated with tic disorders, Tourette's syndrome, mood disorders, and eating disorders. The options for management of OCD are shown in Box 32.5. CBT should be the first-line treatment unless the child can not engage with therapy, in which case an SSRI can be tried first.

Unipolar depression

Depression in childhood is relatively common, with the majority representing a normal response to distressing or adverse circumstances. Children tend to describe themselves as 'grouchy', 'empty', or 'unable to have fun' rather than low or depressed. The diagnostic

Box 32.5 Management of OCD

General measures for all patients

- Psychoeducation for the child and their family
- Problem-solving techniques and relaxation
- Self-help resources

Mild to moderate functional impairment

- CBT

Severe functional impairment

- Combined treatment with CBT and an SSRI (best evidence for sertraline, fluoxetine, or fluvoxamine)
- Family interventions
- Consider clomipramine

criteria for depression in the diagnostic classifications include all ages (p. 261), although there are a number of slight differences in children:

- Mood may be low, but is frequently irritable. Parents may present the child as being easily annoyed, uncaring, and feeling that everything is unfair.

- Atypical features, such as hyperphagia or hypersomnia are more common.

- Sleep is often disturbed, but may not show the classical pattern of early morning awakening.

- Rather than weight loss, children may fail to gain weight or fall off of their growth centile.

- Occasionally, physical symptoms (e.g. abdominal pain, headaches, or fatigue) may be the only presenting complaint.

- Symptoms may vary across different settings; for example, they may be very low at home but able to function slightly better at school.

Aetiology

The aetiology of depression is described in Chapter 21, but in childhood there is often a precipitating stressful event (e.g. bullying, a significant loss). Common environmental factors include:

- abuse or neglect;
- losses or bereavements;
- family discord;
- substance abuse, criminality, or violence within the family;
- bullying;
- living in poverty;
- early attachment difficulties;
- social isolation.

Management

Some children with depression will need treatment within secondary care, but milder cases may be managed by the GP. If any of the following features are present, the child should be referred to a child psychiatrist:

- Moderate, severe, or psychotic depression.

- Mild depression which has not responded to interventions in primary care.

- Recurrence of depression after recovery from a moderate to severe episode.

- Self-neglect.

- Active suicidal ideation (these children may require day or inpatient treatment).

All children and their families should receive adequate psychoeducation, self-help materials, and advice about diet, exercise, and sleep hygiene.

Treatment of mild depression

Initially it may be appropriate to be supportive, undertake the general measures described previously, and arrange a follow-up in 2 weeks ('watchful waiting'). If the child has not improved, offer guided self-help or a short course of CBT.

Treatment of moderate to severe depression

The child should be offered individual CBT, IPT, or brief family therapy. If therapy is not appropriate, unavailable, or ineffective, consider use of an antidepressant. SSRIs are the first line, usually at half the normal adult dose. There is good evidence for fluoxetine, citalopram, escitalopram, and sertraline in those aged 12–18 years. It is important to monitor the child carefully in the first 2 weeks of treatment as there is a higher risk of suicidal thoughts and impulsive acts, as well as the usual side effects.

Post-traumatic stress disorder

Post-traumatic stress disorder (PTSD) is severe psychological disturbance following a traumatic event, characterized by the involuntary re-experiencing of the event combined with symptoms of hyperarousal, dissociation, and avoidance. It is described fully in Chapter 23. Table 32.5 shows some common stressors in childhood, but specific traumatic events (e.g. war and earthquakes) may also play a role. The clinical features

Table 32.5 Stressors in childhood

Chronic	
Poverty	Deprivation
Parental mental illness	Parental substance misuse
Chronic family conflicts	War
Refugee status	Social discrimination
Chronic physical illness	Physical, sexual, or emotional abuse
Acute	
Accidents	Bereavement
Separation from carers	Bullying
Assault	Death of a pet
Change of school	Loss of friends
Physical illness	Illness of a relative

Box 32.6 Physical symptoms commonly relating to somatization in children

Cardiovascular
- Breathlessness
- Chest pain

Gastrointestinal
- Abdominal pain
- Nausea and anorexia
- Vomiting or regurgitation
- Diarrhoea or frequent bowel motions

Genitourinary
- Dysuria
- Frequency
- Copious vaginal discharge
- Odd sensations around genitalia

Neurological
- Headaches
- Tingling or numbness
- Amnesia
- Chronic fatigue

Musculoskeletal
- Aches and pains

are similar to those in adults, and there is frequently co-morbid anxiety, depression, or ADHD. About 50 per cent of children develop PTSD after a major disaster (e.g. plane crash, volcanic eruption), and 25 per cent develop symptoms after lesser events such as road traffic accidents. However, most will recover from the PTSD, with one-third of those diagnosed 3 months after a major disaster being symptom free at 1 year.

Management

The recommended first-line intervention is trauma-focused cognitive behavioural therapy (TF-CBT). Family therapy is usually offered alongside, and young children may benefit from formal art or play therapy. Medication is not recommended, unless there is significant co-morbid depression, in which case an SSRI may be prescribed under close supervision.

Somatization and somatoform disorders

Somatoform disorder is a syndrome of physical symptoms which do not have a known organic cause and

are distressing to the patient. The patient typically attributes the symptoms to a non-psychiatric cause. These are described more fully in Chapter 25. It is extremely common for children to express their distress or unhappiness through physical symptoms, although a disorder fitting standard criteria is relatively rare. The commonest symptoms that children complain of are shown in Box 32.6, but by far the most frequent are abdominal pain and headaches. Co-morbid anxiety or depressive disorders are commonplace.

Prevalence

The prevalence of somatization disorder or somatic symptoms in children is unknown. Abdominal pain accounts for 10 per cent of new appointments with paediatricians, and in very few children is gastrointestinal pathology found. The peak age for unexplained symptoms is 8–12 years, and they are much more common in girls.

Aetiology

Somatoform disorders are multifactorial in origin. There is a genetic component—20 per cent of first-degree relatives of children with somatoform disorder also fit criteria—but psychosocial stressors play a significant role (Box 32.7).

Assessment and management

The aims of assessing a child with a somatic complaint are threefold:

1 To undertake a full psychiatric and social assessment of the child and family.

2 To exclude an organic cause for the symptoms.

3 To produce a management plan.

Box 32.7 Risk factors for somatization in children and adolescents

Child factors

- Previous physical illness
- Oldest child in family
- Low IQ
- Experience of child abuse or neglect
- Personality traits: perfectionism, anxiety, and conscientiousness
- History of depression or anxiety disorder

Family factors

- Familial physical illness, especially chronic disease or disability
- Psychiatric problems, especially depression or anxiety
- Parental somatization
- High expectations of the child
- Poor intrafamily communication and relationships

Social factors

- Lower socioeconomic class
- Poverty
- Life stresses (e.g. bullying or academic pressures)

While a thorough physical examination and basic investigations are appropriate, multiple and specialist investigations should be avoided.

Psychoeducation is the most important aspect of management. It is important to

- acknowledge the symptoms and that they are distressing;
- provide reassurance that no serious organic disorders have been found;
- explain the link between psychological stress and physical symptoms;
- explain that the symptoms can be treated, and that the best way to do this is via a clear treatment plan. The plan should avoid frequent consultations, constant investigations, and unnecessary medications.

Teaching relaxation and problem-solving skills

Family therapy can be extremely helpful in addressing problems such as unsolved conflict within the family, poor communication, and highly expressed emotions.

Individual CBT for the child can allow the links between thoughts, feelings, and physical sensations to be explored. Behavioural techniques may be used to help the child adjust their abnormal illness behaviour; for example, by increasing school attendance.

Practical aspects. Getting the child into school regularly and engaging in social activities is essential, and the family may need education and assistance in order to do this.

Physical interventions may be appropriate for some conditions. Basic approaches such as a hot-water bottle for a stomach ache are usually beneficial. Complex treatment regimens involving medications (especially long-term painkillers) should be avoided.

Antidepressants may be indicated in older children, especially with co-morbid anxiety or depression, as there is evidence in adults that they are efficacious for somatoform disorder. An SSRI (typically fluoxetine) would be the first-line choice.

Sleep disorders

The commonly encountered disorders of sleeping in children are **nightmares**, **night terrors**, and **sleep-walking**. These are all covered in detail in Chapter 28, so what follows are the specific points related to children and adolescents.

The physiology of sleep is very different in children and adults, and is complicated by the fact that it changes throughout development. Some of the differences include:

- the total amount of sleep needed is more than in adults (see Table 32.6);
- the circadian sleep–wake cycle does not become trained until 6–8 months;
- between 5 years and puberty, sleep is very sound at night and children are very alert during the day (there is less of a distinction in adults);
- adolescents have increased daytime sleepiness compared with any other age; the sleep phase often becomes delayed, so that teenagers like to stay up late and lie in during the mornings.

It is important to recognize that sleep disturbance in childhood can have wide-ranging effects, including a direct negative effect upon mood, behaviour, and cognitive function. Adolescents are at particular risk of other psychiatric problems if they have continually inadequate sleep. While adults tend to become slow in mental and physical activities when sleep deprived, children often show increased activity, irritability,

Table 32.6 Average sleep requirements at different ages

Neonate	17 hours
2 years	13 hours
4 years	12 hours
10 years	10 hours
Adolescent	9 hours
Adult	5–9 hours

Box 32.8 Groups at high risk of sleep disturbance

- Anxious children or those with panic disorder
- Traumatic experiences in early life
- Depressive disorders
- ADHD
- ASD
- OCD
- Tourette's syndrome
- Parental mental illness
- Chaotic household and disorganized daily routine
- Homeless children
- Children from lower socioeconomic households
- Learning disorders
- Neurodegenerative disorders
- Acute physical illness (e.g. gastroenteritis)

agitation, and loss of temper control. Groups of children at particularly high risk of a sleep disorder are shown in Box 32.8.

Assessment of a child presenting with a sleep disorder

The general schedule for assessing patients with sleep disorders (p. 406) should be followed, but with a few alterations. It is important to get the parents to record a 24-hour sleep–wake pattern on at least one ordinary day, and then to keep a sleep diary for 2–4 weeks in order to determine the usual routine and sleep disturbances. A full developmental history should be taken and a physical examination done. Investigations can be carried out as for adults (p. 406); actigraphy is well tolerated and validated for use in children.

Insomnia

About 20 per cent of preschoolers and 30 per cent of school-age children either have trouble getting to sleep or wake up repeatedly during the night. Common causes of sleeplessness in children include night-time fears (e.g. monsters), separation anxiety, daytime napping, worries, anxiety, depression, and in teenagers, caffeine, nicotine, and alcohol in the evenings. If a psychiatric or physical disorder is the cause, the best approach is to treat it. For many children, discussing their worries or fears can lessen them, and reassurance to the parents that the problem is likely to resolve by itself. For very young children, basic sleep hygiene and avoidance of reinforcing the problem behaviours are usually effective.

Nightmares

Nightmares are frightening dreams that cause the child to wake up, usually feeling slightly confused. The child may be distressed, and can take time to get back to sleep. They occur during REM sleep, and show a distinctive increase in activity on the EEG. Nightmares are common in childhood, especially around the ages of 5 or 6 years. Frequent nightmares may be accompanied by daytime anxiety. There is no specific treatment, so parents should be reassured that it is likely to improve with time and helped to reduce any stressful circumstances at home.

Night terrors

Night terrors are less common than nightmares. They are characterized by a sudden awakening in which the child sits upright, screams loudly, and has marked autonomic activation. Occasionally, there may be frantic motor activity which can lead to falling out of bed and injury. The episode occurs a few hours after going to bed, and usually lasts about 5 minutes. Afterwards the child goes back to sleep, and is unable to remember the events in the morning. There is no specific treatment, but it is important to reassure the family, make sure the child is safe at night, and ensure good sleep hygiene. Night terrors seldom persist into adult life.

Sleepwalking

Sleepwalking is characterized by complex, automatic behaviours occurring during sleep. In children, this usually involves wandering around the house. The child's eyes are open and they avoid familiar objects. The child may appear agitated, does not respond to questions, and is often difficult to wake, although they can usually be led back to bed. Episodes usually last for a few minutes, although rarely they may continue

for as long as an hour. It is most common between the ages of 5 and 12 years, occurring at least once in 15 per cent of children in this age group. Occasionally, the disorder persists into adult life. There is no specific treatment, but as sleepwalkers occasionally harm themselves, parents should protect the child from injury by fastening doors and windows securely, barring stairs, and removing dangerous objects.

Disorders of elimination

Functional enuresis

Functional enuresis is the repeated involuntary voiding of urine, occurring after an age at which continence is usual and in the absence of any identified physical disorder. The condition may be **nocturnal** (bed-wetting), **diurnal** (occurring during waking hours), or both. Nocturnal enuresis is referred to as **primary** if there has been no preceding period of urinary continence, and **secondary** if there has been a preceding period of urinary continence. There is no absolute period of continence needed to become secondary enuresis, but 6 months is a commonly used timeframe. Most children achieve regular daytime and night-time continence by 3 or 4 years of age, and *5 years is generally taken as the youngest age for the diagnosis*. Nocturnal enuresis can cause great unhappiness and distress, particularly if the parents blame or punish the child, and if the condition restricts staying with friends or going on holiday.

Prevalence

Nocturnal enuresis occurs in about 15 per cent of children at 5 years of age, 7 per cent at 8 years, 1 per cent at 14 years, and 0.5 per cent in adulthood. The condition is more frequent in boys. Daytime enuresis has a very low prevalence by 5 years (outside of the context of more global developmental difficulties).

Aetiology

The majority of cases of nocturnal primary enuresis are idiopathic; there is simply a delay in maturation of the nervous system controlling the bladder. These

Box 32.9 Aetiology of functional enuresis

Common causes of nocturnal primary enuresis

- Idiopathic developmental delay
- Genetics

Less common causes of enuresis (consider in secondary nocturnal or diurnal cases)

- Urinary tract infection
- Diabetes mellitus
- Abnormalities of the urinary tract (e.g. small bladder or vesicoureteric reflux)
- Structural abnormalities of the nervous system (e.g. spina bifida occulta)
- Chronic constipation
- Diuretics: caffeine and alcohol
- ADHD
- Learning disorders or syndromes of developmental delay
- Behavioural: being too engaged in play or 'leaving it too late'
- Psychological: a response to bereavement, stress, abuse, or bullying
- Obstructive sleep apnoea
- Epilepsy

children often have a family history of enuresis, as children who have either one or two parents who were enuretic have a 44 and 70 per cent chance, respectively, of being enuretic themselves. There are a range of other causes of enuresis, but these are more commonly associated with secondary nocturnal or diurnal enuresis (Box 32.9).

Assessment and management

Assessment should be undertaken as in any child presenting to psychiatry. It is important to determine if the enuresis is primary or secondary, any family history, and if there are stressful situations at home or school. Many children will have already had some treatment—find out what this was and why it didn't work. It is essential to exclude a primary physical cause; do a full neurological examination, feel for a loaded colon, inspect for signs of spina bifida, and perform urinalysis.

The majority of children who are bedwetting at 5 years will outgrow it in the next 2 years: a period of conservative management is therefore appropriate. Most clinicians do not start to treat enuresis until 7 years unless it is causing functional, psychological, or social impairment. If a specific physical or psychiatric cause of the enuresis has been found, then it should be treated. Most cases of primary enuresis can be treated successfully in general practice. The treatment options are shown in Box 32.10.

Box 32.10 Management of enuresis

General measures

- Treat any primary physical or psychiatric disorders.
- Psychoeducation and reassurance for parents and child.
- Reduce stressors.
- Practical advice: restrict fluids before bedtime, urinate before bed, use mattress covers, and avoid using pull-up nappies (these can prolong the problem).
- Basic behavioural measures: rewarding success, avoiding punishment, and reducing attention on failure is the most effective approach to reducing enuresis and boosting self-esteem.

For persistent cases

- Enuresis alarms ('bell and pad'): a sensor to detect urine is attached to the child's pyjama trousers and a miniature alarm is carried in the pocket or on the wrist. The child turns off the alarm and rises to complete emptying the bladder while the bed is remade if necessary. In the short term 70 per cent improve, but there is a high relapse rate.
- Desmopressin: a synthetic antidiuretic hormone analogue that is effective at reducing enuresis in 50 per cent of children. Similarly to alarms, there is a high relapse rate upon discontinuation. Frequency used short term (e.g. for a sleepover).
- Tricyclic antidepressants—moderately effective but poorly tolerated.
- Bladder training and pelvic floor exercises.

Functional encopresis

Functional encopresis is an uncommon disorder in which the child passes faeces in inappropriate places after the age at which bowel control is usual. The age at which control is reached varies, but at the age of 3–4 years, 94 per cent of children have control with only occasional accidents. Usually, encopresis would not be diagnosed in a child younger than 4, and have been present for at least 3 months. Encopresis occurs in about 2 per cent of children aged 4 and upwards, but after 5–6 years is much rarer. The condition is more common in boys than girls, by a factor of 6 to 1.

Aetiology

It is important to exclude primary encopresis; this is usually found in a child with learning disabilities or a known physical disorder. The majority of cases of functional encopresis (80 per cent) are associated with underlying constipation. Rarer causes include:

- undiagnosed cerebral palsy or spina bifida;
- progressive neurological disease;
- structural malformations of the colon (e.g. Hirschsprung's disease);
- anal fissures causing pain;
- traumatic or unsettling events;
- deliberate rebellion by the child against the parents (almost never the sole cause);
- associated with anxiety or mood disorder;
- associated with physical, sexual, or emotional abuse (extremely rare).

Treatment

- Treat any primary physical or psychiatric disorder.
- Reassure the parents that the problem occurs in other children and will improve in time.
- Avoid constipation with a high-fibre diet and adequate hydration. Empty the bowel with laxatives, and continue them as maintenance if necessary.
- Encourage normal bowel habits, starting by asking the child to sit on the toilet for 5 minutes after each meal.

- Encourage the parents to reward the child for opening his bowels in the appropriate place, and not to dwell on failure.
- Modify any stressful circumstances if possible.

Eating disorders

An eating disorder is *a disturbance of eating habits or weight control behaviour that results in clinically significant impairment of physical health and/or psychosocial functioning*. A full account of the major eating disorders can be found in Chapter 27; what follows are specific points relating to children and adolescents.

Anorexia nervosa

Anorexia nervosa is a clinical syndrome characterized by an abnormally low body weight, an intense fear of gaining weight, and a distorted perception of body weight and shape. The average age of onset is 15–17 years, although increasingly prepubertal cases are being recognized. Anorexia nervosa can have a devastating impact on the child's pubertal development and on family relationships. Children with anorexia nervosa are more likely to be male (15 per cent) than adults and less likely to have other co-morbid psychiatric disorders than adults.

Clinical features

The features are similar to those found in adults (p. 380). There is more often a definite precipitating event (e.g. change of school, bereavement, physical illness leading to weight loss) and a short illness course. The initial stages of the illness may be general symptoms such as low mood and social withdrawal; later, the child's parents then notice they are avoiding eating. Excessive exercise is common in young children, but laxative abuse and purging are less so.

Prepubertal children do not always show the typical extreme weight loss associated with anorexia nervosa; at first there is a failure to gain weight and a cessation of growth. Later there is weight loss and the usual symptoms and signs of starvation. Primary amenorrhoea is usual, and even in those who recover quickly, onset of menses may be delayed by several years. Other signs of secondary sexual maturation will be absent.

The core psychopathology of anorexia nervosa remains the same, but young children may express their anxieties in different ways. Even very young children will admit to being scared of becoming fat, but less frequently express a distorted body image or self-evaluate in terms of weight and shape. Depressive symptoms and OCD are extremely common co-morbidities.

Assessment and investigations

Assessment should be carried out as for adults (p. 390). Special attention should be paid to identifying any recent stressors at home or school, and to interaction and communication between family members. Weight and height should be recorded on a standard growth curve as BMI is not a reliable measure in those aged under 16. Pelvic ultrasound monitoring of the uterus and ovaries is helpful in monitoring recovery in girls. At a low weight, the volume of the ovaries and uterus will be reduced compared with healthy girls, but this increases into the normal range with good nutrition and weight gain.

Management

Detailed advice can be found on p. 393; the key differences relating to young people are as follows:

- Almost all children can be treated as outpatients. First-line management is family therapy and home refeeding—the Maudsley method (p. 395). All members of the family should be involved.
- The child should also be offered individual therapy sessions based on the principles of CBT.
- Medication (except for a multivitamin supplement) should be avoided unless there is significant co-morbid depression or anxiety.
- More intensive treatment may be needed for severe emaciation, failure of outpatient treatment, or situations where the parents/guardians are unable to manage home refeeding. Admissions should only be to facilities specifically for young people.
- If the child refuses treatment, it is important to assess their competence, and if necessary treat them involuntary under the MHA.

The prognosis in children with a definite precipitating event for the illness and a short illness course is excellent. Those with a more insidious onset and resistance to recovery fare less well, with their illness often continuing into adolescence and early adult years.

Other eating disorders

Bulimia nervosa presents extremely rarely in prepubertal children; the epidemiology and clinical differences from adolescents/adults are therefore poorly defined. Younger children make up the majority of cases of ARFID. They tend to present as described on p. 390, with a high proportion citing prominent anxiety and gastrointestinal symptoms. At present there is a lack of evidence-based treatment for ARFID in children; a combination of behaviour therapy (or CBT for older children) and family therapy are usually used.

Attention deficit hyperactivity disorder

ADHD is a persistent pattern of **inattention**, **hyperactivity**, and **impulsivity** that is more frequently displayed and more severe than is typically observed in individuals at a comparable level of development. Untreated, children with ADHD tend to underachieve academically, struggle in employment, and have difficult interpersonal relationships so it is an important diagnosis to make. Epidemiology is shown in Table 32.1, p. 476.

Diagnostic criteria

The classification and terminology surrounding ADHD have changed in recent years. Under the current ICD-10, the condition is known as hyperactivity disorder, but the upcoming ICD-11 will adopt ADHD to come in line with the DSM-5. The key aspects of the diagnosis are:

- the child must show core symptoms of **inattention**, **hyperactivity**, and **impulsivity**;
- symptoms must have started in early childhood (typically before age 7);
- symptoms are present in at least two settings (e.g. home and school);

- there must be definite evidence of impaired function;

- the symptoms are not caused by or related to another mental health disorder.

The typical clinical features are shown in Box 32.11. These behaviours may vary in severity between places—for example, worse at school than at home—and from day to day. The child's behaviour tends to exhaust their parents and their teachers, alienates

Box 32.11 Symptoms of attention deficit hyperactivity disorder

Symptoms of hyperactivity and impulsivity

- Constant fidgeting (e.g. tapping the hands or feet, or squirming in seat)
- Difficulty remaining seated when sitting is required (e.g. at school, work, etc.)
- Feelings of restlessness or inappropriate running around ('always on the go')
- Difficulty playing quietly
- Excessive talking
- Difficulty waiting turns
- Blurting out answers
- Interruption when others are speaking or doing an activity
- Failure to provide close attention to detail and careless mistakes

Symptoms of inattention

- Difficulty maintaining attention during activities at home, work, or school
- Failure to pay close attention to detail (e.g. makes careless mistakes)
- Seems not to listen, even when directly addressed
- Fails to follow through and complete tasks (e.g. homework, chores, etc.)
- Difficulty organizing tasks, activities, and belongings
- Avoidance of tasks that require consistent mental effort
- Frequently loses belongings (e.g. school books, sports equipment, etc.)
- Easily distracted by irrelevant stimuli
- Forgetfulness in routine activities (e.g. homework, chores, etc.)

other children, and disrupts their school work. This can lead to low self-esteem and sometimes disobedience, temper tantrums, aggression, and other antisocial behaviour.

Co-morbidity

The following conditions are all frequently found in children with ADHD: depression, tic disorders, anxiety, oppositional defiance disorder, substance abuse, and ASD.

Differential diagnosis

It is important to differentiate ADHD from a primary diagnosis of one of the conditions listed under co-morbidities, and from mania. Either condition presents as overactivity, talkativeness, fast thoughts, and irritable mood. In bipolar disorder, these symptoms will be episodic, and there is usually euphoria and grandiosity—ADHD is longer term and without affective disturbance.

Aetiology

The aetiology of ADHD is undoubtedly multifactorial, but has a strong genetic component. Box 32.12 shows the factors that have so far been linked to ADHD.

Genetics. Monozygotic concordance has shown the heritability of ADHD to be very high; 80–90 per cent. The risk of ADHD in a first-degree relative of a sufferer is five times the risk of the general public. ADHD has been linked to a variety of genes related to the action of dopamine; for example, dopamine receptors, dopamine transporters, and the monoamine system.

Brain structure and function abnormalities. MRI scanning of patients with ADHD versus age-matched controls has repeatedly shown that the frontal lobes, striatum, and cerebellum are smaller in those with ADHD. The difference persists into adult life, and is greater in those who have not received stimulants. The restlessness and difficulty in concentration suggest an abnormality in the prefrontal cortex and related subcortical structures since these are involved in guiding and sustaining behaviour, and delaying responses. As these brain regions are rich in catecholamines,

Box 32.12 Aetiology of attention deficit hyperactivity disorder

Biological

- Genetics: heritability 80–90 per cent
- Structural brain abnormalities
- Catecholamine system dysregulation
- Abnormalities in executive and higher brain function
- Low birth weight
- Neurodevelopmental disorders (ASD, tic disorders)

Psychological

- Severe early deprivation (emotional, nutrition, stimulatory)
- Physical, sexual, or emotional abuse
- Institutional rearing
- Poor family communication and interactions

Environmental

- Prenatal exposure to benzodiazepines, alcohol, cocaine, or nicotine
- Perinatal obstetric complications
- Brain injury in early life
- Exposure to high levels of lead
- Low socioeconomic class
- Diet or food intolerances (controversial area)

this observation appears to link with the genetic findings and with the observed therapeutic effect of stimulant drugs.

Prognosis

Longitudinal studies have shown that 50 per cent of patients diagnosed with ADHD in childhood continue to have persisting symptoms into adulthood, but only about 15 per cent still meet diagnostic criteria. In general, overactivity tends to improve with age, while an increase in self-control after puberty helps to reduce the inattention and impulsiveness. However, those who do not lose the overactivity are at high risk of conduct disorder, antisocial behaviour, and juvenile delinquency. It is unclear what the risk factors for continuation of ADHD into adulthood are, but severity of initial ADHD symptoms, a family

history, and co-morbid psychiatric disease are likely contenders. Taken across a lifetime, those given a diagnosis of ADHD in childhood are more likely than the general population to attain poor qualifications, become unemployed, be involved in multiple road traffic accidents, and serve a prison sentence. See Science box 32.1.

Assessment

A full assessment should be carried out as for any psychiatric condition in a child (p. 190). Since the problem behaviours vary in different settings, information should be obtained from teachers and other relevant adults as well as from the parents and the child.

Management

See Table 32.7.

Medication

For unknown reasons, stimulant drugs such as methylphenidate and dexamphetamine have the paradoxical effect of reducing the overactivity in ADHD. These drugs block monoamine transporters, inhibiting uptake of dopamine and norepinephrine (noradrenaline) from the synapse. Atomoxetine, a non-stimulant selective norepinephrine transporter inhibitor, has been shown to be as effective at reducing the symptoms of ADHD as the stimulants.

The indications for offering medication to a child are twofold:

1 Failure of psychosocial interventions to reduce symptoms in ADHD with moderate functional impairment.

2 As a first-line therapy in ADHD with severe functional impairment.

Methylphenidate is the first-line choice for uncomplicated ADHD and can also be used in children with co-morbid conduct disorder, tics, Tourette's, or anxiety disorders. Atomoxetine can be used in children with co-morbid tics, Tourette's, anxiety disorders, or substance misuse.

SCIENCE BOX 32.1

Do food additives exacerbate hyperactivity in children?

The number of children diagnosed with ADHD has increased more than tenfold since the 1970s. In the USA, the prevalence is currently 4–5 per cent of children under 16 years; this represents 4.8 million children, half of whom are taking stimulants.[1] The reason for this change over such a short time period is clearly not genetics. One explanation is that we now have better detection, leading to more diagnoses. The other is that provocative environmental factors are causing or exacerbating hyperactivity in children. One area that has come under scrutiny has been childhood nutrition, specifically artificial food colours and additives (AFCA).

The association between diet and hyperactivity has been investigated since the early 1970s. In 1973, in the first RCT in the area, Feingold published a study claiming that half of all hyperactive children improved after eliminating all AFCA.[2] His 'elimination diet' required the removal of all processed foods and most fruit and vegetables, but it was surprisingly popular. The 1980s/1990s saw a dozen RCTs of AFCA versus placebo, which reported inconsistent results. In 2007, McCann and colleagues published a randomized, double-blinded placebo trial of AFCA in 3- and 8/9-year-old children.[3] These were a sample of the general population, not children diagnosed with ADHD. For the first week all 153 children had an AFCA-free diet; then they were randomly allocated to weeks on supplementation and placebo. The results report that supplementation of AFCA had a significantly adverse effect on behaviour compared with placebo ($P = 0.044$). These results led the European Food Safety Authority (EFSA) to suggest that a comprehensive management plan for ADHD should include trials of dietary elimination.[4]

Nigg et al. published a meta-analysis of AFCA vs placebo in ADHD.[5] Overall they found 35 per cent of patients showed a reduction of hyperactivity symptoms. Taking their evidence and that from the general population studies, they suggested that a subgroup of children, some of whom who have ADHD, were more likely to respond to an elimination diet. Identifying these children in advance of dietary trials is challenging at present. They noted that the literature base remains very small in this area; this is partly because it is extremely hard to conduct trials which control individuals' diet, and even hard to do them double-blinded. Further research is needed, but at present, the best strategy is for clinicians to include dietary elimination trials (with input from a dietician) alongside their other treatment options.

1 Newmark SC. Nutritional intervention in ADHD. *Explore* 2009;5:171.

2 Feingold B. *Why your Child is Hyperactive*. New York: Random House; 1975.

3 McCann D, Barrett A, Cooper A, et al. Food additives and hyperactive behaviour in 3 year old and 8/9 year old children in the community: a randomised, double-blinded, placebo-controlled trial. *Lancet* 2007;370:1560–1567.

4 AFC Panel. Assessment of the results of the study by McCann et al. (2007) on the effect of some colours and sodium benzoate on children's behaviour. *European Food Safety Authority Journal* 2008;660:1–54

5 Nigg JT, Lewis K, Edinger T, Falk M. Meta-analysis of attention-deficit/hyperactivity disorder or attention-deficit/hyperactivity disorder symptoms, restriction diet, and synthetic food color additives. *Journal of the American Academy of Child and Adolescent Psychiatry* 2012;51:86–97.e8

Dexamphetamine should be reserved for children who do not improve on the maximum tolerated dose of methylphenidate or atomoxetine.

The main side effects of stimulants are nausea, appetite (and therefore weight) loss, reduced growth, insomnia, headaches, and stomach pains. It is important to record the height, weight, blood pressure, and pulse rate of the child at each follow-up appointment. Stimulants do lower the seizure threshold, but can be safely used in children with well-controlled epilepsy. There is a very small chance of liver injury, which parents should be warned about, but routine hepatic monitoring is not necessary. If there is no response to all three of the usual drugs, refer the child to a tertiary centre specializing in ADHD. Occasionally, further treatment

Table 32.7 Treatment options for attention deficit hyperactivity disorder

General measures	
Psychoeducation	• The child, their parents, and teachers should be informed about the symptoms of ADHD and different treatment options
School-based interventions	• Schools may have a special educational needs coordinator who can help provide support at school • The child should be assessed for any co-morbid learning difficulties
Psychological treatments	
Parent training and education courses	• First-line intervention for mild to moderate ADHD • Taught courses are the most effective way of delivering psychoeducation and training in behavioural techniques to parents • The groups provide support by allowing parents to meet other families coping with ADHD
Behavioural therapy	• Behavioural therapy is useful to help younger children cope with their symptoms more effectively
Social skills training	• Helps children to learn social norms; good evidence for improving peer relationships long term
CBT	• Beneficial for adolescents with ADHD, especially those with low self-esteem and/or comorbid anxiety and depression
Pharmacological treatments	Drugs are only recommended for moderate to severe ADHD if psychological interventions have been ineffective (see text): • Stimulants: methylphenidate and dexamphetamine • Non-stimulants: atomoxetine • Unlicensed medications: clonidine, modafinil, imipramine

with unlicensed drugs such as clonidine, imipramine, or bupropion may be considered.

Oppositional defiance disorder and conduct disorder

These two conditions are classed as **disruptive behaviour disorders**, and have many similarities; the management strategies are therefore common between the two.

Oppositional defiance disorder (ODD) is defined as a recurrent pattern of negativistic, defiant, disobedient, and hostile behaviour towards authority figures. It is four times more common in boys than girls. Clinical features include:

• frequent loss of temper;

• very easily annoyed—low threshold for becoming angry;

• tendency to argue with adults;

• tendency to deliberately provoke or annoy others;

• ignores or refuses to comply with rules;

• always blames others for the difficulties their own behaviour creates;

• tendency to be vindictive or malicious;

• behaviour does not include delinquency or extreme aggression.

ODD is one of the most common psychiatric disorders of childhood (~4 per cent prevalence), and while a risk factor for the more serious conduct disorder, the majority do not progress to more serious psychopathology or psychopathy.

Conduct disorder (CD) is defined as a persistent pattern of antisocial behaviour in which the individual repeatedly breaks social rules and carries out aggressive acts. The person persistently behaves in a way which is inconsistent with social norms or breaks the law. Examples of behaviours include:

- getting frequently involved in physical skirmishes (which may involve the use of weapons);
- bullies or intimidates others;
- is physically or sexually abusive towards other people or animals;
- steals items from others;
- acts inappropriately towards property: breaks into houses, sets fires, or destroys others' belongings;
- tendency towards lying (especially for personal gain);
- for adolescents: ignores parental rules (e.g. staying out too late), runs away from home or truants from school.

It is usual for children aged less than 10 to attract a diagnosis of ODD rather than conduct disorder. Once an individual reaches 18, if criteria are met they may be considered to have antisocial personality disorder rather than a conduct disorder. Conduct disorders are more common in lower socioeconomic groups.

Co-morbidity

A thorough assessment of a child with ODD or CD is essential as they are commonly associated with other conditions. Any of the following may be present: ADHD, learning disabilities, substance abuse, PTSD, anxiety disorders, depression, or psychoses.

Differential diagnosis

- **ADHD.** A child with hyperactivity, inattention, and impulsivity can be seen as being antisocial. However, those with only ADHD should not show any of the specific behaviours associated with ODD or CD. It is possible for the conditions to coexist.

- **Adjustment reaction to a specific stressful event.** Poor behaviour may occur in the first 3 months after a stressful event, but should resolve by 6 months.
- **Mood disorders.** Depression can present with irritability and oppositional behaviour in children, but mood is usually low, and there are associated biological features.
- **Autistic spectrum disorders.**
- **Learning disorders or specific developmental disorders.**
- **Dissocial/antisocial personality disorder.** This can only be diagnosed from early adulthood. As CD may be diagnosed in adults, there is overlap between the conditions. Antisocial personality disorder refers to a pervasive, severe lack of regard for, and violation of, the rights of others dating back to mid adolescence.
- **Psychosis.** A careful mental state examination should pick up hallucinations and/or delusions, often with associated disorganized behaviour.

Aetiology

At the current time, there is a poor understanding of the aetiology of ODD and CD, although it is clearly a mix of genetics, adverse psychological experiences, and environmental factors. Table 32.8 outlines the potential aetiological factors, but these should be viewed more as risk factors until further research is available.

Course and prognosis

Once ODD or CD is established, it is usually stable throughout the rest of childhood. Of those with early-onset CD (before age 8), 50 per cent will develop antisocial personality disorder in adulthood. Adolescent onset may be just as severe in the teenage years but 85 per cent only have minor problems by their mid twenties. Box 32.13 shows factors predicting a poor outcome in CD/ODD. CD is linked to many problems in later life, including unemployment and dependence on state benefits, divorce, domestic violence, completed suicide, substance abuse, and other mental health problems.

Table 32.8 Risk factors for disruptive behaviour disorders

Biological	Psychological	Social or environmental
• Genetics: twin studies estimate 50% heritability. Adoption studies show children carry their biological parents' risk • Dysregulation of neurotransmitters metabolized by monoamine oxidase • Low IQ • Language disorders or deficits • Minor physical anomalies • Low birth weight • Brain injury or disease • Low resting heart rate	• Irritable temperament as a baby • Institutional care • Poor parent–child relationships • Attachment difficulties • Poor parenting: inconsistent rule setting, criticism, over-punishment, or hostility • Low parental involvement with child • Physical, sexual, or emotional abuse • Neglect • Low self-esteem • 'Unemotional' personality trait	• Maternal smoking in pregnancy • Low socioeconomic class • Poor diet with lack of vitamins and minerals • Bad neighbourhood • Crime in the family • Parental mental illness or substance abuse • Peer influences: associates with other children with OCD/CD

Assessment and management

Assessment should be undertaken as for any child presenting to psychiatry. The management options for children with ODD or CD are outlined in Box 32.14. A key principle is that the whole family need to be involved in treatment.

General measures

The usual scenario is that the child does not feel that their behaviour is unreasonable, and will be resistant to interventions from health services. In some situations it may also be difficult to engage their parents in the process. However, the basis of treatment is psychoeducation; each side needs to understand their own behaviour, how it impacts upon themselves and others, and how they could change it for the better. Providing written and self-help materials is useful, but

Box 32.13 Risk factors predicting a poor outcome in oppositional defiance disorder or conduct disorder

- Male gender
- Co-morbid hyperactivity
- Lower IQ
- Parental criminality
- Parental alcoholism
- Harsh, inconsistent parenting
- Low-income family
- Troublesome neighbourhood
- Poor schools, low achievement
- Lack of parental interest in child
- Severe, frequent antisocial acts
- Early onset

Box 32.14 Treatment of oppositional defiance disorder or conduct disorder

General measures

- Psychoeducation
- Provision of information and self-help materials
- Treat co-morbidities
- Reduce stressful circumstances
- Involve school in treatment plan

Psychological treatments (first line)

- Parental management training course
- Individual or group CBT
- Family therapy
- Anger management skills

Biological treatments (second line)

- Aggression: antipsychotics, lithium, or carbamazepine
- Co-morbid mood disorder: SSRI
- Co-morbid ADHD: stimulants

only if the child is able to read them. Schools can be very helpful in providing extra support if the child has specific difficulties with basic skills, or has dropped behind their peers. Teachers can also be trained in behavioural management techniques, which can reinforce work being done at home.

Psychological treatments

It is recommended that psychological therapies be the first-line management for ODD or CD. In children under 12 years there is good evidence for the efficacy of parental training courses. These are group sessions which teach the child's parents how to manage their child's behaviour in a more effective way. Skills learnt include promoting good behaviour and a positive relationship, setting clear rules and commands, remaining calm, and managing difficult situations. Systematic family therapy can also be beneficial, and may be a good option for older children. For the child themselves, the best approach seems to be providing anger management and interpersonal skills training, rather than more traditional psychotherapies.

Pharmacotherapy

Medications should not be the first-line treatment for ODD or CD, but can be useful adjuncts. There is good evidence that appropriate use of stimulants or an SSRI decrease symptoms in children with co-morbid ADHD or depression. In adolescents with severe aggression, or violent outbursts, an atypical antipsychotic can reduce this behaviour considerably. Compliance with treatment can be a problem, and depot injections are often a good solution.

Tics and Tourette's syndrome

Tics are an important aspect of child and adolescent psychiatry for three main reasons:

1 Tics are extremely common; simple motor tics are found in 1–2 per cent of children.

2 Tics are associated with many other behavioural, learning, and psychiatric disorders.

3 Tics may cause great distress to both the child and their family, and can have a negative impact upon self-esteem, peer relationships, and school performance.

A tic is a **repetitive, individually recognizable, non-rhythmic, stereotyped motor movement or vocalization**. Tics are usually briefly suppressible and may be associated with the awareness of an urge to perform the movement. They can be classified as either motor or vocal (phonic), or as simple or complex:

- **Simple tics** are typically sudden, brief, meaningless movements or sounds that usually involve only one group of muscles. Common examples include neck jerking, eye blinking, grunting, snorting, or throat clearing.

- **Complex motor tics** are typically more purposeful-appearing movements that last for rather longer. Examples include facial movements, jumping, touching, or even self-harming.

- **Complex vocal tics** involve words and phrases, and may include repetition of what was just heard or said (echolalia and palilalia) or socially inappropriate phrases (coprolalia).

It is also usual to define a tic as transient or chronic, the latter being when a tic has lasted for more than 12 months. The number of tics, their frequency, severity, and nature vary widely between patients, and can change over time. Usually, the patient is able to suppress the tic for a short period, but this causes a build-up of tension within the person which eventually can no longer be suppressed. Tics may be triggered or worsened by excitement, fatigue, and visual cues, which tend to be specific to the patient. There are four main tic disorders, shown in Box 32.15.

Clinical features of Tourette's syndrome

The symptoms of Tourette's syndrome are worth a special mention because of the public perception of the condition. Typically, motor tics appear early in life (3–8 years) and are initially simple tics (e.g. blinking) which gradually evolve into more complex movements such as touching, licking, or making obscene gestures (copropraxia). Vocal tics such as grunting, sniffing, and throat clearing are almost universal. The

Box 32.15 Classification of tic disorders

Tourette's syndrome

- Multiple motor tics and at least one vocal tic have been present at some point in the illness
- Tics occur many times a day, nearly every day for more than 1 year

Chronic motor or vocal tic disorder

- Single or multiple motor or vocal tics
- Tics occur multiple times per day, nearly every day for more than 1 year
- Criteria are not met for Tourette's syndrome

Transient tic disorder

- Single or multiple motor and/or vocal tics
- Tics occur many times per day, every day for at least 4 weeks but less than 12 months

more antisocial tics of coprolalia, echolalia, and echopraxia are not seen in every patient, but when they are present, represent a large burden for the patient to manage. The severity of the tics usually peaks at about 20 years and reduces somewhat after this. It is usual for the patient to report that they feel when a tic is about to happen, and that they may be able to suppress them for a short time. Tics are exacerbated by anxiety, boredom, fatigue, and excitement. They may be reduced by sleep, alcohol, and calming surroundings.

Prevalence

Ten to fifteen per cent of school-age children exhibit transient tics at some point, but only about 1 per cent meet criteria for a tic disorder. The mean age of onset of the first tic is typically 4–6 years, but they can occur as late as 15 years. Tics are more common in males than females (ratio 5:1), and do not seem to vary between races or socioeconomic groups.

Co-morbidities

Tics are associated with many other psychiatric conditions, including ADHD, OCD, learning disorders, dyslexia, mood, and anxiety disorders.

Differential diagnosis

- **Abnormal movements due to neurological or neuropsychiatric disorder.** For example, Sydenham's chorea, Huntingdon's disease, Wilson's disease, or tuberous sclerosis.
- **Abnormal movements caused by medications.** Antipsychotics and antiepileptics may cause dystonic movements. Stimulants (e.g. methylphenidate and amphetamine) and opioids may cause or exacerbate tics.
- **ADHD.** Are the movements a failure of impulse control due to ADHD?

Aetiology

Biological factors

1 **Genetics.** The risk of developing Tourette's in a first-degree relative of a sufferer is 15–20 per cent. The figure for any tic disorder is much higher, approaching 50 per cent, although there appears to be incomplete expression and penetrance. Twin studies of monozygotic twins show a 53 per cent concordance. The risk is also substantially increased in those with a family history of ADHD or OCD.

2 **Neuroimaging.** MRI studies have shown various anatomical abnormalities in patients with tic disorders. Imaging consistently shows a reduced volume of the caudate nucleus, and an increased volume of the prefrontal cortex. As tics are likely to be aberration of the cortico–striatal–pallidothalamo–cortical circuit which controls the suppression of unwanted movements and fine control of wanted movements, this would fit well.

3 **Dopamine dysregulation.** The efficacy of antipsychotics to reduce tics highly suggests that there is an excess of dopamine in the brain of those with tics. Postmortem studies that have stained slices of the cerebrum to show dopamine have found increased numbers of dopamine transporter sites in the striatum and prefrontal cortex. Positron emission tomography studies have demonstrated increased dopamine binding in

SCIENCE BOX 32.2

PANDAS: paediatric autoimmune neuropsychiatric disorders associated with streptococcal infections

PANDAS is a group of neuropsychiatric disorders that probably have an autoimmune aetiology and are related to infection with group A beta-haemolytic streptococci. OCD, tic disorders, and Tourette's syndrome are all included in PANDAS. The mechanism of causation proposed is molecular mimicry, similar to that seen in Sydenham's chorea. In the latter, antineuronal antibodies are produced which attack the streptococci but also cross-react with the basal ganglia, producing choreoathetoid movements. The basal ganglia are known to be the site of movement production control and suppression, classically demonstrated in Parkinson's disease. Various studies have attempted to isolate the specific antibodies involved, but as yet have been unsuccessful. The clinical criteria for PANDAS are:

- presence of OCD and/or tic disorder;
- prepubertal onset;
- episodic course of symptom severity;
- abrupt onset or dramatic exacerbations associated with group A beta-haemolytic streptococcal infection (as shown by positive throat cultures and/or elevated anti-group A beta-haemolytic streptococci titres).

The prevalence of PANDAS is currently unknown, as are the factors rendering a child susceptible to developing it. A variety of treatment strategies have been used, including intravenous immunoglobulins, plasma exchange, and long-term prophylactic antibiotics. However, there is no robust evidence for the efficacy of any of these and most children's abnormal involuntary movements simply improve with time.

---

these sites, and correlated the density of dopamine receptors to tic severity.

4 **Autoimmunity.** There has been some suggestion that tics and OCD may be caused by antibodies produced against streptococci cross-reacting in the basal ganglia. This is further discussed in Science box 32.2.

Social and psychological factors

There is little evidence demonstrating that specific psychological vulnerabilities or events predispose to tics. However, tics often start or are exacerbated by a child undergoing life events—this suggests that stress does play some role. Children who were of a low birth weight or exposed to high levels of caffeine, alcohol, or tobacco *in utero* are at higher risk of having a tic disorder. Adverse social circumstances (e.g. poverty) certainly increase the severity of tics, but do not appear to be a direct aetiological factor.

Course and prognosis

In the majority of children, tics are transitory phenomena, and vary in severity over 1–12 months before disappearing. In those with chronic tic disorders, the tics tend to peak in severity in middle children and then gradually reduce. Up to 30 per cent have tics remaining into adulthood, but they are usually simple motor tics. Children with severe tics or Tourette's syndrome often have substantial problems in childhood, but only a minority have long-term mental health problems. Risk factors for a poor prognosis include Tourette's syndrome, co-morbid OCD or ADHD, physical illness, unsupportive home circumstances, and substance abuse.

Assessment

A full assessment should be undertaken of any child presenting with tics. In those with short-lived, non-functionally impairing tics no intervention may be necessary, but it is essential to check for and treat any underlying or co-morbid conditions and to educate and reassure the child and their family. Tics are inherently suppressible for short periods and usually fluctuate in severity throughout the day, so may not be seen in the interview. It may be helpful to ask the family to take a video, which can be played to the assessment team. A formal examination of the child should occur,

Box 32.16 Management of tic disorders

General measures

- Psychoeducation of child, family, and school
- Collaboration with the school
- Good treatment of co-morbidities
- Information about and referral to support groups

Pharmacological treatments

- Alpha-2 agonists
- Antipsychotics

Psychological treatments

- CBT
- Exposure–response prevention
- Habit reversal training
- Relaxation techniques

including a detailed neurological and ophthalmological survey looking for signs of other neurological conditions. The Yale Global Tic Severity Scale can be a useful index by which to measure symptom severity over time.

Management

The most important management of tic disorders is appropriate education of the child, family, school, and anyone else involved. A general outline of treatment options is shown in Box 32.16.

Psychoeducation

It is crucially important to explain to everyone involved with the child that they cannot help making movements or sounds. Knowing that tics can be exacerbated by stress can help others to provide a stress-free environment for the child. Tics tend to fluctuate in severity over time and this should be discussed, and plans made for sudden deteriorations.

Pharmacological treatments

The most effective treatment for tics is medication, but because of the risk of adverse effects these should only be the first-line treatment in the following situations: severely disabling tics, interference with

activities of daily living, risk to self or others, co-morbid ADHD/OCD, or learning disability making therapy impossible. The two effective groups of medications are antipsychotics and alpha-2 agonists. The former are the most efficacious, reducing tics by up to 60 per cent. However, the adverse effects associated with antipsychotics means that the safer alpha-2 agonists are the usual first choice. **Clonidine** and **guanfacine** are the most common drugs used, and they reduce tics by about 30 per cent. The most common side effects are sedation, headache, and irritability. Clonidine is available as a 48-hour transdermal patch, which can be useful in small children who can't swallow tablets. Atypical antipsychotics (risperidone and olanzapine have robust randomized controlled evidence) are a good choice, but they come with the problems of sedation, weight gain, and the metabolic syndrome. Local injection of botulinum toxin has been used in older children and adults with isolated motor tics, and appears to be quite effective.

Psychological treatments

The most effective psychological therapies for tics are habit-reversal training or CBT with exposure–response prevention. These therapies help the child to recognize the signs that a tic is going to occur and try to prevent this from happening. Typically this would be by performing another voluntary movement (that is less socially unacceptable) rather than the tic.

Disorders of adults also seen in adolescents

There are a variety of common psychiatric disorders of adulthood which may begin in adolescence (or rarely childhood), whose presentation may be slightly different to that in adults (Box 32.17. These differences are briefly outlined here, with references to further information in the chapter on each condition. Assessment of all young people should be carried out as outlined in Chapter 17, but also include the specific history/investigations used in adults with the condition.

Box 32.17 Psychiatric disorders in adolescents

- Depressive disorders (Chapter 21, see p. 484 in this chapter)
- Bipolar disorder (Chapter 21)
- Anxiety disorders (Chapter 24, see p. 482 in this chapter)
- Schizophrenia (Chapter 22)
- Eating disorders (Chapter 27)
- Suicide and deliberate self-harm (Chapter 9)
- Substance abuse (Chapter 29)
- Post-traumatic stress disorder (Chapter 23)
- Chronic fatigue syndrome (see p. 349)

Bipolar disorder

Bipolar disorder is rare before puberty, but increases in incidence rapidly in adolescence. The mean age for presentation is 20 years, meaning a large proportion of patients present to child and adolescent services. Diagnostic criteria remain as in adults, but young people may not show the classical alternation between depression and manic episodes. Mixed episodes, where some symptoms of depression and mania are seen at the same time, are quite common, as is rapid cycling—switching between low and elevated moods over short periods. The symptoms of each state are usually allied to those found in older patients.

The prevalence of bipolar disorder in those aged less than 18 is approximately 1 per cent, although almost all of these are in postpubertal children. Males and females are equally affected. One specific tool widely used for assessment is the Young Mania Rating Scale, a questionnaire filled out by parents relating to their child's behaviour.

The younger the presentation of bipolar disorder, the poorer the prognosis; adolescent mania has a 50 per cent relapse rate within 5 years even with maximal treatment. Younger age at presentation, poor family relationships, psychosis, and a family history all carry a poorer prognosis.

Treatment of bipolar disorder in young people initially focuses on mood stabilization, as this is what tends to interfere with function, with emphasis moving towards psychoeducation and relapse prevention

Box 32.18 Treatment of paediatric bipolar disorder

General measures

- Psychoeducation of child and family (including early warning signs for relapse, importance of medication compliance, and avoidance of stressors)
- Appropriate educational setting

Pharmacotherapy

- Lithium (in those over 12 years)
- Atypical antipsychotics
- Sodium valproate (males)
- SSRIs (severe depression)

Psychological treatments

- CBT
- Family therapy

Electroconvulsive therapy

- May be indicated for severe depression or mania.

when this has been achieved. An outline of options is shown in Box 32.18. Most children will be treated as outpatients, but some (especially those with acute mania or severe depression) may need inpatient or day-patient care.

Pharmacotherapy is the mainstay of treatment. If the child is not on any antimanic drugs, an atypical antipsychotic is the first step, but most need a mood stabilizer (lithium or valproate) added in. Before starting medication, bloods including thyroid and renal function should be done, as well as an assessment of height and weight, and an ECG. Sodium valproate should be avoided in women of child-bearing age, as it is teratogenic and can induce polycystic ovary syndrome. Lithium is only licensed in those over the age of 12.

Suicide and deliberate self-harm

This important topic is covered more fully in Chapter 9. In the UK in 2015, Suicide was the second most common cause of death in male adolescents and the sixth most common in females. Together, suicide accounts for about 15 per cent of adolescent deaths.

Around 90 per cent of adolescents who commit suicide have underlying psychiatric disorders. About three-quarters of those who commit suicide are males, and are four times more likely than the general population to have a family history of suicide. The most common co-morbidities are mood disorders, alcohol and substance abuse, anxiety disorder, eating disorders, and chronic physical diseases. About one-third of completed suicides had made at least one previous attempt to end their life. Factors that are thought to be involved in the aetiology of suicide and attempted suicide are shown in Table 32.9. **The strongest predictor of future suicide risk is past suicide attempts.**

Deliberate self-harm (DSH) is any act with a non-fatal outcome, which is undertaken with the intention of causing harm to self. It is hard to obtain accurate figures of the prevalence and incidence of DSH as most young people never present to psychiatric services. Surveys of school-age teenagers suggest 10 per cent of 15–16-year-olds have harmed themselves in the previous year, with the majority of these having done it more than once. Females are four times more likely to self-harm than males. The most common methods of self-harm are cutting and taking overdoses of over-the-counter analgesics.

Assessment

Assessment of a child who has attempted suicide or self-harmed has two aims: a risk assessment and an evaluation of the underlying psychopathology and context in which the act occurred.

A physical examination, routine blood tests, paracetamol and salicylate levels, an ECG, and any special investigations related to the presenting complaint should be carried out immediately. Treatment of any physical effects of the DSH should be the first priority. The history should cover:

- circumstances leading up to the DSH;
- whether the child aimed to end their life (see Chapter 9 for evaluation of intentions);
- current symptoms of mental disorders;
- background: previous DSH, mental and physical disorders;
- current psychosocial functioning (home relationships, peer relationships, bullying, school performance, drug and alcohol abuse, conduct problems, abuse).

The child's parents and other relevant adults should be interviewed to provide further background to the

Table 32.9 Aetiology of completed and attempted suicide

Biological	Psychological	Social or environmental
Family history of suicide or DSH	Psychiatric disorders:	Stressful life events:
Self-harm in close friends	• Depression	• Family discord
Familial mental health problems	• Substance abuse	• Parental divorce
Neurotransmitter dysregulation: low serotonin	• Conduct disorder	• Death of loved one
	• Anxiety disorder	Poor care or neglect
	• Schizophrenia	Imitation—exposure to real or fictional accounts of suicide
	• Past suicide attempt	
	Cognitive factors:	
	• Low self-esteem	
	• Hopelessness	
	• Guilt	
	• Bullying	
	• Confusion regarding sexual orientation	
	Physical, emotional, or sexual abuse	

family situation and co-morbid psychiatric disorders, their account of the DSH event, and their reaction to the event.

Management

Keeping the child safe is paramount. A decision needs to be made as to whether they are at risk of acting upon suicidal thoughts, if there is a safe home environment, and if there is a responsible adult available to find help if the situation deteriorates. Most young people can be treated as outpatients; rarely they may need to be admitted to acute psychiatric wards. The indications for inpatient treatment are active suicidal ideation and intent, a young person not able to promise not to harm themselves, psychosis, impulsivity, and lack of a suitable home environment. Crisis teams who can provide intensive support at home are a good way of providing a safety net. Treatment options depend a lot on the underlying psychiatric diagnosis; specific conditions (e.g. depression or anorexia nervosa) should be treated by standard protocols. A written 'no suicide' contract is usually negotiated at the start of treatment; this usually involves the child promising not to engage in DSH behaviours without informing their parents or therapist. Individual therapy is usually offered; this may be CBT or dialectical behaviour therapy (DBT). The former is particularly useful in depressed teenagers, and the latter in those with borderline personality disorder. Family therapy is often a useful adjunct to address relationship problems and improve communication. There is no good evidence base for the use of medications in reducing suicidal behaviour in adolescents, but in adults both SSRIs and lithium reduce the risk of self-harm in depressed adults. There is some evidence that SSRIs increase suicidal ideation in young people in the first week of treatment; they should be carefully monitored during this period.

Schizophrenia

Schizophrenia is covered more comprehensively in Chapter 22, and is rare in children and adolescents. The diagnostic criteria for schizophrenia are the same in children as in adults. Schizophrenia starting before age 18 is known as early-onset schizophrenia, and before 13 years as very-early-onset schizophrenia. The prevalence of all psychoses in one Scandinavian study was 0.9/10,000 at 13 years, rising to 17/10,000 at 18 years, the majority of which were schizophrenia. It is worth noting that psychotic experiences are relatively common in young people (cross-sectional studies typically report ~15 per cent prevalence in age 11–15-year-olds) but functionally impairing psychosis is rare. Positive symptoms are not pathognomonic of schizophrenia in young people, and the full differential diagnosis of psychosis should be considered. The aetiology of early-onset schizophrenia is similar to that in adults, but children are more likely to have a strong family history of psychosis. An overview of the assessment is shown in Box 32.19, and the differential diagnosis in Box 32.20.

Box 32.19 Assessment of a child with suspected schizophrenia

Psychiatric history

- Symptoms at presentation, including course and co-morbid mood symptoms
- Previous psychiatric and medical history
- Family history
- Personal history and development
- Premorbid personality and level of functioning
- Substance use and abuse
- Self-harm, risk to self and others

Physical examination

- Examine respiratory and cardiovascular systems and abdomen
- Neurology including extrapyramidal movements, tics, and abnormal involuntary movements
- Look for dysmorphic features, and measure height/weight/head circumference

Investigations

- Blood tests (full blood count, U&Es, liver function tests, thyroid function tests, copper, and caeruloplasmin)
- ECG
- Urinalysis including drug toxicology
- Consider neuroimaging and EEG
- IQ testing
- Structured questionnaires for schizophrenia

Box 32.20 Differential diagnosis of childhood schizophrenia

- **Organic conditions:** substance-related psychoses, Wilson's disease, temporal lobe epilepsy, systemic lupus erythematosus, thyroid disease, space-occupying lesions
- **Other psychotic disorders:** mood disorders with psychosis, schizoaffective disorders, brief psychotic episode
- **Developmental disorders:** ASD
- **Other psychiatric disorders:** ADHD, conduct disorders, personality disorders, culture-bound syndromes

Treatment of children with schizophrenia is very similar to that in adults. Early intervention in those with prodromal symptoms and/or a strong family history has been shown to reduce the likelihood of a poor prognosis. Medication use tends to be off licence, with an atypical antipsychotic used first line. After failure of two atypical antipsychotics, clozapine should be considered. It is important to monitor the child for side effects, especially weight gain and extrapyramidal movements. Psychological treatments are important in young people with schizophrenia. Psychoeducation, family therapy to reduce highly expressed emotion, and social skills and communication training have all been shown to improve outcome.

Early-onset schizophrenia has a poorer outcome than the adult-onset disorder. It is associated with a reduced IQ, increased cognitive deficits, increased negative symptoms, and less likelihood of independent living and holding down employment. Young people with schizophrenia often develop illnesses that are very hard to treat by the time they are in middle adulthood.

Substance abuse

Many adolescents take drugs, especially cannabis, and drink alcohol—but only a minority abuse these substances. Full details can be found in Chapter 29.

Juvenile delinquency

Parents sometimes ask GPs for advice about their delinquent adolescents. Delinquency is the failure of a young person to obey the law; it is not a psychiatric disorder, although psychiatric disorder, usually CD, is one of its causes. Delinquency is most common at the age of 15–16 years and in males. Up to a fifth of adolescent boys are found to have carried out an offence, albeit usually a trivial one (e.g. shoplifting). Of these adolescents, only a few continue to offend in adult life and parents can usually be reassured that a single act, especially if carried out as part of a group, is not likely to be of serious significance. Repeat offending is associated with various socioenvironmental factors (Table 32.10).

Management

Delinquency is dealt with by the courts, who generally obtain a social report about the young person's family and social and material environment, an educational report, and, in certain cases, a psychiatric report. Usually, the emphasis is on secondary prevention rather than punishment, with involvement of social, educational, and sometimes psychological or psychiatric services. Rarely, an individual may go to a young offender's institution.

Table 32.10 Risk factors for juvenile delinquency

Patient factors	Family-related factors	Environmental factors
• Poor education or school underachievement	• Parents divorced/separated	• Low socioeconomic class
• Hyperactivity	• Very large families	• Poverty
• Mental health disorders	• Parental criminality/violence	• Poor housing
• Substance abuse	• Familial discord	• Peer group pressure

Further reading

General texts with more detail on child and adolescent psychiatry

Gelder MG, Andreasen NC, López-Ibor JJ, Geddes JR, eds. *New Oxford Textbook of Psychiatry*. 2nd ed. Section 9: Child and adolescent psychiatry. Oxford: Oxford University Press; 2012:1587–1816.

Thapar A, Pine DS, Leckman JF, et al., eds. *Rutter's Child and Adolescent Psychiatry*. 6th ed. Chichester: Wiley-Blackwell; 2015.

Useful resources for specific conditions

Hawton K, Witt KG, Taylor Salisbury TL, et al. Interventions for self-harm in children and adolescents. *Cochrane Database of Systematic Reviews* 2015;12:CD012013.

Cavanna A. Tourette's syndrome. *BMJ* 2013;347:f4964.

Lock J. An update on evidence-based psychosocial treatments for eating disorders in children and adolescents. *Journal of Clinical Child and Adolescent Psychology* 2015;44:707–721.

Pavuluri MN, Birmaher B, Naylor MW. Pediatric bipolar disorder: a review of the past 10 years. *Journal of Clinical Child and Adolescent Psychology* 2005;44:846–871.

Zeanah C, Gleason MM. Annual research review: attachment disorders in early childhood – clinical presentation, causes, correlates, and treatment. *Journal of Child Psychology and Psychiatry* 2015;56:207–222.

Part 6 Psychiatry and you

Chapter 23 — Psychiatry and you 521

33 Psychiatry and you

Keeping yourself well

Improving your *emotional resilience* is a key task for you as a medical student. As a future doctor, your health and well-being are vital to that of your patients: if you are not functioning reliably, you will not be able to help your patients as much as you otherwise would. It is therefore vital that you look after your body and mind and, by implication, adopt a lifestyle that is both healthy and sustainable.

The problem

It is often said that doctors make bad patients. There is some evidence that doctors are slow to seek help for health problems, and comply poorly with advice given by other healthcare professionals. In addition, doctors' lives may be unhealthy, with high levels of stress, low levels of exercise, and excessive consumption of alcohol.

The mental health of doctors is a particular concern. Doctors are at relatively high risk of mental disorder, and female doctors appear to be at higher risk of suicide than women in the general population. The reasons are several, and include the following:

- **The nature of doctors.** Doctors are driven to succeed, and do not tolerate failure well. It is inevitable that some of our patients will die, some treatments will not be successful, and that, in a professional lifetime, some mistakes will be made. Our aim should be to reflect on and learn from these events, and then to move on positively.

- **The nature of doctors' work.** Doctors tend to work hard, work for long hours, and work in challenging, resource-constrained environments.

- **Poor help-seeking.** Doctors may be reluctant to seek help for their medical problems, and this is particularly likely when the problem is psychiatric.

- **Unsupportive and unsustainable lifestyle.** Many doctors have challenging careers and challenging home lives, and allow themselves little time to recharge their batteries away from these ever-present stressors. They may not prioritize the maintenance of important resilience factors, such as the relationship with their partner, or interests outside medicine.

- **Knowledge of and access to the means of suicide.** Doctors (and vets, farmers, and pharmacists, to whom the above-mentioned factors also apply) have special expertise in the use of chemicals which are toxic in overdose.

Increasing your emotional resilience

The following points are intended to encourage you to think about how you will maintain your physical and mental health over your professional lifetime, which is likely to span several decades. As you accumulate responsibilities and commitments, both professional and personal, how will you manage the physical and emotional strains that they inevitably bring?

- **Develop good habits now. And engrain them, so that they become habitual.** These will then stand you in good stead for the future.

- **Prioritize. Ruthlessly.** How many of *you* are there? Just one! How many hours are there in a week? Just 168 (although it usually feels like a lot less). Prioritize your tasks and goals, using a simple system, and be prepared to delete some as not achievable (Box 33.1).

- **Take time off.** Even at your busiest, when you are working long shifts, or preparing for professional exams, make time to get away. There is *always* time for time off, despite what your negative automatic thoughts might be telling you. Planning a holiday or a short break for several weeks' time can help improve spirits and sustain you (and your partner) through a tough time. Holidays don't need to be long—a day or two away from the 'fray' can boost morale, and a 'microadventure' (see Humphreys (2014), in 'Further reading') takes just hours and can help you regain a sense of perspective and purpose.

- **Have interest(s) outside medicine.** As a person, are you defined entirely by your career? Having one or more non-medical interests can help to sustain your professional life.

Box 33.1 Prioritization

1 Do now
2 Do soon
3 Delay/put on back burner
4 Delete/forget about

- **Moderate your use of alcohol, and avoid using other substances.** It is easy to develop the habit of using alcohol to manage your stress or distress, but heavy or regular alcohol use has adverse health impacts and impairs coping.

- **Exercise regularly.** The physical benefits of exercise are clear, but there are emotional benefits too.

- **Manage your thoughts and beliefs.** When we are tired or stressed, the thoughts that we have are less likely to be realistic than when we are rested or calm. These biases in our thinking can help to make our personal situation seem much worse than it actually is. The stress of an imminent and challenging exam, for example, may make us believe we are less capable than we actually are, and that the threat/challenge is greater than it actually is. Learning how to identify and challenge these cognitive biases and negative thoughts is a core self-management skill. When you have mastered it, you will be better equipped to teach your patients!

- **Be wary of seeking meaning.** As the Greek philosopher Epictetus espoused, 'Men are disturbed not by what happens to them, but [by] their opinion of the things that happen.' Medical life brings us into regular contact with challenging events and challenging people which say little about us as individuals, but which we may be tempted to use as evidence about us as individuals.

- **Stop avoiding, and reduce your worry load.** If something has been worrying you, don't delay—sort it out as soon as you can, and then that weight will be lifted from your mind.

- **Cultivate stable and supportive relationships.** Don't neglect your friends and, of course, your boy/girlfriend, or life partner. Relationships outside medicine can help you to maintain a sense of stability, even when other aspects of your life feel 'out of control'.

- **Sleep!** Prioritize it—it's your daily recharge. Regularize it—you sleep best if you go to bed and get up at a similar time each day. Fill the sleep battery when you need to, that is, when you know you are going to be sleep-deprived, get some extra sleep the night or two before. Feeling blue? Consider *sleeping* a little less, and *doing* a little more.

- **Get a diary.** A paper one. And use it to schedule *nice* things in your life, *not* just chores and commitments and 'to dos'.

- **Beware impostor syndrome.** This is when high-achieving individuals, such as medical students and doctors, are concerned that they have succeeded by accident or luck, rather than by talent and hard work, and that at some point they will inevitably be exposed as a fraud or impostor. Reject this hypothesis immediately!

- **Beware clinical perfectionism.** Good is good, and better is better, but best may not be best. Aiming for perfect work or to be a perfect doctor may produce no or minimal return on your investment of time and effort.

- **Beware the proximity paradox.** You're more likely to be able to look after yourself when you're not stressed. But you most need to look after yourself when you are stressed.

- **Believe that you** *can*. Junko Tabei was the first woman to reach the summit of Mount Everest. What a fantastic achievement. She wouldn't even have started her journey if she hadn't believed it was possible. Believe that you can achieve, and that you can cope, even in adversity.

- **Troubled?—Don't get distracted from the power of distraction.** Usually, the most powerful distractor is another person, unless, of course, that person is the problem. It could also be an activity—any activity: don't be perfectionist about your choice of distracting activity!

- **Be a good (enough) doctor.** We all want to be perfect doctors. But is that feasible and sustainable? Better to aim to be a good (enough) doctor, and to sustain that performance level reliably throughout your professional career.

- **Remember that mistakes are inevitable.** The only way to avoid mistakes is to avoid doing anything that is remotely interesting, challenging, or important. Like medicine. The important thing is to be open, with yourself and with others, about your mistakes, and for you and your organization to learn from them. Medicine is gradually changing its attitude to mistakes, but there is much more to be done (see Makary and Daniel (2016), in 'Further reading').

- **Register with a GP! And use them. And don't self-medicate.** Many doctors, especially male doctors, are not registered with a GP or, if they are, they attend rarely. Make sure that you are registered with a GP, that they have up-to-date contact details, and that you change GP when you change location. Don't be tempted to self-diagnose or self-manage your illnesses; get a professional's objective advice and, if necessary, their prescription. Although registered medical practitioners are legally permitted to prescribe for themselves, the General Medical Council (GMC) states that 'doctors should, wherever possible, avoid treating themselves or anyone with whom they have a close personal relationship.'

- **Read more about looking after yourself.** Have a look at Butler et al.'s *Manage Your Mind* (2018), which is an excellent self-help book, written according to cognitive behavioural principles. It is excellent bedtime reading for stressed professionals, but also highly suitable for recommending to patients with common psychiatric disorders.

- **Be prepared to wave the white flag.** All of us get sick from time to time and can't work or need help. There's no shortage of willing helpers—think of your best friend, partner, other friends, family, colleagues you trust, and your GP.

- **Write a stress plan** (Box 33.2).

Box 33.2 My stress plan

- Do
- Do this
- Do the other
- Do that too
- Don't forget to do them
- Remember you **can** do them

- **Finally—prioritize looking after yourself.** Go on, do it! And don't delay—do it now: every effective person requires good-quality self-care.

Professional behaviours

As a medical student, you are in an unusual position. Your non-medical-student colleagues will have considerable flexibility in the way that they live their lives. If they turn up late to a teaching session, and are unable to concentrate due to a hangover, that is an educational matter. However, as a medical student, you need to develop and to demonstrate the kind of professional behaviours that will be expected of you as a qualified doctor. If you turn up late and with a hangover to a teaching session, this may pose a question mark over your ability to function consistently at a high level when you have qualified. Lateness keeps patients and your colleagues waiting, and adverse effects of substances such as alcohol may impair judgement and lead to medical errors.

The UK's GMC and Medical Schools Council (MSC) provide comprehensive guidance on what is expected of medical students, in 'Achieving good medical practice: guidance for medical students' (2016, see 'Further reading'). This is an essential reference for every medical student. Notably, much of this guidance relates to *professional behaviours* rather than to *knowledge* or *skills*, and Box 33.3 summarizes the requirements. We strongly recommend that you take time to familiarize yourself with the actual guidance, and to keep the guidance close to hand throughout your clinical placements. We can do no better than to sum up the exacting behavioural standard required of medical students by using the GMC and MSC's words:

> **Your behaviour at all times, both in the clinical environment and outside of your studies, must justify the trust that patients and the public place in you as a future member of the medical profession.**

Box 33.3 Going above and beyond—taking on the challenge of professional excellence

This guidance explains the standards of professional behaviour expected of you during your studies. True professionalism is about striving for excellence—to achieve this you'll need to learn to:

- develop healthy ways to cope with stress and challenges (resilience);
- deal with doubt and uncertainty;
- apply ethical and moral reasoning to your work;
- work effectively in a team, including being able to give constructive and honest feedback;
- manage your own learning and development;
- be responsive to feedback;
- prioritize your time well and ensure a good work–life balance;
- promote patient safety and be able, where appropriate, to raise concerns;
- work collaboratively with patients and other professionals;
- deal with and mitigate against personal bias.

You may find many of these difficult or challenging to do well but, as with all elements of professionalism, your medical school will help you to develop these skills. Being professional means you'll need to make time to reflect on your experiences, to learn continually, and to apply your learning in practice.

You will need to seek out feedback, remain up to date with professional and ethical guidance, and be able to adapt to changing circumstances.

Your teachers and trainers want you to develop and become an excellent doctor, so you should look to them for guidance and support.

Reproduced from *Achieving good medical practice: guidance for medical students*. © 2016 General Medical Council and Medical Schools Council.

Careers in psychiatry

Undergraduate medical training is dominated by training in general hospital-based specialties. Yet, the WHO (http://www.who.int/topics/global_burden_of_disease/) estimates that, in high-income nations, depressive disorder is a greater contributor to disability than any other disorder, exceeding that arising from heart disease, diabetes, cerebrovascular disease, or respiratory disease. Alcohol misuse and dementia also feature among the top ten causes of disability. In low-income nations, psychiatric disorders are emerging as a major cause of disability as progress is made in conquering infectious disease. It follows that there is a great need for committed and capable psychiatrists, in all areas of the world, and that this need will increase significantly in the coming years.

As you will have seen in these pages, mental disorder is wide ranging in its manifestations, and challenging to treat. Psychiatry offers a stimulating career, not least because of the special skills and attitudes that psychiatrists need to develop, which include:

- being tolerant of, and able to manage, risk;
- being tolerant of, and able to manage, diagnostic and therapeutic uncertainty;
- being able to build relationships over long time periods with patients who lack insight;
- being able to work as part of a multidisciplinary team;
- being able to think in an integrated way about patients' problems;
- being realistic about goals of management.

If you are potentially interested in a career in psychiatry, you should endeavour to find out more, with two aims in mind: first, to help rule in or rule out psychiatry as your chosen career, and second, to develop and sustain your interest until you enter postgraduate training in the field. Talk to your consultant, to one of the trainees, or to your course leader. What made them want to be a psychiatrist? What sustains them now? What do they like about the job? And not like? And what about their subspecialty? What advice would they give you? It is important to talk to more than one individual, to gather different opinions. You can also find out a lot more online, via the Student Associates section of the Royal College of Psychiatrists' website, at http://www.rcpsych.ac.uk/training/studentassociates.aspx. The

website is extensive, and includes details of training pathways, summaries of the main subspecialties, and details of how to become a Student Associate of the College. This is available free of charge to any UK medical student and is highly recommended.

Options for continuing some exposure to psychiatry, after your standard clinical placement, include the following:

- **Undertaking special study modules (sometimes called student-selected components).** These may be established modules, or modules which you arrange yourself, in areas which you find especially interesting.

- **Undertaking your elective, or part of your elective, in psychiatry.** This could be in the UK, at your or another medical school, or overseas. While it is usual to pursue an elective overseas, an elective in your own country may be invaluable, giving you time to pursue your own interests in depth at your own or another university.

- **Submitting entries for prize essay competitions.** In the UK, many are listed under 'Prizes and Bursaries' on the Royal College of Psychiatrists' Student Associates page.

- **Continuing occasional but regular contact with a mental health team.** For example, you might arrange to attend an outpatient clinic or ward round once a fortnight or once a month. Ask a friendly consultant if this might be possible.

If you have a possible interest in academic medicine or psychiatry, it is worth considering the following:

- **Contributing to the work of a research team.** Research is challenging to complete, because it needs considerable time and expertise, and almost all medical research is now done in multidisciplinary teams. A feasible and effective way to learn about psychiatric research is to contribute to the work of a research team, in a modest way, but over a period of several months or more.

- **Helping to develop teaching materials for use by other students.** Working with your course organizer or another active teacher, to help to develop materials for use by other medical students can be highly rewarding.

Further reading

Butler G, Grey N, Hope T. *Manage Your Mind: The Mental Fitness Guide*. 3rd ed. Oxford: Oxford University Press; 2018.

General Medical Council, Medical Schools Council. Achieving good medical practice: guidance for medical students. Published 27 May 2016. http://www.gmc-uk.org/education/undergraduate/achieving_good_medical_practice.asp.

Humphreys A. *Microadventures: Local Discoveries for Great Escapes*. London: William Collins; 2014.

Makary MA, Daniel M. Medical error – the third leading cause of death in the US. *BMJ* 2016;353:i2139.

Index

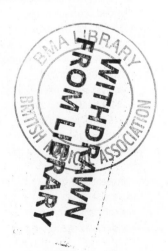